CONTEMPORARY PEDIATRICS

Edited by **Öner Özdemir**

Contemporary Pediatrics
Edited by Öner Özdemir

Published by InTech

Janeza Trdine 9, 51000 Rijeka, Croatia

Publishing Process Manager Irena Voric

Technical Editor Teodora Smiljanic

Cover Designer InTech Design Team

Additional hard copies can be obtained from orders@intechopen.com

Contemporary Pediatrics, Edited by Öner Özdemir
p. cm.
ISBN 978-953-51-0154-3

For EU product safety concerns :
IN TECH d . o . o . , Prolaz Marije Krucifikse Kozulić 3 , 51000 Rijeka , Croatia ,
info@intechopen . com or visit our website at intechopen . com .

Meet the editor

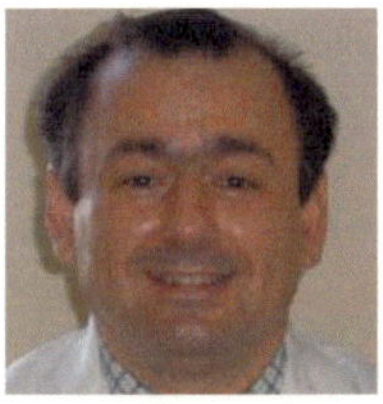

Doc. Dr. Oner Ozdemir was born in Alaplı, Zonguldak, Turkey in 1965. He has graduated from İstanbul Medical School, İstanbul University and become a medical doctor in 1989. Dr. Ozdemir did his pediatric residency at Department of Pediatrics in Children's Hospital, İstanbul Medical School, İstanbul, Turkey. His clinical fellowship training was finished at Pediatric Allergy/Immunology division in Louisiana State University, Health Sciences Centre, New Orleans, LA. Dr. Ozdemir research areas are as follows: LAK-cell generation and cell-mediated cytotoxicity; human mast cell development and mast cell-mediated cytotoxicity; and apoptosis related research. He was the first place winner of Clemens Von Pirquet Award from ACAAI at ACAAI meeting in 2005 for the best research on allergy/asthma/immunology by a fellow in training. Dr. Ozdemir has more than 50 international plus 20 national publications, as well as 90 international and 30 national presentations, and more than 5 chapters related to my research areas. Currently, he works as a chief at the third clinic of pediatrics associated with the division of pediatric allergy/immunology at İstanbul Medeniyet University, Göztepe Teaching and Training Hospital, Kadıköy, İstanbul, Turkey.

Contents

Preface

It is a great pleasure for me to be the editor of the book *Contemporary Pediatrics*. Nowadays; there is lot of classical pediatric text books describing various well-known topics. In these kinds of text books, there have always been similar topics, which are written with the same styles. Nevertheless, in this book volume, beyond classical themes, a different approach was made to current pediatric issues and topics. This volume, as understood from its title, describes nutritional infant health and some interesting topics from pediatric subspecialties such as cardiology, hemato-oncology and infectious diseases.

Book has 17 chapters which will help get us and patients enlightened with the new developments on the contemporary pediatric issues. The introductory section is about the public, politicians and pediatrics. The state and relations between pediatricians and the people as well as politicians in Spain are being told by Labay Matias Miguel, et al.

Nutritional health section depicts the importance of nutrition beginning from newborn period to late childhood. In addition to breastfeeding of infant, growth and development of child is being mentioned. Also, the role of probiotics use in healthy nutrition is discussed under recent literature, in the context of prevention of autoimmune diseases. Probiotics use is a hot topic and draws lots of attention from different medical disciplines.

Pediatric cardiology section enlightens us on cardiovascular changes in fetuses / infants as well as some pediatric cardiovascular surgical procedures needing skill under recent developments. Pediatric hemato-oncology section explains novel developments of well-known diseases such as neuroblastoma and thalassemias. For instance; whole genome searches and molecular basis for diagnosis of neuroblastoma are discussed. However, this section also includes some common complications of oncology e.g. fertility and fatigue seen in these patients. Also, socioeconomic issues related to cancer illness are mentioned in detail. Lastly, pediatric infectious diseases section describes chronic infantile recurrent parotitis and fungal infections during childhood. In conclusion; with the 17 chapters this book volume has, it enlightens us on classical pediatric age diseases as well as different aspects of these diseases such as therapeutic complications.

Before I finish my words here, I am indebted to my mother *Nikâme*, beloved wife *Seval Hülya* and mother-in-law *Sevgi Baş* for their invaluable support during the editing process of time.

Öner Özdemir, MD
Assoc. Prof. of Pediatrics
İstanbul Medeniyet University
Göztepe Research/Training Hospital
3rd Clinic of Pediatrics, Division of Pediatric Allergy/Immunology
Kadıköy, İstanbul,
Turkey

Part 1

The Public and Pediatrics

1

Paediatrics, the People and Politicians in Spain – History, Development, Reality and Future

Miguel Labay Matías
Rural Primary Health Care Services,
Obispo Polanco Hospital,
University of Zaragoza, Teruel,
Spain

1. Introduction

The paper examines the origins of Paediatrics in Spain since 1600. It mentions some of the main pioneers for the speciality highlighting the role of, among others, Jerónimo Soriano, considered the forefather of the speciality in Spain. It looks at the factors that gradually contributed to the beginnings of Paediatrics as a specific branch, distinct from General Medicine and Obstetrics, explaining the slow but spectacular advances in Paediatrics to date. Of particular note are the contributions of Luis Mercado, Andrés Martínez Vargas, Ángel Ballabriga Aguado, Manuel Cruz Hernández and Juan Rodríguez Soriano, among others. It emphasises the late arrival of Institutions to protect and care for children. It examines the beginnings of public healthcare in 1942, analysing the work of the different organisations involved, particularly the National Health Institute. It highlights the quality of the Spanish Public Health System but warns of the risks that it could be facing in the near future, analysing the current reality and circumstances after the transfer of health from the State to the Autonomous Regions. It looks at the achievements of Paediatrics and its specialities, thanks among other things to the self-sacrifice of its professionals and the establishment of the training programme for young doctors, called MIR. It criticises certain aspects of the political management of Paediatrics and healthcare in general. It argues for Paediatrics to be defended to ensure that it remains as currently organised, with its professionals present in Primary Health Care and Hospitals. Finally, it outlines the need for a comprehensive healthcare agreement in Spain, one in which the opinions of the public and professionals are taken into account, to maintain and increase the quality of the current health system, guaranteeing its future.

2. The protohistory

Everything began 1,300 years ago. In 714, Spain was ravaged by a smallpox epidemy. Several arab doctors described it with exactitude and differenced it from other diseases. This is the first evidence of an infant disease written in Spain. Arabs created several medicine schools, the one in Cordoba being the most important with 300,000 medicine texts in its library.

Many Arab doctors wrote about infant diseases in their works. Among them, Garibai-Ben-Said and Kalaph-Ben-Abbas-Abbulcassem published some books in which they described the newborn care, diseases and several techniques as hydrocephalus, amygdalectomy and tracheostomy.

The children protection began in 12th and 13th centuries in Aragón and Castilla after the promulgation of some laws by King Alfonso X "The Wise" of Castilla and King Pedro IV of Aragón. The first of them, in the law "Fuero Juzgo" sentenced the abortion and the infanticide. The second of them, King Pedro IV, created the figure of "Judge and Father of Orphans", whose mission was to look after children's health, to keep them away of begging and to lead them to work. There even were centers where children received food and education. Bernardo Gordonio, in his book published in 1496, dedicated one chapter to newborn care. His work was dedicated to Queen Isabel of Castilla and King Fernando of Aragón, known as 'Catholic Monarchs'. Pedro Díaz de Toledo, Onofre Bruguera and others also discussed children's diseases years later (Laín Entralgo, 1992; García Nieto et al.. 2011).

3. The foundations

We have no way of knowing whether Jerónimo Soriano, a doctor from Teruel, was aware when he published his work: *Methodo y orden de curar las enfermedades de los niños*, "Method to Treat the Diseases of Children" (Arana de Amurrio, 2000; Soriano, 2000; Valle Sánchez et al., 2000) in Spanish in 1600, that he was placing the first building block for a speciality that has become extremely well developed in Spain. After him, other outstanding doctors dedicated their wisdom to the subject: *"it is very dangerous to talk about curing things so dark and uncertain only the basis of conjecture"*. Until then children had been cared for by midwives and the oldest women. Jerónimo Soriano, seeing the lack of attention to children at that time, included original ideas and observations in his book (Figure 1), describing coeliac disease, cradle cap, meningitis, nephritic colic, stomatitis and intestinal malabsorption, distinguishing between febrile *("epilepsy")* and non-febrile convulsions, and examining the difference with sobbing spasms *("twitching"or "pasmo",sic)*. He sensed that there were family hereditary factors behind epilepsy. His recommendation for fever was not wrapping the child up but instead bathing it in lukewarm water. He exactly identified the causes of snoring and breathing difficulties during sleep due to nasopharyngeal obstructions. He established the differences between the various types of intestinal parasites. He talked about dystrophy caused by poor nutrition and advised controlling both the quantity and the quality of food, concepts that would have to wait for the positivist medicine of the 19th century, with the treatises of Albert Czeny and Otto Heubner, to receive their due prominence. In the treatment of diarrhoea, he established the essential rules of fasting for several hours, abstaining from drinking milk *"so as not to curdle in the stomach"* and the administration of small amounts of sugary drinks. He associated cradle cap with the subsequent appearance of eczema and advised having cold drinks with external crystal violet substances in them for mouth ulcers. He described some of the most common psychiatric, respiratory and cardiac problems in his century. In his work he reports findings that were truly novel for that time and that continued to be used, in some cases even into modern times. In addition, his remedies and treatments are always the least aggressive for the children (Arana de Amurrio, 2000; Soriano, 2000; Valle Sánchez et al., 2000).

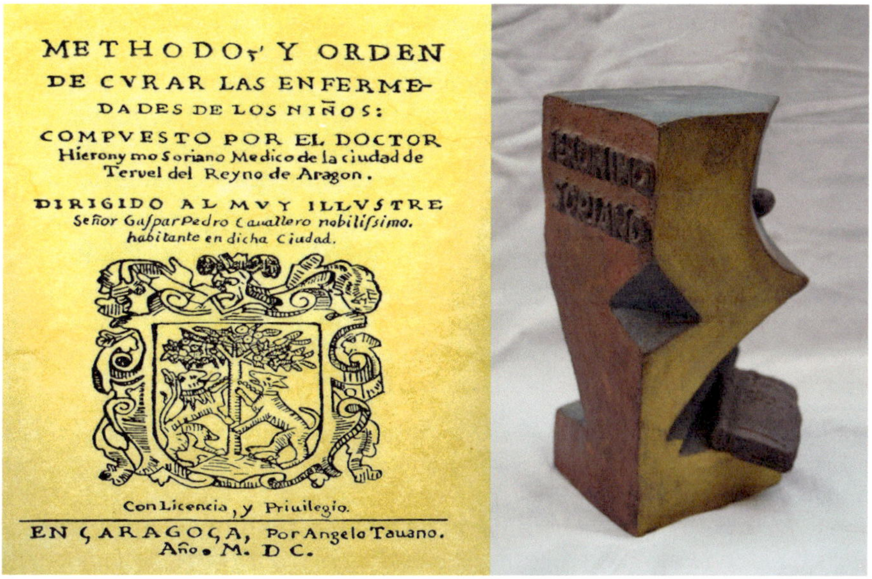

METHODO, Y ORDEN
DE CVRAR LAS ENFERME-
DADES DE LOS NIÑOS:
COMPVESTO POR EL DOCTOR
Hieronymo Soriano Medico de la ciudad de
Teruel del Reyno de Aragon.
DIRIGIDO AL MVY ILLVSTRE
Señor Gaspar Pedro Cauallero nobilissimo.
habitante en dicha Ciudad.
Con Licencia, y Priuilegio.
EN ÇARAGOÇA, Por Angelo Tauano.
Año. M. DC.

Fig. 1. Facsimile of Soriano's Teatrise (front). Allegoric Monument of Jerónimo Soriano by Antonio Cobos, situated in Hospital Obispo Polanco, Teruel, Spain.

To this one must add his complete disinterest in money, his love for even the most helpless child, the opening of a free consulting room for children, the founding at his own expense of the first reported Hospital dedicated entirely to helping children, and his fight against malpractice (Figure 2).

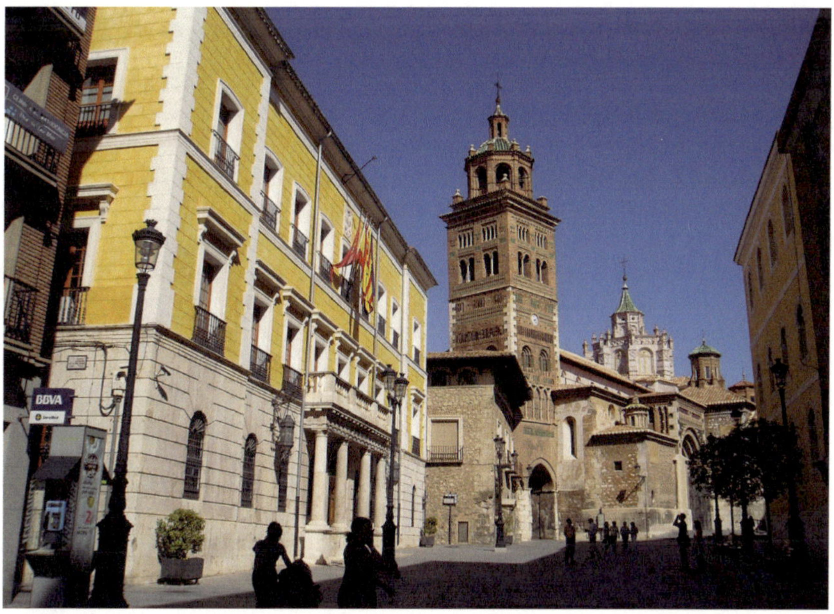

Fig. 2. Santa María de Mediavilla Cathedral, Teruel (Spain). Infant Hospital founded by Jerónimo Soriano in 16th Century was near it.

Jerónimo Soriano had already sensed that medical care for children and adolescents should be different to that provided to adults and the elderly, anticipating by more than 200 years the construction of the first hospital dedicated to children in France. The inhabitants of the city of Teruel called him *"señor san Jerónimo"* (Mister Saint Jeronimo) for his immense human qualities. There were 6 reeditions of his treatise, the last in 1721. So for almost two centuries he had a great scientific influence over many Spanish, European and American doctors.

In 1595 the book *Libro de experimentos médicos, fáciles y verdaderos, recopilados de varios autores* was published. This was the first scientific work written in Spanish with the intention of reaching the largest possible number of readers. It is considered the first medical encyclopaedia whose publication was aimed not only at doctors but also at the general public. It was a great success and it was reedited on 15 occasions over two centuries (Arana de Amurrio, 2000; Soriano, 2000; Valle Sánchez et al., 2000).

As recognition of the person and of his works, the Spanish Paediatric Association has for the last six years been running the Jerónimo Soriano Award for the best article published over the previous year in its official journal *Anales de Pediatría* (Pérez-Yarza, et al., 2009), having created for this purpose the Patronato Jerónimo Soriano Board involving various scientific Institutions and individuals. Seven years ago, the Regional Paediatric Society of Aragón, La Rioja and Soria organised a Jerónimo Soriano Research Project, with a social and humanitarian content, to meet the basic needs of disadvantaged children and adolescents in different parts of the world.

Years earlier, in 1541, Damián Carbó (or Carbón) had tried to provide some guidance on the topic in his text on pregnancy and childbirth called *Libro del arte de las comadres o madrinas y del regimiento de las preñadas y paridas de los niños* (Rodríguez Tejerina, 1981). Other important doctors such as Luis Lobera de Ávila, Luis Mercado, and Francisco Pérez Cascales (between 1551 and 1611) also dedicated their efforts in those olden times, focussing largely on the treatment of malignant diphtheric angina or *"croup"* (García Nieto et al. 2011, Laín Entralgo, 1992; Rodríguez Tejerina, 1981).

In 1611, Luis Mercado published the book *De puerorum educatione, custodia y providentia, atque de morborum, qui ipsis accidunt, curationi, libri duo* (Figure 3). Luis Mercado, professor at the University of Valladolid and doctor to the court of kings Felipe II and Felipe III of Spain, is considered to be the "Saint Thomas of Spanish medicine". His works were known and appreciated throughout Europe. The aforementioned book has specific paediatric content which spiritually was a continuation of Jerónimo Soriano's treatise. Luis Mercado was a true Renaissance man. All of the medicine in this period was characterised by an increase and revaluation of clinical observation. Another of his works *Consultationes morborum complicatorum et gravissimorum* was dedicated to *"croup"* and he also looked at the plague and exanthematic typhus *("typhoid fever" or "tabardillo",* sic.*)* in other publications (García Nieto et al., 2011; Laín Entralgo, 1992; Rodríguez Tejerina, 1981). One of Luis Mercado's great contributions was paving the way, through the synthetic order of his works, for the appearance of paediatric specialities. His fame is reflected in the impressive portrait dedicated to him by the great painter El Greco (García Nieto et al., 2011; Laín Entralgo, 1992) (Figure 4). He dedicated sections of his books to providing advice about basic care for newborns and babies on milk. It included the period of life from cutting the umbilical cord up to teething. He then studied, systematically and analytically, the childhood ailments causing the highest mortality rates at that time. His work is one of the pioneers in the speciality in Spain (García Nieto et al., 2011).

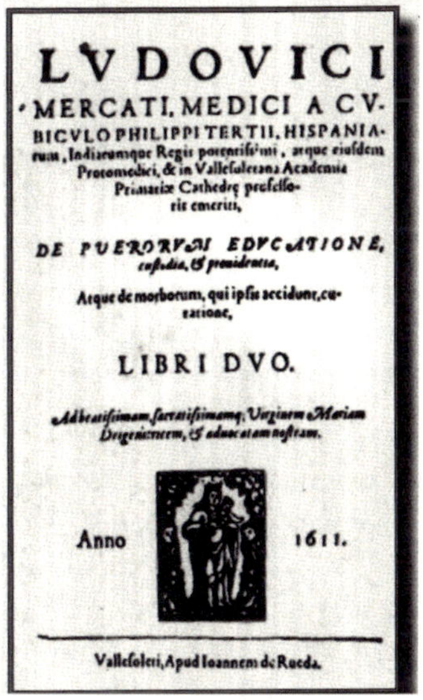
LVDOVICI
MERCATI, MEDICI A CV-
BICVLO PHILIPPI TERTII, HISPANIA-
rum, Indiarumque Regis potentissimi, atque eiusdem
Protomedici, & in Vallesoletana Academia
Primariæ Cathedræ professo-
ris emeriti,

DE PVERORVM EDVCATIONE,
custodia, & providentia,

Atque de morborum, qui ipsis accidunt, cu-
ratione,

LIBRI DVO.

Ad beatissimam, sanctissimamq; Virginem Mariam
Deigenitricem, & advocatam nostram.

Anno 1611.

Vallesoleti, Apud Ioannem de Rueda.

Fig. 3. Front of book by Luis Mercado

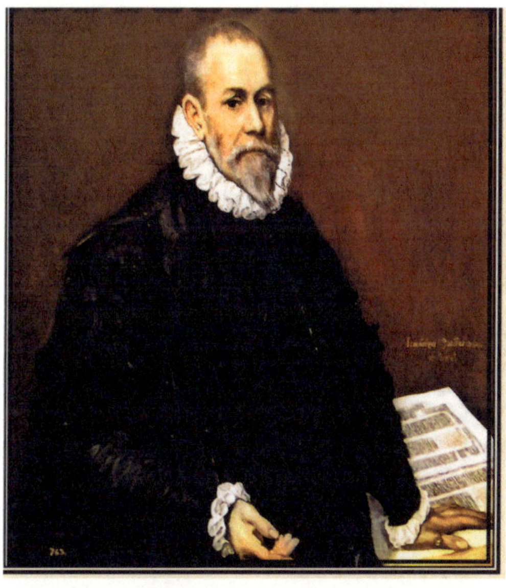

Fig. 4. Luis Mercado portrait by El Greco. Reproduction property of the signer.

Luis Lobera de Ávila and Francisco Pérez Cascales were also very important figures in the foundation of Paediatrics in Spain. Luis Lobera, doctor to Emperor Carlos I of Spain and V of Germany, is the author of *El libro del regimiento de la salud y de la esterilidad de los hombres y las mujeres y de las enfermedades de los niños y otras cosas utilísimas*. Published in 1551, it is viewed as a continuation of the work of Damian Carbó or Carbón. In Europe this book has been considered hugely important. Without detracting from this, it is worth noting that the book is not focused entirely on childhood diseases, although it is an important taster of what would come later and what has already been discussed (Rodrígez Tejerina, 1981). *Liber de affectionibus puerorum, una cum tractatu de morbo illo vulgariter Garrotillo appellatur, cun duabus Quaesttionibus* is the masterwork of Francisco Pérez Cascales. Its more than 300 pages, published in 1611, include a discussion of topics such as: mouth ulcers, epilepsy, scalp infections, rabies, hydrocephalus, coughing, excessive sneezing, conjunctivitis and otitis ("*sanies*"), corneal scarring, intertrigo, suppression of urine, chilblains, smallpox and of course angina, differentiating between malignant and "*croup*". Unlike Luis Mercado, he did not look at issues relating to childcare and he justified the practical nature of his book on the basis of writing it after thirty years of professional practice. Pérez Cascales was particularly influenced by the so called *"Hippocratic-Galenic tradition"*, as can be seen from his written work, and he was Professor of Medicine in the University of Sigüenza in Guadalajara.

In Spain, those condemned to death were killed using a "*garrote vil*". In essence, this involved the complete cutting of the spinal cord in the neck area, as a result of a large screw gradually being introduced into the back of the neck. This produced instantaneous death through suffocation. Francisco de Goya, an exceptional Spanish painter, and like Jerónimo Soriano born in Aragón, depicted this wonderfully in one of his drawings (Figure 5). As a result, childhood malignant diphtheritic angina was known as "*garrotillo*", since the death of the child was caused by suffocation induced by the diphtheritic membranes. Goya also signed the painting in which a doctor has his hands down the throat of a child, trying to pull out the deadly diphtheritic membranes (Figure 6). Pedro Laín Entralgo, born in the province of Teruel, a doctor, great humanist, and author of numerous books, who became President of the Spanish Royal Academy of Language, gave an accurate portrayal of this (Laín Entralgo, 1992).

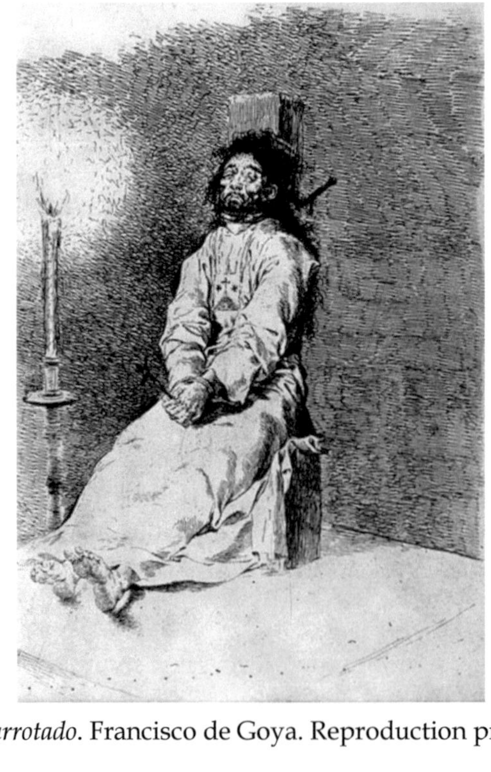

Fig. 5. Garrote vil. *El agarrotado*. Francisco de Goya. Reproduction property of the signer.

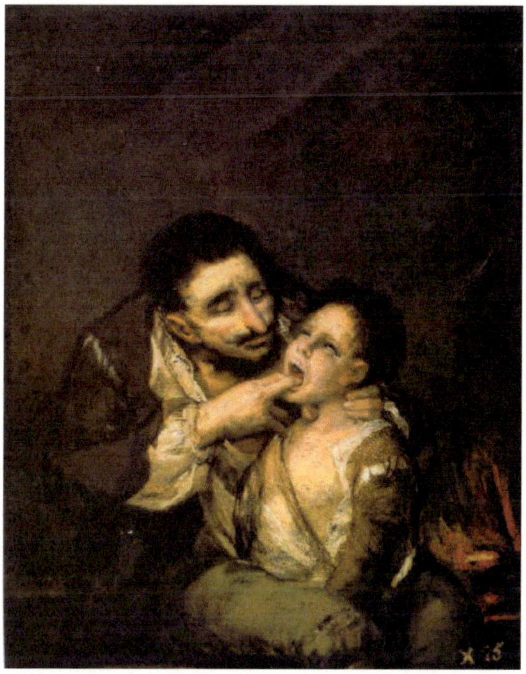

Fig. 6. *El garrotillo.* Francisco de Goya. Reproduction property of the signer.

Almost 300 years would have to pass before our academic authorities created the first Chairs of Paediatrics, uncoupling its teaching from Obstetrics. As ever, the population and the professionals moved with greater speed and more directly than those in power. Apart from some rare exceptions, the great initiatives in Spain have been driven by individuals and the population. As a result of the collapse of the Spanish empire, there was a drop off in scientific works and their publication in Spain during a large part of the 17th and 18th centuries. In Spain, the end of the so called "Golden Age" for Spanish arts, which accompanied the decline of its political role in the world, also negatively affected science. There are no known paediatric works by Spanish authors from the mid-17th century to the start of the 18th century (García Nieto et al. 2011; Laín Entralgo, 1992; Rodríguez Tejerina, 1981; Valle Sánchez et al., 2000).

For centuries children were one of the marginalised groups, along with women, old people and the mentally ill. Medical history paid them little attention. After several attempts in the 18th, 19th and early 20th centuries, involving, among others, Lorenzo Hervás y Panduro, Andrés Martínez Vargas, Manuel Tolosa Latour, Francisco Criado Aguilar, Rafael Ulecia y Cardona and Francisco Vidal Solares, attention for children became a completely medicalised area, where the only possible approach was medical. In 1789, Lorenzo Hervás (Arana de Amurrio, 2000; García Nieto et al. 2011, Laín Entralgo, 1992; Rodríguez Tejerina, 1981; Soriano, 2000; Valle Sánchez et al., 2000), following the doctrine laid down by Jerónimo Soriano, set out the need for there *"to be doctors dedicated to curing children's diseases, to educate the children well about physical matters"*.

During the 18th century, there was a re-emergence of interest in childhood diseases. Gaspar Casal masterfully described "pellagra", a disease caused by deficiencies due to the diet in his native Asturias which was based almost exclusively on corn. This deficiency in the intake of niacin, or nicotinic acid, which he called *"mal de la rosa"*, devastated the North of Spain until 60 years ago. In 1762 he also carried out an exhaustive study of whooping cough and its complications (Arana de Amurrio, 2000; Laín Entralgo, 1992). In 1787 we start to see the first glimpses of Paediatrics becoming organised in Spain. An ordinance to control the courses given at the San Carlos School of Surgery in Madrid proposed breaking childhood pathology training into three parts: processes relating to newborns, diseases suffered by babies from 40 days after birth to teething, and the pathology of children up to seven years old (Laín Entralgo, 1992). The foundations for the study of Paediatrics in Spain were laid in the period known as "The Enlightenment". In this era the governing class made famous the phrase "everything for the people, nothing by the people". Even so, it was an interesting era, with the Borbon dynasty now in power, in which Spain recovered part of the prestige lost during the reign of the two final kings from the Austrian dynasty, Felipe IV and Carlos II, so far and so different from their brilliant predecessors, particularly Carlos I and Felipe II, who inherited the incisiveness and shrewdness of Fernando "The Catholic", the first King of Spain.

The greatest change during this century was the introduction of practices to prevent infections, with the discovery by the Englishman Edward Jenner (1749-1823) of a vaccination against smallpox. Spain was the most enthusiastic nation in welcoming this discovery. In 1803 the ship *"María Pita"* left the Spanish coast on an expedition led by the doctors Francisco Javier de Balmis and Francisco Salvany. Their sole aim was to take the prized vaccine to the Spanish overseas territories. This expedition was supported by King Carlos IV de Borbon. Given the long duration of the journey they needed to have enough people to inoculate with the vaccine lymph over the period. This is because the only way they knew of conserving it was direct person to person inoculation. The solution to this was to use children from the *"Inclusa"* (Orphanages) in Madrid and other Spanish cities. The Inclusas were centres that took in the children of single mothers and those whose families could not look after them. They took on board 22 children and when the pustules of one child were about to clear up they would take material from them and inoculate another child. Thanks to this inventive idea they were able to carry out the wide scale vaccination of the indigenous, Creole and Spanish populations in all the Spanish territories in America, the Philippines, and the Visayas, Macau and Canton islands, in China (Arana de Amurrio, 2000; Laín Entralgo, 1992). Although from a modern perspective many of Spain's actions when it conquered the Americas were reprehensible, this does not mean that everything it did was bad. Far from it, examples such as the mixing of races and cultures between the two worlds and Doctor Balmis' expedition are proof of this. A decade ago the Spanish Paediatric Association quite rightly organised the "Balmis Award" in memory of what was a hugely important scientific event in its era. This was created by Prof. Alfonso Delgado, Professor of Paediatrics and at that time President of the Spanish Paediatrics Association.

In the 18th century people started to see children as the seeds of society and this led to the view forming that they needed to be looked after. The education, feeding and care of abandoned children and awareness of the source of many diseases were the four basic areas of concern among the most enlightened and humanistic people of the era. Among these, the aforementioned Jesuit Priest Lorenzo Hervás y Panduro stands out. The abandoned children, the *"expósitos"*, are a cause of debate. The fact that Children's Homes, called *"Hospicios"*, existed, and that they survived in Spain until half a century ago, is commendable, but their conditions and the lack of financial resources to maintain them were horrendous. The treatment received by the children was dreadful and they were subjected to all sorts of abuse. Some intellectuals and politicians finally became involved in trying to pass laws to protect children and adolescents. These laws were never put into practice. Once again the ruling classes ignored the reality of their people. There were even attempts, to avoid the terrible morbidity and mortality rates in the "*Hospicios*", to home children in private houses in return for a financial payment, but the abuses and mistreatment continued to take place in these houses. They also tried to recruit a large number of *"nodrizas sanas" (healthy wet nurses)* to feed the abandoned newborns and babies still on milk. These *"nodrizas"* were initially required to be healthy and upright citizens, but in the end women of all types ended up entering the *"Hospicios"*: sick women, prostitutes, etc. They transmitted serious illnesses and caused the death of more than half of the children admitted (Arana de Amurrio, 2000; Laín Entralgo, 1992).

4. The early stages

Modern Paediatrics did not start in Spain until the early 19th century. Scientific advances influencing the professionals of that era, combined with their exemplary dedication, drive and courage, ensured that the "flame" of Paediatrics, kept alive over the preceding centuries, with caring for children as its hallmark, came to fruition and the authorities became involved. In 1802 the *"Hôpital des Enfants Malades"* was founded in Paris, but we would have to wait until 1876 for the *"Hospital del Niño Jesús"* to open in Madrid. This is still a first-class hospital today. Its patron was the Duchess of Santoña and it was officially opened by King Alfonso XII de Borbón. The institutions were finally present at an event of this sort, one which was a breakthrough and a new development: the authorities began to involve themselves in childcare. However, the initial drive still came from the professionals and wealthy benefactors. In Barcelona, the *"Hospital de Niños Pobres"* was built thanks to the concerns of Doctor Francisco Vidal y Solares, the *"San Rafael"* was opened in Madrid and staffed by members of the Order of "San Juan de Dios", and one was built in Chipiona (Cádiz), at the request of Doctor Manuel Tolosa Latour.

Worthy of special mention is Doctor Francisco Vidal y Solares who founded the *"Gota de leche"* in Barcelona in 1890. The idea was a success and fourteen years later, at the initiative of Doctor Rafael Ulecia y Cardona, another similar institution was opened in Madrid, after which these centres were gradually opened all across Spain. The idea was great. These centres were involved in caring for children, which they did by collecting milk from donors and *"nodrizas sanas"*, with the maximum health guarantees. The milk was then stored at the correct temperature and subjected to a sterilisation process before being placed in bottles and fed to the children in need. They also educated mothers on how to look after their children. In those days, if the families could not afford to pay for a wet nurse, almost all of the children from humble families whose mothers could not breast feed or had died in childbirth would themselves die. Infant mortality at that time in Spain, during the first year of life, was 250 for every one thousand born alive: terrifying but real statistics. Doctor Francisco Criado Aguilar was the first Professor of Paediatrics at the University of Madrid and ran a clinic in San Carlos Hospital toward the end of the 19th century. Doctor Manuel Tolosa Latour, a tireless campaigner, was behind the first official guidelines to protect children (Laín Entralgo, 1992).

After more than 100 years, this idea is now being reintroduced and several Spanish regions have seen the arrival of "*Bancos de leche materna*" (Breast milk banks), as if it were a new idea, an advance, and without public acknowledgement of its inventors who in technically very difficult conditions, without financial support and with great generosity, started and disseminated the idea over many years.

Reviewing some medical books published during the 19th century, there were already chapters dedicated to attending to and looking after children, with a description of the main illnesses known. What draws the attention is the clinical clarity with which the symptoms and signs of the childhood diseases are described. This all has the added value of them being general medical and surgical books. So children were considered as different from adults from a medical point of view, which was a great advance and new development (Baldivieso, 1871; Ramos y Luengo, 1821). The author has even been able to find from that era prescriptions for children signed by doctors who were practicing in the towns of the province of Teruel (Figure 7). What draws our attention is the main active ingredients used: opiates and vegetable extracts. In another prescription we can find digitalis. Few pharmaceuticals were effective in those days.

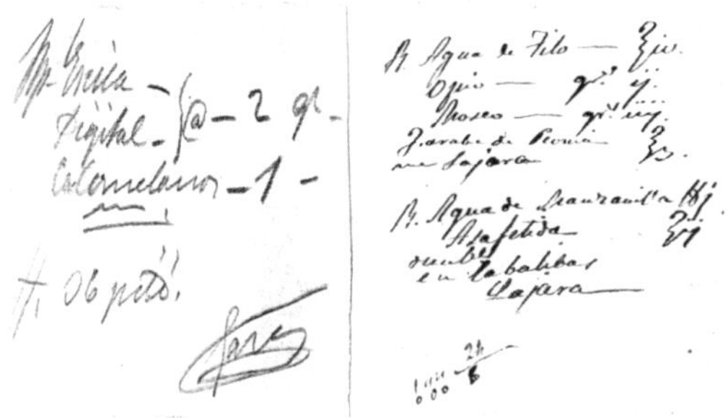

Fig. 7. Prescriptions for children. 19th Century. Provided by Ms. María José Doñate

One great scientific individual is Andrés Martínez Vargas, born in Barbastro, in the province of Huesca (Aragón), in 1861. After studying at the University of Zaragoza, he went to the United States to specialise in Paediatrics under the supervision of Professor Jacobi. He was appointed Professor of Paediatrics at Granada and subsequently performed the same role in Barcelona. He was a fascinating person, but controversial to some. His love of Spain did not please some members of the Catalan bourgeoisie. His activity was vast and ground breaking until his death in 1948. Gifted with a great intellectual capacity and a boundless curiosity, he worked intensively in this speciality. Author of numerous books and treatises, of countless articles published in first-class journals, and founder of many journals for his speciality, kindergartens, he was the first Spanish paediatrician to travel to many international conferences, sharing his knowledge (Figure 8). He even founded the *"Instituto Nipiológico"* in his native city in order to educate fathers and mothers in the comprehensive care of their children. As a result of this Institute, infant mortality in Barbastro reduced by 50% in seven years. It is also acknowledged that he was the first Spanish paediatrician to regularly publish in English. In fact, in April 1890, in "The Archives of Paediatrics", from Philadelphia, he published the first known article by a Spanish paediatrician written in English ("Adherent vesical calculus in a child. Clinical history and general study of the question"). His *"Tratado de Pediatría"* and *"La Historia de la Pediatría en España"*, along with others of his works, were used as teaching resources for his students and for many generations of doctors in Spain and Spanish speaking America. He also founded the Spanish

Paediatric Association in 1901 and was the president of the three first Paediatric National meetings. He had an excellent relationship with many of his colleagues, particularly with Professor Sarabia Pardo, another great figure. Jerónimo Soriano amazed him and after reading his treatise he wrote a long article about his work, dated 1901, which appeared in the "Anales de Medicine et Chirurgie Infantiles" in Paris. From the start of his hospital activity, he managed to find specific rooms in the hospitals that could be used to see children and adolescents. He is considered to be the father of modern Paediatrics in Spain (Laín Entralgo, 1992; Grupo de Trabajo de Historía de la Pediatría de la AEP., 2010) His energy, strong character and ability to fight meant that he was not always understood, as is the case with all innovators who are ahead of their time. This makes his legacy all the more impressive and increases our gratitude for his masterwork.

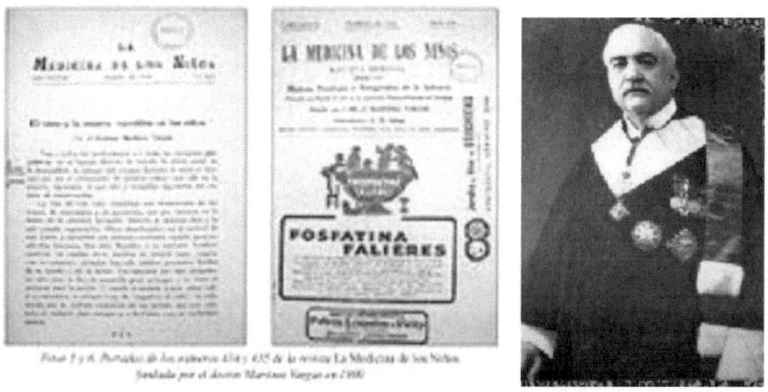

Fig. 8. Fronts of journals founded by Dr. Martínez Vargas. Portrait of him.

5. Early development

The first Spanish Paediatrics Professorship in San Carlos Hospital in Madrid, created in 1866, the enactment of the "Child Protection Law" in 1904, and the first three Paediatrics Conferences in Palma de Mallorca (1914), San Sebastian (1923) and Zaragoza (1925), confirmed the arrival of our speciality (Labay Matías,2010). Later on, academics such as Arce, Laguna, Ramos, Lorente Sanz and Suárez, among others, kept alive the flame of Paediatrics under difficult circumstances. After the unfortunate Spanish Civil War, from 1936 to 1939, there was widespread poverty among the population. There were insufficient resources and the Clinical Hospitals, reliant on the Universities, did not have the appropriate technology. Many children would die due to a lack of medical care. However, in 1908 the *Instituto Nacional de Previsión* (National Institute of Social Welfare) had been founded so that the working and lower classes could receive some financial support on retirement. In 1942 they added *"Seguro Obligatorio de Enfermedad" (SOE)* (Compulsory Health Insurance), which was the start of medical care for all Spaniards. For example, rural doctors were originally paid their monthly salary by the local Councils: with the SOE, the system changed and they were paid by the State. Hospital care was provided in charitable hospitals, in those connected to the Universities, or in private clinics. The 1950s saw the start of the construction of newly built hospitals in all the provincial capitals and heavily populated areas in Spain, paid for by the SOE. For the first time in the history of Spanish medicine these hospitals were given the appropriate human and technical resources for that time. The Hospital Obispo Polanco in Teruel, the second constructed in Spain, was opened in 1953 by the SOE (Figure 9). An old manager at the Hospital in Teruel told how a famous German professor, invited to Valencia in 1954 to give a couple of conferences, was driven to Teruel so that he could see a modern hospital, since those in Valencia were not presentable. Valencia is the third largest Spanish city in terms of population, but its new hospital was still being constructed. It is true that initially children were not included in the hospital care system. It looked after mothers during childbirth and the only specialities included were the surgical ones for adults. Farmers were excluded, but it was a start. Only some Centres such as the "Casa de Salud of Valdecilla" in Santander, and the old hospitals mentioned above, cared for children in a way that was appropriate for that time. In this context it is worth mentioning Professor Guillermo Arce, who disseminated his wisdom from Santander, creating a school of paediatrics which was very well known for its quality. Apart from some exceptions, there was no guarantee of "excellence" in the training of paediatricians: They would acquire qualifications as best they could. One should also mention the foundation, at this time, of the Childcare Schools which at least guaranteed that doctors had some basic ideas about children (Fleta Zaragozano, 2009; Sánchez Martín, 2007). From 1960 many brilliant specialists, many happily still with us, have been focussing all their energy and thinking on providing an extraordinary service to society in general and to Paediatrics in particular.

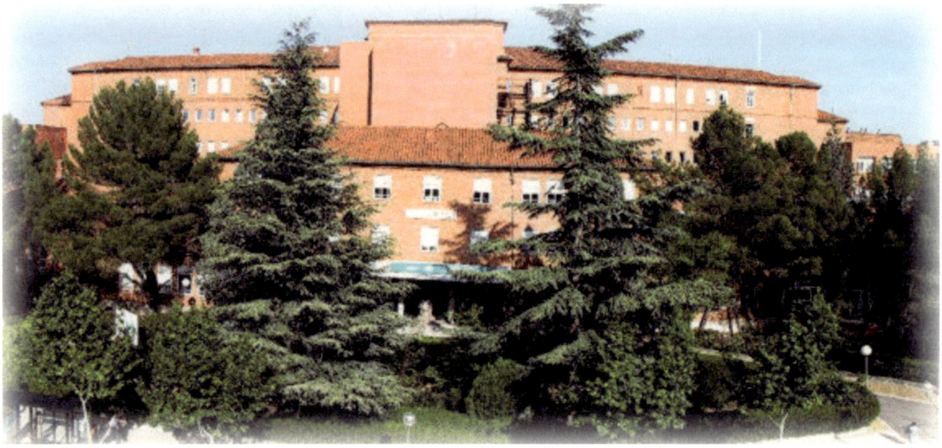

Fig. 9. Hospital Obispo Polanco, inaugurated in 1953. Teruel, Spain

6. The golden age

When analysing the past we can identify five fundamental events that have contributed to the development of paediatric care in Spain: the creation of the old National Institute of Social Welfare (1908), with the establishment of the aforementioned Compulsory Health Insurance (SOE) in 1942, the predecessor of the National Health Institute (INSALUD); the implementation of the Medical Residency Training (MIR) system for training graduates in Medicine and Surgery (1974); the creation of children's hospitals with the beginning of the paediatric specialities (1964-80); the General Health Law (1986); and the design of the Primary Health Care System (1986), which was largely the brainchild of the academic Segovia de Arana. These events led to a change from the "quota" of outpatient paediatricians, with a consultation time of two and a half hours and 10 hours on alert for home visits, to the situation that exists today. In the new care model we have Paediatric specialists working alongside the family doctors in the health centres (Labay Matías, 2010). Curiously, in Teruel Jerónimo Soriano founded, and maintained at his own expense, the first recorded hospital dedicated entirely to disadvantage children: another great action by this exceptional person (Labay Matías, 2010). The creation of the Children's Hospitals in the main Spanish cities was a giant leap forward in terms of caring for children. The paradox was that these Hospitals were much better equipped than those attached to the Universities. In addition, with them we saw the start of the paediatric specialities that led to unstoppable advances in the level of care. The best specialists trained in Spain and oversees were attracted by the potential for professional development. These Hospitals began during the Franco dictatorship and culminated with the happy arrival of democracy in Spain, brought about by the efforts of the public, by intellectuals and by politicians full of generosity such as Adolfo Suárez. They were all protected by King Juan Carlos I de Borbón.

The aforementioned INSALUD turned out to be a highly effective organization and contributed decisively to the development of Spanish medicine and paediatrics. It was also concerned about ensuring that the University Hospitals and their Paediatric Services had the necessary resources.

The author can remember the first National Meeting of the Society of Intensive Paediatric Care, held in Bilbao in 1977, and led by Dr. Xavier Allué and Dr. María Teresa Hermana. This decade saw the spectacular development of all the paediatric skills in the INSALUD network Children's Hospitals.

In this golden era for our speciality, the people who stand out, among many others, are Ernesto Sánchez Villares (Professor at the University of Valladolid), Ángel Ballabriga Aguado (Head of Paediatrics and Professor at the University of Barcelona in the Valle de Hebrón Hospital in Barcelona) and Juan Rodríguez Soriano (Head of Department and Professor at the University of the Basque Country in the Hospital Infantil de Cruces in Bilbao). The first of these instilled in his students the need to specialise in the different paediatric areas (Sánchez Martín, 2007). The second, born in Naval, a province of Huesca, (Aragón), was tireless in his efforts to introduce into his hospital and others the new child-related trends and techniques. Professor Ballabriga, who had great intelligence and vision of the future, wrote 20 years ago: "The development of paediatrics in Spain since 1975 has been enormous thanks to the generosity of the professionals. However, we have not been able to achieve all the milestones initially planned, and what we need is for our administrative systems, both central and regional, to be less arrogant, less dogmatic, less bureaucratic, more flexible, more capable of accepting criticism and more cooperative with the professionals who still maintain a scientific spirit and enthusiasm". He also, with his characteristic sarcasm, complained about the official recognition of the paediatric specialities, when in 1992 he wrote about our healthcare system: "...in spite of all of this we still feel happy!, because for the moment when we are sick we can go to our National Heath System (NHS) doctor. Perhaps in the near future we will be obliged to go first to our NHS economist!" (Argente Oliver, 2011). These assertions are still the reality at the current time, but the outlook has become even worse.

Few people know that Professor Juan Rodríguez Soriano (Figure 10) was coincidentally born in Zaragoza because at a very young age he moved to Barcelona. He always considered himself to be Catalan, but he had a special fondness for his city of birth. It is safe to say that, of all the Spanish paediatricians throughout time, he is the most famous in the scientific world thanks to his contributions to Paediatric Nephrology. After graduating he trained in Paris and the United States. He described renal tubular acidosis, contributed to improving awareness about Bartter's Syndrome, published more than 100 highly-rated scientific articles in English, and took part in many editions of Nelson, being involved in the nephrological aspects. An ardent defender of the paediatric specialities, his Paediatric Department was the prototype for modern medicine, involving collaboration with great minds coming from all over the world. Gifted with easy and forceful eloquence, with a superlative intelligence and with a personality that affected all who met him, he devoted himself body and soul to his work. The author was lucky enough to train as a resident doctor (MIR) in his hospital. All of us resident doctors were impressed by his knowledge, which spanned the whole of Paediatrics. The daily clinical sessions were a pure intellectual delight. Towards 1980 we saw the introduction into Spain and Europe of a new baby milk formula. After a few months babies started to arrive in the emergency rooms at the hospitals showing signs of neurological affection and some died. Professor Rodríguez Soriano observed that all of them were suffering from metabolic alkalosis, with very noticeable changes in blood electrolytes and in gasometries. All of them were being fed that milk formula. With the help of his team of collaborators he analysed its composition, detecting significant imbalances in the ions. He contacted the laboratory that manufactured it, explaining his findings and asking for the milk formula to be removed from sale. Given the refusal of the company and the treatment he received, he published his findings immediately. He received the unanimous support of the entire international scientific community and of the Spanish Paediatric Association. The formula was then withdrawn from the market. As a result, many babies around the world owe him their life. His career was an example of what science must be, which is always there to serve society. The entire international scientific community lamented his death. His friend Professor Manuel Bueno, another great name in Paediatrics, dedicated an accurate and moving article to him in 2011 (Bueno Sánchez, 2011).

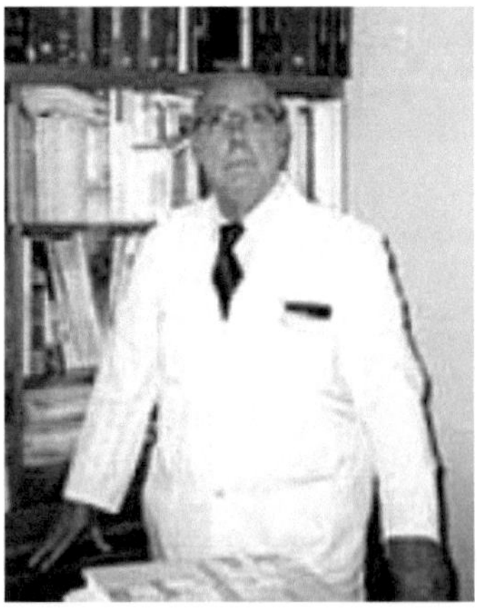

Fig. 10. Prof. Dr. Juan Rodríguez Soriano (1933-2010)

We cannot forget to mention Professor Cruz Hernández, professor at the University of Barcelona and author of the best modern Treatise on Paediatrics in the Spanish language.

His scientific work is of the first order. His book is the Spanish Paediatric Association's official treatise.

The system for training specialists in Spain, which as has been mentioned was very deficient, changed radically with the introduction across Spain in 1974 of the post-graduate training system, for those graduating in Medicine, known as the training plan for resident physicians (MIR). Thanks to that, the quality of the qualifications available in Spain has reached enviable heights. The current system involves, after a testing entry exam, 4 or 5 years of training for a speciality. Since its implementation it has resulted in very high quality healthcare in Spain. Infant mortality during the first year of life is currently around 3 per thousand born alive. The Spanish National Health System is considered one of the five best and most efficient in the world. This is true to such an extent that we have what is called "health tourism", where people from many countries throughout Europe come to have their complaints treated in Spain.

The transfer of health care to the Autonomous Regions, which culminated at the start of this century, is another factor to take into account. The much missed Minister Ernesto Lluch, Julián García Vargas and Ana Pastor are three politicians who in their time helped to develop Spanish medicine. The General Health Act, created twenty five years ago by Minister Lluch, resulted in the extension of high quality healthcare to the entire Spanish population, subsidised by the General Spanish State Budget. Among other things, it ensured that children would be seen by paediatricians up to the age of 14, instead of the previous 7. Years later Ernesto Lluch was sadly assassinated by the terrorist group ETA. Julián García Vargas understood his work as an act of service to the Spanish population. During his years in charge he periodically organised meetings in the Teruel Parador Hotel, in which he met with social and political representatives so that he could listen to suggestions and keep in touch with the reality. This was called *"the spirit of Teruel"*. Both belonged to the Spanish Socialist Worker's Party (PSOE). Ana Pastor, of the Popular Party (PP), was capable of fulfilling her role during the difficult period in which health issues were being transferred to the Autonomous Regions, despite not being very convinced that this was the best solution for healthcare (Labay Matías, 2010). To summarise, from the end of the 1960s to the arrival of the 21st century, healthcare in general, and paediatrics in particular, experienced the golden age of the Spanish National Health System.

The increase in the level of Primary Care meant the creation in almost all Spanish hospitals of paediatric specialities. These have become indispensable to society due to the excellent work of the paediatricians in the health centres.

Today Spanish society has a high quality paediatric service which can comfortably address the needs of children and adolescents. The generosity and self-sacrifice of its professionals is the cornerstone to this situation (Labay Matías, 2010).

7. The future and its uncertainties

On the horizon we can make out some concerns, certain changes, and the risk of not improving on what we already have (Cruz Hernández, 2010; Labay Matías, 2010). The impression is that paediatric care is more highly valued by the public than by the politicians and administrators (Pérez Tirado et al, 2010). Our speciality does not have the waiting lists seen by others, and the number of admissions of children and adolescents into the hospitals are limited and involve brief stays. The main focus is always the wellbeing of the child, and they are allowed home early, providing the results of the tests carried out in the hospital appointments. We are probably the most clinical of all the specialities. As soon as the symptoms and signs improve, the child is sent home. This does not happen in other medical areas, where the patients remain in hospital until the final complementary tests have been completed. The right thing is done, but this is not appreciated by the health authorities who are guided by the number of people admitted, the occupation index, the reduced waiting lists, etc.: quality is not taken into account. Not taking time off after being on call so that they can continue working or providing consultations, interrupting holidays to look after children.....these are common practices for many Spanish paediatricians. Primary Care is visited by many children outside normal surgery hours and as a result there are no delays in receiving care. Each day high quality medicine is provided in all possible areas: curative, preventive and social (Fernández Pérez et al., 2003; Haagan, 2009; Martínez González, 2010; Pérez Tirado et al., 2010). The paediatricians involved in this form the very heart of our heath care model. It has been shown that paediatricians in health centres request less complementary tests and write less prescriptions for medicines for children than are requested and written when the children are seen by other professionals (Buñuel Álvarez et al., 2010).

This dedication and self-sacrifice, following the path carved out by Jerónimo Soriano, is starting to count against our speciality. In many Paediatric Services, severely ill children and those that are complicated to manage come on demand to the hospitalisation floor to receive medical attention, which generates a considerable "hidden care" which is not taken into account by the administrators (Labay Matías et al., 1994).For the politicians, our speciality is a minor issue because it does not cause them any problems. In the Spanish Public Health System there seems to be an unwritten rule that penalises its most loyal and hard working professionals.

The transfer of health care to the Autonomous Regions has improved certain aspects of care, but only at the cost of a considerable increase in the political, management and administrative structure, which we consider unnecessary and excessive. They have become impervious to each other and to professionals. In some, if comments made by colleagues are to be believed, the health care politicians in charge do not know the range of services offered in the hospitals by the Paediatric Services. This range of services has been repeatedly mentioned to the administrators. *"Primun non nocere deinde filosofare"*, said Aristotle. It is dangerous for politicians to make decisions about our speciality without being aware of the current reality. They must justify their positions and actions to society as a whole and to the health care professionals. Without these premises they do not have enough credibility. As a result of all this they could cause irreparable damage to Paediatrics. With the transfer of healthcare from the State to the 17 autonomous governments in Spain, finalised in 2003, the healthcare system in Spain became very peculiar. Each Autonomous Region decides on its own IT system (each incompatible with the rest), children's medical cards, calendar of vaccinations and range of services offered to the public which vary depending on the Region. To receive attention in another Community people must deregister their health card in their place of residence and register in the other place where they are a patient, even if this is just for one day. In Spain there is an expression used when everything divides up:

"Son reinos de taifas", which can be roughly translated as "they are taifa kingdoms". This alludes to the fact that the Muslims in Spain were powerful while the Caliphate of Cordoba kept them united, up to the 11th century. Once cracks appeared, small Muslim kingdoms, called "taifas", sprung up throughout their territories. This decline of the Muslims allowed the Christian Kingdoms at that time to reconquer the whole of Spain. The same has happened with school education, with the negative consequences being borne by Spanish children and young people.

In the light of the risks that could be faced by Spanish Paediatrics in the future, one must act sensibly and vigorously (Cruz Hernández, 2010; Labay Matías, 2010). All paediatricians, regardless of ideology, professional activity or residency, have to be capable of uniting behind a sole common objective: to preserve and improve the care of Spanish children and adolescents. I am convinced that the Management Board of the Spanish Association of Paediatrics, with the Regional and Paediatric Speciality organisations, are the most qualified to act as spokespeople representing us in the face of public opinion, and to the politicians and unions. Our President, the academic Serafín Málaga Guerrero, must be able to rely on our unconditional support when it comes to some basic areas. His successors will deserve the same support.

In the opinion of the undersigned, close cooperation between the Primary Care and Specialist professionals is fundamental. The specific core subject of Paediatrics must be respected. The MIR medical post-graduate training system in untouchable: it can be improved but never reduced. Having shown its effectiveness over the decades, it would be a huge error to dispense with it or limit its duration and content. The specialities are vital for the development of Paediatrics and as a result must be strengthened as much as possible (Cruz Hernández, 2010; Labay Matías, 2010; Martín Mateos, 2010). There is probably no risk for those looking after seriously ill children: Neonatology, Neonatal Intensive Care, Paediatric Intensive Care, Paediatric Surgery and Oncology. Very sick children scare people and will be left in our hands. Other branches of Paediatrics could be swallowed up by other specialities or see themselves reduced to a bare minimum. This goes against the current approach taken in Europe, to which Spain belongs (Cruz Hernández, 2010; Labay Matías, 2010; Martín Mateos, 2010). It is impossible to forget the efforts made in this field by academics such as Sánchez Villares, Ballabriga, Peña, Cruz Hernández, Rodríguez- Soriano, Bueno, Delgado, Crespo, Málaga, Argente, Pérez-Yarza and many more. This entire brilliant generation has set out an unalterable path for us. The paediatricians trained through their teaching are the current leaders in our specialty. The undersigned remembers meetings chaired by the lecturer Rodríguez-Soriano and Doctor Bezanilla Regato in the Hospital Infantil Universitario de Cruces children's hospital, and involving residents finishing their second or third year of MIR, at the point of selecting a speciality. Many of these students are now well known experts in different branches of paediatrics. That vision of the future, which existed in the children's hospitals during that time, has raised the level of the specialities and paediatrics in Spain and allowed professional excellence to be attained. This scientific treasure cannot under any circumstances be lost. It is essential for the future and for progress.

People with other qualifications cannot be allowed to hold posts in paediatrics as they do not have enough knowledge of the area. The politicians, in Primary Care, may be assessing the option of importing health care models in which paediatricians do not play a full part because they do not exist: the care of children and adolescents would be taken out of our hands. In fact, if the important thing is efficiency and results, we should be offering and exporting our health care system to other countries. If paediatricians gradually disappear from health centres it would result in a drastic reduction of the current quality and the start of the dismantling of an exemplary health care system, which is less expensive than in other parts of Europe because of the salaries of the Spanish doctors. Who would benefit from this?: not the public of course, but private medicine would. It would mean turning back the clock 60 years in terms of the social benefits and what we call the welfare state.

It is surprising that there is no common Children's Health Book for all Spanish children, with calendars of specific vaccinations in keeping with the guidelines in the 17 Autonomous Regions making up the country. The IT system in the Autonomous Regions must be the same. In the list for access to posts, medical knowledge must take precedence over all other aspects in all Communities. Even when it comes to medical positions of responsibility, such as heads of service and section, politics with a small p is interfering. The Ministry of Health's Inter-Regional Board must make some decisions and cease to be a fictitious organisation without a real role. The Ministry of Health must justify its existence and its actions. The Inter-Regional Board has currently been reduced to a mere consultative body, without any decision making or coordinating powers, and the Ministry of Health lacks control, with practically everything being in the hands of the Autonomous Regions. This is what leads to its zero control of management and decision making. A health care agreement must be imposed in Spain; one in which all the political parties and professionals have a say. There must be a debate on many issues and decisions need to be taken, including those on the joint financing and creation of a new health model which more effectively meets current and future needs. The health system does not belong to any one political party; it belongs to the public who pay for it through their taxes. The politicians are there to serve the people they represent and to whom they are accountable for the running of the country. Health care administrators must be professional posts and not political ones. It is incomprehensible for the Hospital and Primary Care Directors, for example, to be appointed and removed on the basis of the political party in power in the Autonomous Regions.

The age for receiving Paediatric care must be increased to 18 years: we are more familiar with the problems of these young people than other specialities (Labay Matías et al., 2006). Demands must be made for the Ministry of Health to provide real figures about the current and future need for paediatricians and doctors, and for the Universities to act on this information. It is difficult to accept that such data is not available and that there are no figures on the short, medium and long term requirements for professionals within the existing bureaucratic structure: what are the politicians and administrators doing with their time?

Foreign doctors are currently needed and they are welcomed with affection and respect. Almost 16,000 work in Spain, as a result of the Spanish Universities producing very few doctors (Labay Matías, 2010). Many of them take advantage of their time in our country to specialise while they work, putting themselves forward for the MIR exam. Have they all faced the difficulties that the Spanish students have in accessing our Universities? In the 2010 exam almost 50% of the doctors registering were from outside the EU and in 2011 the figure was 35%. Many of them go back to their countries after finishing their MIR. In the meantime, the Spanish State has invested €200,000 in training each of them, which in these cases is a waste of financial resources. As a result, there is a risk that the Spanish students finishing their medical degrees will have problems in accessing MIR training and obtaining a specialist position in Spain. It is also hard to understand why, with the real need for doctors in Spain, the Universities do not increase the number of degree course places for this profession in such high demand in our country. The percentage of paediatric posts unfilled or being carried out by a doctor without the appropriate qualifications is 33%. The real reason is that the Ministry of Education is almost entirely powerless, since it has assigned it powers to the Autonomous Regions whose politicians do not normally have enough personal or intellectual capacity or a vision of the future. Unfortunately, politics in Spain is in the hands of many people whose main merit is following the orders of their superiors, since there are many who have no previous profession or studies to demonstrate their worth. They are bound to the senior members of their political parties, but not to the population.

Of the Spanish population, 13% are immigrants. As many are without resources or work, they receive financial aid from the Government and have the right to receive the full range of healthcare services. This has led to the healthcare system becoming overstretched at every level. The author has complete respect for immigrants, who he sees and helps as best he can. This does not stop him from understanding that the immigration policy in Spain has been mistaken over the last few years and that it may result in some unforeseen consequences.

According to published data, the Spanish healthcare system owes €15bn to suppliers and is on the point of financial meltdown. This is partly due to the Autonomous Regions taking on much more debt than they can cope with, often without good reason. People are starting to understand that what we call the "welfare state" has to be maintained by everyone, and that the politicians are responsible for misspending public money received from the taxpayers' pockets. There is now talk of the transfers in education and health having been a political and financial mistake[25]. In Spain, another democratic State was built on the structures of General Franco's totalitarian state, superimposed on the original one. This has led to administrative and political infrastructures that are overloaded and unsustainable for the Spanish population. What might have made good sense thirty years ago needs a wholesale review at this time. As a result, all the political parties must plan to completely remodel the current State system. According to official polls, politics is the third most worrying thing for the Spanish population, after the terrible unemployment problem and the management of the financial crisis by the Government (Usera et al. 2011).

The Official State Bulletin of 23 May 2011 contained a Ministry of Employment and Immigration Order (TIN/1362/2011) which has specifically prohibited, since 1 July, without any alternative, professionals who retire from continuing to provide services on their own behalf. This affects doctors, architects, lawyers and other groups. This means that 500,000 Spanish professionals aged 65 years old and upwards, in full possession of their mental faculties, have to stop working and cannot contribute to the State through their private activities. As a result, many clinics, consulting rooms and offices will close, with the result that the employees will lose their jobs and swell the numbers of the unemployed. Since 1986, doctors and paediatricians working for the public system who also have their own private practice, which they run in the evenings while strictly complying with their public duties and schedules, receive €12,000 a year less than their counterparts who work exclusively for the public sector. The aforementioned Ministerial Order, which has caused outrage, has been widely challenged by the political parties, Professional Bodies and other organisations, but this Ministerial Order has been suppressed in order to avoid massive resignations of brilliant professionals. It is yet another example of the fact that in Spain some politicians do not think sensibly or wisely. The Spanish present politic scenario has been masterfully analized wy Arturo Pérez- Reverte, extraordinary writer and member of Spanish Royal Academy of Language in a recent article (Pérez-Reverte, 2011).

8. Conclusion

As argued by Varela (Varela el al., 2010): *"to advance in terms of continuous improvement everything must be negotiated and shared between professionals and managers"*. This is not common in Spain. We must be united in defending Paediatrics in Spain, which means defending top quality care for our children and young adults but still thinking about the future, not being afraid of change as long as it results in an improvement to what already exists. This must be our legacy, what we leave for those who are coming after us. More than 400 years of history and effort must motivate us to continue along the path shown by our grand masters. In defence of Paediatrics (Cruz Hernández, 2010; Labay Matías, 2010; Martín Mateos, 2010), united to the end. Not everything was better in the past, but the future must be (Cruz Hernández, 2010). Children and adolescents always have the right to receive care from paediatricians and specialists from the different areas of paediatrics (Elías Pollina et al., 2011; Labay Matías, 2010; Málaga Guerrero 2011). Between all the groups: the public, politicians, managers, professionals and the unions, a way must be found to ensure that Spain continues maintaining and improving its enviable National Health System, for children and the entire population. I am convinced that the spirit of Jerónimo Soriano is with us, encouraging us to complete the wonderful adventure that he began: caring for children.

9. Acknowledgements

Professor Serafín Málaga Guerrero, President of the Spanish Paediatric Association, for his tireless work representing Spanish paediatricians; to Professor Eduardo G. Pérez-Yarza, Chief Editor of "Anales de Pediatría" for his friendship and work in favour of the speciality; to Professor Alfonso Delgado Rubio, ex-President of the Spanish Paediatric Association for his involvement in the Jerónimo Soriano Award; to Dr. Ángel Ferrández and Dr. Juan Elías, ex-presidents of the Aragon, La Rioja and Soria Paediatric Association, for the same reason; to Dr. Víctor García Nieto, a great paediatric nephrologist, history expert and friend; and to Dr. Francisco Valle, an extraordinary person and wonderful colleague, who introduced me to the Jerónimo Soriano path of knowledge. To Miguel Labay Guerrero, my elder son, for his help with ofimatics.

10. References

Arana de Amurrio, J. I. (2000). Evolución de los saberes pediátricos en España desde el tratado de Gerónimo Soriano hasta la actualidad. Cuatro siglos de historia. *An Esp Pediatr*, Vol. 52, Supl. 5, (June 2000), pp. 1-6, ISSN 1695-4033

Argente Oliver, J. (2011). Perspectivas presentes y futuras de la endocrinología pediátrica en España. *An Pediatr (Barc)*, Vol. 74, No. 2, (February 2011), pp. 69-71, ISSN 1695-4033

Baldivielso M. (1871). *Manual del Estudiante de Medicina,* Moya y Plaza editores, Madrid, Spain

Bueno Sánchez, M. (2011). In memoriam: Prof. Dr. Juan Rodríguez Soriano (1933-2010). *An Pediatr (Barc),* Vol. 74, No. 1, (January 2011), pp. 1-2, ISSN 1695-4033

Buñuel Álvarez, J. C.; García Vera, C.; González Rodríguez, M. P.; Aparicio Rodrigo, M.; Barroso Espadero D.; Cortés Marina, R. B.; et al. (2010). ¿Qué profesional médico es el más adecuado para impartir cuidados en salud a niños en Atención Primaria en países desarrollados? Revisión sistemática. *Pediatría Atención Primaria,* Vol. 12, Supl. 18, (March 2010), pp. 9-72, ISSN 1139-7632

Cruz Hernández, M. (2010). En defensa de la Pediatría. *An Pediatr (Barc),* Vol. 72, No. 3, (March 2010), pp. 163-164, ISSN 1695-4033

Cruz Hernández, M. (2010) *Sesenta años de Pediatría inacabada,* Ergón, ISBN 978-848-473-589, Madrid, Spain

Elías Pollina, J.; Bastarós García, J. C.; Olivares López, J. L.; Ferrández Longás, A.; Labay Matías, M.; García Vera, C.; Ruiz Echarri, M. & Romero Gil, R. (2011). ¿Quo vadis Pediatría?: Problemas actuales; soluciones de futuro. Zaragoza, 25 de marzo de 2010. *Boletín de la Sociedad de Pediatría de Aragón, La Rioja y Soria,* Vol. 41, No. 1, (January 2011), pp. 19-24, ISSN 1696-358X

Fernández Pérez, M.; López Benito, M. M. & Franco Vidal, A. (2003). Consultas de alta resolución desde Pediatría de Atención Primaria: una apuesta por la calidad asistencial. *Pediatría Atención Primaria,* Vol. 5, No. 17, (January 2003), pp. 133-144, ISSN 1139-7632

Fleta Zaragozano, J. (2009). Hace 50 años: acontecimientos y avances médicos en 1960. *Boletín de la Sociedad de Pediatría de Aragón, La Rioja y Soria,* Vol. 39, No. 3, (September 2009), pp. 78-83, ISSN 1696-358X

García Nieto, V.; Málaga Guerrero, S.; Arana de Amurrio, J. I.; Fernández Menéndez, J. M.; Fernández Teijerio, J. J.; Gorrotxategi Gorrotxategui, P. J.; Ponte Hernando, F. & Zafra Anta, M. (2011). *IV centenario de los libros de Pediatría. Cuadernos de historia de la pediatría española. Vol. 1,* ISBN 978-84-615-1197-6, Asociación Española de Pediatría, Madrid, Spain

Grupo de Trabajo de Historia de la Pediatría y Documentación Pediátricas de la Asociación Española de Pediatría (Ed.). (2010). *Crónicas de la Pediatría Española (1888-1913), Historia de la Pediatría en España de Andrés Martínez Vargas,* Facsimile edition, Privierno S.L.L., Madrid, Spain

Haagan, J. F. (2009). Reflenting on "Reflections on Were-Child Care Practice". *Pediatrics,* Vol. 124, No. 3 (September 2009), p. 990, ISSN 0210-5721

Labay Matías, M. (2010). Pediatría, ciudadanos y políticos. *An Pediatr (Barc),* Vol. 73, No. 2, (August 2010), pp. 67-69, ISSN 1695-433

Labay Matías, M.; De Miguel Pardo, C.; Valero Adán, M. T.; Buñuel Álvarez, C.; Martín Calama, J. & Valle Sánchez, F. (1994). Asistencia oculta en un Servicio de Pediatría. *An Esp Pediatr,* Vol. 40, No. 4, (November 1994), pp. 386-387, ISSN 1695-4033

Labay Matías, M.; Valero Adán, M. T.; Miralbés Terraza, S.; Valle Sánchez, F.; Martín Calama, J. & De Miguel Pardo, C. (2006). A partir de los 14 años, la Pediatría existe. *Boletín de la Sociedad de Pediatría de Aragón, La Rioja y Soria,* Vol. 36, No. 2, (March 2006), p. 61, ISSN 1696-358-X

Laín Entralgo, P. (1992) *Historia universal de la medicina*, Masson, ISBN 978-80-45-80-2427, Barcelona, Spain

Málaga Guerrero, S. (2011). ¡Salvemos la Pediatría!, In: *Asociación Española de Pediatría*, (08/09/2011), Available from http://www.aeped.es/noticias/nota-prensa-sobre-campaña-salvemos-pediatria

Martín Mateos, M. A. (2010). Acreditación europea de las especialidades pediátricas. *An Pediatr (Barc)*, Vol. 72, No. 1, (January 2010), pp. 1-3, ISSN 1695-4033

Martínez González, C. (2010). La mirada social del pediatra. *An Pediatr (Barc)*, Vol. 73, No. 5, (November 2010), pp. 229-232, ISSN 1695-4033

Pérez-Reverte, A. (2011). Sobre imbéciles y malvados. XLSemanal. N° 1243 (21-28 August 2011), Available from www.xlsemanal.com and www.xlsemanal.com/perezreverte ISSN 1835-5865. Madrid, Spain

Pérez Tirado, L.; Hernández Blanco, M.; Nogales Cortés, M. D. & Sánchez Sánchez, M. J. (2010). Evaluación de la satisfacción de los familiares en las urgencias pediátricas. *Revista de calidad Asistencial*, Vol. 25, No. 2, (March 2010), pp. 58-63, ISSN 1134-282 X

Pérez-Yarza, E. G.; Cabañas, F.; García-Algar, O. & Valverde Molina, J. (2010). Año 2009: Anales de Pediatría estrena factor de impacto. *An Pediatr (Barc)*, Vol. 73, No. 3, (September 2010), pp. 113-114. ISSN 1695-4033

Ramos y Luengo, F. (1821). *Manual Médico-Quirúrgico o elementos de Medicina y Cirugía práctica*, José Santa María, Murcia, Spain

Rodríguez Tejerina, J. M. (1981). *Historia de la Medicina en Mallorca*, Ramón Balmes, ISBN 978-84-300-500-43, Palma de Mallorca, Spain

Sánchez Martín, J. (2007). Semblanza de los profesores Arce y Sánchez Villares. *Boletín de Pediatría*, Vol. 47, No 202/4, (June 2007), pp. 307-309, ISSN 0214-2597

Soriano, J., (2000). *Methodo y orden de curar las enfermedades de los niños, con un estudio preliminar de los doctores Jesús Sarabia Pardo y José Ignacio de Arana Amurrio*, Facsimile edition, ISBN 84-95136-40-6, Alhulia, Granada, Spain

Usera, V. & Martín, J. (2011). La sanidad pública roza el colapso. *El Mundo*, Mercados No. 178 (6 June 2011)

Valle Sánchez, F.; Labay Matías, M.; De Miguel Pardo, C.; Valero Adán, M. T.; Martín Calama, J. & Muñoz Albillos, M. (2000). Jerónimo Soriano: Cuatrocientos años de su obra. *Boletín de la Sociedad de Pediatría de Aragón, La Rioja y Soria*, Vol. 30, No. 3, (October 2000), pp. 56-57, ISSN 1696-358-X

Varela, J.; Craywinckel, G.; Esteve, E. & Picas, J. M. (2010). Implicación de los médicos en la gestión basada en el profesionalismo y en el liderazgo de equipos multidisciplinares. *Med Clin (Barc)*, Vol. 134, No. 1, (January 2010), pp. 35-39, ISSN 0025-7753

Part 2

Nutritional Health

2

Feeding and Fluids in the Premature and Sick Newborn in the Low-Middle Income Countries

Tina Slusher, Yvonne Vaucher,
Tara Zamora and Beverly Curtis
Center for Global Pediatrics,
University of Minnesota, Minneapolis,
USA

1. Introduction

1.1 Overview of the feeding principles in premature and sick infants

There are many appropriate feeding regimes in neonatal nurseries around the world. (Adamkin, 2005; Chan, 2001; Gomella,2004; Eyal, & Zenk, 2004; Klingenberg, Embleton, Jacobs, O'Connell, & Kuschel, 2011; McCormick et al, 2010; WHO, 2007) Exact regimes are not as important as following basic principles of feeding these fragile infants. These principles include the following components below.

Start feedings as early as it is safe to do so. This is especially important because most nurseries in low-middle income countries (LMICs) do not have access to total parenteral nutrition (TPN). Although controversial and not consistently practiced in high-income countries (Klingenberg, et al., 2011) infants in LMICs who are stable should begin feedings on day 1 or 2 at the latest. In very low birthweight infants, who are too ill to feed on day 1, it is helpful to give intravenous (IV) fluids on day 1 and then begin an intravenous to enteral titration on day 2. Generally feeds should be advanced as rapidly as tolerated, especially in locations without TPN. Once on full feeds and off intravenous fluids, most infants will require about 160-200 ml/kg/day (and occasionally more) to meet their caloric needs and ultimate weight gain goals of about 15g/kg/day (Gomella, et al., 2004). As stressed, later in the chapter, the first feedings ideally should be colostrum. The exact volume needed for adequate weight gain after the initial expected drop in weight in the first 7-14 days of life (up to 21 days in very small infants) will depend on the caloric content of the mother's breastmilk or substitute feedings. Mothers' breastmilk can vary in caloric content from about 14 to 35 calories per ounce depending on the fat content of her breastmilk (Meier et al., 2002). For detailed information on how to determine the caloric content of breastmilk see the Textbook of Global Child Health (AAP) (Slusher T et al, 2012) .

Preterm infants less than 1200 grams require gavage feedings every 2 hours; ≥ 1200 g-1500g generally require gavage feedings every 2-3 hours; infants >1500-2000 grams can be given a combination of gavage and oral feedings (cup and spoon or dropper) every 3 hours. Infants greater than 2000 grams who are neurologically intact can generally be fed at the breast or via cup and spoon if unable to feed at the breast due to either infant or maternal problems (guidelines adapted from Gomella et al for LMICs) (Gomella, et al., 2004). When first beginning feeding at the breast, most premature infants will require supplementation with cup and spoon feeds because of insufficient milk transfer to support adequate weight gain. Bottle feedings should be strongly discouraged in LMICs because of the difficulty of keeping them clean and their association with diarrheal diseases and death in these environments (Alrifai et al, 2010; Eshete, 2008; Ghosh et al., 1997).

Advance feedings as rapidly as is safe to do so. Generally this works best if there is a specific protocol that the nurses can follow without additional orders. Guidelines about when to deviate from these protocols and when to call the physician for feeding problems should also be in place. For infants less than 1000 grams birthweight, begin at 1cc every 1-2 hours and advance by 1-2cc every 24 hours if tolerated; for birth weight 1000g-1500 grams start at 1-2cc every 2 hours if possible (every 3 hours may be required depending on nursing shortages) and advance by 1-2cc every 12 hours; for birth weight greater than 1500 grams to 2000 grams start at 2-3cc/feed every 3 hours and advance every 8-12 hours; for birth weight greater than 2000 grams-2500 grams and unable to feed at the breast start at 5cc and advance by 5cc every 6-8 hours; for birth weight greater than 2500 grams and unable to feed at the breast start at 10cc every 3 hours and advance by 10-15cc every 3-6 hours (adapted from Zlatkin and Perman) (Zlatkin, 1988).

All breastfeeding babies should get Vitamin K_1 at birth and be supplemented with Vitamin D (Leung & Sauve, 2005). Additionally, iron supplementation should be started in all breastfed premature infants as soon as they are tolerating feeds and in term breastfed infants by four months of age(Baker & Greer, 2010).

1.2 Addressing feeding problems

Observe for signs of feeding intolerance including signs of necrotizing enterocolitis (NEC). Some of the signs of feeding intolerance include increasing abdominal distention, increasing gastric aspirate (especially if > than 30% the previous feeding), bilious vomiting and bloody stools (Gomella, et al., 2004). Isolated delayed gastric emptying should not be used as the only criteria for initiating, advancing, or withholding feeds (Adamkin, 2005). This practice can lead to excess delays in reaching appropriate caloric goals with consequent poor weight gain. If the infant has only increasing abdominal distention or gastric aspirate, without other signs of NEC, it may be appropriate to hold 1-2 feedings and then resume feedings at a smaller volume and increase slowly to reach caloric goals. If the infant has other signs of NEC or a surgical abdomen such as abdominal tenderness, edema of the gut wall, thrombocytopenia, X-ray changes consistent with NEC or a surgical abdomen, feedings will need to be held, IV fluids and/or total parental nutrition (if available) started along with other appropriate care as indicated by the disease process including antibiotics, nasogastric decompression and surgical consults.

Recognize the importance of distinguishing between swallowed blood and true gastrointestinal bleeding. Feedings do not need to be held for swallowed blood. Bloody gastric aspirates are not a sign of NEC but may be associated with swallowed maternal blood, gastric irritation, hypothermia, thrombocytopenia, and gastric ulcers. However, if available, it is appropriate to begin ranitidine and give Vitamin K_1 (if not previously given) in infants with gastrointestinal bleeding not of maternal origin. Consider a second dose of Vitamin K_1 if bleeding is severe.

Recognize contraindications for beginning enteral feeds and/or continuing or advancing feeds. Absolute contraindications include a complete obstruction at any level unless the obstruction is caused from a meconium ileus, which may be alleviated non-surgically; severe hemodynamic instability, and confirmed necrotizing enterocolitis. In the absence of TPN, supporting these infants for more than 1-2 weeks on IVF's alone is difficult. Therefore, feedings should be started or re-started as soon as it is safe to do so. Signs that it is safe to attempt feedings include a soft, non-distended, non-tender abdomen with bowel sounds present and minimal gastric drainage.

2. Routes of feeding (gastric tube verses cup verses at the breast)

Oral feeding of the preterm infants is a challenge to the provider, the mother and the family. The maturation of feeding skills occurs in the last trimester of pregnancy and therefore, preterm infants are born deficient in the skills necessary for effective feeding including the ability to latch, to suck effectively, and to coordinate sucking, swallowing and breathing. Due to early delivery and complicated by interventions including suctioning, intubation, and ventilation, as well as neurologic, gastroenterological and cardiac status, the development of appropriate skills may be delayed, or significantly affected. The motor activities necessary for feeding, sucking, swallowing and breathing, develop in utero and are observed developing as early as 10-12 weeks gestation with the infant opening the jaw and 3-4 weeks later beginning suckling with fingers in the oral cavity. Breathing movements and swallowing begin as early as the 12th week of life. By the 28th week of gestation the jaw is observed in rhythmic movements with alveolar ridge stimulation. As the infant matures in utero, so do the behaviors necessary to sustain feeding. By the 28th-33rd week of gestation, suckling bursts can appear erratic and non-rhythmical. A mature suck, swallow, pause pattern is not observed until 35 to 36 weeks of gestation. This consistent rhythmic organization of suckling coordinated with swallowing and respirations is often considered a hallmark for neurologic maturation (adapted from Delaney and Anderson)(Delaney & Arvedson, 2008). Even when able to suckle, preterm infants have limited fat suckling pads in the cheeks, which impact the ability to maintain suction and duration of feeding.

Prior to initiating oral feeding, an evaluation of the infant's feeding skills should be performed by an experienced observer (Nightlinger, 2011). The respiratory rate during rest and sleep in the past several days should be noted. Infants who are tachypneic or have frequent apneic spells are at risk during oral feedings. Presence of excessive oral secretions with drooling or choking spells may be an indication of poor swallowing or anatomical abnormalities that need to be evaluated. Any abnormalities of the tongue, palate or lips should be noted as they may affect the method of feeding.

An oral-digital exam may be helpful in assessing readiness for feeding. The examiner presents his or her gloved finger in the mouth of the infant, with the pad of the examiners finger toward the palate. It is not unusual to find the tongue elevated posteriorly pressed against the hard palate. As the jaw opens wide for feeding, this initiates a drop in the tongue and one can observe central grooving as the side of the tongue elevates, surrounding the nipple or examiner's finger. The observer should see or feel the tongue move in a peristalsis motion not retracting and protruding. There should be a smooth peristaltic rhythm to the suckle with pausing, while suction is felt on the finger. Persistent retraction of the tongue, lack of seal or suction, sustained milk leakage, during oral feedings, hyperactive gag reflex, jaw gapping with loss of suction, or jaw tightening, and jaw or tongue undulations are adversely affect feeding. If persisting, these may be signs of neurologic deficits or swallowing disorders rather than prematurity (Nyqvist et al, 2001;Guilleminault et al, 1984).

Feeding regimens typically begin with gastric tube feeding in infants under 1500 grams. The determination of when to transition to oral feeds and how to begin oral feeding depends on the clinical status of the infant and the nursery specific protocols. Studies have shown that many neonatal units have no set policy for breastfeeding and that neonatal nurses have not received training in breastfeeding techniques (Cricco-Lizza, 2009; Siddell & Froman, 1994). This lack of training translates into poor and erroneous feeding information, lack of guidance for mothers and families, introduction of artificial feeds, and ultimately the possibility of breastfeeding failure for the mother and infant (Buckley & Charles, 2006; Grossman et al., 2009; Manganaro et al., 2009).

Work has been done by Nyqvist and Anderson (Nyqvist et al,2010) and de Aquino(de Aquino & Osorio, 2009) identifying a developmental care approach to feeding. This involves teaching staff and mothers to identify behavioral cues, stress cues, periods of wakefulness, feeding readiness and alertness. Reactions to overstimulation including excessive crying or staying asleep are behavioral cues of disorganization of state. Identifying these cues helps mothers and caregivers to adjust the environment and the feeding as needed for the infant. Thus feeding success is on a continuum of small developmental increments beginning with early tube feeding with gradual introduction of the breast through Kangaroo Mother Care (KMC) (Nyqvist, 2004) [see Figure 1.]. Skills are acquired slowly and will likely be associated with ups and downs, which should not be regarded as a failure. Mothers should be actively encouraged during this process. It is appropriate to allow the infant to lick or suckle the breast at each feeding even before effective suckling develops. This continuum begins with the preterm infant in developmentally appropriate positioning from the day of birth, which affords the infant the best opportunities to develop physiologically appropriate skills for readiness for feeds.(de Aquino & Osorio, 2009) Kangaroo Mother Care [i.e. the infant unclothed except for a hat and skin to skin against the mother's chest with the infants back covered with a blanket] should be initiated as soon as possible. KMC promotes temperature stability, steady growth, early and prolonged duration of breastfeeding, parental ability to respond to infant cues and enhanced attachment. KMC also reduces length of hospital stay, maternal postpartum depression symptoms, pain and incidence of infection.(Hake-Brooks & Anderson, 2008; Nyqvist et al, 2010) KMC allows the mother to spontaneously offer her breast and the infant to readily feed when awake and alert (Kliethermes et al, 1999; Nyqvist, 2010). Nyqvist noted that some very preterm infants have the capacity for early development of oral motor competence that it sufficient for establishment of full breastfeeding even at a low post-menstrual age(Nyqvist, 2008). De Aquino (de Aquino & Osorio, 2009) evaluated feeding retrospectively for infants who were tube fed at breast with expressed breastmilk. At discharge, 100% of the infants who were tube fed at the breast, were exclusively breastfed with appropriate weight gain, supporting breast feedings supplemented with oral gastric tube feedings as an efficient method in the feeding transition of preterm infants (de Aquino & Osorio, 2009).

The impact of cup feeding or bottle feeding on weight gain, oxygen saturation, and breastfeeding rates of preterm infants was examined in 34 bottle-fed and 44 cup-fed preterm infants (Rocha et al, 2002). No significant differences between groups were found with regard to time spent feeding, feeding problems, weight gain, or breastfeeding prevalence at discharge or at 3-month follow-up. Possible beneficial effects of cup feeding were lower incidence of desaturation episodes and a higher prevalence of breastfeeding at 3 months of age (Rocha, et al., 2002).

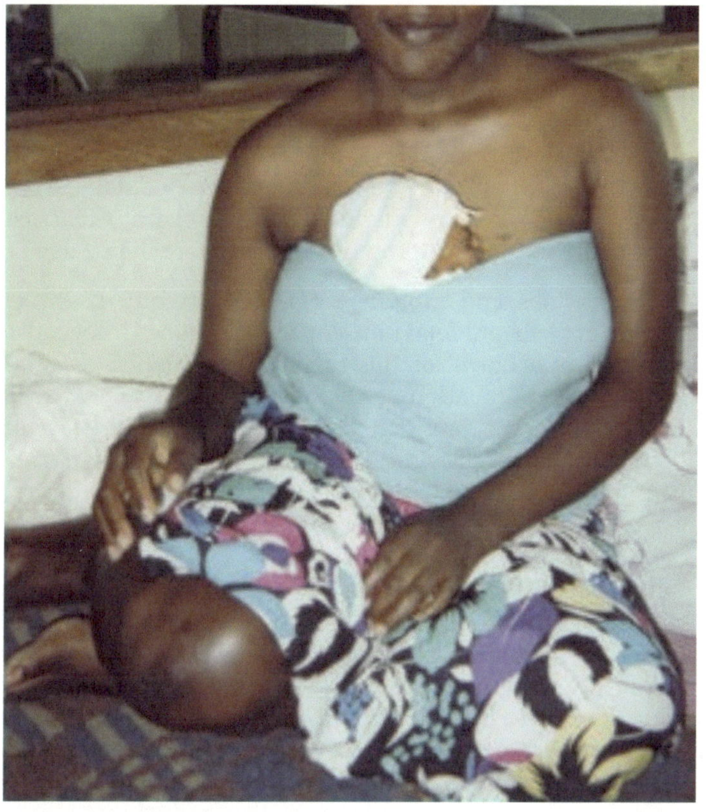

Fig. 1. Kangaroo Mother Care

In another study Abouelfettoh (Abouelfettoh et al, 2008) evaluated the use of cup feeding as an exclusive method of feeding preterm infants during hospitalization and its impact on breastfeeding outcomes after discharge. Sixty preterm infants averaging 35weeks gestation and birth weight of < 2150 grams participated in the study. Control group infants received only bottle feedings during hospitalization and the experimental group received only cup feedings during hospitalization. At six weeks of life the cup fed infants had significantly more mature breastfeeding behaviors than bottle fed infants and had a significantly higher proportion of breast feedings one week after discharge (Abouelfettoh, et al., 2008).

Meier (Meier et al., 2000) reported outcomes for 34 preterm infants whose mothers used silicon nipple shields during breast feedings. The mean milk transfer was significantly greater for feedings with the nipple shield (18 vs. 4 ml), with all 34 infants consuming more milk during breastfeeding. Major factors limiting the use of breast shield in LMIC are availability of shields, costs, concerns about cleanliness, and promoting bottle-feeding. However, as with many technologies used in high-income countries, it may be appropriate to have shields available in the special care baby nurseries for use before discharge of the infant from the nursery.

3. Monitoring for appropriate growth and responding appropriately to poor weight gain and growth

Observe for adequate weight gain which is generally about 15g/kg/day. However, the smaller the baby the slower the initial weight gain and the longer it is expected to take to get back to birth weight. In LMIC's where TPN is generally not available using the older growth chart from Dancis et al (Dancis et al, 1948) (see Figure 1.) may be more appropriate than using newer growth charts included in current neonatal handbooks and textbooks. Premature infants should ideally be weighed on the same scale daily (or at a minimum of every 2-3 days) and plotted on their individual growth chart. Adjustments to feedings should be made if the infant falls off the growth curve for more than 2 days.

Preterm nutritional guidelines and growth goals are currently based on the reference standard of intrauterine growth and fetal nutrient accretion rates (McLeod & Sherriff, 2007). This standard is difficult to achieve for this high-risk population especially in LMICs. If postnatal growth fails, preterm infants are at higher risk for adverse neurological outcomes and compromised health. The nutrient deficit occurring in the early weeks post delivery, when the infant is medically fragile, is difficult to overcome. Weight, length and head circumference measurements remain important clinical indicators of growth, but composition of weight gain is emerging as a necessary measure in determining the adequacy of nutrition intake and growth (McLeod et al, 1994). The need to monitor weight for estimation of fluid balance is a different task than monitoring for growth, and the practitioner needs to be aware of both issues. As noted on the growth chart (Dancis, et al., 1948), most preterm infants have a precipitous drop in weight in the first 7-14 days of life due to diuresis; the smaller the infant, the greater the percent of weight loss and the longer the time to regain birth weight. It is helpful to document this weight loss on a growth chart and establish the rate of growth from the lowest weight's plotting point(Zorlu, 2011). If early weight loss is not plotted, weight gain in the first several weeks of life appears inadequate. Inadequate growth is also identified by a lower growth rate than that required to follow the growth curves on the chart (Pridham et al., 2011).

If growth is poor, it is important to evaluate the cause. It may simply be that the infant is getting inadequate calories. This can be addressed as noted below by increasing the volume and/or fat content of the breastmilk, ideally by improved breastmilk expression techniques and/or increasing the fat content of the feeds or lacto-engineering (discussed later in this chapter). Rarely, it may be appropriate, if available, to add breast milk fortifiers and/or supplemental artificial feeds. Additionally, fat malabsorption, chronic lung disease, fluid restrictions and increase in energy expenditure may all contribute to poor growth. In infants feeding at the breast, weighing the infant pre-feed and post-feeds has been discussed in the literature and used in clinical practice for the last decade (Funkquist et al, 2010). Data by Hasse supported the use of pre- and post-feeds weighing as accurate, and an objective assessment of breastmilk intake (Haase et al, 2009), although this requires very accurate scales, not usually available in LMICs.

4. Breast milk use in premature and sick infants

4.1 Advantages of breastmilk

Breastmilk is the best food available for infants and should be strongly supported and encouraged worldwide. No substitute provides the same benefits as breastmilk to the infant. The many benefits are appropriately summarized in this table adapted from a wall hanging in Swaziland (Table 1.). These benefits of breastfeeding are also summarized in an article by Leung et al(Leung & Sauve, 2005) that highlights nutritional, immunological, anti-infective advantages of breastmilk, as well as the enhanced cognitive development and prevention of allergies, obesity, diabetes, and possibly sudden infant death and later hypertension.

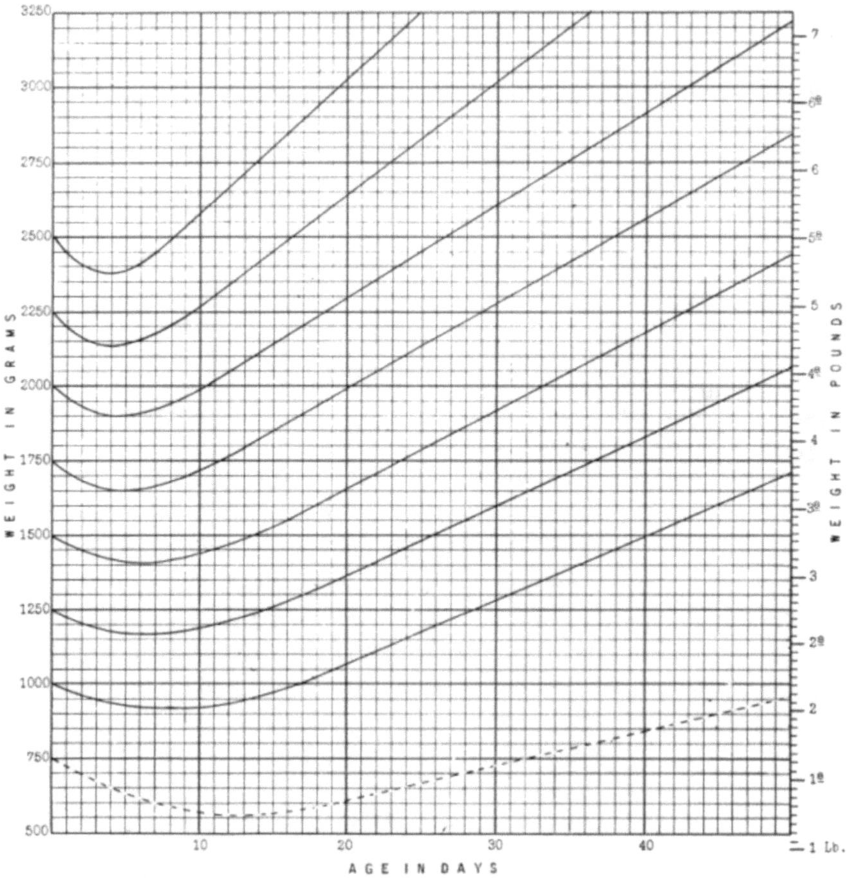

From: Dancis J, O'Connell JR, and Holt LE. J Pediatrics 1948; 33:570-572.

Fig. 1. Expected Neonatal Weight Changes based on Birth Weight.

For the premature infant the benefits are even more numerous and as summarized in an article by Meier, et al (Meier , 2010) the use of breastmilk also reduces the risk of a multitude of problems including necrotizing enterocolitis, nosocomial infections and re-hospitalizations in this vulnerable population.

Breast Feeding is BEST	
Best for Baby	Fresh milk never goes off (never spoils)
Reduces Allergies	Emotionally bonding
Economical	Easy, once established
Antibodies-greater immunity	Digested well
Stool inoffensive-rarely constipated	Immediately available-no mixing required
Temperature ideal	Nutritionally optimal
	Gastroenteritis greatly reduced

Table 1. Breast Feeding is BEST

When using breastmilk, use the colostrum first. Do not dilute breastmilk. In many cultures, discarding colostrum is common (Okolo et al, 1999; Rogers et al., 2011; Tiwari et al,, 2009). Education regarding the importance of giving the colostrum and not discarding the colostrum should be emphasized. As also noted in these studies (Okolo, et al., 1999; Rogers, et al., 2011; Tiwari, et al., 2009) and many others, pre-lacteal feedings are also common,(Ahmed et al, 1999; Chandrashekhar et al., 2007; Darmstadt et al., 2007; Lakati et al, 2010) are associated with increased morbidity and mortality(Engebretsen et al, 2008;Leach et al., 1999) and should be discouraged.

4.2 Breastmilk production

The challenge of producing sufficient quantities of breastmilk to support the growth of the preterm infant falls largely on the mother of the medically fragile infant. However, health care providers can help educate these mothers in improved expression techniques and thus, relieve some of this burden. Some mothers presented with the challenge of providing expressed breastmilk for their fragile infant have feelings of helplessness, powerlessness and inadequacy arising in an extremely vulnerable period for the mother-baby breastfeeding pair(Boucher et al, 2011; Rossman et al., 2011). The importance of initiating early breastmilk expression by hand and/or pumping cannot be emphasized enough. Creating nursing routines that document breastmilk expression and frequency into the regular record of care for the postpartum mother, legitimizes this cause and empowers the nurse to begin helping the mother down the lactation pathway. This journey of providing milk, a life saving substance for the infant, is one the entire nursery must take part in. Protocols and procedure as well as policies regarding breastfeeding, milk expression including pumping, milk storage and handling, will clarify each participants role in providing this life saving white gold to fragile infants (Dougherty & Luther, 2008). Breastmilk expression regimens that mimic the feeding behaviors of full term infants are best for establishment of lactogenesis (Slusher et al., 2007). This includes frequent expression of milk every two hours beginning as soon after delivery as possible, ideally within the first two hours. Recovery from birth can be arduous and pumping is often viewed as something a mother does once she feels healthy. This attitude, thereby, delays breastmilk expression by hours or days and mothers lose the natural window and hormonal levels necessary for ease of transition from colostrum to mature milk (Chen et al, 2001). When breastmilk expression is begun in the second hour of life or as soon thereafter delivery as is possible, mothers experience prolactin surges and prolactin cell receptor proliferation that promotes quick and efficient milk flow (Meier et al 2011). Trophic feeds for sick infants can then be managed with mothers' own milk, thereby avoiding the risk of artificial feeds in the immature gut. As noted by Slusher et al (Slusher, 2011) many mothers can express enough breastmilk by hand expression and this method should be supported and encouraged for most mothers. If a mother's milk supply is inadequate or decreasing over time, high quality hand pumps are also useful, especially in hospitals without consistent electricity. However, breastmilk expression protocols should include procuring a hospital grade pump (double pump) especially in referral hospitals as they do increase total maternal milk volume expressed (Slusher, et al., 2007; Slusher, et al., 2011) and can prove to be invaluable in those mothers who have an inadequate or decreasing milk volume with hand expression and hand pumps. Teaching the mother to combine hand expression and breast massage with pumping helps increase the expression of hind milk and avoids the problem of overly full breasts (Renfrew MJ, 2009). A combination of techniques, hand expression along with pumping may actually prove to be optimal (Morton et al., 2009). Fitting the pump breast shield to the mother's breast is an important part of providing the proper equipment for the mother who is expressing milk for her infant via an electric breast pump. The breast shield, the portion of the pumping kit that actually fits on the breast, must have adequate room for the nipple to move easily in the tunnel portion of the shaft. If this opening is too small or too large, then the mother may experience trauma to the breast or nipple and reduced milk flow. Persistent use of inappropriate breast shields may limit milk production and lead to early weaning. Mothers should be advised to pump regularly every 2-3 hours, as well as given advice that if it appears that they will be traveling or busy during the scheduled pumping time to pump early rather than miss the pumping session. If mother's feel they cannot pump the entire pumping session of 15- 20 minutes or two minutes beyond the time she no longer sees milk, then she should pump as long as possible for that pumping and then try to pump more frequently and more efficiently later to make up for the limited pumping session earlier in the day. Mothers who have prolonged pumping sessions beyond 20 minutes typically do not produce more milk and may have more nipple soreness. It is the repeated removal of milk from the breast that creates the stimulus for higher milk yield. There are large variances of how much milk the breast is able to store as well as how much milk the mother is able to pump. Mothers who appear to have plenty of milk but pump limited amounts may have mechanical problems with the pump, the wrong size breast shield, may be more successful hand expressing or need a different environment to promote let down.

4.3 Breastmilk storage

Milk storage containers are best when made of polypropylene, hard sided plastic or glass with a solid lid. Avoid open containers, containers closed with a bottle nipple, and polyethylene soft-sided storage bags (Cossey et al, 2011; Manohar, Williamson, & Koppikar, 1997). These bags often sequester nutrients and may split or tear. Concern has been expressed about regarding bacterial contaminant in breastmilk and the need for random culturing of milk. A recent analysis by Schandler demonstrated that breastmilk cultures are not predictive of infection in premature infants (Schanler et al., 2011) and therefore, are not recommended. Ideally, storage facilities in the nursery should be readily available for refrigerating freshly pumped milk and freezing extra milk while the infant is nil per os (NPO) or not consuming the amounts the mother is pumping. Even when such facilities are not available, or when her infant is taking only small volumes of milk at each feeding, the mother still needs to express until the breast is emptied. Emptying or nearly emptying the breast at each expression session increases milk production and increases the likelihood that the mothers of these infants will continue to be able to have enough milk to exclusively breastfeed their infants after discharge from the nursery (Chapman & Perez-Escamilla, 2000; Daly et al, 1996; Neville, 1999). Breast feeding mothers know when most of the milk has been extracted as the breast feels soft and lighter in weight.

Unrefrigerated breastmilk can be generally be given to infants for up to 3-4 hours (6 hours if very clean conditions) when stored at room temperature (ABM, 2010). Breastmilk may be safely refrigerated however, the suggested times vary widely depending on the study and the conditions of refrigeration from 3-8 days (ABM, 2010). If facilities exist for freezing expressed breast milk and keeping it frozen (consistent power), it may be frozen in the back of the freezer for at least 3 months (ABM, 2010). If fresh milk is not available, then refrigerated mother's milk should be given. Give frozen milk to infants who have exhausted both fresh and refrigerated supplies.

4.4 Increasing the caloric content of breastmilk

One major advantage of having extra milk at each breastmilk expression session is the opportunity to alter the caloric content of the milk by pumping the milk in two or even more aliquots. The first milk that the mother expresses is low fat, low calorie foremilk and can be set aside or stored for later use if those facilities are available. The later milk is higher fat, higher calorie milk or hindmilk and can be fed to the infant preferentially and improves the growth rate of the infant. This process is called "lacto-engineering" and is described in detail in the AAP book "Textbook of Global Child Health"(Slusher T, 2012). If time for teaching and staffing allow, both mothers and health care providers can be taught to determine the caloric content of breastmilk using a simple hematocrit spinner and reader. This process determines the creamatocrit or cream content of the milk and is discussed in detail by Slusher and Lucas (Lucas, 1978; Slusher et al, 2012). If this is not possible, mothers can be taught to watch their milk as they express it and to change containers when it begins to thicken and feed the second milk to their infants. For infants feeding at the breast, the first milk extracted from the breast is high in lactose, is sweet to the infant and entices the infant to feed more. The last milk in the breast or expressed near the end of the pumping or feeding session is high in fat and can be over 30 calories per ounce (Bishara et al 2008; Ogechi et al, 2007; Slusher et al., 2003). Feedings of hind milk alone contribute to weight gain in the infant (Ogechi, et al., 2007). Hind milk feeding is often employed for the infant unable to tolerate advancing volumes of feed or who demonstrates inadequate growth (Griffin et al, 2000; Lucas, 1978). Other additives have been utilized to promote growth in breastfed infants. These additives include human milk fortifiers, powdered formula and exogenous oil to improve caloric and nutrient intake. Each of these has disadvantages especially in LMICs. The cost of commercial breastmilk fortifiers is prohibitive in LMICs, artificial milk is expensive and easily contaminated during mixing, and oils may be poorly absorbed and adhere to tubing (Hamosh, 1987; Mehta, Hamosh et al, 1988). Supplementing breast milk involves not only the direct cost of the formula or supplement but also that of training the mothers in techniques for feeding their infants without compromising breastfeeding or increasing the risk of infectious diseases (Griffin, et al., 2000; Lucas, 1978; Ruiz et al, 2002).

4.5 Increasing breastmilk volumes

Bishara (Bishara et al, 2009) determined factors associated with foremilk volume (milk produced in the first 3 minutes of pumping), hindmilk volume (remainder of milk produced), and total milk volume produced by mothers of very preterm infants at 3 weeks postpartum. Milk volumes were not associated with mother's age, race or ethnic background, education, parity, reported pre-pregnancy body mass index, previous breastfeeding experience, frequency of milk pumping, longest time between pumps, infant birth weight, or multiple births. However, degree of pre-maturity (<26 weeks vs. 26 to 27 weeks) was significantly related to the relative proportion of foremilk/hindmilk volumes (Bishara, et al., 2009).

Increasing breastmilk volume is a challenge to all mothers who provide milk for their infants. The best practice is to prevent low milk supply by expressing breastmilk as soon as possible after delivery preferably within 2 hours. During the early hours after birth this may require the assistance of nursing personnel, depending on the physical condition of the mother. Slusher and her research team physically assisted mothers who were too sick to hold the pumping equipment or physically participate in the pumping (personal communication). Instruction in assisting mothers should be included in training protocols for obstetric and neonatal staff. Some mothers of preterm infants express minimal milk volumes in the first few days of life and will need encouragement to continue expressing until their milk volume increases. Documentation of breastmilk expression, including method, by nursing staff and giving data in report to oncoming staff helps to establish a team approach to pumping and milk collection. Inadequate milk production needs to be investigated. Most mothers experience inadequate production due to improper removal of milk or a number of reasons which may include: infrequent pumping, shortened pumping, inadequate removal of hind milk, medications including birth control commencement, uterine hemorrhage, and thyroid conditions. Inadequate breast pumps and mechanical pump problems may also be at fault for inadequate milk removal and subsequent limited production. Correcting these problems may increase milk production (Hill et al., 2009). Mothers need encouragement, support, and an observation of breastmilk expression techniques to establish and build a supply. Advise the mother to eat as nutritious and high caloric diet as feasible, and drink fluids to thirst.

Galactogogues (ABM 2011) have been used to help preterm and term mothers create more milk. These include both herbal remedies and prescribed medications that stimulate milk receptor cells or prolactin surges. Galactogogues typically will not produce more milk if the regular removal of milk is not occurring. Establishing a good milk removal routine is paramount in addressing low milk supply. Combining hand expression and pumping may increase milk expression (Morton, et al., 2009). Many mothers find that seeing more milk with pumping or hand expression is the best motivator for pumping more. Galactogogues based on herbs and other natural substances include fenugreek, galega (goat's rue) and milk thistle (Zuppa et al., 2010). Mothers with ragweed and peanut allergies should be advised to avoid fenugreek. Principle prescription medications contributing to increased milk supply include metoclopramide (Betzold, 2004) and domperidone (Wan et al., 2008). The latter is more effective, is associated with fewer side effects, and is preferred throughout much of the world. Galactogogues may be started at any time during the pumping process and should not be withheld as a last resort. The use of galactogogues should be limited to those situations in which reduced milk production from treatable causes has been excluded.

Occasionally hormonal imbalances in conditions such a polycystic ovarian syndrome, thyroid disorders, insufficient glandular development of the breast, breast reduction surgeries or breast lumpectomy may reduce the ability for the breast to make milk (Andrade et al, 2010).

4.6 Alternate feedings in premature and sick infants

As previously noted, the preferential milk for the preterm infant is, of course, his or her own mother's milk fed fresh to the infant. Options if the mother does not wish to breastfeed or has an absolute or relative contraindication to breastfeeding include primarily donor milk, wet nurses and artificial feeds. Donor breastmilk is considered an important adjunct to infant feeding in many high-income countries where donor milk is both screened carefully and stored properly making it an unlikely source of feedings in LMICs. Likewise, wet nurses should be screened for infections to ensure their breast milk is safe. Wet nurses cannot be recommended in LMICs when this screening is unavailable. Preterm formula, if available, can be offered if breastmilk feedings are not an option. Milk based formula is preferred. Special nutrient and caloric enriched formulas that support good growth and development are available for use in preterm infants in the first six months of life (Jeon et al., 2011). In most LMICs, availability and cost mean that powdered artificial feedings designed for term infants are the only alternate infant food available to both premature and term infants for whom breastmilk is not an option. When using powdered formula it is essential that it be prepared hygienically with good hand washing, clean water (ideally boiled) and clean utensils. There is a very small risk of bacterial contamination in powdered milk formula with Enterobacter sakasakii, a rare opportunistic pathogen associated with meningitis, necrotizing enterocolitis and sepsis (Gurtler et al, 2005; Palcich et al., 2009). As pointed out in a study in Tanzania, this is of particular concern in the preterm, but can occur at any age (Gurtler, et al., 2005; Mshana et al., 2011). Therefore, breastmilk is preferred in the neonatal period particularly for preterm infants. Most other homemade formulas, including animal milks, are less ideal for the neonate than formula designed for infant feedings and should only be used as a last resort, especially during the neonatal period. As mentioned earlier, cups and spoons should be encouraged instead of bottles in any LMIC where hygiene is often not ideal.

4.7 Breastmilk and the HIV positive mother

Breastmilk was recognized to be a leading cause of maternal-to-child transmission (MCTC) of HIV early in the epidemic (Kreiss, 1997; Ogundele & Coulter, 2003; Ruff, 1994). Initial efforts to curtail this mode of transmission were focused heavily on substitute feedings for breast milk. Breastfeeding was strongly discouraged and heroic efforts were made to get breastmilk substitutes into LMICs. Unexpectedly, this effort was met with at least as many infants dying in the substitute feeding group as were dying in the breastmilk group due to an unacceptably high incidence of illnesses including diarrhea in the substitute feeding group.(Horvath et al., 2009; Rollins, 2007; Thior et al., 2006) In some studies (Shapiro et al., 2007) discontinuing breastfeeding was considered to be the primary risk factor for death. Additionally, mothers may choose to breastfeed because breastfeeding is culturally acceptable: and not breastfeeding can lead to discrimination or stigmatization (Cavarelli & Scarlatti, 2011; Sadoh & Sadoh, 2009) Unfortunately, women given breastmilk substitutes often choose to give mixed feedings with breastmilk and breastmilk substitutes. This combination of mixed feedings is identified as the most risky choice with the highest incidence of maternal to child transmission (MTCT) of HIV (Coutsoudis et al., 2001).

Researchers and clinicians alike continue to struggle with the best feeding options and other interventions in low-resource settings to curtail MTCT of HIV (Kuhn et al., 2008). Significant strides have been made in recent years. All involved continuing to emphasize educating mothers on their infant feeding choices and supporting those choices whatever they are. If the mother concurs, the current recommendation is to support breastfeeding unless breastmilk substitutes are acceptable, feasible, affordable, sustainable and safe (AFASS)(WHO, 2010). Because exclusive breastmilk feedings are associated with the lowest incidence of HIV transmission, exclusive breastmilk feedings are recommended for the first six months of life (WHO, 2010). After six months of life complimentary foods should be added as appropriate. Breastmilk feeding should continue along with these complimentary foods unless breastmilk substitutes are now AFASS. At any point during the breastfeeding period that breastmilk substitutes become AFASS, the transition to breastmilk substitutes should be supported. This approach still has a significant ongoing risk of MTCT of HIV unless antiretroviral drugs are included in the regime (Cavarelli & Scarlatti, 2011; Horvath, et al., 2009; McIntyre, 2005). Additionally, boiling expressed breastmilk may be an option for some mothers where artificial feeds are not available (Cavarelli & Scarlatti, 2011; Savage & Lhotska, 2000).

Recent advances in making antiretroviral drugs available and affordable to HIV+ mothers who choose to breastfeed have decreased the risk of transmission of HIV through breastmilk. If fully implemented, the WHO recommendations could potentially reduce the risk to 5% or less from the background risk of 35% in breastfeeding infants (WHO, 2010). The risk of MTCT of HIV can be reduced by using either maternal ARV prophylaxis (WHO Option A) initiated as early as 14 weeks gestation and then daily infant nevirapine throughout the period of breastfeeding and one week beyond or maternal ARV treatment (WHO Option B) of HIV during pregnancy and continuing through breastfeeding and 1 week beyond as recommended by the WHO publication "Antiretroviral Drugs for Treating Pregnant Women and Preventing HIV Infection in Infants: Recommendations for a Public Health Approach" 2010 version (summarized in table 2. below) (WHO, 2010). However, it is agreed that all HIV infected pregnant women with CD4 cell count < 350 cells/mm^3 should receive antiretroviral treatment for their own health and for prevention of MTCT (WHO, 2010). Some protocols include an option B+ in which mothers who don't meet the criteria for ARV treatment themselves, are continued on ARV's for life after beginning ARV's during pregnancy and breastfeeding instead of stopping them one week after weaning from breastfeeding (Ciaranello et al., 2011). For many LMICs daily nevirapine is more economical and therefore, more feasible than treating the mothers with ARV's but either regime decreases MCTC and can be supported with current evidence-based studies. For details of these regimes and others consult a pediatric HIV specialist and an up to date source of recommendations of ARV's for the prevention of MCTC. All recommendations regarding MCTC are frequently changing, therefore, all health care providers treating HIV+ mothers and their infants should check current recommendations from WHO, UNICEF and other updated sources.

Antiretroviral (ARV)-prophylaxis options recommended for HIV-infected pregnant women who do not need treatment for their own health	
Maternal AZT + Infant ARV prophylaxis **(Option A)**	Maternal triple ARV prophylaxis **(Option B)**
Mother	Mother
Antepartum twice-daily AZT starting from as early as 14 weeks gestation and continued during pregnancy. At onset of labour, sd-NVP and initiation of twice daily AZT + 3TC for 7 days postpartum (Note: If maternal AZT was provided for more than 4 weeks antenatally, omission of the sd-NVP and AZT + 3TC tail can be considered; in this case continue maternal AZT during labor and stop at delivery).	Triple ARV prophylaxis starting from as early as 14 weeks of gestation and continued until delivery, or if breastfeeding, continued until 1 week after all infant exposure to breast milk has ended. Recommended regimes include: ATZ + 3TC + LPV/r or AZT + 3TC + ABC or AZT + 3TC + EFV or TDF + 3TC (or FTC) + EFV
Infant	Infant
For breastfeeding infants Daily NVP from birth for a minimum of 4 to 6 weeks, and until 1 week after all exposure to breast milk has ended.	Irrespective of mode of infant feeding Daily NVP or twice daily AZT from birth until 4 to 6 weeks of age
Infants receiving replacement feedings only Daily NVP or sd-NVP + twice daily AZT from birth until 4 to 6 weeks of age	
ARV-antiretroviral; AZT-zidovudine; 3TC-lamivudine; NVP-nevirapine; sd-NVP-single dose nevirapine; LPV/r- lopinavir/ritonavir; EFV-efavirenz; FTC-emtricitabine;	

WHO. Antiretroviral Drugs for Treating Pregnant Women and Children and Preventing HIV Infection in Infants Recommendations for a public health approach 2010 version. 2010; http://www.who.int/hiv/pub/mtct/PMTCTfactsheet/en/

Table 2.

4.8 Contraindications and relative contraindications to breastmilk feeding

There are few conditions in which breastfeeding is not recommended for the infant or for the mother. Unless alternate feedings are acceptable, feasible, affordable, sustainable, and safe (AFASS), HIV positive mothers are encouraged to breastfeed. An infant diagnosed with galactosemia, a rare metabolic disease should not breastfeed. Mothers with certain untreated infections (e.g. tuberculosis) should not breastfeed at the breast but may be able to use expressed breastmilk depending on the particulars of their disease. Infants of mothers with Hepatitis B carriage may breastfeed provided their newborns are immunized against Hepatitis B immediately after birth as soon as dry and stable(IOM, 2011) . For specific situations consult an infectious disease specialist or the Red Book(AAP, 2009). Any mother using illicit drugs, taking cancer chemotherapy agents such as antimetabolites, or undergoing radiation therapy, generally should not breastfeed. Nuclear medicine studies vary in their components and advice should be sought in particular for the radioactive component of the scan (AAP, 2001; Hale, 2010).

4.9 Team approach and education: Supporting and encouraging breastfeeding

Breastfeeding incidence and duration rates are significantly affected by maternal educations and staff education (Brent et al, 1995). It is important to focus on providing evidenced based education and support regarding breastfeeding practices in special care baby units to mothers as well as all staff interfacing with the mother and baby (Meier, 2010). In a USA study, Hallbauer found that infants with a lower weight and gestational age, who had prolonged stays in the neonatal intensive care unit were less likely to be breast-fed after discharge (Hallbauer et al, 2002). This suggests that efforts to promote breast-feeding in the neonatal unit were ineffectual or inadequate. The author suggests that in order to remedy this situation it is necessary to keep the mother-infant pair together, to promote breastfeeding before and immediately after delivery and to train staff in the management of lactation (Hallbauer, et al., 2002). Family-centered care has been implemented in many neonatal intensive care units throughout the U.S. and is invaluable in helping families, whose infants require hospitalization, cope with the stress, fear, and altered parenting roles that may accompany their child's condition and hospitalization (Mulasky, 2005). In high-income countries, a combination of breastfeeding management and family centered training for neonatal intensive care unit staff enhances the care of these medically fragile infants and their families. In LMICs family centered care is the norm and essential in providing care for their family members. Mothers already play a vital role in the care of their premature and sick infants and in many of these LMICs and stay either with the infant in the nursery or nearby. However, education and support in the feeding and care of their infant is crucial to providing optimal growth, development and exclusive breastfeeding for these most vulnerable infants.

Statistics specific for infants graduating from special care baby units in low-middle income countries is lacking. However, since breastfeeding is the norm in these countries it is likely that most infants go home with at least partial breastmilk feeds. The larger problem is promoting exclusive breastmilk feedings for the first six months of life. This is challenging especially in HIV positive mothers. Mixed feedings are common and misconceptions about the adequacy of mothers' own milk are widespread. There is an ongoing need to continually promote and reinforce the Baby Friendly Hospital Initiatives (UNICEF, 2009). Abolyan found the Baby Friendly training among staff increases breastfeeding rates as well as maternal satisfaction (Abolyan, 2006). Breastmilk is the life saving choice for infant feeding in high-risk special care baby nurseries and should be the standard of care for these infants. However, this must be balanced with the needs of the individual infant and, when appropriate, alternative feedings recommended (i.e. some infants of HIV+ mothers, orphaned or abandoned infants, infants who are failing to thrive despite their mothers efforts to produce adequate breastmilk). All policies, procedures and training regarding infant feeding should promote, protect and support breastfeeding for the mother and their infants whenever possible.

5. Indications for and appropriate intravenous fluids in premature and sick infants

The goals of IV fluid therapy are to maintain adequate hydration, appropriate electrolyte balance and sufficient carbohydrate intake to support basic metabolic processes and avoid hypoglycemia. Fluid and electrolyte requirements for newborns change with advancing gestational age and postnatal age as total body water decreases, extracellular fluid volume contracts, renal tubular reabsorption of free water, sodium, and bicarbonate improves, and skin matures. Extremely preterm infants are at especially high risk for excessive rate of water loss through their very thin skin. Transepidermal water loss immediately after birth at 26 weeks gestation is 60 $g/m^2/h$ decreasing to approximately 25 $g/m^2/h$ by 32 weeks and to 10 $g/m^2/h$ by 40 weeks post-menstrual age (Seri I, 2005). A 25-27 week gestation infant placed in 50% humidity on the first day after birth may lose 129 ml of water/day through the skin alone (Modi, 2005). The skin matures quite rapidly so that even in the most immature infants born at 26 weeks gestation, the transepidermal fluid loss has decreased to about 43 ml/day by one week after birth. Antenatal steroids accelerate skin maturation in the preterm infants, thereby reducing postnatal transepidermal water loss.

In the healthy term infant the immediate post-delivery period is characterized by a negative fluid and sodium balance. Hormonal changes associated with labor and delivery initiate a postnatal diuresis over the first 2-3 days at which time fluids should be limited so as not to impede this process. Normally during the first 1-3 days oral intake via breastfeeding is limited. Consequently, isotonic contraction of extracellular fluid volume occurs. The result in the healthy term newborn is an appropriate weight loss over the first several days after birth of 1-2% per day for a total weight loss of 5-10%(Kalhan , 2001). Birth weight is usually regained by day 7. Preterm infants are born with relatively more total body water to excrete, immature renal function, and greater transepidermal water loss. Therefore, they have a substantially greater initial weight loss, up to 15% over the first week, and regain birth weight between the second and third week after birth. In both term and preterm infants, weight gain over the first few days is abnormal and represents fluid and sodium retention due either to excessive administration of fluid or to neonatal conditions which compromise organ function or increase capillary leak.

5.1 Fluid requirements

Fluid requirements are influenced by clinical and environmental conditions. Insensible, evaporative fluid losses are increased by low humidity environments (<50%), care under radiant warmers, high ambient temperature, phototherapy, non-humidified respiratory gases, skin defects or breakdown (e.g., omphalocele, gastroschisis, burns), fever, and tachypnea. Gastrointestinal losses are readily evident when due to diarrhea or nasogastric drainage, but may be unapparent when due to third spacing associated with necrotizing enterocolitis or to large evaporative losses during GI surgery. Environmental factors such as clothing, high humidity, care in a double walled incubator, skin ointments, and humidified respiratory gases all decrease insensible losses. Some clinical problems decrease fluid requirements due to organ injury (e.g., birth asphyxia) or the underlying pathophysiology (RDS, PDA).

Taking the normal adaptive changes into account, IV fluid administration in the first few days should be limited and then gradually increased to maintenance volumes over the next several days. Urine output should normally be at least 2 ml/kg/hour after the first day. Daily fluid intake will vary depending upon gestational age and medical condition. Extremely preterm infants have very high insensible water loss due to epidermal immaturity and will need a higher fluid intake to compensate for their transepidermal water loss. However, excessive fluid and sodium administration at this time is associated with complications, particularly in preterm infants, such as pulmonary edema, increased respiratory distress, patent ductus arteriosus and a greater risk of bronchopulmonary dysplasia. Because of the contraction of total body water, Na supplementation is not needed until 3-4 days after birth.

For term infants begin IV infusion rates at 60-80 ml/kg/day on days 1-3, increasing slowly by 10-20 ml/kg/day to 100 ml/kg/day. On days 3-7, if clinically stable with appropriate weight loss of 1-2% per day, continue increasing total fluid intake (IV + PO) by 20 ml/kg day up to a maximum of 180 ml/kg/day. After day 7, do not exceed a maximum fluid intake (IV plus PO) of 180 ml/kg/day until the infant is off IV fluids and entirely on ad lib oral feeds.

The fluid requirement for premature infants varies depending upon the degree of prematurity, as well as environmental factors and clinical problems that increase or decrease insensible fluid loss. In general, on days 1 and 2 after delivery, infants with birth weights < 1000 g require 100-150 ml/kg/day; infants with birth weights 1001-1500 require 60-100 ml/kg/day ; and infants with birth weights >1500 require 60-80 ml/kg/day. For all infants total fluids (IV + PO) are gradually increased by 10-20 ml/kg/day to reach 150-160 ml/kg/day by 7-10 days of age. When growing, and without medical complications, premature infants may tolerate up to 180 ml/kg/day. Providing preterm infants with humidified incubators or placing them under small plastic tents will decrease insensible loss and total fluid requirements. Fluid intake should be based on birth weight until birth weight is regained. In general, too much fluid is more deleterious than too little fluid It is better to err on the side of cautious fluid administration.

For all infants, be sure to include the volume of oral feeds when calculating the daily total intake/day. If receiving only intravenous (IV) fluids write the order to indicate how much is to be given each hour. If the infant is also receiving oral feeds, an IV+ PO order will avoid inadvertently giving too much or too little fluid as IV and/or PO volumes are changed (ex. if the infant is receiving a total of 360 ml of fluid/day and is being fed every q 3 hours: "Give 20 ml D5W IV + 25 ml breastmilk PO/NG every 3 hours = 45 ml q3 hours= 360 ml/day total.") Rewrite the order to maintain the appropriate interval volumes as IV and PO intakes change.

5.2 Glucose

Begin with a glucose infusion rate of 6 mg/kg/min given as D5W if birth weight is < 1000g and 8 mg/kg/minute as D10W if birth weight is greater than 1000 g. Increase the glucose infusion rate by 3-6 gm/kg/day (10-20 kcal/kg/day) to a maximum of 12-14 mg/kg/min. Keep the serum glucose less than 150 mg/dL. It is helpful to calculate the glucose infusion rate (GIR) in mg/kg/minute [(% glucose X ml/kg/day) /24 hours per day/60 minute per hour] and the caloric intake (Cal/kg/day) provided (IV glucose =3.4 Cal/gm). A GIR of 4-6 mg/kg/minute approximates basal hepatic glucose production. About 50 Cal/kg/day are needed for maintenance of weight and basic metabolic function (Kalhan SC, 2001). This level of caloric intake is barely achievable using D10W at maximum fluid volumes. Initiation of enteric feeds is necessary as soon as possible in order to provide enough calories and nutrients for growth.

5.3 Electrolytes

In the first 3 days after birth, electrolytes are not needed and IV fluids containing only 5% or 10% glucose (D5W or D10W) are adequate. Sodium (Na) supplementation (3-4 mEq/kg/day) should be started by day 3 to avoid hyponatremia and help establish the positive sodium balance needed for growth. Nasogastric and ostomy drainage contain a considerable amount of NA (45-140 mmol/L) which can generally be replaced with equal amounts of 1/3-1/2 NS. Potassium (K) can also be added (1-2 mEq/kg/day) on day if urine output is adequate and the infant is not yet taking enteric feeds. Adding 10 mEq K/1000ml of IV fluid provides 1 mEq K/100 ml which is adequate for most infants. Since inadvertent administration of excess potassium may be fatal, potassium should be added to IV fluids only when necessary and the preparation carefully checked by two nurses.

5.4 Types of IV fluids

If stock IV solutions are not available, adding 25 ml of Ringers Solution or Ringers Lactate to 100 ml of D5W or D10W will approximate ¼ NS and deliver 3-4 mEq Na/100ml (Slusher et al, 2011). If only D5W is available, an appropriate amount of D50W can be added to the D5Wsolution to make D10W as described in detail in the AAP book"Textbook of Global Child Health" (Slusher T, 2012). Care must be taken to maintain sterility when mixing IV solutions together. All fluids except for acute volume expansion should contain glucose.

Total parenteral nutrition (TPN) containing protein and lipid in addition to glucose, is necessary to achieve adequate intravenous caloric and nutrient intake when enteric feeds are not possible. TPN has dramatically improved the survival following neonatal surgical procedures such as diaphragmatic hernia, tracheoesophageal fistula, omphalocele, gastroschisis and bowel resection associated with prolonged inability to take enteric feeds. However, TPN is associated with a much higher risk of sepsis because the solution itself is an excellent culture medium and infusion lines, especially if centrally placed, are at high risk for contamination. Although used routinely to support nutrition for sick newborns in developed countries, TPN solutions require preparation and administration under strictly controlled, aseptic conditions with appropriate facilities and staff.

5.5 Methods of fluid administration

IV fluids are best given continuously by infusion pumps. Alternatively a non-mechanical drip set with a buretrol may be used. Accidental acute fluid overload may be life threatening. It is therefore critical to limit the amount of fluid that can be rapidly infused by filling the pump syringe, pump chamber or buretrol with only 2-4 hours of IV fluid. When continuous infusion is not possible, IV fluid can be given intermittently as frequent, small boluses every 2 hours. However, intermittent bolus administration of glucose increases the risk of hyperglycemia and hypoglycemia, acute changes in serum osmolality and risk infection from frequent entry into the IV line. This method of IV fluid administration should be used only if safer methods of IV infusion with pumps or drip sets are unavailable.

5.6 Routes of fluid administration

IV fluids may be given by peripheral or central lines. Do not exceed D12.5W when using a peripheral IV or D20W if using a central venous line. NS, 1/2NS or D5W can be used in central arterial lines; hypertonic solutions should be avoided.

5.7 Monitoring fluid status and electrolytes

Monitoring fluid and electrolyte balance is essential. All fluid intake should be systematically recorded including IV infusions, medications, blood products, and feeds. Passage of urine and stool should also be recorded. Whenever possible urine output should be measured. Any drainage from NG tubes and chest tube should be measured and recorded. Vital signs including heart rate, respiratory rate, temperature and blood pressure should be recorded at least once or twice per day. A careful daily physical exam should include evaluation of capillary refill, skin turgor, mucous membranes, and the anterior fontanel. An accurate, unclothed, daily weight is one of the best ways of assessing overall fluid balance in the first several days after birth. Obtaining a daily weight in preterm infants, especially those who are extremely immature, must be balanced against the difficulty of doing so, the accuracy of the scale and potential complications which may occur during the process of weighing (e.g., hypoxia, hypothermia, exposure to contaminated surfaces). If possible, serum electrolytes should be checked using small capillary blood samples every 24-48 hours during the first week or until stable. At a minimum Na and K should be checked on days 3 and 7. The normal serum sodium level is Na 132-144 mmol/L; the normal K level is 3.8-5.7 mmol/L(Modi, 2005).

5.8 Complications

Common complications of IV fluid therapy include hyponatremia (< 130 mmol/L), hypernatremia (> 150 mmol/L), hyperglycemia (> 150 mg/dl), hypoglycemia (< 40 mg/dl) if fluids are abruptly discontinued, accidental fluid overload, and skin injury due to IV infiltration. Avoiding severe burns due to IV infiltration requires frequent inspection of the IV infusion site. Treat IV infiltration in an extremity by elevating the limb. If circulation to an area on the infiltrated extremity is compromised, warm the opposite extremity which will help reflexly dilate blood vessels in the affected limb without increasing oxygen demand. If the skin is broken down, the area should be treated as a burn.

5.9 Fluid requirements in common neonatal conditions

Birth asphyxia is often associated with renal insufficiency due to acute tubular necrosis resulting in severe oliguria or anuria. In this circumstance, fluid intake should be limited to insensible loss, approximately 30 ml/kg/day on day 1 in term infants. Fluids intake is liberalized slowly as urine output improves. A tight nuchal cord may result in hypovolemia when venous return from the placenta to the fetus via the umbilical vein is obstructed. Affected infants have poor capillary refill, tachycardia, may have weak pulses, and often have respiratory distress. These infants usually respond promptly with improved perfusion and resolution of respiratory distress and tachycardia after volume expansion with boluses of 10 ml/kg normal saline IV boluses up to a total of 20-30 ml/kg. A symptomatic patent ductus arteriosus is common in preterm infants, especially if fluid administration has been excessive. Indomethacin, used to pharmacologically close the ductus, is associated with transient oliguria, fluid retention and hyponatremia. Extremely premature infants (24-27 weeks gestation) have very high transepidermal free water loss and renal immaturity in the first several days after birth that increase the risk of hypernatremia and hyperkalemia. Changes in weight and electrolytes must be closely monitored and fluid intake adjusted accordingly. Respiratory distress syndrome is associated with increased pulmonary fluid and failure to diurese until 3-4 days after birth at which time the respiratory disease improves. Use of diuretics is ineffective in hastening the spontaneous diuresis. Immediately after gastrointestinal surgery, infants are often oliguric or anuric. Usually this is due to intravascular volume depletion from large, intraoperative insensible fluid losses from the exposed gut and/or post-operative third. The appropriate treatment is volume expansion, not administration of a diuretic. In shock, due to acute blood loss, the best treatment is immediate volume expansion with blood products.

6. Diagnosis and treatment of hypoglycemia in sick and premature infants

Glucose production in the fetus is normally very low, and most glucose for fetal energy utilization is obtained from the maternal circulation via facilitated diffusion across the placenta (Hay, 2006). Under normal circumstances, birth represents the beginning of a transition period when the neonate will develop the ability to maintain glucose homeostasis independently. Serum glucose levels fall initially, reaching a nadir around 2-3 hours of age. Catecholamine release, cortisol surge, insulin production, enhanced glycogenolysis and gluconeogenesis are a few of the important hormonal and metabolic events taking place that ultimately lead to activation of independent glucose production in the normal neonate. Serum glucose concentrations will rebound within the first 4 hours after birth from this physiological nadir. With established feedings, the serum glucose level will continue to stabilize over the first 24 hours of life.

Routine glucose monitoring is not recommended in the normal, healthy, term neonate (Committee on Fetus and Newborn, 2011). However, there are specific neonatal populations that are at increased risk of developing hypoglycemia and warrant close observation and monitoring. Glucose homeostasis is the result of a balance between energy production and energy utilization. When this balance is skewed, hypoglycemia results. Preterm infants, small for gestational age (SGA) infants, and very low birth weight (VLBW) infants have an impaired ability to produce glucose due to limited hepatic stores available for glycogenolysis. Illness in any neonate increases metabolic demand and energy utilization. Infection, asphyxia, and hypothermia thus increase the risk of neonatal hypoglycemia. Infants of diabetic mothers (IDM) and large for gestational age infants have increased metabolic demands secondary to macrosomia. Prolonged hyperglycemia in utero leads to abnormal glucose metabolism in the IDM after birth. IDMs have higher levels of circulating insulin, lower serum glucose levels, lower availability of alternative fuels, and impaired counter-regulatory hormones, all of which contribute to a high risk of neonatal hypoglycemia, often developing immediately after birth earlier than what is seen in other at risk populations (Martin, 2011; Peace O, 2010).

The overall incidence of neonatal hypoglycemia is difficult to define. Studies have reported incidence rates from 0.4% to 29% during the first 24 hours of life depending on the study population and level of serum glucose used to define clinically significant hypoglycemia (Burdan DR, 2009; Depuy AM, 2009; Johnson, 2010; Najati N, 2010). The risk of hypoglycemia is higher in resource poor countries, even in populations not characteristically thought of at risk. A study in Nepal among term infants born by uncomplicated delivery in a hospital setting found 10% with serum glucose <37 mg/dl (<2.0 mmol/l) and over 50% with at least mild hypoglycemia <50 mg/dl (<2.8 mmole/L) within the first 24 hours of life (Pal Deb, 2000). Contributing factors that are often more common place in resource poor countries include lack of prenatal care, poor maternal nutrition, and delayed feeding practices.

Neonatal hypoglycemia may have long-term sequelae. Hypoglycemia is often associated with hypoxemia, respiratory compromise, prematurity and other problems of the ill or premature infant. This can make it difficult to associate neurodevelopmental outcomes with hypoglycemia alone. Generally, transient hypoglycemia in an otherwise healthy neonate has a good prognosis whereas recurrent, severe, or prolonged hypoglycemia has been associated with poor developmental outcomes ranging from attention disorder to cerebral palsy (Martin et al, 2011).

6.1 Signs and symptoms of hypoglycemia

Signs and symptoms of neonatal hypoglycemia are subtle and nonspecific. Jitteriness, irritability, feeding difficulty, apnea, hypothermia, cyanosis, tachycardia, lethargy, floppiness, eye rolling or tachypnea could all be signs of symptomatic neonatal hypoglycemia. Diagnosis is confirmed with the identification of a low serum glucose, and resolution of symptoms after glucose administration. Because the symptoms are nonspecific, consideration should be given to other diagnoses as well, including sepsis and asphyxia. More severe signs, including seizures and coma, often result from recurrent and/or prolonged hypoglycemia. Seizures and coma are not as quickly or easily reversed with glucose administration (Martin et al, 2011).

Serum glucose levels are among the most common laboratory tests performed on neonates. Hypoglycemia is common, easily confirmed by laboratory testing, and the symptoms are reversible if intervention occurs in a timely manner. Any infant with nonspecific signs of illness should raise concern for possible neonatal hypoglycemia.

6.2 Glucose values and Interpretation

The definition of clinically significant hypoglycemia is not known. There is no current research to indicate a level of serum glucose that consistently leads to permanent neurologic injury. Instead, general consensus and an operational approach guides management and treatment decisions in neonatal hypoglycemia.

Serum glucose levels between 40-50 (2.2-2.7 mmol/l) during the first 4 hours of life is generally regarded as normal, less than 35 mg/dl is regarded as abnormal. After reaching a physiologic nadir, infants' serum glucose levels should stabilize. As a result, glucose levels >45 mg/dl is considered normal in infants 4-24 hours of age (Martin et al, 2011).

6.3 Treatment options for hypoglycemia

Treatment begins with prevention and screening of at risk infants. Early breastfeeding, ideally within the first hour following birth, and frequent feedings every 2-3 hours, can avoid severe neonatal hypoglycemia. Delayed neonatal feedings for up to several days is sometimes practiced in developing countries. This places all infants, but especially the ill and preterm infant at risk for significant and prolonged hypoglycemia. Known at risk infants should be screened for hypoglycemia by 3 hours of age and sooner if clinical concerns arise.

Neonatal hypoglycemia is treated by replenishing the substrate supply. The preferred method is by breastfeeding. As mentioned, frequent feeding helps maintain euglycemia. Infant formula, or expressed breastmilk, can also be given by bottle, cup or gavage as necessary. This provides immediately accessible glucose through carbohydrate metabolism, as well as fats and protein for glycogenesis and maintenance of glucose stores during times of fasting. Enteral glucose administration via breastmilk, formula, or D5W should be used in mild to moderate neonatal hypoglycemia.

The goal is to achieve a balance of energy production with energy utilization through frequent bolus feeds occurring every 2-3 hours, for a total fluid goal of 60 ml/kg on the first day of life. Once feeds become well established, continued persistent hypoglycemia is an indication of an underlying metabolic or endocrine disorder.

Intravenous glucose should be used if the neonate is symptomatic or if moderate to severe hypoglycemia is identified, which can be defined as a serum glucose <25 mg/dl during the first 4 hours of life, <35 mg/dl from 4-24 hours of age. Intravenous dextrose should also be given to the infant manifesting late stage symptoms of coma and/or seizures. Intravenous dextrose is given as a small bolus of 2 ml/kg of D10W followed by a maintenance glucose infusion rate (GIR- see Equation I for calculating) of 5-7 mg/kg/minute. Although suboptimal, in the rare occasion that intravenous fluids are not available for the treatment of symptomatic or moderate to severe hypoglycemia, D5W at 10 ml/kg by gavage can be given orally or by naso-gastric tube. Hyperosmolar glucose solutions (D25 and D50) should not be used in neonates and have been associated with intracranial hemorrhage and rebound hypoglycemia (Marx JA, 2010). Available solutions should be diluted to a concentration of D10.

$$\text{GIR}\ (\text{mg / kg / minute}) = \frac{(\%\ \text{dextrose concentration x total ml / kg / day})}{144}$$

6.4 Summary

Neonatal hypoglycemia is the result of abnormal glucose metabolism after birth. It is a manifestation of the imbalance between energy production and energy utilization. While the incidence of hypoglycemia is unknown, it is potentially more common in resource poor countries, and known to occur at higher rates in susceptible populations such as the ill or preterm neonate. The neonatal brain is the primary consumer of serum glucose, and is at risk during periods of energy depletion. As such, prolonged, recurrent, or severe hypoglycemia may result in neurologic sequelae. Identification of at risk infants, close monitoring and prevention strategies, prompt recognition and effective treatment can be achieved in the developing world.

7. References

AAP. (2001). The transfer of drugs and other chemicals into human milk. Pediatrics, 108, 776-789.

Academy of Breastfeeding Medicine Protocol Committee, Clinical Protocol #8: Human Milk Storage Information for Home Use for Full-Term Infants (Original Protocol March 2004; Revision #1 March 2010). (2010). Breastfeeding medicine, 5(3), 127-130.

Academy of Breastfeeding Medicine Protocol Committee, Clinical Protocol #9: Use of Galactoguogues in Initating or Augmenting the Rate of Maternal Secretion (First Revision, January 2011). (2011). Breastfeeding medicine, 6(1), 41-46.

Abolyan, L. V. (2006). The breastfeeding support and promotion in Baby-Friendly Maternity Hospitals and Not-as-Yet Baby-Friendly Hospitals in Russia. Breastfeeding medicine : the official journal of the Academy of Breastfeeding Medicine, 1(2), 71-78.

Abouelfettoh, A. M., Dowling, D. A., Dabash, S. A., Elguindy, S. R., & Seoud, I. A. (2008). Cup versus bottle feeding for hospitalized late preterm infants in Egypt: a quasi-experimental study. International breastfeeding journal, 3, 27.

Adamkin, D. H. (2005). Pragmatic approach to in-hospital nutrition in high-risk neonates. [Review]. Journal of perinatology : official journal of the California Perinatal Association, 25 Suppl 2, S7-S11.

Ahmed, S., Parveen, S. D., & Islam, A. (1999). Infant feeding practices in rural Bangladesh: policy implications. Journal of tropical pediatrics, 45(1), 37-41.

Alrifai, S. B., Al Saadi, A., & Mahmood, Y. A. (2010). Nosocomial diarrhoea in relation to sanitation state: a study in Tikrit, Iraq. Eastern Mediteranean Health Journal, 16(5), 546-552.

American Academy of Pediatrics Red Book 28th Edition. (2009). American Academy of Pediatrics.

Andrade, R. A., Coca, K. P., & Abrao, A. C. (2010). Breastfeeding pattern in the first month of life in women submitted to breast reduction and augmentation. [Comparative Study]. Jornal de pediatria, 86(3), 239-244.

Baker, R. D., & Greer, F. R. (2010). Diagnosis and prevention of iron deficiency and iron-deficiency anemia in infants and young children (0-3 years of age). *Pediatrics, 126*(5), 1040-1050.

Betzold, C. (2004). Galactagogues. Journal of Midwifery & Women's Health, 49(2), 151-154.

Bishara, R., Dunn, M. S., Merko, S. E., & Darling, P. (2008). Nutrient composition of hindmilk produced by mothers of very low birth weight infants born at less than 28 weeks' gestation. [Research Support, Non-U.S. Gov't]. Journal of human lactation : official journal of International Lactation Consultant Association, 24(2), 159-167.

Bishara, R., Dunn, M. S., Merko, S. E., & Darling, P. (2009). Volume of foremilk, hindmilk, and total milk produced by mothers of very preterm infants born at less than 28 weeks of gestation. [Research Support, Non-U.S. Gov't]. Journal of human lactation : official journal of International Lactation Consultant Association, 25(3), 272-279.

Boucher, C. A., Brazal, P. M., Graham-Certosini, C., Carnaghan-Sherrard, K., & Feeley, N. (2011). Mothers' breastfeeding experiences in the NICU. [Research Support, Non-U.S. Gov't]. Neonatal network : NN, 30(1), 21-28

Brent, N. B., Redd, B., Dworetz, A., D'Amico, F., & Greenberg, J. J. (1995). Breast-feeding in a low-income population. Program to increase incidence and duration. Archives of pediatrics & adolescent medicine, 149(7), 798-803.

Buckley, K. M., & Charles, G. E. (2006). Benefits and challenges of transitioning preterm infants to at-breast feedings. International breastfeeding journal, 1, 13.

Burdan DR, B. V., Teodorescu D. (2009). Neonatal hypoglycemia- the incidence of the risk factors in salvator vuia obstetrics-gynecology hospital, Arad. TMJ, 9, 77-80.

Cavarelli, M., & Scarlatti, G. (2011). Human immunodeficiency virus type 1 mother-to-child transmission and prevention: successes and controversies. Journal of internal medicine.

Chan, D. K. (2001). Enteral nutrition of the very low birth weight (VLBW) infant. [Review]. Annals of the Academy of Medicine, Singapore, 30(2), 174-182.

Chandrashekhar, T. S., Joshi, H. S., Binu, V., Shankar, P. R., Rana, M. S., & Ramachandran, U. (2007). Breast-feeding initiation and determinants of exclusive breast-feeding - a questionnaire survey in an urban population of western Nepal. [Multicenter Study]. Public health nutrition, 10(2), 192-197.

Chapman, D. J., & Perez-Escamilla, R. (2000). Maternal perception of the onset of lactation is a valid, public health indicator of lactogenesis stage II. [Research Support, Non-U.S. Gov't]. The Journal of nutrition, 130(12), 2972-2980.

Chen, C. H., Shu, H. Q., & Chi, C. S. (2001). Breastfeeding knowledge and attitudes of health professionals and students. Acta paediatrica Taiwanica July-Aug 2001, 42(4), 207-211.

Ciaranello, A. L., Perez, F., Maruva, M., Chu, J., Engelsmann, B., Keatinge, J., et al. (2011). WHO 2010 guidelines for prevention of mother-to-child HIV transmission in Zimbabwe: modeling clinical outcomes in infants and mothers.PLoS One. 6(6), e20224..

Committee on the Fetus and Newborn, Adamkin DH. Postnatal glucose homeostasis in late preterm and term infants. (2011). Pediatrics, 127(3), 575-579.

Cossey, V., Jeurissen, A., Thelissen, M. J., Vanhole, C., & Schuermans, A. (2011). Expressed breast milk on a neonatal unit: A hazard analysis and critical control points approach. American journal of infection control.

Coutsoudis, A., Pillay, K., Kuhn, L., Spooner, E., Tsai, W. Y., & Coovadia, H. M. (2001). Method of feeding and transmission of HIV-1 from mothers to children by 15 months of age: prospective cohort study from Durban, South Africa. AIDS Feb 16, 2001, 15(3), 379-387.

Cricco-Lizza, R. (2009). Formative infant feeding experiences and education of NICU nurses. MCN. The American journal of maternal child nursing, 34(4), 236-242.

Daly, S. E., Kent, J. C., Owens, R. A., & Hartmann, P. E. (1996). Frequency and degree of milk removal and the short-term control of human milk synthesis. Experimental physiology, 81(5), 861-875.

Dancis, J., O'Connell, J., & Holt, L. (1948). A grid for recording the weight of premature infants. J Pediatrics 33, 570-572.

Darmstadt, G. L., Hussein, M. H., Winch, P. J., Haws, R. A., Lamia, M., El-Said, M. A., et al. (2007). Neonatal home care practices in rural Egypt during the first week of life.

[Research Support, U.S. Gov't, Non-P.H.S.]. Tropical medicine & international health : TM & IH, 12(6), 783-797.
de Aquino, R. R., & Osorio, M. M. (2009). Relactation, translactation, and breast-orogastric tube as transition methods in feeding preterm babies. Journal of human lactation, 25(4), 420-426.
Delaney, A. L., & Arvedson, J. C. (2008). Development of swallowing and feeding: prenatal through first year of life. [Review]. Developmental disabilities research reviews, 14(2), 105-117.
Depuy AM, C. K., Som DA, Simulian JC. (2009). Neonatal hypoglycemia in term, nondiabetic pregnancies. Am J Obstet Gynecol, 200, e45-51.
Dougherty, D., & Luther, M. (2008). Birth to breast--a feeding care map for the NICU: helping the extremely low birth weight infant navigate the course. [Review]. Neonatal network : NN, 27(6), 371-377.
Engebretsen, I. M., Tylleskar, T., Wamani, H., Karamagi, C., & Tumwine, J. K. (2008). Determinants of infant growth in Eastern Uganda: a community-based cross-sectional study. [Research Support, Non-U.S. Gov't]. BMC public health, 8, 418.
Eshete, W. B. (2008). A stepwise regression analysis on under-five diarrhoael morbidity prevalence in Nekemte town, western Ethiopia: maternal care giving and hygiene behavioral determinants. East African journal of public health, 5(3), 193-198.
Funkquist, E. L., Tuvemo, T., Jonsson, B., Serenius, F., & Nyqvist, K. H. (2010). Influence of test weighing before/after nursing on breastfeeding in preterm infants. [Comparative Study]. Advances in neonatal care : official journal of the National Association of Neonatal Nurses, 10(1), 33-39.
Ghosh, S., Sengupta, P. G., Mondal, S. K., Banu, M. K., Gupta, D. N., & Sircar, B. K. (1997). Risk behavioural practices of rural mothers as determinants of childhood diarrhoea. The Journal of communicable diseases, 29(1), 7-14.
Gomella, T. L., Cunningham, M. D., Eyal, F. G., & Zenk, K. E. (2004) (Ed(s)). Neonatology: Management, Procedures, On-Call Problems, Diseases, and Drugs: McGraw-Hill. ISBN 007-138918-0, New York.
Griffin, T. L., Meier, P. P., Bradford, L. P., Bigger, H. R., & Engstrom, J. L. (2000). Mothers' performing creamatocrit measures in the NICU: accuracy, reactions, and cost. J Obstet Gynecol Neonatal Nurs, 29(3), 249-257.
Grossman, X., Chaudhuri, J., Feldman-Winter, L., Abrams, J., Newton, K. N., Philipp, B. L., et al. (2009). Hospital Education in Lactation Practices (Project HELP): does clinician education affect breastfeeding initiation and exclusivity in the hospital? Birth, 36(1), 54-59.
Guilleminault, C., Souquet, M., Ariagno, R. L., Korobkin, R., & Simmons, F. B. (1984). Five cases of near-miss sudden infant death syndrome and development of obstructive sleep apnea syndrome. [Case Reports]. Pediatrics, 73(1), 71-78.
Gurtler, J. B., Kornacki, J. L., & Beuchat, L. R. (2005). Enterobacter sakazakii: a coliform of increased concern to infant health. [Review]. International journal of food microbiology, 104(1), 1-34.
Haase, B., Barreira, J., Murphy, P. K., Mueller, M., & Rhodes, J. (2009). The development of an accurate test weighing technique for preterm and high-risk hospitalized infants. Breastfeeding medicine : the official journal of the Academy of Breastfeeding Medicine, 4(3), 151-156.

Hake-Brooks, S. J., & Anderson, G. C. (2008). Kangaroo care and breastfeeding of mother-preterm infant dyads 0-18 months: a randomized, controlled trial.Neonatal network : NN, 27(3), 151-159.

Hale, T. (2010). Medications and Mother's Milk: A Manual of Lactational Pharmacology (14th ed.): Hale, ISBN-13 978-0982337998, Amarillo, Tx.

Hallbauer, U., Grobler, J. M., & Niemand, I. (2002). Factors influencing a mother's choice of feeding after discharge of her baby from a neonatal unit. South African medical journal,, 92(8), 634-637.

Hamosh, M. (1987). Lipid metabolism in premature infants. Biology of the neonate, 52 Suppl 1, 50-64.

Hay, W. W., Jr. (2006). Recent observations on the regulation of fetal metabolism by glucose. the Journal of physiology, 572(Pt 1), 17-24.

IOM (Institutes of Medicine). Hepatitis and Liver Cancer: A National Strategy for Prevention and Control of Hepatits B and C. (2011). from http://www.nap.eud/catalog.php?record_ed=12793

Hill, P. D., Aldag, J. C., Demirtas, H., Naeem, V., Parker, N. P., Zinaman, M. J., et al. (2009). Association of serum prolactin and oxytocin with milk production in mothers of preterm and term infants. Biological research for nursing, 10(4), 340-349.

Horvath, T., Madi, B. C., Iuppa, I. M., Kennedy, G. E., Rutherford, G., & Read, J. S. (2009). Interventions for preventing late postnatal mother-to-child transmission of HIV. [Meta-Analysis Review]. Cochrane database of systematic reviews(1), CD006734.

Jeon, G. W., Jung, Y. J., Koh, S. Y., Lee, Y. K., Kim, K. A., Shin, S. M., et al. (2011). Preterm infants fed nutrient-enriched formula until six months show improved growth and development. Pediatrics international, 53(5):683-688.

Johnson, T. (2010). Hypoglycemia and the full term newborn: how well does birth weight for gestational age predict risk. J Obstet Gynecol Neonatal Nurs, 32, 48-57.

Kalhan SC, Price PT. (2001). Nutrition and Selected Disorders of Gastrointestional Tract. In F. A. Klaus MH (Ed.), Care of the High Risk Newborn (5th ed.),Saunders, ISBN: 0721677290. Philadelphia, Pa.

Kliethermes, P. A., Cross, M. L., Lanese, M. G., Johnson, K. M., & Simon, S. D. (1999). Transitioning preterm infants with nasogastric tube supplementation: increased likelihood of breastfeeding. [Clinical Trial Randomized Controlled Trial]. Journal of obstetric, gynecologic, and neonatal nursing : JOGNN / NAACOG, 28(3), 264-273.

Klingenberg, C., Embleton, N. D., Jacobs, S. E., O'Connell, L. A., & Kuschel, C. A. (2011). Enteral feeding practices in very preterm infants: an international survey. Archives of disease in childhood. e-pub ahead of print.

Kreiss, J. (1997). Breastfeeding and vertical transmission of HIV-1. Acta paediatrica, 421, 113-117.

Kuhn, L., Aldrovandi, G. M., Sinkala, M., Kankasa, C., Semrau, K., Mwiya, M., et al. (2008). Effects of early, abrupt weaning on HIV-free survival of children in Zambia. The New England journal of medicine, 359(2), 130-141.

Lakati, A. S., Makokha, O. A., Binns, C. W., & Kombe, Y. (2010). The effect of pre-lacteal feeding on full breastfeeding in Nairobi, Kenya. East African journal of public health, 7(3), 258-262.

Leach, A., McArdle, T. F., Banya, W. A., Krubally, O., Greenwood, A. M., Rands, C., et al. (1999). Neonatal mortality in a rural area of The Gambia. Annals of tropical paediatrics, 19(1), 33-43.

Leung, A. K., & Sauve, R. S. (2005). Breast is best for babies. [Review]. Journal of the National Medical Association, 97(7), 1010-1019.

Lucas, A. (1978). Creamatocrit: simple clinical technique for estimating fat concentration and energy value of human milk . British Medical Journal, 1, 1018-1020.

Manganaro, R., Marseglia, L., Mami, C., Paolata, A., Gargano, R., Mondello, M., et al. (2009). Effects of hospital policies and practices on initiation and duration of breastfeeding. [Multicenter Study]. Child: care, health and development, 35(1), 106-111.

Manohar, A. A., Williamson, M., & Koppikar, G. V. (1997). Effect of storage of colostrum in various containers. [Comparative Study]. Indian pediatrics, 34(4), 293-295.

Martin RJ, Fanaroff AA, Walsh MC. (Ed(s),).(2011)Fanaroff and Martin's Neonatal Perinatal Medicine: Diseases of the Fetus and Infant. Vol Two. 9th ed. St. Elsevier, ISBN 078-0-323-065445-0, St Louis, MO.

Marx JA Hockenberger R, Walls RM. (Ed(s).) (2011) . Rosen's Emergency Medicine Concepts in Clinical Practice. 7th ed. Mosby Elsevier, ISBN 032305472, Philadelphia, PA.

McCormick, F. M., Tosh, K., & McGuire, W. (2010). Ad libitum or demand/semi-demand feeding versus scheduled interval feeding for preterm infants. [Meta-Analysis Review]. Cochrane database of systematic reviews(2), CD005255.

McIntyre, J. (2005). Prevention of mother-to-child transmission of HIV: treatment options. [Review]. Expert review of anti-infective therapy, 3(6), 971-980.

McLeod, G., & Sherriff, J. (2007). Preventing postnatal growth failure--the significance of feeding when the preterm infant is clinically stable. [Review]. Early human development, 83(10), 659-665.

McLeod, M. K., Kothary, P. C., & Farrell, C. M. (1994). Molecular and functional studies of inhibitory G protein in RINm5F cells. J Surg Res, 57(5), 619-624.

Mehta, N. R., Hamosh, M., Bitman, J., & Wood, D. L. (1988). Adherence of medium-chain fatty acids to feeding tubes during gavage feeding of human milk fortified with medium-chain triglycerides. [Research Support, U.S. Gov't, P.H.S.]. The Journal of pediatrics, 112(3), 474-476.

Meier PM, E. J., Patel AL, Jegier BJ, Bruns NE. (2010). Improving the Use of Human Milk During and After the NICU stay. Clin Perinatol, 37(1), 217-245.

Meier, P. P., Brown, L. P., Hurst, N. M., Spatz, D. L., Engstrom, J. L., Borucki, L. C., et al. (2000). Nipple shields for preterm infants: effect on milk transfer and duration of breastfeeding. [Journal of human lactation, 16(2), 106-114; quiz 129-131.

Meier, P. P., Engstrom, J. L., Janes, J. E., Jegier, B. J., & Loera, F. (2011). Breast pump suction patterns that mimic the human infant during breastfeeding: greater milk output in less time spent pumping for breast pump-dependent mothers with premature infants. Journal of perinatology, E-pub ahead of print.

Meier, P. P., Engstrom, J. L., Murtaugh, M. A., Vasan, U., Meier, W. A., & Schanler, R. J. (2002). Mothers' milk feedings in the neonatal intensive care unit: accuracy of the creamatocrit technique. J Perinatol, 22(8), 646-649.

Modi, N. (2005). Fluid and Electrolyte balance. In Rennie, JM (Ed.), Roberston's Textbook of Neonatology (4th ed.), Elsevier, Churchill LIvingston, ISBN 0443073554, Philadelphia, Pa.

Morton, J., Hall, J. Y., Wong, R. J., Thairu, L., Benitz, W. E., & Rhine, W. D. (2009). Combining hand techniques with electric pumping increases milk production in mothers of preterm infants. J Perinatol, 29(11), 757-764.

Mshana, S. E., Gerwing, L., Minde, M., Hain, T., Domann, E., Lyamuya, E., et al. (2011). Outbreak of a novel Enterobacter sp. carrying blaCTX-M-15 in a neonatal unit of a tertiary care hospital in Tanzania. International journal of antimicrobial agents, 38(3), 265-269.

Mulasky, S. (2005). A concept analysis of family-centered care in the NICU. Neonatal network : NN, 24(6), 25-32.

Najati N, S. L. (2010). Prevalence and underlying etiologies of neonatal hypoglycemia. . Pakistan Journal of Biological Sciences, 13(15), 753-756.

Neville, M. (1999). Physiology of lactation. Clin Perinatol, 26, 251-279.

Nightlinger, K. (2011). Developmentally supportive care in the neonatal intensive care unit: an occupational therapist's role. Neonatal network : NN, 30(4), 243-248.

Nyqvist, K., Anderson GC, Bergman N, Cattaneo A, Charpak N, Davanzo R, Widstrom AM. (2010). Toward universal Kangaroo Mother Care: recommendations and report from the First European conferences and Seventh International Workshop on Kangaroo Mother Care. Acta paediatrica, 99(6), 820-826.

Nyqvist, K. H. (2004). How can kangaroo mother care and high technology care be compatible? Journal of human lactation, 20(1), 72-74.

Nyqvist, K. H. (2008). Early attainment of breastfeeding competence in very preterm infants. Acta paediatrica, 97(6), 776-781.

Nyqvist, K. H., Farnstrand, C., Eeg-Olofsson, K. E., & Ewald, U. (2001). Early oral behaviour in preterm infants during breastfeeding: an electromyographic study. Acta paediatrica, 90(6), 658-663.

Ogechi, A. A., William, O., & Fidelia, B. T. (2007). Hindmilk and weight gain in preterm very low-birthweight infants. Pediatrics international : official journal of the Japan Pediatric Society, 49(2), 156-160.

Ogundele, M. O., & Coulter, J. B. (2003). HIV transmission through breastfeeding: problems and prevention. [Review]. Annals of tropical paediatrics, 23(2), 91-106.

Okolo, S. N., Adewunmi, Y. B., & Okonji, M. C. (1999). Current breastfeeding knowledge, attitude, and practices of mothers in five rural communities in the Savannah region of Nigeria. Journal of tropical pediatrics, 45(6), 323-326.

Pal Deb K, M. D., Sajbhandari S, Land JM, Patel N, Costello AM de L. (2000). Neonatal hypoglycemia in Nepal 1. Prevalence and risk factors. Arch Dis Child Fetal Neonatal Ed, 82, F46-F51.

Palcich, G., Gillio Cde, M., Aragon-Alegro, L. C., Pagotto, F. J., Farber, J. M., Landgraf, M., et al. (2009). Enterobacter sakazakii in dried infant formulas and milk kitchens of maternity wards in Sao Paulo, Brazil. Journal of food protection, 72(1), 37-42.

Peace O, T. J., Uche OC (2010). Morbidity and mortality amongst infants of diabetic mothers admitted into a special care baby unit in Port Harcourt, Nigeria. . Ital J of Ped, 36(77).

WHO Pocket Book for Hospital Care for Children Guidelines for the Management of Common Illnesses with Limited Resources. (2007). World Health Organization. ISBN 92 4 154670 0, Geneva, Switzerland.

Pridham, K., Brown, R., Bamberger, J. M., Wells, J., Greer, F., & Mounts, K. (2011). Graphical exploration of dimensions of preterm infant growth in weight in association with biological, nutritional, and energy expenditure conditions. [Comparative Study]. Biological research for nursing, 13(3), 260-273.

Renfrew MJ, C. D., Dyson L, McCormick F, Rice S, King SE, Misso K, Stenhouse E, Williams AF. (2009). Breastfeeding promotion for infants in neonatal units: a systematic review and economic analysi. Heatlh Technol Assess, 13(40), 1-146.

Rocha, N. M., Martinez, F. E., & Jorge, S. M. (2002). Cup or bottle for preterm infants: effects on oxygen saturation, weight gain, and breastfeeding. Journal of human lactation : official journal of International Lactation Consultant Association, 18(2), 132-138.

Rogers, N. L., Abdi, J., Moore, D., Nd'iangui, S., Smith, L. J., Carlson, A. J., et al. (2011). Colostrum avoidance, prelacteal feeding and late breast-feeding initiation in rural Northern Ethiopia. Public health nutrition, 1-8.

Rojahn A, L. C. (2001). Enteral feedings in infants <1250 g starting within 24 h post-partum. Eur J Pediatr, 160(10), 629-632.

Rollins, N. C. (2007). Infant feeding and HIV. BMJ, 334(7592), 487-488.

Rossman, B., Engstrom, J. L., Meier, P. P., Vonderheid, S. C., Norr, K. F., & Hill, P. D. (2011). "They've walked in my shoes": mothers of very low birth weight infants and their experiences with breastfeeding peer counselors in the neonatal intensive care unit. Journal of human lactation, 27(1), 14-24.

Ruff, A. J. (1994). Breastmilk, breastfeeding, and transmission of viruses to the neonate. [Review]. Seminars in perinatology, 18(6), 510-516.

Ruiz, J. G., Charpak, N., & Figuero, Z. (2002). Predictional need for supplementing breastfeeding in preterm infants under Kangaroo Mother Care. [Research Support, Non-U.S. Gov't]. Acta paediatrica, 91(10), 1130-1134.

Sadoh, W. E., & Sadoh, A. E. (2009). Experiences of HIV positive mothers who chose not to breastfeed their babies in Nigeria. African journal of reproductive health, 13(1), 27-35.

Savage, D. F., & Lhotska, L. (2000). Recommendations on feeding infants of HIV positive mothers. WHO, UNICEF, UNAIDS guidelines. Adv Exp Med Biol, 478, 225-230.

Schanler, R. J., Fraley, J. K., Lau, C., Hurst, N. M., Horvath, L., & Rossmann, S. N. (2011). Breastmilk cultures and infection in extremely premature infants. [Research Support, N.I.H., Extramural]. Journal of perinatology : official journal of the California Perinatal Association, 31(5), 335-338.

Seri I, e. a. (2005). Acid-Base, Fluid and Electrolyte Management. In B. R. Taeusch HW, Gleason CA (Ed.), Avery's Diseases of the Newborn (8th ed.). Philadelphia: Elsevier, Saunders.

Shapiro, R. L., Lockman, S., Kim, S., Smeaton, L., Rahkola, J. T., Thior, I., et al. (2007). Infant morbidity, mortality, and breast milk immunologic profiles among breast-feeding HIV-infected and HIV-uninfected women in Botswana. J Infect Dis, 196(4), 562-569.

Siddell, E. P., & Froman, R. D. (1994). A national survey of neonatal intensive-care units: criteria used to determine readiness for oral feedings. Journal of obstetric, gynecologic, and neonatal nursing, 23(9), 783-789.

Slusher, T., Hampton, R., Bode-Thomas, F., Pam, S., Akor, F., & Meier, P. (2003). Promoting the exclusive feeding of own mother's milk through the use of hindmilk and increased maternal milk volume for hospitalized, low birth weight infants (< 1800 grams) in Nigeria: a feasibility study. J Hum Lact, 19(2), 191-198.

Slusher, T., Slusher, I. L., Biomdo, M., Bode-Thomas, F., Curtis, B. A., & Meier, P. (2007). Electric breast pump use increases maternal milk volume in African nurseries. J Trop Pediatr, 53(2), 125-130.

Slusher T, Vaucher Y, Greenwood C, Powell C, Nakakeeto-Kijjambu M. (2012). Newborn Care. In Fischer P, Kamut DM (eds.) Textbook of Global Child Health, 1st Edition. Elk Grove American Academy of Pediatrics. 425-530.

Slusher TM, S. I., Keating EM, Curtis BA, Smith EA, Orodriyo E, Awori S, Nakakeeto MK. (2011). Comparison of Maternal Milk (Breastmilk) Expression Methods in an African Nursery. Breastfeeding medicine. E-pub ahead of press.

Swai M, O. R., Kinabo G. (2009). Paediatric Management Schedules at Hospital Level (7th ed.). Moshi: New Millennium Books.

Thior, I., Lockman, S., Smeaton, L. M., Shapiro, R. L., Wester, C., Heymann, S. J., et al. (2006). Breastfeeding plus infant zidovudine prophylaxis for 6 months vs formula feeding plus infant zidovudine for 1 month to reduce mother-to-child HIV transmission in Botswana: a randomized trial: the Mashi Study. JAMA : the journal of the American Medical Association, 296(7), 794-805.

Tiwari, R., Mahajan, P. C., & Lahariya, C. (2009). The determinants of exclusive breast feeding in urban slums: a community based study. Journal of tropical pediatrics, 55(1), 49-54.

UNICEF. (2009). Baby-Friendly Hospital Initiative Revised, updated and expanded for integrated care. from <http://www.who.int/nutrition/publications/infantfeeding/9789241594950/en/>

Wan, E. W., Davey, K., Page-Sharp, M., Hartmann, P. E., Simmer, K., & Ilett, K. F. (2008). Dose-effect study of domperidone as a galactagogue in preterm mothers with insufficient milk supply, and its transfer into milk. [Randomized Controlled Trial]. British journal of clinical pharmacology, 66(2), 283-289.

WHO, UNAIDS, UNFPA, unicef. Guidelines on HIV and Infant feeding 2010 Principles and Recommendations for Infant Feeding in the Context of HIV and Summary of the Evidence. (2010). ISBN 978 92 4 159953 5 hiv-aids_infantfeedingguidelines.pdf

WHO. (2010). Antiretroviral Drugs for Treating Pregnant Women and Children and Preventing HIV Infection in Infants Recommendations for a public health approach 2010 version. ISBN 978 92 4 159981 8 from http://www.who.int/hiv/pub/mtct/PMTCTfactsheet/en/

Zlathkin SH, Perman M. Feeding the preterm infant.(1988) In: Jeejeebhoy, KN. (Ed.), Current therapy in nutrition, BC Decker, Inc, Toronto, Ontartio, Canada.

Zorlu, G. (2011). New WHO child growth standards catch on. [News]. Bulletin of the World Health Organization, 89(4), 250-251.

Zuppa, A. A., Sindico, P., Orchi, C., Carducci, C., Cardiello, V., & Romagnoli, C. (2010). Safety and efficacy of galactogogues: substances that induce, maintain and increase breast milk production. [Review]. Journal of pharmacy & pharmaceutical. 13(2), 162-174.

3

The Long-Term Effects of Breastfeeding on Development

Wendy H. Oddy[1], Jianghong Li[1,3],
Monique Robinson[1] and Andrew J.O. Whitehouse[1,2]
*[1]Telethon Institute for Child Health Research,
Centre for Child Health Research,
The University of Western Australia, Perth,
[2]Neurocognitive Development Unit,
School of Psychology,
The University of Western Australia, Perth,
[3]Centre Population Health Research,
Curtin Health Innovation Research Institute,
Curtin University, Perth,
Australia*

1. Introduction

The link between breastfeeding duration and subsequent development, cognition, educational, mental, psychomotor and behavioural functioning of the infant has been the subject of much scientific enquiry. Indeed, the effect of feeding on infant health and development was first discussed more than half a century ago when breastfed babies were reported to have better cognitive outcomes in childhood than artificially fed babies (Hoefer and Hardy 1929).

Some studies have found striking results pertaining to the relative advantages that breastfeeding can confer on child neurodevelopment (Oddy, Kendall et al. 2003; Vohr, Poindexter et al. 2006; Kramer, Aboud et al. 2008). Breastfeeding has previously been associated with improvements across neurodevelopmental domains for low birthweight babies in comparison with not breastfeeding at all (Vohr, Poindexter et al. 2006). One study reported results from a large randomized controlled trial and found that breastfeeding for a longer duration and exclusive breastfeeding were associated with significant increases in the child's IQ by age six years (Kramer, Aboud et al. 2008).

Breastfeeding is more common among women of social advantage and confounding complicates study interpretation (Bauchner, Leventhal et al. 1986). The question of whether breastfeeding and formula feeding have differential effects on development, cognitive and language has not yet been comprehensively answered (Drane and Logemann 2000), largely due to lack of sample size resulting in inadequate statistical power and failure to obtain prospective data on a wide range of variables. These include infant feeding, the relevant covariates and validated outcome tests later in childhood. While language development in humans is under substantial genetic control (Stromswold 2001; Spinath, Price et al. 2004), there is accumulating evidence that environmental factors such as early nutrition can alter the expression of the genome and lead to enduring phenotypic changes.

Breastfed infants have cognitive advantages over formula-fed infants in a meta-analysis of 20 studies of children, after adjusting for confounders (Anderson, Johnstone et al. 1999). Studies that examined developmental time points have observed advantages of breastfeeding in comparison with not breastfeeding for infant development that can be observed from the neonatal period (Hart, Boylan et al. 2003), through to infancy (Vestergaard, Obel et al. 1999), early childhood (Fergusson, Beautrais et al. 1982), mid-childhood (Oddy, Robinson et al. 2011), adolescence (Oddy, Kendall et al. 2010) and into midlife (Richards, Hardy et al. 2002). Some reviews and individual studies have found the protective effect of a longer duration of breastfeeding on child behaviour and cognition to be an artifact of sociodemographic confounding rather than a true association. Zhou and colleagues (Zhou, Baghurst et al. 2007) suggested that the benefits of breastfeeding were diminished when improvements in the home environment were taken into consideration and concluded that socioeconomic factors mediate the relationship between breastfeeding and child cognitive development. The authors of a meta-analysis of studies on breastfeeding and child intelligence argued that the relationship between breastfeeding and child development is heavily mediated by maternal IQ and studies that do not adjust for maternal IQ will observe biased results (Der, Batty et al. 2006). However, other studies have found that controlling for maternal education and IQ does not eliminate the positive effects of breastfeeding, suggesting that maternal IQ is not always an alternative explanation for results (Bartels, van Beijsterveldt et al. 2009).

To ascertain the true effect of breastfeeding on infant development, adequate study design is essential. A review of 24 studies found that almost all studies contained a methodological flaw; either inadequate control for confounders; insufficient definition of outcomes; or inconsistent definition of breastfeeding (Drane and Logemann 2000) concluding that the benefits of breastfeeding for development and cognitive IQ could not be determined due to study design limitations. Many studies are limited by insufficient methodological rigour, as suggested by a review of 40 studies on breastfeeding and intelligence between 1929-2001 that concluded no convincing evidence existed regarding the effects of breastfeeding versus formula feeding in relation to intelligence. The major challenge is to adequately control for the considerable confounding of parental and family characteristics also strongly associated with both breastfeeding for longer periods and good developmental outcomes for children. Given controversy in this area, efforts must be concentrated towards study design that allows for the appropriate determination of any relationship between breastfeeding and early developmental outcomes whilst allowing adjustment for factors that are closely associated with both. Future investigations must use more rigorous methods and criteria in the design of breastfeeding studies (Drane and Logemann 2000; Jain, Concato et al. 2002).

Breastfeeding is promoted as beneficial to both the mother and newborn and exclusive breastfeeding for at least six months is recommended (World Health Organisation 2003). Although there are many reasons to encourage breastfeeding, its benefits for cognitive ability, intelligence and academic achievement have received increasing scientific scrutiny (Horwood and Fergusson 1998; Der, Batty et al. 2006; Silva, Mehta et al. 2006; Kramer, Aboud et al. 2008).

Neurobehavioural development is an essential aspect of childhood development and an estimated one in five children have some mental health problem in Australia (Zubrick, Silburn et al. 2000). Between ten and twenty percent of children globally have emotional or behavioural problems and these have been listed as one of the six priority areas for future strategic directions for improving the health and development of children and adolescents (Belfer 2008). Although evidence shows that family, social, economic and psychological disadvantages associated with poverty, low parental income and education, single-parenthood and living in deprived areas are key risk factors for child mental health problems (Robinson, Oddy et al. 2008), little is understood about the potential impact of early infant feeding on subsequent mental health.

Compelling evidence exists for a relationship between breastfeeding, developmental milestones (Sacker, Quigley et al. 2006) and cognition from longitudinal (Drane and Logemann 2000), experimental (Koletzko, Aggett et al. 1998) and neurodevelopmental studies (Farquharson, Cockburn et al. 1992). However there has been conflicting evidence as to the psychological and behavioural outcomes associated with breastfeeding, potentially caused by inherent methodological challenges in this area including inadequate adjustment for confounding factors and problems with study design (Der, Batty et al. 2006; Kramer, Aboud et al. 2008).

1.1 Aims of our study

The aim of our study was to overcome some of the main methodological challenges that have limited previous research and in so doing determine whether independent effects of breastfeeding on early child development, cognitive IQ, academic attainment and mental health were apparent using data collected from the Western Australian Pregnancy Cohort (Raine) Study, a large prospective pregnancy cohort study followed to fourteen years of age.

We examined the association between early infant feeding and developmental outcomes at ages one, two and three years after adjusting for confounders. We hypothesized that developmental outcomes would be improved for children who were breastfed for a longer duration (Oddy, Robinson et al. 2011).

We examined the association between the duration of full breastfeeding and cognitive outcome (cognitive IQ) measured at six (Oddy, Kendall et al. 2003) and at ten years (Whitehouse, Robinson et al. 2011), taking into account perinatal, social and family factors. We conducted a longitudinal follow-up investigation of previous positive findings of breastfeeding (Oddy, Kendall et al. 2003) on language ability among children, whether the association persists until middle childhood, and whether any effect was of comparable magnitude at ten years (Whitehouse, Robinson et al. 2011).

We aimed to determine if the duration of breastfeeding was associated with numeracy and literacy achievement in children at ten years (Oddy, Li et al. 2011). We hypothesised that children breastfed for longer compared to those breastfed for a shorter duration would achieve higher scores in numeracy and literacy, independent of maternal and demographic factors, and early cognitive stimulation received in the home.

Finally, we aimed to investigate the duration of breastfeeding with child and adolescent mental health (Oddy, Kendall et al. 2010). We hypothesised that infants breastfed for longer would have improved mental health outcomes throughout childhood and adolescence.

2. Methods

2.1 Study population

The Western Australian Pregnancy Cohort (Raine) Study commenced as a randomized controlled trial to study the effects of repeated ultrasound during pregnancy in which 2,900 pregnant women were enrolled from the public antenatal clinic at the major obstetric hospital in Perth, Western Australia, and nearby private practices. This became a longitudinal study following 2,868 children born over a three year period with approximately 100 women per month enrolled from May 1989 to November 1991 (Newnham, Evans et al. 1993). The criteria for enrolment were gestational age between 16 and 20 weeks, sufficient proficiency in English to understand the implications of participation, an expectation to deliver at the hospital and an intention to remain in Western Australia so that follow-up would be possible.

2.2 Data collection during pregnancy and subsequent follow-ups

Comprehensive data on social and demographic factors, and medical and obstetric history were obtained from the parent at enrolment and, in the mother's case, updated during the 34th week of pregnancy. The babies were examined at two days of age by a paediatrician or midwife. Follow-ups at the first (N=2,441), second (70% follow-up; N=1,988) and third years (N=2,280) involved a structured interview and clinical examination of participating children in the cohort. A questionnaire was administered and information from a clinical examination was collected at around the intended age of one (mean age= 14 months), two (mean age= 26 months) and three years (mean age= 37 months) and at six (mean age= 71 months), eight (mean age=97 months), ten (mean age=126 months) and fourteen (mean age=168 months) years. For all follow-up assessments, parents were contacted and a questionnaire was posted for completion as soon as possible. Parents were asked to return the questionnaire at the time of the physical examination. The questionnaire collected information about parental sociodemographic factors (housing, family structure, employment, income), family functioning, and information about their child such as the development of speech and language, cognitive development, behaviour and history of illnesses, injuries and admissions to hospital.

2.3 Infant feeding

Infant feeding data were collected at one, two, and three years. Information about 'age at which milk other than breast milk was introduced' was applied to obtain a continuous measure of predominant breastfeeding in months. In a similar way, information about the age at which breastfeeding stopped was used to obtain measures of any breastfeeding. These data were categorised as 'less than four months' versus 'four months or longer', and 'less than six months' versus 'six months or longer'.

2.4 Covariate measures

We considered a wide range of pregnancy, antenatal, obstetric and postnatal variables throughout the child's life. Perinatal covariates included gender; gestational age (weeks) and; percentage of expected birthweight,. Social covariates were maternal age at child's birth; parental smoking; and presence of other siblings. In addition we considered fathers education, family income and parental employment status. Language stimulation was measured at three and five years by asking the parent how often she reads a story to the child. Maternal postnatal depression, diagnosed by a doctor, was measured retrospectively at the ten year follow-up.

2.5 Outcome measures

2.5.1 Infant/Child Monitoring Questionnaires (IMQ)

The IMQ (now known as the Ages and Stages Questionnaire (ASQ)) is a series of parent completed questionnaires designed to be used as a screening tool to assist in the monitoring of child development in the early years (Squires, Bricker et al. 1990). Each questionnaire measures communication, gross and fine motor, adaptive and social/personal development. IMQ was administered at 12, 24 and 36 months and scored as per the manual (Squires, Bricker et al. 1990). Scoring below the cutpoint was classified as having an "atypical score" for that domain. We also created a variable representing the presence of any atypical score across domains for each age and categorised the outcomes according to the total number of atypical scores for all follow-ups in each domain

2.5.2 Cognitive IQ

At both the six and ten year follow ups, children completed a clinical assessment that included administration of the Peabody Picture Vocabulary Test - Revised (PPVT-R). This was an achievement test of receptive vocabulary in English that provides an estimate of one major aspect of verbal ability for subjects who have grown up in an English speaking environment (Dunn and Dunn 1981). The PPVT-R was administered by the two child health nurses according to the manual and supervised by a registered psychologist. A child with a score less that the first negative standard deviation for the group was deemed to have a "below average verbal ability" irrespective of the language spoken at home. There were significant tester effects and these were adjusted in all analyses.

2.5.3 Educational assessment

The Western Australian Literacy and Numeracy Assessment (WALNA) was administered annually to all students across Western Australia in grades three, five and seven (approximately 75% of West Australian children from public schools completed the assessment). The assessment consists of multiple-choice, short-response, and open-response questions in four areas: mathematics, reading, writing and spelling. WALNA records were linked for 1,038 Raine study children who were in grade five and attending government schools at the time of assessment.

2.5.4 Mental health measures

We focused on the parent-report Child Behaviour Checklist (CBCL/4-18) (Achenbach 1991) as the mental health outcome variable at the two, five, eight, ten and fourteen year follow-ups. The CBCL/2-3, validated for use with two year old children, was applied at the two-year follow-up (Achenbach, Edelbrock et al. 1987). The CBCL/4-18 is a 118-item instrument that assesses behavioural psychopathology in children according to syndrome scales. The scales of withdrawn, anxious/depressed and somatic complaints are grouped and scored as internalizing problems while the syndrome scores of delinquent behaviour and aggressive behaviour are grouped and scored as externalizing problems. A total score of overall mental health morbidity, representing the sum of all the items, is derived for the entire scale. Higher scores represent more disturbed behaviour. In accordance with the normative criteria, we applied the recommended clinical cut-off scores ($T \geq 60$) to total, internalizing, and externalizing T-scores to distinguish those children with a 'mental health problem' of clinical significance (Achenbach 1991). Therefore we were able to analyse mental health outcomes at all years using continuous CBCL T-scores and a binary variable reflecting clinical significance.

2.6 Statistical analysis

(See references (Oddy, Kendall et al. 2003; Oddy, Kendall et al. 2010; Oddy, Li et al. 2011; Oddy, Robinson et al. 2011; Whitehouse, Robinson et al. 2011) for detail)

Numerous statistical methods were used for these analyses. They included T-tests to assess differences in mean scores for each of the early developmental outcomes of gross motor skills, fine motor skills, adaptability, sociability and communication at ages one, two and three according to breastfeeding status. The predictor variables were entered into a multivariable logistic regression model, with an outcome of any atypical scores at each age, adjusting for the confounding factors. Finally, we examined IMQ outcomes as total atypical scores across follow-ups in a multinomial logistic regression model with a reference category of no atypical scores at any follow-up. For the cognitive IQ investigation, basic chi square tests for association, Spearman's correlations and multiple linear regression were conducted. Adjustment was made for the factors correlated with each outcome and breastfeeding (gestational age, maternal age, maternal education and presence of other siblings). PPVT-R scores across breastfeeding groups were compared and hierarchical multivariable linear regression analyses were conducted.

Associations between breastfeeding duration and educational outcomes were estimated using linear models with adjustment for gender, family income, maternal factors and early stimulation at home through reading. For mental health, chi-square tests for trends were conducted using standard bivariate models between the primary exposure and the outcomes. To look at the estimated effect of breastfeeding on child mental health over time, we constructed binary outcomes, which provided information on clinical relevance. Factors were adjusted as potential confounders (maternal age, education, smoking in pregnancy, stress in pregnancy, proportion of optimal birthweight, family income, and family structure) (Robinson, Oddy et al. 2008). Chi square tests and generalised estimating equations that generate odds ratios, confidence intervals and p-values are given.

3. Results

3.1 Development at one, two and three years

The frequency characteristics for our predictor and control variables are presented for the cohort who provided data at the one-year follow-up (n=2,375). Approximately 63% of the cohort was breastfed for four months or longer, 41% of mothers had completed high school education, and 29% had a family income below the poverty line during pregnancy. When the baby was one year, more than one in five infants had at least one atypical score for an early developmental domain, increasing to 32% with at least one atypical score at age two and reducing to 29% at age three. Infants breastfed for four months or longer had significantly higher mean scores for fine motor skills at one, two and three years (Table 1).

N=2,375	Breastfeeding Mean (SD)		Sig 2 tailed*	Cohen's D
Year 1	<4months	4+ months		
Gross Motor	5.39 (1.10)	5.41 (1.10)	0.647	-0.02
Fine Motor	5.33 (0.90)	5.44 (0.80)	0.002	-0.13
Adaptability	4.84 (1.27)	5.14 (1.09)	<0.001	-0.25
Sociability	4.72 (1.14)	4.81 (1.12)	0.058	-0.08
Communication	4.08 (1.49)	4.25 (1.38)	0.005	-0.12
Year 2				
Gross Motor	5.58 (0.72)	5.59 (0.71)	0.645	-0.01
Fine Motor	5.35 (0.75)	5.44 (0.74)	0.009	-0.12
Adaptability	5.02 (1.00)	5.14 (0.90)	0.007	-0.13
Sociability	4.51 (0.99)	4.52 (0.95)	0.888	-0.01
Communication	5.24 (1.16)	5.34 (1.09)	0.076	-0.09
Year 3				
Gross Motor	5.57 (0.68)	5.60 (0.75)	0.356	-0.04
Fine Motor	5.19 (1.07)	5.38 (0.92)	<0.001	-0.19
Adaptability	5.46 (0.84)	5.51 (0.83)	0.198	-0.06
Sociability	5.16 (0.81)	5.22 (0.77)	0.121	-0.08
Communication	5.34 (0.80)	5.44 (0.73)	0.007	-0.13

*equal variances not assumed

Table 1. Mean Infant Monitoring Questionnaire (IMQ/ASQ) scores (with standard deviations) and breastfeeding for less than four months and four months or longer (Oddy, Robinson et al. 2011)

The risk of any atypical score for all developmental outcomes was significantly increased for infants who were breastfed for less than four months at age one (OR=1.49, 95%CI= 1.16, 1.92), two (OR=1.29, 95%CI= 1.01, 1.65) and three years (OR=1.34, 95%CI= 1.06, 1.70) (Table 2).

The results of multinomial logistic regression analyses showed that breastfeeding for less than four months increased the risk for two or more atypical scores across all domains over the three years of the study except for gross motor skills (Table 3).

	Breastfeeding duration <4 months[μ]		
	Atypical score at year 1, 2 or 3		
	Year 1	**Year 2**	**Year 3**
	OR (95% CI) § p-value		
Atypical score on 1 or more domains	**1.49**** 1.16, 1.92 .002	**1.29*** 1.01, 1.65 .041	**1.34*** 1.06, 1.70 .016

* p<0.05, ** p<0.005 [μ] Reference category breastfeeding 4+ months
§ Adjusted for child's age at examination, maternal age at conception, maternal education, total stress events experienced during pregnancy, maternal smoking during pregnancy, biological father living with family, family income, Apgar scores at 5 minutes, gestational age and child gender

Table 2. Adjusted binary logistic regression analyses for the risk of any atypical scores on the total score of the IMQ/ASQ by breastfeeding < 4 months compared to breastfeeding 4+ months (Oddy, Robinson et al. 2011)

	Breastfeeding duration <4 months[μ]		
	No atypical scores (reference category)	**One atypical score at any time point**	**Atypical scores at two or more time points**
IMQ Domains	OR (95% CI) § p-value		
Gross motor	1.00	**1.52*** 1.03, 2.23 .035	1.23 0.60, 2.51 .577
Fine Motor	1.00	1.35 0.96, 1.90 .085	**1.81*** 1.05, 3.15 .034
Adaptability	1.00	**1.49*** 1.07, 2.07 .019	**1.91*** 1.10, 3.31 .021
Sociability	1.00	1.11 0.82, 1.50 .492	**2.09**** 1.31 3.33 .002
Communication	1.00	**1.53*** 1.10, 2.14 .013	**1.97*** 1.22, 3.17 .006

* p<0.05, ** p<0.005

[μ] Reference category breastfeeding 4+ months
§ Adjusted for child's age at examination, maternal age at conception, maternal education, total stress events experienced during pregnancy, maternal smoking during pregnancy, biological father living with family, family income, Apgar scores at 5 minutes, gestational age and child gender

Table 3. Adjusted multinomial logistic regression analyses for the risk of atypical scores at one or two or more time points compared with no atypical scores for domains of the IMQ/ASQ by breastfed< 4 months compared to breastfed 4+ months (Oddy, Robinson et al. 2011)

3.2 Cognitive development

Table 4 gives the adjusted mean IQ scores for each level of breastfeeding, the F test for linearity from the fitted model and corresponding significance test at six years. After adjustment for covariates there remained a significant association between duration of breastfeeding and cognitive IQ (F=8.59 p=0.003) with a 3.56 point advantage for those children fully breastfed for more than six months compared with children never breastfed.

	Duration of full breastfeeding							
Measure	Total group	Never breastfed (n=117)	Fully breastfed < 4 months (n=495)	Fully breastfed 4-6 months (n=378)	Fully breast-fed > 6 months (n=412)	F test for linearity	p-value	max-min
Cognitive IQ†	106.88 (12.86)	105.19 (12.98) (n=79)	105.55 (12.73) (n=348)	107.18 (12.44) (n=272)	108.67 (13.15) (n=299)	8.59	.003	3.56

† Cognitive IQ measured by 'Peabody Picture Vocabulary Test – Revised' at six years adjusted for gestational age, maternal age, maternal education, parental smoking and older siblings.

Table 4. Mean (SD) standardised cognitive IQ scores at six years by duration of full breastfeeding after adjustment for covariates (Oddy, Kendall et al. 2003)

There was a strong positive association between PPVT-R scores at six and ten years for the 1067 children who provided data at both time-points, $r = 0.601$, $p < 0.01$. A one-way ANOVA revealed a significant difference between the PPVT-R scores of the groups representing different predominant breastfeeding durations, $F(3,1193) = 12.32$, $p < 0.01$. Bonferroni post-hoc tests found that the children who had been breastfed predominantly for between 4 and 6 months or for greater than 6 months, had greater language scores than children who had been breastfed predominantly for 0 to 4 months or not at all (for all comparisons, $p < 0.05$) at ten years.

	B (95%CI)	P*
Duration of predominant breastfeeding		
< 4 months	2.94 (0.51, 5.36)	0.02
4 to 6 months	3.98 (1.45, 6.5)	<0.01
> 6 months	4.39 (1.88, 6.9)	<0.01

*Significant covariates only are presented
†Adjusted for maternal age at conception, gender, maternal education, smoking during pregnancy, alcohol during pregnancy, parity, reading to child

Table 5 Adjusted† multivariate linear regression models showing the effect of the duration of predominant breastfeeding on receptive vocabulary at ten years (Whitehouse, Robinson et al. 2011).

Children who had been breastfed predominantly for less than four months had higher language scores than children never breastfed ($B = 2.33$, 95% CI = 0.51, 5.36, $p = 0.02$), while the effect was stronger for children breastfed predominantly for between 4 to 6 months ($B = 3.98$, 95% CI = 1.45, 6.5, $p < 0.01$) (Table 5), and stronger still for children who were breastfed predominantly for more than 6 months (B = 4.39, 95% CI = 1.88, 6.9, p <0.01). Of the confounders included in the

model, a higher maternal age at conception, male gender and low levels of alcohol during pregnancy were associated with small increases in language scores. Lower levels of maternal education, maternal smoking of 11+ cigarettes per day during pregnancy, and having at least one older sibling were significantly associated with poorer language scores at ten years. A progressively stronger positive association was observed between the frequency of reading to the child at three years and language ability in middle childhood.

3.3 Educational outcomes

Data for 1,038 children were matched with West Australian Literacy and Numeracy Assessment (WALNA) grade five records. Of 1,038 children, complete data were available on most key outcome and exposure variables for 980 children.

In univariate associations between breastfeeding and educational outcomes at ten years, parameter estimates from linear regression showed that continuous breastfeeding was associated with an increase in scores with each additional month of breastfeeding for mathematics (Beta 1.21; 95% CI 0.30, 2.13; P=0.010), reading (Beta 1.68; 95% CI 0.78, 2.58; P<0.001), writing (Beta 2.13; 95% CI 0.68, 3.59; P=0.004) and spelling (Beta 1.46; 95% CI 0.44, 2.48; P=0.005). Results were attenuated when adjusted for confounding factors and we concluded that breastfeeding as measured in months was weakened in multivariate models.

Predominant breastfeeding for six months or longer was a significant predictor for improved academic scores in multivariable models for mathematics, reading and spelling and approaching significance for writing (Table 6).

	Mathematics			Reading			Writing			Spelling		
	Beta	95% CI	P value†	Beta	95% CI	P value †	Beta	95% CI	P value†	Beta	95% CI	P value†
Predominant breastfeeding 6+months**	**15.79**	**1.04, 30.55**	**0.036**	**18.28**	**3.92, 32.64**	**0.021**	**18.00**	**5.68, 41.67**	**0.136**	**15.60**	**-0.03, 31.24**	**0.050**

* Adjustment was made for child gender, maternal age, maternal education, family income, marital status, parent looks at book with child; also adjusted for maternal race: Aboriginal, Asian/other, or Caucasian.

** Reference for predominant breastfeeding for 6 or more months was predominant breastfeeding for less than 6 months.

† Test of between-subjects effects

Table 6. Multivariable linear regression model between predominant breastfeeding for six months or longer and educational outcomes at 10 years of age* (N=980) (Oddy, Li et al. 2011)

We observed increased mathematics, reading, writing and spelling scores for boys but no effect of breastfeeding was apparent on the educational attainment of girls. Significant observed interactions for mathematics (p=0.007) and spelling (p=0.047), revealed that boys were more likely than girls to have improved academic scores if they were breastfed for longer (Oddy, Li et al. 2011).

3.4 Mental health outcomes

Children breastfed for six months or longer had significantly lower mean behavioural scores (meaning improved behaviour) across total, internalizing and externalizing domains of mental health morbidity (Table 7). Younger mothers, those with 12 years education or less, those who were stressed, with low incomes, or who smoked during pregnancy were more likely to breastfeed for less than six months. Postnatal depression and inappropriate fetal growth were associated with a shorter duration of breastfeeding. There were significant downward trends in the proportions of children above the behavioural cut-off score at all ages as duration of breastfeeding increased. These trends were most pronounced in the total and externalizing domains.

Multivariable generalized estimating equations with binary mental health outcomes across the years revealed similar trends (Table 8), with a shorter duration of breastfeeding being consistently associated with increased risks for mental health problems of clinical significance through childhood and into adolescence. Prenatal risk factors such as smoking, experience of multiple stress events, low family income, younger maternal age and the absence of the biological father in the family home, plus postnatal depression, were also associated with increasing CBCL scores and in some cases mental health morbidity, as has been previously identified (Robinson, Oddy et al. 2008).

Breastfeeding duration	Age 2 N=1899	Age 5 N=2036	Age 8 N=1938	Age 10 N=1895	Age 14 N=1695
Total morbidity					
Never breastfed	16.1	26.3	19.4	15.2	16.7
<3 mo‡	16.4	31.2	29.8	20.9	18.9
3 mo - <6 mo	9.6	20.6	20.3	16.4	12.6
6 mo-<12 mo	9.3	18.4	16.2	12.1	12.6
12+ mo	9.6	16.0	13.5	12.6	10.9
Test for trend*	0.001	<0.001	<0.001	0.004	0.004
Internalizing morbidity					
Never breastfed	12.8	21.6	18.9	18.2	19.4
<3 mo	11.3	21.8	25.6	21.2	16.4
3 mo - <6 mo	5.6	17.6	20.6	19.9	11.3
6 mo-<12 mo	7.3	16.7	15.8	15.1	12.2
12+ mo	7.2	16.0	18.0	15.8	9.3
Test for trend*	0.007	0.013	0.022	0.037	<0.001
Externalizing morbidity					
Never breastfed	16.7	21.1	20.0	13.3	20.8
<3 mo	21.2	30.9	25.6	18.4	20.4
3 mo - <6 mo	10.5	18.4	18.6	13.2	14.6
6 mo-<12 mo	12.1	17.9	16.0	10.4	13.2
12+ mo	9.8	16.4	12.2	9.4	12.3
Test for trend*	<0.001	<0.001	<0.001	0.001	0.001

*P-value for linear by linear association; ‡ mo= month

Table 7. Percentage of children in mental health morbidity groups (total, internalizing and externalizing) and breastfeeding duration (never, < 3 mo, 3 mo- <6 mo, 6 mo -<12 mo, 12+ mo) (Oddy, Kendall et al. 2010).

Multivariable Generalised Estimating Equation Model- Years 2 to 14 Inclusive			
	Total Morbidity	**Internalizing Morbidity**	**Externalizing Morbidity**
Exposure variables	Odds Ratio 95% Confidence Interval p-value		
Breastfeeding duration < 6 months: 6+ months	1.33 1.09, 1.62 0.005	1.21 1.00, 1.46 0.054	1.23 1.01, 1.49 0.044

** Adjusted for maternal age, education, marital status, smoking in pregnancy, family income, life stress events, postnatal depression. Also adjusted for proportion of optimal birth weight and child gender.

Table 8. Association between breastfeeding duration and mental health morbidity of clinical significance † (Oddy, Kendall et al. 2010)

4. Discussion

We have shown convincing evidence that breastfeeding for less than four months was associated with lower developmental scores in the first three years of life. We observed a clear and significant dose response relation between duration of full breastfeeding in infancy and cognitive IQ as measured at six and ten years of age. The magnitude of the association at ten years was comparable to the effect observed at six years and indicates long-term advantages of breastfeeding. Predominant breastfeeding for six months or longer was associated with significantly higher scores for mathematics, reading and spelling in ten-year-old children when adjusted for the socio-demographic characteristics of the mother and family, and early stimulation of the child in the home at age five through reading. However, significant interaction effects were shown between gender and breastfeeding. We showed that a shorter duration of breastfeeding (less than six months) compared with a longer duration (≥ six months) was associated with increased mental health morbidity from early childhood to adolescence. This association was evident for the continuous measures of total, externalizing and internalizing behaviours as well as for dichotomous measures of morbidity which reflect clinically significant behavioural problems. Further, these associations persisted after adjustment for social, economic, birth and psychological factors in early life. Hence, we suggest that breastfeeding impacts on development, cognitive IQ, educational attainment and mental health from infancy to adolescence and potentially beyond.

A number of domains of early child development were sensitive to a longer duration of breastfeeding, following adjustment for confounding factors. In particular, we observed that the developmental domains of adaptability and communication were most responsive to the effects of breastfeeding duration, with children breastfed for longer than four months being more likely to have higher scores in these domains. Our findings pertaining to the communication domain of early development are consistent with a previous study that has found a link between an increased length of breastfeeding and mastery of developmental milestones including polysyllabic babbling (Vestergaard, Obel et al. 1999). These results also support findings from a New Zealand cohort study that demonstrated benefits for infants breastfed for four months or longer in the domains of intelligence, comprehension and expression (Fergusson, Beautrais et al. 1982). A recent study of infants from the Millennium Cohort Study (Sacker, Quigley et al. 2006) found that those who were never breastfed were 30% more likely to have developmental delays for gross motor skills (Montgomery, Ehlin et al. 2006). Unexpectedly, we found that gross motor skills were least sensitive to duration of breastfeeding and a shorter duration of breastfeeding was associated with an increased risk of atypical gross motor scores for boys at age one and two years.

Gender differences are apparent in the effect of breastfeeding on early development whereby girls appear to be less responsive to extended breastfeeding than boys. A longer duration of breastfeeding remained predictive for academic achievement in ten-year-old boys for mathematics and spelling with a small but insignificant benefit for reading in girls. We suggest that gender ought to be considered in explanations of the link between breastfeeding and neuro-cognitive development. Boys may be more vulnerable to adversity during critical periods than girls (Catalano, Bruckner et al. 2005), possibly due to the neuro-protective effect of estrodiols (Garcia-Segura, Azcoitia et al. 2001) at higher concentration in females. The neuro-protective components in breast milk - and the downstream consequences for development - may have greater benefits for boys. Compelling evidence exists for sexual dimorphism in the developing brain, giving rise to gender differences in cognition and behaviour (Baron-Cohen, Knickmeyer et al. 2005). For example, males generally do better on tests of mental rotation, map reading, targeting, and embedded figures, whereas females do better on tests of emotional recognition, social sensitivity, and verbal fluency and they start to talk earlier than males (Baron-Cohen, Knickmeyer et al. 2005). Only one previous study has examined gender differences in the association between breastfeeding and child development. Breastfeeding was associated with improved clarity of speech in boys and girls but significantly more so in boys and better speech was associated with improved reading ability (Broad 1972). The effect of breastfeeding on speech and reading in boys was reported in a later follow-up, suggesting that breastfeeding accelerates the rate of maturation of boys (Broad 1972; Broad 1975). Significant gender differences were observed in the association between breastfeeding and educational outcomes in our study. Therefore we analysed our data by boys and girls separately.

Our studies were based on a prospective birth cohort study reasonably representative of the general population and has a number of strengths. Firstly, although controlling for every potential confounding in the child's developmental trajectory is not possible, we were able to adjust for a range of socio-demographic, biological and psychological factors that share a relationship with breastfeeding duration and child developmental, in particular maternal education, family income and maternal stress (Jain, Concato et al. 2002; Der, Batty et al. 2006) to minimise the possibility of confounding being responsible for any observed results.

The ten year findings extend those of a previous investigation in the same cohort (Oddy, Kendall et al. 2003), and have implications for our understanding of the longitudinal effects of breastfeeding on development. At six years, children breastfed predominantly for more than six months had an adjusted increase in PPVT-R scores of 3.56 points compared with children who were never breastfed. This increase in PPVT-R score at ten years was 4.39 points. We suggest that our findings provide evidence for a beneficial effect of breastfeeding on language development in middle childhood of at least equivalent magnitude to the association in early childhood at six years.

A growing literature suggests that a relationship between breastfeeding and cognitive development exists (Silva, Buckfield et al. 1978; Clandinin, Chappell et al. 1980; Fergusson, Beautrais et al. 1982; Taylor and Wadsworth 1984; Doyle, Rickards et al. 1992; Wharton 1992; Makrides, Neumann et al. 1994; Michaelson, Larsen et al. 1994; Malloy and Berendes 1998; Quinn, O'Callaghan et al. 2001; Oddy, Kendall et al. 2003). In a recent critical evaluation (Drane and Logemann 2000) of the three methodological standards described by Bauchner(Bauchner, Leventhal et al. 1986), definition of outcome, correct classification of infant feeding type and control of potential confounding variables were determined in relation to cognitive development. The evaluation found that adherence to an infant feeding standard was poor with most studies classifying partial and exclusive breastfeeding together and only five considering feeding as a continuous variable (Taylor and Wadsworth 1984; Morrow-Tlucak, Haude et al. 1988; Bauer, Ewald et al. 1991; Lucas, Morley et al. 1992; Horwood and Fergusson 1998). Most studies adjusted for confounding factors including maternal education, socioeconomic status, birthweight and birth order. Few studies had well-defined and consistent outcome measures. Only five studies met all three methodological standards (Lucas, Morley et al. 1992; Lucas, Morley et al. 1994; Pollock 1994; Horwood and Fergusson 1998; Malloy and Berendes 1998); three of these found consistent advantages to breastfed infants (Lucas, Morley et al. 1992; Lucas, Morley et al. 1994; Horwood and Fergusson 1998) but two did not find significant associations (Lucas, Morley et al. 1994; Pollock 1994). The lack of association in these two studies may be explained by design issues. One study found differences for the Bayley Scale Psychomotor Index but not for Mental Development Scale Scores, when comparing infants fed donor breast milk with infants fed formula milk. In this study the low birthweight breastfed infants were fed 'drip' milk rather than own mothers' milk, which had a higher calorific value and fat content (Lucas, Morley et al. 1994). In relation to intelligence, the breastfed infant has been shown to have an advantage over the non breastfed infant (Pollock 1994), although some studies have been criticised for neglecting the possible genetic influence of maternal intelligence (Der, Batty et al. 2006).

In prospective studies after adjustment for numerous confounding variables, children breastfed for longer performed better on tests of cognition, verbal ability and school performance. Similar results have been observed in term and pre-term infants (Horwood and Fergusson 1998; Horwood, Darlow et al. 2001) and extend beyond adolescence (Lucas 2005). In a study to examine the association between duration of breastfeeding and cognitive ability at 7-8 years in a birth cohort of very low birthweight infants (Horwood, Darlow et al. 2001), increasing duration of breast milk feeding was associated with increases in both cognitive IQ ($p<0.001$) and performance ($p<0.05$). The effects on cognitive IQ are in the range of 2-5 points and may be as large as 10 points in low birthweight babies (Lucas, Morley et al. 1992; Lucas, Morley et al. 1994; Horwood, Darlow et al. 2001). The results of our study agree with this and other reports and adds to a growing body of evidence for an association between breastfeeding and cognitive development.

An early study showed small but significant increases in later intelligence and educational attainment between breast and formula-fed infants (Rodgers 1978). Fergusson et al combined males and females and tested for differences in intelligence, comprehension, expression and articulation and found significantly increased scores in infants breastfed for four months or longer for intelligence and comprehension at three, five and seven years, and expression at three and five years (Fergusson, Beautrais et al. 1982). Quinn et al speculated the observed that cognitive differences between breast- and formula-fed infants observed in their birth cohort of 3,880 infants followed to five years was due to unique constituents of breast milk (Quinn, O'Callaghan et al. 2001).

Available meta-analyses reflect a less conclusive pattern of breastfeeding effect on developmental outcomes. A meta-analysis of studies published up to 1996 found that breastfed children had higher cognitive scores, compared to bottle-fed children (Anderson, Johnstone et al. 1999) although some studies adjusted for few confounders. Another meta-analysis showed that only two studies met stringent criteria for inclusion, such as adequate adjustment for socioeconomic status of the family and stimulation of the child (Jain, Concato et al. 2002). Of these two studies, one reported a positive association between breastfeeding and intelligence (Johnson, Swank et al. 1996), while the other found no benefit (Wigg, Tong et al. 1998).

The majority of previous studies have focused on the association between breastfeeding and cognitive ability, and only a few have examined academic achievement. Where this has been studied, positive associations have been observed (Horwood and Fergusson 1998; Anderson, Johnstone et al. 1999; Jain, Concato et al. 2002). For example, Richards (Richards, Hardy et al. 2002) found a positive impact of breastfeeding on educational attainment in midlife independent of early background in 1,739 participants from the British 1946 birth cohort. Further analyses found that the association was largely mediated through adolescent cognition and educational attainment.

Despite the evidence for an impact of breastfeeding on cognitive development, there have been few published papers on mental health outcomes since the early theorists working within a developmental psychopathological framework (Hoefer and Hardy 1929) which is surprising given the popularity of attachment theory in relation to healthy psychological development (Rutter 2006). There is reluctance to suggest an association between breastfeeding and later mental health partly due to the possibility of alternative explanations such as parenting behaviours and cognitive ability (Anderson, Johnstone et al. 1999) and concern for creating guilt in women who do not breastfeed. In developed nations breastfeeding is more likely in communities with greater economic and social resources (Pollock 1994; Vohr, Poindexter et al. 2006), and the confounding socioeconomic effects complicate interpretation of this association (Li, Kendall et al. 2008). Our study addresses this issue by adjusting for many of these underlying factors, although we acknowledge that not all potential confounders (such as maternal IQ) were measured with sufficient validity and precision to fully control for all potential confounding effects.

Existing research tends to focus on infant and early childhood behaviour (Golding, Rogers et al. 1997) and consistent with our findings, infants who are breastfed for at least six months have a distinct developmental advantage over non breastfed infants and infants breastfed for a short period of time (Horne, Parslow et al. 2004). One study found that low birthweight infants fed breast milk had significantly higher scores for engagement and emotional regulation on the Bayley Developmental Scale than low birthweight infants not given breast milk (Vohr, Poindexter et al. 2006). However, this study did not differentiate the effects of feeding at the breast versus feeding of breast milk through a tube or bottle (Lucas, Morley et al. 1994). Another study found that breastfed infants were more able to face adverse stimuli with greater degrees of control, show more appropriate amounts of change in arousal levels, and were more able to return to moderate states of arousal than formula fed infants (Hart, Boylan et al. 2003). However, much of this research is based on small and non-random samples with a few exceptions to this (Sacker, Quigley et al. 2006). One exception includes the results from a large, cluster-randomized trial, whereby the authors did not find significant differences in behavioural outcomes at age six for those infants whose mothers were encouraged to breastfeed exclusively and for longer durations; however, the age at follow-up was considerably less than in our study, the children were only assessed at one point in time and a short form behavioural measure was used (Kramer, Aboud et al. 2008). Later childhood outcomes in breastfed children include greater resilience against stress and anxiety associated with parental separation and divorce at ten years in a study of 8958 children (Montgomery, Ehlin et al. 2006).

Breastfeeding may influence children's academic achievement by promoting brain development and general health. Nutrients in breast milk that are essential for optimum brain growth, such as long-chain polyunsaturated fatty acids (LCPUFA), may not be contained in formula milk (Larque, Demmelmair et al. 2006). LCPUFAs are structural elements of cell membranes and are essential in the formation of new tissue, including neurons. Makrides et al. noted an increased docosahexanoic acid (DHA; 22:6n-3) content of brain cortex with breastfeeding (Makrides, Neumann et al. 1994). Breastfed infants had a greater proportion of DHA in their erythrocytes and brain cortex and scored better on visual and developmental tests than did formula-fed infants. Crawford highlighted arachidonic acid (AA; 20:4n6) and DHA as vital components of breast milk that support development of the newborn brain (Crawford 1993) and research supports this (Crawford, Bloom et al. 1999; Crawford, Bloom et al. 2001).

Animal studies have found that LCPUFA may also play a neuroprotective role in early development, eliminating the build-up of neurotoxic levels of certain molecules (e.g., Ca^{2+}) and inhibiting glutamatergic synaptic transmission (Lauritzen, Blondeau et al. 2000). Further studies (Das 2002; Farkas, de Wilde et al. 2002; Das 2003) have identified that certain LCPUFAs, including eicosapentaenoic acid, docosahexaenoic and arachidonic acid, act as secondary messengers, inducing the release of acetylcholine and noradrenaline, which are neurotransmitters known to be involved in cognitive development (Sarter and Bruno 1997; Dalley, McGaughy et al. 2001). The specific fatty acid content of breast milk is essential for central nervous system development, including the brain in the neonate. Breastfeeding may have long-term consequences for child mental health outcomes because of the maternal fatty acids and other bioactive components essential for neurodevelopment (Keating and Hertzman 1999; McCain and Mustard 1999; Yehuda, Rabinovitz et al. 1999). Further, breast milk may contain elements relevant to the stress response. For example, the hormone leptin in breast milk may reduce stress in infants through its action on the hippocampus, hypothalamus, pituitary gland, and adrenal gland (Montgomery, Ehlin et al. 2006), whereas formula milk may have a depressant effect on newborn behavior (DiPietro, Larson et al. 1987).

Breastfeeding may also promote growth and development by facilitating the mother-child bonding, interaction and, indirectly, cognitive growth (Quinn, O'Callaghan et al. 2001). Positive maternal contact may induce a biological response in offspring. In rats, variations in maternal licking and grooming have been shown to promote the development of neural systems that mediate hypothalamic–pituitary–adrenal axis and behavioral responses to stress in offspring as well as certain forms of learning and memory (Caldji, Tannenbaum et al. 1998; Liu, Diorio et al. 2000). Stimulation associated with maternal contact during breastfeeding may have a positive effect on the development of neuroendocrine aspects of the stress response, which may affect development (Huizink, Robles de Medina et al. 2003). There is some evidence to date in human studies (Strathearn, Mamun et al. 2009), but this hypothesis is largely informed by rat models (Uvnäs-Moberg 1998). Rat pups who experienced a greater frequency of maternal contact during nursing in the first ten days after birth (licking and grooming) exhibited a more controlled response to acute stress as adults (e.g. a lower magnitude of hypothalamic-pituitary-adrenal (HPA) response) (Liu, Diorio et al. 2000). In humans the pattern of mother-infant interaction differs between breastfeeding and bottle-feeding. The amount of mutual touch, tactile stimulation and mother's gaze to infant were significantly elevated during breastfeeding compared with bottle-feeding (Lavelli and Poli 1998). Breastfeeding helps promote attachment between the mother and the infant which is known to have a positive influence on the child's psychological development into adulthood (Crowell and Waters 2005).

4.1 Directions for future research

More rigourous research is required to investigate the plausible biological mechanisms discussed above and any other factors we have not considered, eg, since we have not adjusted for maternal IQ in any of the studies, there is a possibility that this factor confounds or mediates some of the breastfeeding effects we have shown.

4.2 Conclusion

Breastfeeding for a longer duration appears to have significant benefits for the development, cognitive IQ, educational attainment and mental health of the child into adolescence. Our study has demonstrated that following adjustment for socioeconomic, psychological and maternal exposures in early life, a longer duration of breastfeeding was positively associated with the developmental, cognitive, educational and psychological health and wellbeing of children and adolescents. Therefore, public health programs aimed at increasing breastfeeding duration could be of long-term benefit for child and adolescent health.

5. Key findings

Breastfeeding for six months or longer is preferable to shorter breastfeeding or formula feeding because it is independently and longitudinally associated with better development, cognition, educational attainment and mental health throughout childhood and into adolescence.

Mothers should be encouraged, enabled and supported to continue breastfeeding for six months and longer in order to promote the optimum developmental health and well-being of their infants into childhood and adolescence

6. Information on contributors

Professor WH Oddy developed the hypotheses, statistical analyses, wrote the main drafts of the manuscript, and is responsible for correspondence and requests for reprints. Associate Professor Li played a lead role in the conceptualisation of the chapter, undertook statistical analyses and with Associate Professor Whitehouse and Dr Robinson contributed to the interpretation and discussion of the results and other sections.

We declare that none of the co-authors have competing interests.

7. Abbreviations

AA	Arachidonic acid
DHA	DocosaHexanoic acid
LCPUFA	Long-Chain Polyunsaturated Fatty Acids
PPVT	Peabody Picture Vocabulary Test
WALNA	Western Australian Literacy and Numeracy Assessment

8. Acknowledgments

Acknowledgments are extended to the study investigators and staff responsible for the collection of the data presented here, the Raine Medical Research Foundation at the University of Western Australia and the Telethon Institute for Child Health Research. Sincere thanks are extended to all study families without whose participation this research could not have been conducted. We thank Peter Jacoby for his statistical advice.

9. Funding for the research

WH Oddy was supported by a National Health & Medical Research Council Population Health Career Development Award. J Li was supported by a Curtin University of Technology Research Fellowship Award. The Western Australian Pregnancy Cohort Study is funded by project and program grants from Raine Medical Research Foundation, the National Health & Medical Research Council of Australia, Western Australian Health Promotion Foundation and Australian Rotary Health Research Fund, National Heart Foundation of Australia and Beyond Blue.

10. References

Achenbach, T. M. (1991). Manual for the Child Behavior Checklist/4-18 and 1991 Profile. Burlington, University of Vermont, Department of Psychiatry.

Achenbach, T. M., C. Edelbrock, et al. (1987). "Empirically based assessment of the behavioural/emotional problems of 2- and 3-year-old children." Journal of Abnormal Child Psychology 15(4): 629-650.

Anderson, J. W., B. M. Johnstone, et al. (1999). "Breast-feeding and cognitive development: a meta-analysis." American Journal of Clinical Nutrition 70(4): 525-535.

Baron-Cohen, S., C. Knickmeyer, et al. (2005). "Sex Differences in the Brain: Implications for Explaining Autism." Science 310(5749): 819-823.

Bartels, M., C. E. M. van Beijsterveldt, et al. (2009). "Breastfeeding, maternal education and cognitive function: a prospective study in twins." Behavior Genetics 39(6): 616-622.

Bauchner, H., J. M. Leventhal, et al. (1986). "Studies of breast-feeding and infections. How good is the evidence?" Journal of the American Medical Association 256(7): 887-892.

Bauer, G., L. S. Ewald, et al. (1991). "Breastfeeding and cognitive development of three-year-old children." Psychological Reports 68((3 Pt 2)): 1218.

Belfer, M. L. (2008). "Child and adolescent mental disorders: the magnitude of the problem across the globe." Journal of Child Psychology and Psychiatry 49(3): 226-236.

Broad, F. E. (1972). "The effects of infant feeding on speech quality." New Zealand Medical Journal 76(482): 28-31.

Broad, F. E. (1975). "Further studies on the effects of infant feeding on speech quality." New Zealand Medical Journal 82(553): 373-6.

Caldji, C., B. Tannenbaum, et al. (1998). "Maternal care during infancy regulates the development of neural systems mediating the expression of fearfulness in the rat." Proceedings of the National Academy of Sciences of the United States of America 95(9): 5335-40.

Catalano, R., T. Bruckner, et al. (2005). "Population stress and the Swedish sex ratio." Paediatric and Perinatal Epidemiology 19(6): 13-20.

Clandinin, M. T., J. E. Chappell, et al. (1980). "Intrauterine fatty acid accretion rates in human brain: implications for fatty acid requirements." Early Human Development 4: 121-129.

Crawford, M. A. (1993). "The role of essential fatty acids in neural development: implications for perinatal nutrition." American Journal of Clinical Nutrition 57(5 Suppl): 703S-709S.

Crawford, M. A., M. Bloom, et al. (1999). "Evidence for the unique function of docosahexaenoic acid during the evolution of the modern hominid brain." Lipids 34(Supplement 1): S39-S47.

Crawford, M. A., M. Bloom, et al. (2001). "Docosahexaenoic acid and cerebral evolution." World Review of Nutrition and Dietetics 88: 6-17.

Crowell, J. and E. Waters (2005). Attachment representations, secure-base behavior, and the evolution of adult relationships : the Stony Brook Adult Relationships Project. Attachment from infancy to adulthood : the major longitudinal studies. K. E. Grossmann, K. Grossmann and E. Waters. New York, Guilford Press.

Dalley, J. W., J. McGaughy, et al. (2001). "Distinct changes in cortical acetylcholine and noradrenaline efflux during contingent and noncontingent performance of a visual attentional task." Journal of Neuroscience 21(13): 4908-14.

Das, U. N. (2002). "The lipids that matter from infant nutrition to insulin resistance." Prostaglandins, Leukotrienes and Essential Fatty Acids 67(1): 1-12.

Das, U. N. (2003). "Long-chain polyunsaturated fatty acids in the growth and development of the brain and memory " Nutrition 19(1): 62-65.

Der, G., G. D. Batty, et al. (2006). "Effect of breast feeding on intelligence in children: prospective study, sibling pairs analysis, and meta-analysis " British Medical Journal 333(945).

DiPietro, J. A., S. K. Larson, et al. (1987). "Behavioral and heart rate pattern differences between breast-fed and bottle-fed neonates." Developmental Psychology 23(4): 467-474.

Doyle, L. W., A. L. Rickards, et al. (1992). "Breastfeeding and intelligence.[comment]." Lancet 339(8795): 744-5.

Drane, D. L. and J. A. Logemann (2000). "A critical evaluation of the evidence on the association between type of infant feeding and cognitive development." Paediatric and Perinatal Epidemiology 14: 349-356.

Dunn, L. and L. Dunn (1981). PPVT-R. Circle Pines, Minnesota, 55014-1796, American Guidance Service.

Farkas, E., M. C. de Wilde, et al. (2002). "Dietary long chain PUFAs differentially affect hippocampal muscarinic 1 and serotonergic 1A receptors in experimental cerebral hypoperfusion." Brain Research 954(1): 32-41.

Farquharson, J., F. Cockburn, et al. (1992). "Infant cerebral cortex phosholipid fatty-acid composition and diet." Lancet 340: 810-813.

Fergusson, D. M., A. L. Beautrais, et al. (1982). "Breast-feeding and cognitive development in the first seven years of life." Social Science and Medicine 16: 1705-1708.

Garcia-Segura, L. M., I. Azcoitia, et al. (2001). "Neuroprotection by estradiol." Progress in Neurobiology 63(1): 29-60.

Golding, J., I. S. Rogers, et al. (1997). "Association between breast feeding, child development and behaviour." Early Human Development 49(Suppl): S175-S184.

Hart, S., L. M. Boylan, et al. (2003). "Brief report: breast-fed one-week-olds demonstrate superior neurobehavioral organization." Journal of Pediatric Psychology 28(8): 529-34.

Hoefer, C. and M. C. Hardy (1929). "Later development of breastfed and artificially fed infants." Journal of the American Medical Association 92: 615-619.

Horne, R. S., P. M. Parslow, et al. (2004). "Comparison of evoked arousability in breast and formula fed infants." Archives of Disease in Childhood 89(1): 22-5.

Horwood, L. J., B. A. Darlow, et al. (2001). "Breast milk feeding and cognitive ability at 7-8 years." Archives of Disease in Childhood 84(Fetal Neonatal Edition): F23-F27.

Horwood, L. J. and D. M. Fergusson (1998). "Breastfeeding and later cognitive and academic outcomes." Pediatrics 101: E91-E97.

Huizink, A. C., P. G. Robles de Medina, et al. (2003). "Stress during pregnancy is associated with developmental outcome in infancy." Journal of Child Psychology and Psychiatry and Allied Disciplines 44(6): 810-8.

Jain, A., J. Concato, et al. (2002). "How good is the evidence linking breastfeeding to intelligence?" Pediatrics 109(6): 1044-1053.

Johnson, D. L., P. R. Swank, et al. (1996). "Breastfeeding and children's intelligence." Psychol Rep 79: 1179-1185.

Keating, D. and C. Hertzman (1999). Developmental Health and the Wealth of Nations. New York, Guildford Press.

Koletzko, B., P. J. Aggett, et al. (1998). "Growth, development and differentiation: a functional food science approach." British Journal of Nutrition 80(Suppl 1): S5-S45.

Kramer, M. S., F. Aboud, et al. (2008). "Breastfeeding and child cognitive development: new evidence from a large randomized trial." Arch Gen Psychiatry 65(5): 578-584.

Larque, E., H. Demmelmair, et al. (2006). "Perinatal supply and metabolism of long-chain polyunsaturated fatty acids: importance for the early development of the nervous system." Annals of the New York Academy of Sciences 967: 299 - 310.

Lauritzen, I., N. Blondeau, et al. (2000). "Polyunsaturated fatty acids are potent neuroprotectors." Science Signalling 19(8): 1784-1793.

Lavelli, M. and M. Poli (1998). "Early mother-infant interaction during breast- and bottle-feeding." Infant Behavior and Development 21(4): 667-684.

Li, J., G. E. Kendall, et al. (2008). "Maternal psychosocial well-being in pregnancy and breastfeeding duration." Acta Paediatrica 97(2): 221-225.

Liu, D., J. Diorio, et al. (2000). "Maternal care, hippocampal synaptogenesis and cognitive development in rats." Nature Neuroscience 3(8): 799-806.

Lucas, A. (2005). "Long-Term Programming Effects of Early Nutrition [mdash] Implications for the Preterm Infant." J Perinatol 25(S2): S2-S6.

Lucas, A., R. Morley, et al. (1994). "A randomised multicentre study of human milk versus formula and later development in preterm infants." Archives of Diseases in Childhood 70: F141-F146.

Lucas, A., R. Morley, et al. (1992). "Breast milk and subsequent intelligence quotient in children born preterm." Lancet 339: 261-264.

Makrides, M., M. A. Neumann, et al. (1994). "Fatty acid composition of brain, retinea and erythrocytes in breast- and formula- fed infants." American Journal of Clinical Nutrition 60: 189- 194.

Malloy, M. H. and H. Berendes (1998). "Does breast-feeding influence intelligence quotients at 9 and 10 years of age." Early Human Development 50: 209-217.

McCain, M. and J. F. Mustard (1999). Early Years Study: Reversing the Brain Drain. Toronto, Canada, Canadian Institute for Advanced Research. 0-7778-8953-6.

Michaelson, K. F., P. S. Larsen, et al. (1994). "The Copenhagen Cohort Study on Infant Nutrition and Growth: breast-milk intake, human milk macronutritent content, and influencing factors." American Journal of Clinical Nutrition 59: 600-611.

Montgomery, S. M., A. Ehlin, et al. (2006). "Breast feeding and resilience against psychosocial stress." Archives of Disease in Childhood 91 (12): 990-4.

Morrow-Tlucak, M., R. H. Haude, et al. (1988). "Breastfeeding and cognitive development in the first 2 years of life." Social Science and Medicine 26(6): 635-639.

Newnham, J. P., S. F. Evans, et al. (1993). "Effects of frequent ultrasound during pregnancy: a randomised controlled trial." Lancet 342: 887-891.

Oddy, W., J. Li, et al. (2011). "Breastfeeding duration and academic achievement at 10 years." Pediatrics. 127: e137-45.

Oddy, W. H., G. E. Kendall, et al. (2003). "Breastfeeding and cognitive development in childhood: a prospective birth cohort study." Paediatric and Perinatal Epidemiology 17(1): 81-90.

Oddy, W. H., G. E. Kendall, et al. (2010). "The long-term effects of breastfeeding on child and adolescent mental health: a pregnancy cohort study followed for 14 years." The Journal of Pediatrics 156(4): 568-74.

Oddy, W. H., M. Robinson, et al. (2011). "Breastfeeding and early child development: a prospective cohort study." Acta Paediatrica 100(7): 992-999.

Pollock, J. I. (1994). "Long-term associations with infant feeding in a clinically advantaged population of babies." Developmental Medicine and Child Neurology 36(5): 429-440.

Quinn, P., M. O'Callaghan, et al. (2001). "The effect of breastfeeding on child development at 5 years: A cohort study." Journal of Paediatrics and Child Health 37(5): 465-469.

Richards, M., R. Hardy, et al. (2002). "Long-term effects of breast-feeding in a national birth cohort: educational attainment and midlife cognitive function." Public Health Nutrition 5: 631-635.

Robinson, M., W. H. Oddy, et al. (2008). "Pre- and post-natal influences on preschool mental health: A large-scale cohort study." Journal of Child Psychology and Psychiatry In Press.

Rodgers, B. (1978). "Feeding in infancy and later ability and attainment: a longitudinal study." Developmental Medicine and Child Neurology 20: 421-426.

Rutter, M. (2006). "Attachment from infancy to adulthood. The major longitudinal studies." Journal of Child Psychology and Psychiatry 47(9): 974-977.

Sacker, A., M. A. Quigley, et al. (2006). "Breastfeeding and developmental delay: findings from the millennium cohort study." Pediatrics 118(3): e682-9.

Sarter, M. and J. P. Bruno (1997). "Cognitive functions of cortical acetylcholine: toward a unifying hypothesis." Brain Research Reviews 23(1-2): 28-46.

Silva, A. A. M., Z. Mehta, et al. (2006). "Duration of breast feeding and cognitive function: population based cohort study." Eur J Epidemiol 21: 435-441.

Silva, P. A., P. M. Buckfield, et al. (1978). "Poisoning, burns and other accidents experienced by a thousand Dunedin three year olds: a report from the Dunedin Multidisciplinary Child Development Study." New Zealand Medical Journal 87: 242-244.

Spinath, F. M., T. S. Price, et al. (2004). "The genetic and environmental origins of language disability and ability." Child Development 75(2): 445-54.

Squires, J., D. Bricker, et al. (1990). Infant/Child Monitoring Questionnaires Procedures Manual, University of Oregon, Center on Human Development.

Strathearn, L., A. A. Mamun, et al. (2009). "Does breastfeeding protect against substantiated child abuse and neglect? a 15-year cohort study." Pediatrics 123(2): 483 -493.

Stromswold, K. (2001). "The heritability of language: A review and metaanalysis of twin, adoption, and linkage studies. ." Language 77(4): 647-723.

Taylor, B. and J. Wadsworth (1984). "Breast feeding and child development at five years." Developmental Medicine and Child Neurology 26(1): 73-80.

Uvnäs-Moberg, K. (1998). "Oxytocin may mediate the benefits of positive social interaction and emotionsBottom of Form 1" Psychoneuroendocrinology 23(8): 819-835

Vestergaard, M., C. Obel, et al. (1999). "Duration of breastfeeding and developmental milestones during the latter half of infancy." Acta Paediatrica 88(12): 1327 - 1332.

Vohr, B. R., B. B. Poindexter, et al. (2006). "Beneficial effects of breast milk in the neonatal intensive care unit on the developmental outcome of extremely low birth weight infants at 18 months of age." Pediatrics 118(1): e115-123.

Wharton, B. A. (1992). "Food for the brain." Proceedings of the Royal College of Physicians of Edinburgh 22: 336-346.

Whitehouse, A. J. O., M. Robinson, et al. (2011). "The effects of breast-feeding duration on language ability to middle childhood." Paediatric and Perinatal Epidemiology 25(1): 44-52.

Wigg, N. R., S. Tong, et al. (1998). "Does breastfeeding at six months predict cognitive development?" Australian and New Zealand Journal of Public Health 22(2): 232-236.

World Health Organisation (2003). Global strategy for infant and young child feeding. Geneva, Author.

Yehuda, S., S. Rabinovitz, et al. (1999). "Essential fatty acids are mediators of brain biochemistry and cognitive functions." Journal of Neuroscience Research 56(6): 565-570.

Zhou, S. J., P. Baghurst, et al. (2007). "Home environment, not duration of breast-feeding, predicts intelligence quotient of children at four years." Nutrition 23(3): 236-241.

Zubrick, S. R., S. R. Silburn, et al. (2000). "Mental health disorders in children and young people: scope, cause and prevention." Australian and New Zealand Journal of Psychiatry 34(4): 570-578.

4

Breastfeeding and Infant Growth

Luiz Antonio Del Ciampo
Department of Pediatrics
Faculty of Medicine of Ribeirão Preto
University of Sao Paulo,
Brazil

1. Introduction

Although it would be appropriate to consider various aspects related to the historical, social and cultural contexts, in a simplified manner it is possible to understand the child as a human being who is in a phase of life characterized by rapid growth and development. Thus, during this phase that starts with conception and continues until the beginning of adolescence, a child needs appropriate feeding, physical and emotional hygiene conditions, safety and protection, so that its genetic expression will fully manifest.

Growth, more than representing an increase in body mass size and in the number of cells, should be understood as a complex, continuous and dynamic process of interaction between the child and its environment, influenced by countless factors of a biological, environmental, emotional, cultural and social nature. Thus, growth represents an adaptation of body composition that results from all vital processes involved in the construction of the human body (1,2,3).

During the nursing phase, mainly during the first year of life, growth is directly related to nutrition and to various environmental factors. Thus appropriate feeding in terms of quantity and quality is a fundamental element for growth since the child will derive from it all the energy and the approximately fifty essential nutrients that will be used for the transformation and differentiation of structures, the consolidation of reserves, the repair of tissues, as well as for the protection of the organism against infectious and chronic-degenerative diseases (4,5).

2. The nutritional requirements of nursing infants

Due to their intense metabolism and rapid growth during the first two years of life, infants have high nutritional requirements. At 4 months of age, about 30% of the energy ingested is utilized for growth, with a reduction to 5% at the end of the first year of life and to 2% at 3 years. At birth, for example, the brain is responsible for about 65% of the basal metabolic rate, with this rate being reduced to 50% at the end of the first year of life (6).

To fulfill the requirements of an organism that grows from about 3.5 kg of weight and 50 cm in length at birth to almost 13 kg and 87 cm at the end of two years of life, macro- and micronutrients of appropriate quantity and quality are necessary. In general, a child in good health and well fed should gain 25 to 30 grams per day in the first trimester of life, with its birth weight doubling between 4 and 5 months, tripling by 11 months to 1 year, and quadrupling by 2 years to 2 years and 3 months. Regarding length, a child should gain 15 centimeters in the first year of life and 10 centimeters in the second year [7,8].

For an appropriate occurrence of these somatic changes some recommendations should be followed in order to meet the nutritional requirements of the child during each growth phase in association with its life characteristics, since the period from six months to three years of life is the one during which a child is more subjected to nutritional risks.

The necessary quantity of daily calories may vary from 125 kcal/kg/day for newborns to 110 kcal/kg/day at six months of age and from 95 to 100 kcal/kg/day from six months to two years of age [9,10]. The distribution of this energy consumption is presented in Table 1.

Energy consumption	kcal/kg/day
basal metabolism	50 - 55
growth in the 1st year of life	15 - 20
growth in the 2nd year of life	8 - 10
physical activity	20 - 30
specific dynamic action of food	5 - 8
excretions	8 - 10

Table 1. Daily energy consumption of nursing infants

The protein requirements range from 1.8 g/kg/day for the first six months to 1.5 g/kg/day in the second semester and 1.2 g/kg/day in the second year of life, considering proteins of high biological value that should account for about 15% of the total daily calorie intake.

Lipids should account for about 30% to 35% of the total daily calorie intake, supplying appropriate amount of the essential fatty acids, linoleic and linolenic acids, and carbohydrate should account for about 50% to 55% of the daily calorie intake. In addition to these nutrients, the feeding of an infant should also satisfy the requirements of water (150 ml/kg/day), vitamins and minerals [48], as specified in Table 2 [7,9,10]

3. Breastfeeding and growth

There is an intimate relationship between physical growth and nutritional status which can be understood as the quantitative reflex of the food consumed daily by the child. According to the World Health Organization (WHO)[11], appropriate infant feeding should provide a sufficient quantity of food to cover the nutritional needs and to protect the airways against the aspiration of foreign substances and should not exceed the metabolic and functional capacity of the digestive tract and the renal system of the child.

There is a current consensus that breast milk as the exclusive food and offered freely satisfies all the needs of an infant during the first six months of age, being the only ideal food for the child's growth and development [8,12,13]. Universally supported and disseminated by the World Health Organization, the practice of breast-feeding finds important allies in Brazil in the National Program of Encouragement of Breast-feeding (PNIAM in the Portuguese acronym) of the Health Ministry and in the Departments of

Nutrient	Nutritional recommendations/day		Breast milk (quantity/100 ml)
	0 - 6 m	7 - 12 m	
Energy (kcal/kg/day)	110	100 - 110	71 kcal
Protein (g)	2.1	2.1	1.2 g
Fat*	35 %	35 %	3.8 g
Carbohydrates **	50 %	50 %	7 g
Water (ml/kg/day)	150	150	87.6 g
Calcium (mg)	400	600	33 mg
Iron (mg)	6	10	0.07 - 0.15 µg
Iodine (µg)	40	50	7 µg
Copper (mg)	0.4 - 0.6	0.6 - 0.7	40 µg
Chromium (mg)	10 - 40	20 - 60	50 ng
Manganese (mg)	0.3 - 0.6	0.6 - 1.0	0.6 µg
Selenium(mg)	10	15	1 µg
Fluorine (mg)	0.1- 0.5	0.2 - 1.0	16 µg
Zinc (mg)	5	5	300 µg
Magnesium (mg)	40	60	3 mg
Potassium (mg)	500	700	58 mg
Sodium (mg)	120	200	15 mg
Chlorine (mg)	180	300	42 mg
Phosphorus mg/dl	300	500	15 mg
Vitamin A (µg)	375	375	53 µg
Vitamin D (µg)	7.5	10	0.04 µg
Vitamin E (mg)	3	4	0.34 mg
Vitamin K (µg)	5	10	0.2 µg
Vitamin C (mg)	30	35	4.0 mg
Vitamin B1 (mg)	0.3	0.4	0.02 mg
Vitamin B2 (mg)	0.4	0.5	0.03 mg
Vitamin B6 (mg)	0.3	0.6	0.01 mg
Vitamin B12 (mg)	0.3	0.5	0.3 µg
Pantothenic acid (mg)	2	3	0.25 mg
Folic acid (µg)	25	35	5 µg
Niacin (mg)	5	6	0.2 mg

* 35% of total daily calories
** 50% of total daily calories

Table 2. Nutritional recommendations for infants younger than one year and biochemical composition of breast milk

Breast-Feeding and Nutrology of the Brazilian Society of Pediatrics. Thus, it is understood that breast milk, because of its quality, completeness, biological complexity and appropriate nutrient balance, guarantees the nutritional status, the growth and the development of nursing infants during the first months of life (14,15,16,17,18). This is the case even in the presence of unfavorable conditions (19), with no benefits having been found that compensate for the risks and the disadvantages of introducing complementary foods before six months of life, which, in addition to being of poorer nutritional quality compared to breast milk, may be associated with contamination and the triggering of allergic diseases, interfering with the absorption of essential nutrients such as iron and zinc and therefore increasing infant morbidity and mortality [20]

The protective effects of breastfeeding are also evident in relation to other situations or diseases such as celiac disease, sudden infant death, neonatal hypocalcemia, acrodermatitis enteropathica, Crohn's disease, diabetes and cardiovascular disease, among many others, that every day is more described.

Although it is recognized that allergic diseases are related to various genetic and environmental components, in recent years breastfeeding has also been studied with respect to protective effects against atopic eczema, asthma and hay fever [21,22,23,24,25].

Bringing the infant to the breast has not only for mother and child the sense of satisfying hunger, there is much more, because the contact of the mouth with the breast and the child's body with the body of his mother bring warmth and comfort. This contact is very important to the child’s psychological development in the first months of life. Mother, well aware of the reasons to breastfeed the child with pleasure, will release the endogenous beta-endorphin more reason, in this case pharmacologically demonstrated, to enhance this pleasure. Thus, it can be argued that breastfeeding promotes a strong bond between mother and child, with benefits for both stimuli, full of affection and bonuses and leading to a mother-child interaction at its most elevated and perfectly natural. Also, the infant has his sucking needs met, without the use of pacifiers, which can deform the teeth and palate, as well as facilitating contamination of the oral cavity. In addition, the breast feeding acts as a positive factor in the development of speech through early and continuous exercise of facial muscles. Studies suggest that learning ability and IQ of children exclusively breastfed, and adequate time, are higher than those not breastfed. Although these studies still need to proof, is visible to those who work and live with infants the distinct impression that those who are exclusively breastfed are more calm and smiling, and have more restful sleep than those who do not breastfeeding [26,27,28].

Several studies published in the specialized literature have shown a positive association between the duration of the breast-feeding period and infant growth [29,30,31,32,33,34]. Motil et al [35] did not observe significant differences between infants exclusively breast-fed or receiving milk formulas, and concluded that the quantity of protein found in breast milk did not limit growth. Kramer et al [33] demonstrated that infants who are exclusively breast-fed for a longer period of time can experience accelerated weight and length gain during the first months of life, showing no growth deficit at one year of age, or even growing more than infants fed artificial milk during adolescence [16,36].

By being a species-specific food, balanced and equilibrated in order to satisfy the needs of the infant and containing all the essential nutrients for growth and development, breast milk is one of the priorities in the fight against infant malnutrition[37,38], with the practice of breast-feeding being established and widely disseminated as one of the Basic Actions for Infant Health since the Alma-Ata Conference in 1978.

Still in terms of nutritional disorders and being invested with great importance in the prevention of health problems in infancy and in future life, breast milk plays an important role regarding the problem of excessive weight gain. Studies by different investigators have demonstrated the protective role of breast milk against obesity in infancy and adolescence (39,40,41) and have detected an association of a reduced prevalence of overweight and obesity with different feeding practices, demonstrating the protective effect of mother's milk (42,43,44,45,46,47). An adequate duration of breastfeeding is associated with low prevalence of obesity during school age. Also, the excess of protein contained in infant formulas and consumed by early children may influence weight gain, indicating that as excessive increase of weight would be associated with high amount of protein of infant formulas (48,49).

Although breast milk has low levels of iron, its high bioavailability makes it much more absorbed than other infant formulas. The finding of iron deficiency is not common in full-term children and breastfed, according to the Nutrition Committee of the American Academy of Pediatrics, although this fact is much more common in breastfed infants with cow's milk. Should be considered the possibility of iron supplementation after the sixth month of life for full-term children and when introducing complementary feeding. For those born prematurely or underweight, will be given iron supplements, even two years old (50). Calcium and phosphorus have lower levels in human milk, but the Ca / P in (around 2.2) is very favorable to the absorption of calcium. Breastfeeding and child's sun exposure in areas with good sunlight conditions are essential in the prevention of vitamin D deficiency.

Human growth, understood as a seasonal and pulsatile phenomenon characterized by different rates along time, can be assessed with the use of growth curves that provide references both for body growth as a whole and for the growth of different parts of the organism such as the head, the length of the limbs, the length of the trunk etc.

The instruments used to assess growth have been modified over time in order to better fit the conditions of infant populations since there is still discordance among authors about what should be used as reference or standard of infant growth. The various growth curves classically used, constructed for widely varying pediatric groups, when taken as reference do not always reflect the reality of each particular child since questions such as type of feeding, birth and health conditions during the first years of life, for example, can modify the parameters analyzed.

Starting in 2006, with the publication of the new growth curves of the WHO for children younger than 5 years, constructed with better defined criteria (singletons born at term to a non-smoking mother, with no diseases, exclusively breast-fed during the first six months of life and living under appropriate environmental and economic conditions) and therefore permitting to consider that all of these children will develop in a similar manner, we are able use an instrument that better represents the description of the physiological growth of these children from the beginning of life. More than a reference, these curves represent a growth pattern for children in this age range.

4. References

[1] Wolansky N. Genetic and ecological factors in human growth. Hum Biol 1970;42:349-56.

[2] Spyrides MHC, Struchiner CJ, Barbosa MTS, Kac G. Effetct of a predominant breastfeeding duration on infant growth: a prospective study using nolinear mixed effect models. J Pediatr (Rio J) 2008;84(3):237-43.

[3] Lawson M. Contemporary aspects of infants feeding. Paediatr Nurs 2007;19:39-46.
[4] Longo GZ, Souza JMP, Souza SB, Szarfarc SC. Growth of children up to six months of age and breast feeding practices. Rev Bas Saúde Matern Infantil 2005;5(1):109-18.
[5] Law C. Early growth and chronic disease: a public health overview. Matern Child Nutr 2005;1:169-76.
[6] Lissaur T & Clayden G. Illustrated Textbook of Paediatrics. London, Mosby International, 3ª ed. 2007.
[7] Ricco RG, Del Ciampo LA, Almeida CAN. Puericultura. Princípios e Práticas. Atenção Integral à Saúde da Criança e do Adolescente. Editora Atheneu. São Paulo. 2ª. ed. 2008.
[8] WHO. Infant and Young Child Nutrition. Geneva: World Health Organization; 2002.
[9] Calil VMTL, Vaz FAC. Composição bioquímica do leite materno. In: Issler H. O Aleitamento Materno no Contexto Atual. Políticas, Prática e Bases Científicas. Editora Sarvier, 2008. São Paulo.
[10] Rego JD. Aleitamento Materno. Editora Atheneu. 2ª ed. 2006. São Paulo.
[11] WHO. Working Group on Infant Growth: an evaluation of infant growth: the use and interpretation of anthropometry in infants. Bull World Health Org 1995;73:165-74.
[12] WHO. Expert Consultation on the Optimal Duration of Exclusive Breastfeeding. Conclusions and Recommendations. World Health Organization. Document A54/Inf.Doc./4. Geneva. 2001.
[13] Spyrides MHC, Struchiner CJ, Barbosa MTS, Kac G. The effect of breastfeeding practices on infant growth. Rev Bas Saúde Mater Infant 2005;5(2):145-53.
[14] Marques RFSV, Lopez FA, Braga JAP. Growth of exclusively breastfed infants in the first 6 months of life. Rev Chil Pediatr 2006;77(5):529-30.
[15] Rautava S., Walker WA. Academy of Breastfeeding Medicine Founder's Lecture 2008: Breastfeeding - An extrauterine link between mother and child. Breastfeed Med 2009;4(1):3-10.
[16] Kramer MS, Guo T, Platt RW, Sevkovskaya Z, Dzikovich I, Collet JP et al. Infant growth and health outcomes associated with 3 compared with 6 mo of exclusive breastfeeding. Am J Clin Nutr 2003;78:291-5.
[17] Del Ciampo LA, Ricco RG, Almeida CAN. Aleitamento Materno. Passagens e Transferências Mãe-Filho. São Paulo. Editora Atheneu, 2004.
[18] Augusto RA, Souza JMP. Growth of children in exclusive breastfeeding in their first semester of life. Rev Bras Crescimento Desenvolv Hum 2007;17(2):1-11.
[19] Ricco 73:165-74. Del Ciampo LA, Almeida CAN, Daneluzzi JC. Aleitamento exclusivamente ao seio, morbidade e utilização de serviços de saúde pediátrico em uma unidade básica de saúde. Pediatria (S. Paulo) 2001;23(2):193-8.
[20] Monte CMG, Giugliani ERJ. Recommendations for the complementary feeding of the breastfed child. J Pediatr (Rio J) 2004;80(5 supl):S131-S141.
[21] Gdalevich M, Mimouni D, David M, Mimouni M. Breast-feeding and the onset of atopic dermatitis in childhood: a systematic review and meta-analysis of prospective studies. J Am Acad Dermatol 2001;45:520-7.
[22] Gdalevich M, Mimouni D, Mimouni M. Breast-feeding and the risk of bronchial asthma in childhood: a systematic review with meta-analysis of prospective studies. J Pediatr 2001;139:261-6.
[23] Kramer MS. Breast is best: The evidence. Early Hum Dev 2010;86:729-32.

[24] Scholtens S, Wijga AH, Brunekreef B. Breast feeding, parental allergy and asthma in children followed for 8 years. Thorax 2009;64:604-9.
[25] Silvers KM, Frampton CM, Wickens K. Breastfeeding protects against adverse respiratory outcomes at 15 months of age. Matern Child Nutr 2009;5:243-50.
[26] Petherick A. Mother's milk: a rich opportunity. Nature 2010;468:S5-S8.
[27] Quigley MA, Hockley C, Carson C, Kelly Y, Renfrew MJ, Sacker A. Breastfeeding is Associated with Improved Child Cognitive Development: A Population-Based Cohort Study. J Pediatr. 2011 Aug, on line.
[28] Chapman DJ. Breastfeeding, brain imaging, and maternal behavior. J Hum Lact. 2011;27(3):304-5.
[29] Piwoz EG, Creed de Kanashiro H, Lopes de Romana GL, Black RE, Brown KH. Feeding practices and growth among low-income Peruvian infants: a comparision of internationally-recommended definitions. Int J Epidemiol 1996;25:103-14.
[30] Galler JR, Ramsey FC, Harrison RH, Brooks R, Weiskopf-Bock S. Infant feeding practices in Barbados predict later growth. J Nutr 1998;128:1328-35.
[31] Onyango AW. Breast feeding and growth in rural Kenyan toddlers. Adv Exp Med Biol 2000;478:151-62.
[32] Diaz S, Herreros C, Aravena R, Casado ME, Reyes V, Schiappacasse V. Breastfeeding duration and growth of fully breast-fed infants in a poor urban Chilean population. Am J Clin Nutr 1995;62:371-6.
[33] Donma MM, Donma O. Infant feeding and growth: A study on Turkish infants from birth to 6 months. Pediatr Int 1999;41(5):542-8.
[34] Martin RM, Smith GD, Mangtani P, Frankel S, Gunnell D. Association between breast feeding and growth: the Boyd-Orr cohort study. Arch Dis Child Fetal Neonatal 2002;87:F193-F201.
[35] Motil KJ, Sheng HP, Montandon CM, Wong WW. Human milk protein does not limit growth of breast-fed infants. J Pediatr Gastroenterol Nutr 1997;24:10-7.
[36] Kramer MS, Guo T, Platt RW, Shapiro S, Collet JP, Chalmers B et al. Infant breastfeeding and infant growth: biology or bias? Pediatrics 2002;110(2 Pt 1):343-7.
[37] Ricco RG, Almeida CAN, Del Ciampo LA, Daneluzzi JC, Ferlin MLS, Muccillo G. Growth of exclusively breast-fed infants from a poor urban population. Arch Latioamerican Nutr 2001;51(2):122-6.
[38] Escuder MCL, Venâncio SI, Pereira JCR. Estimativa de impacto da amamentação sobre a mortalidade infantil. Rev Saúde Pública 2003;37(3):319-25 319
[39] Chen A, Rogan WJ. Breastfeeding and the risk of postneonatal death in the United States. Pediatrics 2004;113;e435-e439.
[40] Butte NF. Impact of infant feeding practices on childhood obesity. J Nutr 2009;139:412S - 416S.
[41] Gillman MW, Rifas-Shiman SL, Camargo CAJr. Risk of overweight among adolescents who were breastfed as infants. JAMA 2001;285:2461-7.
[42] Owen CG, Martin RM, Whincup PH. Effect of infant feeding on the risk of obesity across the life course: a quantitative review of published evidence. Pediatrics 2005;115:1367-77.
[43] Kramer MS, Barr RG, Leduc DG, Boisjoly C, McVey-White L, Pless IB. Determinants of weight and adiposity in the first year of life. J Pediatr 1985;106:10-14.

[44] von Kries R, Koletzko B, Sauerwald T, von Mutius E, Bamert D, Grunert V et al. Breast feeding and obesity: cross sectional study. Br Med J 1999;319:147-50.
[45] Tulldahl J, Pettersson K, Andersson SW, Hulten L. Mode of infant and achieved growth in adolescence: early feeding patterns in relation to growth and body composition in adolescence. Obes Res 1999;7:431-7.
[46] Toschke AM, Vignerova J, Lhotska L, Osanvoca K, Kolezko B, von Kries R. Overweight and obesity in 6 to 14 year-old Czech children lin 1991: protective effect of breast-feeding. J Pediatr 2002;141:764-9.
[47] Balaban G, Silva GAP. Efeito protetor do aleitamento materno contra a obesidade infantil. J Pediatr (Rio J) 2004;80(1):7-16.
[48] Koletzo B, Von Kries R, Closa R. Lower protein in infant formula is associated with lower weight up to age 2 y: a randomized clinical trial. Am JmClin Nutr 2009;89(6):1836-45.
[49] Koletzo B, von Kries R, Closa R. Can infant feeding choices modulate later obsity risk? Am L Clin Nutr 2009;89(5):1502S-1508S.
[50] Gartner LM, Morton J, Lawrence RA. Breastfeeding and the use of human milk. Pediatrics 2005;115(2):496-502.

5

Nutrition in Healthy Children

Şenay Çetinkaya
Pediatric Nursing,
Adana School of Health,
Çukurova University,
Turkey

1. Introduction

The most significant factor in the development and growth of a country is providing effective health care services to society. The purpose of each health care application is different. Among these applications, the factor that accelerates the growth and development, living healthy, protection from diseases, and healing is nutrition (Baysal, 1993; Perk, 1992).

Nutrition is a basic need that affects the lives of individuals and societies, and is affected from all biological, social, cultural and economic factors. Adequate and balanced nutrition is unquestionably a precondition for the generation of healthy societies (Allen & Gillespie, 2001).

Ensuring the existence of the living organism, putting his/her losses into place, getting the needed food stuffs, by means of digestion to fulfill the necessary physiological functions for survival is called *nutrition*. *Healthy nutrition* means the use of food to maintain the growth-development and survival and to protect health (Perk, 1992).

Nutrition has a very important role in the development of both individual's and society's health. Good nutrition is necessary for the individual to grow and develop, maintain his/her physical and mental health and resist to diseases, especially infectious diseases (Bilgel, 1997).

Nutrition in the family is related to whether the sources required by the family are adequate or not to meet their nourishment, the manner of their food preparation and consumption, their socio-cultural and economic level, the environment that they live, the size of the family, their birth rate, age of the mother and personal characteristics of the individual (Inanc & Hatipoglu, 1995).

Nutrition has more significance in terms of the child's health (Baysal, 1993; Bilgel, 1997), because the period of life in which development and growth occur most intensively and most rapidly is the childhood period (Bilgel, 1997). The most significant factor having positive or negative effects on the development and growth of the child after birth is his/her nutritional status (Kavaklı, 1992). Majority of the children comes into the world healthy. In order to sustain the healthy status and enable the organism to complete its normal development and growth, the child should be nourished adequately in terms of the food's composition and amount beginning from the first days and at every period of the childhood (Baysal, 1993).

Accomplished nutrition plays a major part in healthy growth and development of a newborn infant. Infants in various countries of the world are exposed to malnutrition because of social, economic and cultural reasons. Inadequate and unbalanced nutrition leads growth and development failures and deaths among children (Yapicioglu et al, 2002).

Whereas neonatal mortality rate per a thousand live births is 26 in the world, 40 in Africa, 7 in Europe, 35 in East Mediterranean countries according to the report of 2010 World Health Organization (WHO), this rate is 14 in Turkey (WHO, 2010). With regard to 2010 WHO report it is stated that infectious diseases such as diarrhea, pneumonia and bronchitis are the leading diseases that cause infant deaths in developing countries, and one of the easiest ways to prevent these infections is breastfeeding (WHO, 2010). Death rates of infants who are not breastfed are 4-6 times more than the breastfed ones. According to WHO, the high ratio of nursing mothers contributes to survival of infants at an annual average of 1.5 million (Baysan et al, 2009). In a research conducted by Wilson and his colleagues it is determined that the probability of catching respiratory diseases among infants who are at least 15 weeks old and regularly breastfed is low. The probability of catching respiratory diseases is 17% for the infants at least 15 week old and particularly breastfed, it is 26.8-35.2% for those partially breastfed, and it is 30.7-33.7% for those only bottle-fed (Wilson et al, 1998).

According to Turkey Demographic and Health Survey (TDHS 2008), the 68.9% of the infants between 0-1 months are exclusively breastfed. When they are 2-3 months-old this ratio decreases to 42%. Moreover, the ratio in which the newborn infants are breastfed within the first 1 hour is 39%, that within the first day is 73.4%, and the ratio of those who are fed with other nutrients before mother's milk is 23.2% (www.scribd.com/doc/ 21717405/ TNSA-2008-ana -Rapor-tr, 172).

Malnutrition problems in Turkey are particularly observed during the infancy. The 12.2% of the infants under the age of five suffer acute and chronic malnutrition (TDHS 2003). Anemia can also be considered among malnutrition problems. In our country an average of 50% in preschool age, the 30% of school children, and 50% of the pregnant or breastfeeding women are anemic. Primary causes of anemia are the iron deficiency, vitamin B6, vitamin B12 and folic acid intake or their low bioavailability (TUIK, 2006). Furthermore, unbalanced nutrition is an important health concern in the World as it is in Turkey. The widespread availability of fast-food style, nutrition with monotype food, and sedentary lifestyles led the increase in adiposity caused by unbalanced nutrition (Aslan, 2007; TDHS, 2003). Adiposity in childhood period draws attention as a growing concern both in the world and in our country.

To raise healthy and productive generations, the childhood period that lasts from impregnation to the end of adolescence along with the growth-development within this period are crucial for the future of societies. While Maslow places nutrition to forefront among required physical needs (in Hierarchy of Basic Human Needs) Henderson underlines the importance of the subject by claiming that adequate and balanced nutrition comes in the first place among 14 basic needs (Birol, 1997).

Whatever the long-term benefits of nutrition are, ensuring people they would have good nutrition falls to the international laws. This law issue has been expressed in various ways at international declarations and documents about human rights since the Declaration on Rights of the Child was adopted in 1924 (Bellamy, 1998).

The requirements stated below should be met in order to determine the adequateness of nutrition, and to discuss clinical adequacy of the nutrition:

1. Providing the energy that is spent by basal metabolism, and that is used to maintain life functions,
2. Providing the energy that is spent in daily activity as a result of muscle movements,
3. Providing with the building blocks that is needed by organism and required for regeneration and synthesis process,
4. Letting an infant who has a growing and developing organism take the nourishment in ideal quality and quantity for sustaining this feature (Arcasoy et al, 1994).

As the concept of adequateness in nutrition is searched, the problem of what kind of nutrition the human organism needs in various age periods under the environmental and living conditions has come up. The most practical standard to determine the adequateness in nutrition is that the child keeps his/her birth weight and height within the percentile channel where he/she begins to live (Arcasoy et al, 1994).

In order to overcome the nutrition problems, the importance of eliminating social inequalities which are the basic source of the problem should be emphasized by highlighting that health services constitute an equal, costless, qualified and reachable right. Also preventive health services should be prioritized among the health services.

2. Nutrition requirements

The foods include 3 essential nutrients which are protein, carbohydrate and fat, in different ratios. All the energy (calorie requirement), building blocks (amino acids, fatty acids), vitamins and minerals are taken to the organism by means of the nutrients. Requirement of each one changes depending on the environment where the individual lives and his/her daily activity. The suggested values in numerical expression of the requirement are given according to the age, body surface (m^2), weight (kg) and height (cm) of the individual. Although it is advocated that the ideal evaluation is the rating of body surface to weight or to height and the second rank belongs to m^2, the most commonly used one is the criteria of age-weight in practice. Example: The calorie requirement of 0-3 month-old infant is 120 Kcal/kg (Arcasoy et al, 1994).

In the first 4-6 months of life, breast milk and various infant formulas can provide with the complete nutrition to a growing infant. Still, breast milk is recommended nearly for all infants as the source of nutrient. However, very few numbers of infants are fed through only breastfeeding for more than 2-3 months. In this regard, all kind of efforts should be made to encourage breastfeeding. Another option is iron-fortified formulas which support sufficient growth of infants. These formulas are not the only ways to give nutritional supplements. Following the months 4-6, solid foods and fruit juice are being introduced in a manner such that they will gradually substitute the nutrients and calories that came from breast milk or formula. Because infants' activities increase in this period (despite a decrease in growth rate) their energy requirements also increase. A diet (milk) which has relatively high fat content and high calories is required to provide them with adequate energy. Nutritional supplements start forming a source for some important nutrients (iron) within the second 6-months. Genetic coordination of neoplasm is remarkable. However, a variety of nutritional deficiencies may be restrictive on one of these growth functions. Energy and nutrition requirements are generally proportional to Body Muscle Mass (BMM); as the child grows up, these requirements increase and reach to higher BMM. These requirements are very low for women compared to men, because mass of fat is higher and BMM is lower in women. In terms of some nutrients, the requirements of girls may be more than the requirements of boys or they may be equal like iron or vitamin C. In order to meet the requirements of suggested daily nutrients, a girl should have a richer diet in terms of nutrients compared to a boy. Hence the deficiency risk of some nutrients is higher for girls (Tershakovec, & Stallings, 1996).

Nutrition requirements: The minimum nutrition requirement of any food is determined as the amount below the consumed level that would show deficiency. It is determined that the daily nutrient requirement is 2-6 times of the minimum requirement, and the daily nutrient requirement is calculated by taking weight, gender, age and the requirements in pregnancy and lactation into consideration. Calorie requirement is calculated more frequently depending on the requirements below: 100 kcal/kg for the first 10 kg, 50 kcal/kg for 10-20 kg and 20 kcal/kg for over 20 kg (Tershakovec, & Stallings, 1996).

2.1 Energy requirement

The measure of the organism's energy requirement is the units of "calorie" or "joules". "Kcal" is practically used both in the world and in our country (Arcasoy et al, 1994). One kilocalorie is the required energy amount to raise the temperature of one kilogram of water from 15°C to 16 °C. Fats, carbohydrates and proteins are used as the source of energy. 1 gram of oils, 1 gram of carbohydrates and 1 gram of proteins generate 9 kcal, 4 kcal and 4 kcal, respectively. It is desired in a well-balanced prepared diet that each contribution of the carbohydrates, fats and proteins to total energy is 50%, 35% and 15%, respectively (Coskun, 1996).

In general, 4 criteria are used to determine either the energy requirement or other requirements.

1. The requirement for basal metabolism (BM): is calculated according to $m^{2'}$. The shares that the organs take from BM according to the age period are different in childhood period. For example: the brain of an infant uses 2/3 of BM energy, whereas this ratio is 1/4 for adults.
2. A requirement obedient to physical activity should be calculated.
3. Specific-dynamic effect (SDE) of the nutrients: While the energy use of the organism is calculated, SDE of the nutrients accounts for a low ratio such as 5-10%.
4. The required energy for growth-development (G/D): It is calculated that 3.5-5 Kcal are needed in order to increase the weight of an organism by one gram. Rapid growth during infancy requires rapid energy consumption. It is estimated that 1/4-1/3 of the total energy taken within the first months of life is used for G/D (Arcasoy et al, 1994).

Since the growth rate is high in the first years of the childhood period, the requirements for energy and the other nutritional elements are unexpectedly higher than the body mass. For example, whereas the energy and protein requirement of a moderately active woman at a weight of 40 kg is 40 kcal/kg and 1 g/kg, respectively, these requirements for an infant in the first six months of life are three times of the stated values (Coskun, 1996).

2.2 Nutrition types for infants

1. *Nourishment through breastfeeding:* It is the most ideal diet for the newborn infant (Coskun, 1996). World Health Organization (WHO) and American Pediatry Association (APA) suggest that the newborn infants should be breastfed exclusively, nutritional supplements should start as of the sixth month, and the breastfeeding period should last beyond two years and more (1 year and more-APA) (APA, 2003).

The ingredients of breast milk make mother milk as the most suitable nutrient for infants. This is due to the fact that the ingredients of mother milk change according to the requirements of newborn, besides it is protective against the infections, while it is affordable, as well. Mother milk, thus, meets all the physiological and psychosocial requirements of an infant alone by itself within the first 4-6 months (Dallar et al, 2007; Tuncel et al, 2005).

- *Exclusively breastfeeding:* The infant is fed only with breast milk of its mother or a wet nurse. Otherwise, any liquid food (except vitamin drops and syrups, drugs) or solid food is not given (Beaudry, 1995; Coskun, 1996).
- *Nutrition in which breastfeeding is dominant*: The essential nutrition source of the infant is breast milk. Additionally, liquid beverages, sugared water, tea, fruit juice, vitamin drops and syrups, medicine can also be given (Beaudry, 1995; Coskun, 1996).
- Mixed Nutrition: In addition to breast milk, semi-solid and solid foods are given to child.
- *Nutrition in weaning period:* It is the period which follows the breastfeeding for 4-6 months, breastfeeding is kept but nutritional supplements are also newly added to meet the infant's requirements.

2. *Artificial Nourishment:* It is the diet in which the infant cannot be breastfed due to the problems arising from itself or its mother as a result of misfortune (Coskun, 1996). If it is possible in this nutrition, infant formula milk (industrial milk) which is very similar to breastmilk should be used. Under the clean and proper preparation conditions, digestion problems are seen scarcely and the drawbacks of artificial nutrition are minimized in use of infant formula milk. However, it should be known that these nutrients will create economic burden for the family.

Age	Amount	Meal/day
1-2 weeks	50-70 ml.	7-8
2-6 weeks	75-110 ml.	6-7
2 months	110-180 ml.	5-6
3 months	170-220 ml.	5
6 months	220-240 ml.	4

Table 1. Artificial nourishment (Tuncdogan & Tuncdogan, 2005).

The infant should pass 3 consecutive periods which have the terms and characteristics compatible with the growth physiology of the child. These are: Exclusively breastfeeding, weaning, nutrition with modified foods for adults (Ozalp, 1996).

2.2.1 Energy and nutrient needs of infants

Nutrient and energy needs of the children differ from the adults'. Due to the generation of new tissues within infant's body, the need for proteins, minerals and vitamins is high. Significant amount of energy is necessary in growth period. Because the children have not learnt eating food by themselves yet, the diets that will be prepared for their nutrition should be in conformity with the child and include definite nutrient elements (Netsel, 2003).

Energy Needs of Infants:

- 120 calories per kilogram between 1-3 months
- 110 calories per kilogram between 4-9 months
- 105 calories per kilogram between 10-12 months (Netsel, 2003).

Majority of the calories are provided from fats and carbohydrates. The carbohydrate (lactose) and fats within the breast milk are absorbed easily (Netsel, 2003).

Infant's need for protein is substantially high. Intake of qualified and adequate protein is a requirement, since the growth of body tissues requires continuous protein synthesis. Breast milk has the characteristics of sample protein. The digestion rate of the sample protein accounts for 95%.

2.2.2 Vitamins and minerals

The daily average need of an infant for vitamins and minerals are:

Vitamin A : 1500 I.U.
Vitamin D : 400 I.U.
Vitamin C : 20- 30 mg
Vitamin B 6 : 0.3-0.6 mg
Vitamin B12 : 1- 2 mcg
Folic acid: 40- 60 mcg

Calcium: 500 mg
Iron: 5-10mg (after 6th month)
Iodine : 50 mcg
Phosphorus : 400 mg
Zinc : 5–10 mg
Potassium: 4- 8 mg (Koksal, 2007).

Breast milk can meet an infant's need for vitamins and minerals up to 4th-6th month under normal conditions. Afterwards the need should be met by means of the nutritional supplements (Koksal, 2007).

2.2.3 Nutrition of infants in the first 6 months

The ideal nutrition for infants is exclusively breastfeeding the first 6 months, then starting to get proper nutritional supplements and the continuation of breastfeeding for two years. It is estimated that breastfeeding will be able to prevent 1.3 million infants from dying every year. If inartificial nutrition cannot be provided, artificial nutrition or mixed nutrition are applied (APA, 2003).

2.2.3.1 Breastfeeding

With respect to "*The Innocenti Declaration*" that WHO and UNICEF published in 1990, it is suggested that the conditions are created to enable the women to breastfeed commonly, the necessary information about this subject can be reached easily, to begin breastfeeding within half an hour following the birth is encouraged, anything like fake breast or infant pacifier is not given to the breastfeeding infant, exclusively breastfeeding is kept up to the first 4-6 months and then breastfeeding with nutritional supplements is applied in the following period (Arcasoy et al, 1994; Bellamy, 1998; T.R. Ministry of Health General Directorate of MCH/FP, 1997; Tuncel et al, 2005).

2.2.3.2 Characteristics of the breast milk

Breastfeeding is the most appropriate diet for infants to let them grow and develop healthily. The first year of the infant is extremely important in terms of laying the foundations of a healthy life. Adequate and balanced nutrition is provided in infanthood period through the breast milk of each infant's own mother. It is exclusively sufficient for 4-6 months to give the infant breast milk of its mother without giving water beginning from the birth and observe the growth (Bertan & Guler, 1995). Since 87% of breast milk consists of liquid, in the first six months the infant does not need anything like water or similar liquid nutrients, except the breast milk (Gokcay & Garibagaoglu, 2002).

We can summarize the superiorities of breast milk: it is suitable for the growth rate of the infant in terms of its composition, it is digested easily and there is not any loss in digestion, it is non-allergic, economic, clean and sterilized, furthermore it does not require special preparation, it has protective elements against the microbes, toxic elements that will give harm to the infant are at minimum level in breast milk, it strengthens the affection relation between the mother and the child, it assists the mental health of both to be protected (Baysal, 1993; Ozalp, 1996). In breast milk, there are different growth factors having effects in infant's growth that are demonstrated by means of in vivo and in vitro studies. Tiny molecules such as taurine, ethanolamine, phosphoethanolamine, and proteins such as "epidermal growth factor", "nerve growth factor" which look like hormones and interferon affect the growth and development by affecting the mammary gland or distinct organs of infants (Ozalp, 1991). Besides that taurine is one of the factors in breast milk that orders the growth, it is known that it provides the coherence of cell membrane and prevents the destruction of retina (Ozalp, 1996).

2.2.3.3 Content of breast milk

Breast milk is the unique ideal and physiological nutrient for the newborn. It supplies all feeders according to requirement of the infant in an organized and sterilized manner. Moreover when breast milk is compared with the infant formulas which are sterilized but "inert" because of enabling the mother to adapt to the microbial environment where she is, and providing the infant both general and specific anti-infective factors, breast milk is a "living" biological liquid. Even though macro-feeders are imitated for their concentration and content in the sense of "static", supplying the micro-feeders at-will cannot be always guaranteed. For example, the existence of a different whey casein ratio in the formula affects the infant's cholesterol levels in blood. While whey casein ratio in breast milk is 63:37, this is 18:82 in cow's milk. Although the ratio of 60:40 in infant formulas that are regarded as "humanize" is adopted nowadays, rich formulas (20:80) have been generated from the casein within last 10 years because of its affordability. It was found that blood cholesterol levels of the infants who had been fed with these formulas were high, in which only the protein ratio was modified and lipids remained the same (Civi et al, 1997).

2.2.3.a Colostrum

The breast milk which is lactated within the first 4-5 days following the birth is called *colostrum.* The milk turns into *transitional milk* in the next days by changing its structure. It takes the form of *mature milk* within thirty days (Arcasoy et al, 1994).

Colostrum is a yellowish liquid having pH 7.7 approximately. Its structure is different from the mature milk and it has the characteristics of retention liquid (Arcasoy et al, 1994; Ok, 1991; Ozalp, 1996).

Colostrum has a rich content in terms of minerals, vitamin A, IgA. Its sugar and fat content is lower compared to the following milk (Ok, 1991; Özalp, 1996).

Protein: Its rate is an average of 2.2% g.

Carbohydrate: Lactose rate is lower than it is in mature milk due to the resorption of lactated liquid from the breast again. Its rate is an average of 4-5% g (Arcasoy et al, 1994). The concentration of breast milk is not affected from the mother's diet. Lactose is influential in the absorption of calcium within the milk. The compounds of lactose's galactose component with lipids are essential for the development of brain tissue (Ozalp, 1996).

Fat: The fat rate is low in the first days; afterwards it is 3% g approximately (Arcasoy et al, 1994).

As lactation increases, the total protein and mineral levels decrease and the level of fat, lactose and frequently vitamin B1 increase (Arcasoy et al, 1994).

Energy: It is 570 Kcal per liter approximately (Arcasoy et al, 1994).

Immunoglobulins: All structural factors for the development and protection of the newborn are available in colostrum. Colostrum is very rich in terms of the immunoglobulins. After the first breastfeeding, the mouth and gastrointestinal mucous is covered by secretory lgA. These interlink the toxins, bacteria and macromolecular agents and prevent their absorption from intestinal epithelium. Moreover, they have the function of stimulating infant to form its own lgAs. In the first days most of the cells in the colostrum comprise of neutrophils, and macrophages in the next days. Both cell types protect the infant from infections through the synthesis of phagocytosis and interferon. Half of the lymphocytes in colostrum are T-lymphocytes. B lymphocytes constitute lgA and also it is discovered that they are able to generate interferon when they are stimulated by viruses (Arcasoy et al, 1994).

As the volume of milk decreases through the end of lactation, immunoglobulins increase again. Thus, both the infant and the breast are protected (Arcasoy et al, 1994).

The amount of *taurine* in colostrum which is a necessary amino acid for the newborn, is 7-8 times more than the cow's milk in 3th-7th days (Arcasoy et al, 1994).

Rather than for the nutrition of newborn (in any case, the energy and water requirements of a 3-day-old infant is minimal), colostrum is beneficial for protecting the newborn from the microbes in external environment and preparing it for the function of gastro-intestinal system (Ok, 1991).

Breastfeeding within the first half an hour after the birth is a crucial factor for not delaying the increase in the amount of milk, and it affects the total breastfeeding period positively (Richard, 2001; TR Ministry of Health, 1996; Yurdakok, 2004).

2.2.3.b Temporary milk

The milk in the period of 5-10 day-old infant is the temporary milk. The concentration of phosphorus is higher in transitional milk than it is in the colostrum or mature milk (Ok, 1991). It contains fat, lactose and vitamin in higher rates than the colostrum and its calorie value is also higher (Taskin, 1997).

2.2.3.c Mature milk (breast milk)

Color of the breast milk is white and its pH is 6.97 (Arcasoy et al, 1994).

Lactose is the most important component of the carbohydrates in breast milk. Its rate is higher in breast milk than it is in cow's milk (7.1 g/dl and 4.1 g/dl). The compounds of lactose's galactose component with lipids have a significant role in the development of brain. Also, it facilitates the calcium absorption and affects the bone mineralization positively. The indigestible part of lactose has role in the development of acidophilic bacterial flora (*Lactobacillus bifidus*) in intestines as fermented, and prevents reproduction of the pathogen microorganisms (Gokçay & Garibagaoglu, 2002; Oran & Yurdakok, 1996).

Whey protein, which is digestible and rich in biological value, constitutes the 60% of the protein content (which is almost 18% in cow's milk). Alfa-lactalbumine makes up the significant part of the whey proteins and has a function in the lactose synthesis in the breast alveoli. Most of the whey proteins are anti-infective proteins and protects the infant from infections. Lactoferrin, lysozyme, emunctory immunoglobulin-A and other types of immunoglobulin, nucleotides, and growth factors play key role in immunity. The rate of casein that is less digestible is lower in breast milk than it is in cow's milk (40% and 80%) (Gokcay & Garibagaoglu, 2002; Oran & Yurdakok, 1996).

The protein content in breast milk is less than it is in cow's milk (1.1 g/dl and 3.2 g/dl), but its biological value is higher and it meets the protein requirement of the infant alone (Oran & Yurdakok, 1996).

The nucleotides in breast milk increase the protein utilization. When amino acids are insufficient through diet, nucleotides are used in the synthesis of proteins and non-essential amino acids. It is known that there are 12 distinct nucleotides in the breast milk and inosine phosphate among these increases the absorption of iron in the breast milk (Ozalp, 1996).

Carbohydrate: Lactose within the breast milk is almost 7% at average. Lactose of the breast milk is more digestible than the lactose in cow's milk (Arcasoy et al, 1994). Lipids which supply 50% of the calories in breast milk are more in breast milk than they are in cow's milk (4.5 g/dl and 3.8 g/dl) and they exist in the form of fat globules. Lipase in breast milk promotes the digestion of fat even in low bile level. Furthermore, the breast milk has a rich content in terms of long chain poly unsaturated fatty acids such as arachidonic acid, docosahexaenoic acid, linolenic acid and alfa linoleic acid all of which are in the structure of nerve cell and retina cell and have role in the development of the nervous system and optical functions. Particularly, milk of the mothers of premature infants has higher amounts of long chain unsaturated fatty acids. The fat rate in breast milk changes during the breastfeeding period. The fat rate which is low at the beginning of breastfeeding rises through the end of breastfeeding. This situation creates the feeling of fullness for the infant and prevents the adiposity to occur. Phospholipid and cholesterol contents in the breast milk are high in the early lactation period. It is argued that this situation can be influential on the early activation of lipid enzyme system and the prevention of hyperlipidemia and atherosclerosis (Gokcay & Garibagaoglu, 2002; TR Ministry of Health, 1996).

Lipid: The fat level is quite variable depending on mother's diet. Its structure has the characteristics of vegetable oil, its level changes between 3.5-4.5% g (Arcasoy et al, 1994).

Minerals: While the level of minerals in breast milk is 3 g in the first 15 days following the birth, it falls gradually afterwards. The absorption of the calcium in breast milk is more than it is in cow's milk. Ca/P ratio in the milk is 1/2. The levels of Zn, Co, Cu and Se are higher than they are in cow's milk. The lower level of mineral in breast milk creates less osmotic pressure on the kidney and supplies safe nutritional source in the first months for the infant who has functional defects. The celitis load of kidney is 75-90 mOsm/L for the breastfed infants, whereas this is 228 mOsm/L for the ones who are fed with cow's milk. Thus, maintaining the fluid balance is a lot easier among breastfed infants (Arcasoy et al, 1994; Gokcay & Garibagaoglu, 2002; Ozalp, 1996; Schack & Michaelsen, 2006).

Immunoglobulin types and enzymes: IgA in the breast milk has antibody activity against many gram (+) and gram (-) bacteria, various viruses and *Candida albicans*. IgM and lgG pass immediately from the mother's serum to the infant (Arcasoy et al, 1994).

Lysozyme level in the breast milk is approximately 5000 times higher than the Lysozyme level in cow's milk. Similarly, this enzyme has protective function against gram (+) bacteria and some virus infections. Some of the enzymes in the milk have immunological function and some of them affect the cell ripening indirectly (Arcasoy et al, 1994).

Lactobacillus bifidus flora that reproduces within the intestines of breastfed infants prevents the pathogenic bacteria to reproduce. The nutritional supplements that are given soon after the birth destroy the protective mechanism by preventing these bacteria to reproduce (Arcasoy et al, 1994; Coskun, 1996).

Breast milk is vitally important for the protection, nutrition and development of 4-6 month-old infants. In addition to that the breast milk in every period is not the same at every meal, it undergoes modification in the periods in which the infant starts breastfeeding and ends. The milk of the premature infant's mother is different from the milk of mother who has a infant in time, and it is adjusted for the growth of little infant more rapidly and healthily. Depending on that how early this infant was born, the breast milk is ideally adjusted; at first protein, calcium and iron are increased, all the other nutrients, except phosphorus are adjusted nearly for that infant (Ok, 1991).

Fat and water soluble vitamins in breast milk, except vitamin K and vitamin D are at adequate level for infants. Since the intestine flora has not developed exactly yet, vitamin K is applied through parenteral or oral passage in order to prevent the hemorrhagic disease of the newborn. 400 IU of vitamin D supplement is required daily beginning from 15th day up to the end of the first year to meet vitamin D requirement (Gokcay & Garibagaoglu, 2002; Oran & Yurdakok, 1996).

Studies about the breastfeeding physiology demonstrated the existence of the hormones in the breast milk such as adipokine, leptin, adiponectin, Insulin-Like Growth Factor I (IGF-I), ghrelin, obestatin and resistin. Human milk is a complicated liquid. Leptin and ghrelin hormones are synthesized and secreted to breast milk by mammary gland. Leptin and ghrelin hormones protect the child against the obesity in his/her childhood and adulthood periods particularly by giving the feeling of fullness to infant, and organizes the infant's energy metabolism (Gokcay & Garibagaoglu, 2002; Savino et al, 2009).

2.2.4 Scala of breastfeeding diagnosis

The researchers have developed various tools that measure the effective nursing behavior of the infant exactly and clearly, and they measured successful breastfeeding through the effectiveness of nursing and lactating behavior. Some of these tools are MBA (Mother Infant Assessment tool), IBFAT (Infant Breastfeeding Assessment Tool) and LATCH Breastfeeding diagnosis measurement (LATCH Assessment tool) (Jensen et al, 1994).

2.2.4.1 LATCH (LATCH assessment tool) breastfeeding diagnosis measurement tool

LATCH Breastfeeding diagnosis measurement tool is a tool that is developed in 1986 by assimilating to Apgar score system in terms of scoring method. The evaluation of LATCH Assessment Tool is fast and easy like Apgar score. The development purposes of this assessment tool are classified below:

- Being able to conduct the breastfeeding diagnosis objectively,
- Determining the breastfeeding problems and making the training plan,
- Creating a common language among the health care personnel,
- It is developed to be used in surveys (determining the breastfeeding achievement in longitudinal studies) (Hamelin & Mcleman, 2000; Jensen et al, 1994).

This assessment tool consists of five evaluation criteria. LATCH generates from the combination of first letters of these five criteria in English. These criteria are listed below:

- **L:** Latch on breast
- **A:** Audible swallowing
- **T:** Type of nipple
- **C:** Comfort breast/nipple
- **H:** Hold

Each term is evaluated between 0-2 points. The total is 10 points (Adams & Hewell, 1997; Hamelin & Mcleman, 2000).

The reliability of LATCH Breastfeeding diagnosis measurement tool is determined in America by means of the studies of Adams and Hewell in 1997. The concordance percentage between three breastfeeding consultants and researchers, and independent observers is found out 94.4%. The concordance percentage of each term between the observers changes between 85-100% (Adams & Hewell, 1997; Hamelin & Mcleman, 2000).

Evaluation criteria	0+	1	2
Latch on breast	It sleeps or reluctant; it cannot achieve to latch on the breast	It tries again, only latches on the nipple, nursing activity is observed.	It holds nipple by also latching on the areola, sucks rhythmically, its lips are extraverted.
Audible swallowing	No	Some nursing movements	Short term strong expirations are observed while swallowing.
Type of nipple	Dented	Smooth	Discharge through stimulation
Mother's Comfort regarding to breast and nipple	Blocking of duct; swelling, bleeding, bruise of breast	Reddish color, small bruises, decrease in comfort	Soft breasts and comfortable mother
Hold	Completely through assistance	Minimal assistance	Without assistance

Table 2. Evaluation of the effective breastfeeding (LATCH breastfeeding scale) (Yenal & Okumus, 2003).

2.2.5 Weaning

It is difficult to say when the infant should be weaned. Following the 6th month, which is an obligation to breastfeed, the mother may last this period by adding nutritional supplements up to the 1st year. Children breastfed for longer terms tend to abandon nutritional supplements and prefer breast milk.

Some principles in weaning:

a. Weaning is never carried out suddenly. It is most appropriate to start weaning by reducing meals and waiting for child to adapt nutritional supplements.
b. If the infant is ill, weaning is not made.
c. Weaning should not be tried in hot seasons unless there is a significant reason.
d. Weaning before the 4th month carries risks to the life of the infants (Arcasoy et al, 1994).

2.2.6 Artificial nutrition

The role of the breast milk in infant's nutrition is no contestable. The most important duty of health care personnel should be not to deprive the infant of this irreplaceable natural nutrient and to do the necessary. However in case of the existence of some health problems stated before, the mother cannot feed her infant with her milk (Ozalp, 1996).

The terms to consider in artificial nutrition are:

- Choosing the substitute nutrient for breast milk,
- Informing mother about how to prepare the nutrient and its amount to give the infant,
- Teaching the requirements to prepare it in a hygienic manner,
- Observing the growth and development of the infant (Ozalp, 1996).

Name of the Assessment Tool	Focused Point or Person	Evaluator	Criteria Used in the Assessment
LATCH	Mother and infant	Mother or nurse	Latch on breast Audible swallowing Type of nipple Comfort breast/nipple Hold
IBFAT (Infant Breastfeeding Assesment Tool)	Infant	Mother or nurse	Readiness to feed Rooting Fixing (latching on); Sucking
MBA (Mother Infant Assesment Tool)	Mother and infant	Nurse	Signaling Position Fixing Milk transfer Ending
SAIB (Systematic Assessment of the Infant at the Breast)	Infant	Mother or nurse	Alignment Areolar grasp Areolar compression Audible swallowing
BAPT (Breastfeeding Attrition Prediction Tool)	Information of mother and her manner about breastfeeding shows the risk of giving up breastfeeding early	Mother	Manner Subjective norm Control
H&H Lactation Scale	Mother and infant	Nurse	Insufficient milk supply (Has 3 subscales) Saturation and confidence of mother Satisfaction of child Adequacy of mother-infant breastfeeding
Evaluation Scale of Breastfeeding Manner	Mother	Nurse	Mother's own manner about breastfeeding Mother's manner about breastfeeding related to other people (husband, family and immediate vicinity, health care personnel) Society's manner about breastfeeding as a function special to woman
MBFES (The Maternal	Mother and infant	Nurse	Satisfaction of mother /Gaining the role of maternity

Name of the Assessment Tool	Focused Point or Person	Evaluator	Criteria Used in the Assessment
Breastfeeding Evaluation Scale)			Infant's capacity/development Life style /body image
Breastfeeding Observation Form (WHO/UNICEF)	Mother and infant	Nurse	Body position Infant's behavior Emotional commitment Anatomy Sucking Spent time for sucking

Table 3. Various breastfeeding assessment tools and their properties (Hamelin & Mcleman, 2000).

Artificial nutrition can be applied through industrial formulas or cow's milk which has modified content.

When the socio-economic conditions of the family are suitable, industrial formulas should be preferred especially in early months.

According to their features, industrial formulas can be classified in three groups which are adapted, semi-adapted and follow-on-formulas (Ozalp, 1996).

Adapted Milk Formulas: This milk is in the form of liquid and powder. It is made from cow's milk and shows compliance with the composition of breast milk. Protein and minerals (Na, K, Cl, Ca, P) of cow's milk are reduced, their fats are modified and enriched with the vegetable oil supplement. Fat contents supply half of the total energy and they have rich content in terms of essential fatty acid-linoleic acid. Amylase enzyme is physiologically low. As the infant grows up, it begins to secrete the amylase enzyme in normal amounts. Adapted formulas do not contain starch in accord with the physiological growth of the infant. Their carbohydrate contents include the invert sugar-lactose in breast milk. The ratios and osmolarities of whey protein/casein, protein/ carbohydrate are made familiar to breast milk. Also vitamin D and some other vitamins are added and some of them contain nucleoproteins, carnitine, taurine and additional iron. It is recommended for the infant to be fed with the adapted formulas in neonatal period and in the first months of life (Ozalp, 1996).

Semi-adapted Formulas: Protein content and energy densities of these formulas are higher. Their complex carbohydrate structures that are comprised of lactose and corn syrup essence accustom the infant to nutrition. With respect to their contents, they also show some of the characteristics of the adapted formulas. Similarly, the osmolality of the semi-adapted formulas are made similar to the breast milk. When they are given in proper amounts, they are adequate for the infant's nutrition up to 4th-6th month (Ozalp, 1996).

Follow-on-Formulas: These are the industrial formulas having the content to meet or support the infant's needs after the month 4-6. They are recommended for the infants that are breastfed after the month 4-6 (Ozalp, 1996).

2.2.6.1 Artificial nutrition technique

Before starting any usage of formula, the information about financial aspects of this decision must be given to mothers. Tolerating selected formula by infant and ease of preparing are the essential criteria for deciding on which type of formula will be selected (Arcasoy et al, 1994; Turkish Republic Ministry of Health AÇS/AP General Directorate, 1997).

Readymade formulas contain enough calories for newborn when it's diluted with warmed water in a recommended way. There exist some formulas that are prepared for the infants that are allergenic to cow's milk and must have a special diet (Cavusoglu, 2000).

Formulas with prebiotics are of a big advantage to the infants. Especially during the lack of mother milk these formulas with the closest probiotic and prebiotic to the mother milk should be given. In asthma and atopic dermatitis, there are also numerous benefits if given to infants. In addition, there are studies about which the probiotics prevent allergic diseases (Pehlivanoglu, 2007).

Formulas are prepared for a time period of 24 hours and are kept in the fridge. If they are not used in this term, they must be thrown away. The opened powder-type formulas can be maintained in the fridge for 4 weeks. After this period, the remaining part should be disposed.

To prevent the contamination by pathogenic microorganisms, great caution is given to the sanitation rules during the preparation of infant's formula. The chance of contamination is relatively low if the mother boils chlorinated water and makes use of hygiene techniques. Before its use, the feeding-bottle is kept for 25 minutes in boiling water for the sterilization purpose.

An hour before the nutrition, the bottle is taken out of the fridge and kept at the room temperature. Although some parents chose to heat the feeding-bottle for 20 seconds in microwave oven, this is often considered to be risky. The milk at the middle of the heated bottle will be hotter than the milk on the sides. To prevent the infants' tongue getting burnt, parents may shake the bottle and test the milk (temperature) on their wrists.

Alternatively, the feeding-bottle can be heated by placing it inside of a larger container which is filled with water. In any case, parents are strongly advised to check the temperature of milk before using the formula.

During nutrition the infant is taken onto lap holding its head a little high above so that the aspiration risk can be reduced. To prevent infant to swallow air instead of formula, it is important to check if the nipple is filled with milk. Since the infants are particularly subject to accumulation of gas in their stomach during feeding, the infant should be burped after nutrition (Çavuşoğlu, 2000).

Infants that are nourished with feeding-bottle or spoon are generally held at the horizontal position. Connected with the negative pressure occurring at the rear pharynx during nursing, otitis media is observed more often in the infants who are nourished with feeding-bottle. Otitis media is rarely observed in infants who are nourished with breast milk because they are not held at that position.

Although the infants who are nourished with formula put on more weight than those who were breastfed, such growth is no natural (Yurdakök, 1991).

It was observed that mothers had a tendency of preparing condense formulas believing this way would be more nutritious for their infants. However, if the industrial formulas are not watered down with sufficient cow's milk, the osmolar burden at kidneys significantly increases. In this case, the infant dehydrates more while attempting to rid the solid load at the urine. To make the things worse, the infant's crying at this time might be (mis)interpreted as the sign of hunger, not thirst! Loading infant with the same regimen might result in a negative water-balance for infants to develop, not to mention the risk of obesity due to the excessive food intake.

Fever of the infants fed with hyperosmolar nutrients goes up. Depending on the oral solid load diarrhea may follow. Abdominal distension and vomiting can also happen. The infant is seen disturbed at these times. Such findings in relation to feeding infants with concentrated formulas are often considered as "gastroenteritis" caused by infection.

At inadequate socio-economic conditions, the tendency of mothers on giving diluted infant formula was also observed. Affecting the growth of infant, it may result in other health problems should the infant also have malnutrition (Özalp, 1996).

According to a study by Egemen et al (1997) in which the formulas given in Izmir were determined if they had been prepared watery or not, it was found that 80% of the mothers prepared infant formulas either too less or too much watery, and the 50% prepared with different amounts of water at two separate meals (Egemen et al, 1997).

Mothers should be well-educated on preparing formulas, and if possible, having the formulas prepared demonstratively at home is needed (Egemen et al, 1997; *Özalp, 1996)*

The Amount of Milk to be given during Artificial Nourishment: By calculating the calorie and protein of nourishment, it is prepared according to the required amount that would be given.

If there is no chance of giving breast milk to a newborn -8 or 10 hours after the birth, this type of nourishment is started as 8 meals a day, and to give 10 ml of milk each time. By the seventh day, it is increased by 60 – 70 ml a day. After the seventh day, 60 – 70 ml a week is added until the end of the first month. The milk to be given is an adapted version of genuine breast milk; the watering of milk can be increased to 8%, 10%, or even 12%. These amounts at meals are not constant. Sometimes the infant can take more or less of it. While seven meals are generally enough, 8 meals can be given to those who get tired easily or who were born with low weight.

A normal infant sleeps if it is full, wakes up when it is hungry. Although it cannot find rhythm following the first few days after delivery, it starts focusing its requisitions on the daytime. It's suggested to prepare a infant bottle of 110-120 ml, and to let the infant start nursing as much as it wants. The remaining milk in the bottle is measured, afterwards. By checking for 2-3 days, whether the infants take a proper ration is examined. The period between two meals shouldn't be less than 2 hours. The infant becomes full after 7 meals at first, and with 6 meals, later on. Night infant bottle is at the end of the first month in general.

Some infants never have regular nutrition. After 15 or 20 days of trying, a strict behavior should be preferred after 15-20 days. 7 glasses at the first, 6 of which should be given between 07-22, and the seventh should be given at night; 6 infant bottles at the 2nd month. The sleeping infant must not be woken up for nutrition after the first month.

Weekly weight controls should be done, and the rations of the infants who didn't put on weight should be gently increased. Some children require more than enough nutrition even though they grow well. Therefore, Adding water rather than increasing the ration would be of a better course of action (Arcasoy et al, 1994; Çavuşoğlu, 2000).

2.2.6.2 Nutrition with cow's milk

It is necessary to give milk with making watery at first months of life in which cow's milk, especially lots of enzymatic functions and kidneys are immature. Basically, in first 4 months, feeding the infant with industrial milks called adapted milk whose composition is liken to breast milk is truer. But in truly necessary cases, children of the families with bad economic condition cannot drink breast milk either; hence, nutrition with cow's milk partially or completely starts. Cow's milk is not appropriate nourishment for the first months of life (Arcasoy et al, 1994).

Composition	Breast milk	Cow's milk
Calcium mg/dl	34.0	120.0
Phosphorus mg/dl	15.0	95.0
Iron mg/dl	0.5	0.5
Iodine UG/L	30.0- 70.0	47.0
Flour UG/L	5.0- 50.0	70.0- 220.0
A vitamin IU/L	1988.0	1025.0
C vitamin IU/L	43.0	11.0
D vitamin IU/L	22.0	14.0
K vitamin IU/L	16.0	60.0

Table 4. Ingredients of Breast Milk and Cow's milk (Kliegman & Marcdante, 2008)

If giving cow's milk is necessary, milk is made watery with boiled water. Between 1st and 4th months, it's prepared as 2 parts water 1 part milk, between 4th and 5th months, there are 2parts milk 1part water. For the children above 6 months, it's unnecessary to make cow's milk watery (Arcasoy et al, 1994; Baysal, 1993; Çavuşoğlu, 2000).

Cow's milk is sweetened on the purpose of preventing constipation and increasing energy with 5%rate of sucrose, which means sugar used at home; because of the fact that cow's milk lactose is less than breast milk. It must be defined to mothers as one tea spoon granulated sugar for 100 cc milk (Arcasoy et al, 1994).

2.2.7 Starting additional supplements for infants

As of the month 4 - 6 breast milk becomes deficient in satisfying some of the infant's needs. Additional supplements are added slowly to start the transition from newborn breastfeeding to adult feeding. All nutrients given to infant except the breast milk are called additional supplement. They provide energy, protein, fat and other nutrient elements. This early period is called the period of starting additional supplements or *"weaning period"* (Bertan & Ozcebe, 1995; Tokatli, 1996). The word weaning comes from the Anglo-Saxon word *"wenian"* which means getting used to something new (Coşkun, 1991). Weaning is a period in which breastfeeding continues for another year while additional supplements are being served in an appropriate fashion (Bertan & Özcebe, 1995; Tokatlı, 1996).

Considering that breast milk can still be enough for an infant during the months 4-6, additional supplements may start at any time in this period. The deviations in the growth curve are often the best indicators showing that there is a need for additional supplements. The time of starting, therefore, can be determined by observing the infant's growth (Bertan & Özcebe, 1995; Coşkun, 1991).

In fact, the level of growth for the infant's gastrointestinal and metabolic functions determine this time. Neurological and psychosocial developments have also their share in that determination.

The completion of head-neck control, the development of hand-eye coordination, starting to interact with mother and the surroundings, starting to sit, the development of mastication-swallowing coordination are of the required steps for an infant to start additional supplements. Neurological and psychosocial developments within this period also enable additional supplements for an infant in 4-6 months (Tokatlı, 1996).

Since weaning is an orientation term for infants, whether or not the infant is ready should be considered. For instance, starting to additional supplements may be postponed for a while when the infant grows teeth, has fewer, or is sick (Coskun, 1991).

There are complications and inconveniences regarding whether the infant starts additional supplements too early, or too late (Bertan & Özcebe, 1995; Taskin, 1997).

Early Starting to Additional Supplements (Before the month four)

- The given supplements may be contaminated (even in small amounts) which increases the risk of infection in infants.
- Early supplements cause too much solute load-up for the kidneys, hyperosmolarity and dehydration become imminent.
- Due to the diminishing demand for breast milk, the breastfeeding rate drops and milk production decreases; eventually this affects the growth rate.
- Malnutrition.
- May reveal allergic reactions.
- Increases the obesity risk for the coming ages.
- Coeliac disease emerges at younger ages (Bertan & Özcebe, 1995; Tokatlı, 1996).

Late Starting to Additional Supplements (After the month six):

- May lead to growth retardation due to having food less than what infant needs.
- May lead to diarrhea, other infectious diseases, and decrease in immunity.
- May lead to nutritional deficiency and related illnesses, such as iron deficiency anemia and malnutrition.
- Micronutrient deficiency may develop.

The 4th and 6th months are the terms when infant learns mastication. If the ability is not gained, this may lead to significant nutrition problems in the future (Bertan & Özcebe, 1995; Tokatlı, 1996).

Breast milk cannot satisfy the calcium needs of infant after 4th or 6th months. That's why yoghurt is given as the first additional supplement with breast milk. Secondly; breast milk cannot satisfy the needs of C vitamin and carotene and fruit, vegetable juices and after purees of these foods are given as additional supplements. Thirdly; breast milk and additional supplements cannot satisfy the needs of B vitamin and energy. For being able to provide these, floury foods, vegetable soups with flour and especially tarhana soup is given. Fourthly, breast milk and additional supplements cannot satisfy the iron need of infant and nonfat ground meat, meat or lentil is added to infant's soup. After adding meat, egg also takes place in the infant's nutrition (Bertan & Guler, 1995).

In selecting the additional supplement will be given, some features like the needs of infant, motor and mental improvements, capacity of GIS digestion and absorption, kidneys' capacity, sensibility to allergens must be considered (Taşkın, 1997).

The most allergenic foods: Sugared foods with additives inside, chocolate, egg, milk, peanut, walnut, horse-bean, green peas, lentil, game animals, various fishes, shellfishes, wheat, corn, rye, chees, brewer's yeast, melon, water-melon, strawberry, fig, tomato, grapefruit, etc.

Gluten enteropathy (coeliac disease - CD): What is recommended today is to give the mother-milk ideally long, and to start supplementary nutrition containing gluten between the months 4-7. As a protective measure for infants against meeting early with the gluten rice can be a good substitute (and a fine starter of cereals) since it is already a part of the traditional infant nutrition. Even there could be genetic susceptibility it depends on the nutrition habits of societies and individuals, to the qualitative and quantitative characteristics of the gluten taken, and whether the clinical symptoms were distributed on a large spectrum. Unless there is gluten in the diet CD does not develop, which is why countries like Japan and China are the best examples to it for their traditional nutrition habits (Demirceken, 2011).

Feeding the infants with formulas lacking iron (formulas with rice flour) and starting to cow's milk (in larger quantities than half a liter) before age 1 is a major reason for iron deficiency anemia to develop. The iron in mother milk, however, is absorbed better than that in cow's milk. To overcome this matter, additional iron supplements in small amounts (such as 1-2 mg/kg) as of the 2nd month are recommended to the mothers who have delivered their premature newborns with a low birth infant weight; as to those who had in-term deliveries the supplement is suggested after the 4th month. In general mother milk should be given for the first 6 months, while formulas rich in the iron should be supplied until the age 1.

Nutrition habits with ready convenience foods, insufficient food intake in the name of diet, vegetarianism, bad socio-economic conditions all contribute to iron deficiency anemia, especially for the elder children.

It was observed that the nutrition habits even at our rural areas are changing; for instance, our traditional nutrient-rich foods "*tarhana soup*" and "*bulgur*" (rice in the form of cracked wheat cooked with tomatoes) were being replaced by fried potatoes in all three meals, in which case, the iron intake through potatoes would be very inadequate and, thus, iron deficiency anemia has increased in recent years in our country (Cetin, 2011).

2.2.7.1 Subjects to take into consideration when starting additional supplements

- Socio-economic and cultural conditions of parents, relations with the infant must be considered.
- If it's not needed, not been started to additional supplements before 3rd after 6th month.

- When the infant is 6-month-old, energy comes from the additional supplements mustn't exceed 50% of the total energy.
- Every additional supplement must be started to give alone and must be followed whether the infant tolerates or not. Do not start more than one additional supplement for the infant in a week.
- Additional supplements will be given are started at most 1 or 2 dessert spoons and must be increased as the infant tolerates.
- While preparing the additional supplements, pay attention to hygienic measures. Before preparing the foods and feed the infant, hands must certainly be cleaned.
- All nutrients must be tried by spoon.
- Infant may not eat some new nourishment. In this case, do not insist and try it again soon after.
- New nourishments must be tried while the infant is hunger and foods must clean and be pureed, ragged puree must be given as the infant is getting used to eat (Bertan & Güler, 1995; Coşkun, 1991; Tokatlı, 1996).

2.2.8 Mixed nutrition

It means giving other milks or milky nourishments to the infant who drinks breast milk. Major indication for mixed nutrition is lagging in weight gain of infant that is nourished with breast milk and has not any health problem and not recovering in spite of measures taken. This condition can only be determined by weekly or frequent measuring. For being able to reach this decision, the infant must be followed for 1 or 2 weeks (Kliegman & Marcdante, 2008).

Mixed nutrition is started as one meal a day. Meals that contain the least breast milk is evening times. For this reason, in the meal at 18:00-19:00 pm milk recipe or cow's milk prepared appropriately is given by spoon with the intended amount of infant after nursing for 5 or 10 minutes. If it's not enough, mixed nutrition is applied in two or more meals. In the infants facing with mixed nutrition, fruit juice is given after 4 weeks and pudding is given after 4 months (Kliegman & Marcdante, 2008).

2.2.9 Nutrition program of nursling at different months

0-6 TH Months

For the first 6 months, only breast milk (Köksal, 2007). Breast milk must be given at every infant crying in first days, afterwards it must be given at every 2 or 4 hours if infant wants (Baysal & Arslan, 1997; Turkish Republic Ministry of Health AÇS/AP General Directorate, 1991; Turkish Republic Ministry of Fundamental Health General Directorate of Health Services, 1997).The growth by month of infant must be followed (Köksal, 2007).

6TH Months

4 or 5 meals Breast Milk + Every Second Days 1 Egg Yolk+ 1 meal Yoghurt+1 meal Fruit Puree /+1 meal Vegetable Puree (Baysal & Arslan, 1997; Köksal, 2007; Turkish Republic Ministry of Health AÇS/AP General Directorate, 1991; Turkish Republic Ministry of Fundamental Health General Directorate of Health Services, 1997). Pudding without sugar can also be given (milk + rice flour). Cow's milk can be used a little for preparing nourishments (Köksal, 2007).

7-9Th months

7th Month: Continue to breast milk, yoghurt, fruit juice, vegetable juice, grape molasses, rice flour, rice, egg yolk (all), meat (fish, chicken meats and red meat), vegetal oils, vegetable puree or vegetable soup (Köksal, 2007).

8th Month: Continue to breast milk, yoghurt, fruit juice, vegetable juice, grape molasses, meat (fish, chicken meats and red meat), lamb liver or chicken liver, vegetal oils, well mashed home meals (with ground meat and vegetable), all egg or pasteurize cheese, cereal - red lentil, haricot bean, chickpea purees (Köksal, 2007).

Sample Menu:

At Morning 8 am: Breast Milk, One or Two Biscuits, + One Egg Yolk or White Cheese sized with Matchbox.

At 10 am: Fruit Puree+ A Biscuit

At 13 pm: Vegetable Soup with Meat or Puree (Farci and Similar Home-made Vegetable Meals).

At 16 pm: Breast Milk or Yoghurt (With little sugar or Plain).

At 20 pm: Breast Milk. 150 ml milk or Pudding (for the infants having meal four-times-a-day, fruit puree is given after the vegetable soup at 13 pm). If needed, Breast Milk at night (Baysal & Arslan, 1997; Turkish Republic Ministry of Health AÇS/AP General Directorate, 1991; Turkish Republic Ministry of Fundamental Health General Directorate of Health Services, 1997).

10-11Th months

Sample Menu:

Morning At 8 am: Breast Milk, Honey or Grape Molasses + One All Egg (Instead of every second days White Cheese) + A Thin Slice of Bread+ One Tea Spoon of Butter.

At 12 am: Vegetable Puree + Two Dessert Spoons of Wigged Liver Pate Mixed to the Vegetable Puree, Chicken or Meatloaf. Instead of vegetable puree normal homemade mashed food is given Pieces of food must be given. If there isn't any bread taken in the morning, it is given in this meal.

At 16 pm: 150-200 gram Pudding or Fruit Puree with Yoghurt

At 20 pm: Pudding or Yoghurt (1 or 2 Spoons Pastry; For Instance it can be mixed with macaroni). + 2 or 3 Soup Spoons of Vegetable Puree. Milk can be given to the infant that doesn't eat yoghurt (Baysal & Arslan, 1997; Turkish Republic Ministry of Health AÇS/AP General Directorate, 1991; Turkish Republic Ministry of Fundamental Health General Directorate of Health Services, 1997).

12Th months

12th Month: Continue to breast milk, yoghurt, fruit or fresh-squeezed fruit juice, vegetable juice, grape molasses, egg (all) or pasteurize cheese (Köksal, 2007).

Sample Menu:

Morning, 150 ml Milk + 30 Gram White Cheese or Egg + 1 or 2 Biscuit or A Thin Slice of Bread + A Dessert Spoon of Jam, Honey or Grape Molasses.

Midday, Vegetable Meals with Meat at home or Vegetable Puree, If there is not, A meatloaf + Macaroni or Fruit Puree.

Midday-Afternoon, 150 ml. Cow's milk or Yoghurt or Rice Pudding + Two Biscuits.

Evening, 2 or 3 Soup Spoon of Vegetable Puree+ Mashed Macaroni or Rice+ Yoghurt (or other soups or vegetable meals prepared for family members) (Baysal & Arslan, 1997; Turkish Republic Ministry of Health AÇS/AP General Directorate, 1991; Turkish Republic Ministry of Fundamental Health General Directorate of Health Services, 1997).

2.3 Nutrition of game chıld

In order to avoid occult gastrointestinal bleeding, cow's milk should not be given until the age of 1. It is essential to avoid excessive milk consumption (>24 oz/day, 1 oz=30 ml) among game children (age of 1-3) because doing so causes decrease in the solid and nutrient-rich intake, which later results in overweighting. Fruit-juice consumption should be limited to 4-6 oz/day for those and younger children, while it should be 8-10 oz/day for the elder ones (up to the age of 18). Infants should be present at the dinner table as soon as they are 1-year-old, so they could start having regular meal. They should have a refreshments list, and they should be encouraged to eat food by themselves, especially the foods which are edible by use of their hands. Generally, the required amount of food is satisfied by filling up one spoon from every nutriment in every meal; more can be supplied should the infant require or demand otherwise (Kliegman & Marcdante, 2008).

In spite of having one or two meals a day some children may have all the energy they needed. The required energy of a game child is 80-90 kcal /kg/day, and the important point here is that a regular nutritional habit should be gained (Tunçdoğan & Tunçdoğan, 2005; Weisstaub et al, 2003).

The Food Groups to be Present in their Menu:

In the first group: Meat, chicken, fish, egg, legume, etc. This group has high quality of protein for

- Strengthen of Muscles
- Blood-forming
- Healthy growth and healthy life (2 or 3 portions a day).

In the second group: Milk, yoghurt, cheese, and so forth belong to here. Besides high quality of protein, there are

- Enough CA
- Vitamin A and
- Vitamin B for bone and teeth development.

400-500 ml. milk or yoghurt, and cheese in the size of a match-box should be consumed in a day.

In the third group: There are cereals, vegetal proteins and Vitamin B. It is needed to take three or four portions a day from this group.

In the fourth group: Vegetables, Fruits, and the Vitamins A-B-C. Three or four portions should be taken every day.

In the fifth group: Sugars and Fats: foods made of sugar or rich in saccharides, grape molasses, honey, jam, butter, olive oil and other vegetal oils, fatty foods, all of these provide huge energy (Kliegman & Marcdante, 2008; Tuncdogan & Tuncdogan, 2005).

2.4 Nutrıtıon of school chıld

While nutrition during the term -sometimes called- nursing infancy (roughly the age of 0-1) is the determining factor of growth and development, it gains more importance for the aging children with respect to learning or developing nutritional habits and the prevention of future health-problems. Especially during the school childhood, making the habit of regular age-appropriate physical activities is also essential next to the nutrition in order to maintain a healthy life in the adulthood. Parents who send their children to the school may readily feel comfortable about the nutrition times of their children. The fact is, however, children at school need family supervision as much as before. Of the areas parental control has a crucial role are the child's ability to choose nourishments, the likelihood of becoming influenced by friends, and their tendency of skipping meals (Süoğlu et al, 1999).

School children are still at the growing period. Growth requirements are determined by the physical activities, genetic features, and body structures, which all affect the overall nutritional needs. While the qualitative characteristics of the required nutrition for this age group are the same as adults, the required amounts differ significantly. Appetite increases especially during rapid growth periods; likewise, if the growth slows down the nutrient amount that is taken decreases. Carbohydrates and fats provide energy for growth and physical activities. Proteins which form and repair the body tissues are essential for healthy growth. It is strongly recommended that every school children should consume foods rich in protein, such as meat, fish, or poultry 2-3 portions a day in addition to milk and dairy products, which are also good sources of protein (Tunçdoğan & Tunçdoğan, 2005).

Although there is enough calcium in milk and dairy products, or the dark green vegetables to satisfy the daily requirements of young children, the need for increasing amounts at the adolescence cannot be satisfied. Iron requirements increase with the increase in blood volume during this period. With the start of menstruation girls should compensate their iron loss. Among the best sources of iron are meat, fish, barnyard fowl, and bread and cereals which are prepared rich in iron (AAP, 2003).

In most of the developing countries, insufficient nutrition and inability to provide additional supplements at the weaning period lead to malnutrition and short stature as an outstanding health problem. On the other hand, obesity, hypercholesterolemia, atherosclerosis and type-II diabetes risk are major concerns in developed countries caused by the same problem. (Jinabhai, 2003; Weisstaub et al, 2003). This situation draws attention to the nutrition types present at schools, and leads to studies about exercise habits and ways of correcting. The fatty ingredients of the food offered in schools, school canteens and mass-rooms with high saturated fat rate, appears to be a serious risk factor (Lytle et al, 2002; Stitzel, 2004).

One other problem related to the malnutrition of school children is skipping of breakfast (Lytle et al, 2002; Stitzel, 2004).

Analyzing the data in nurseries in our country, vitamin and mineral deficiencies were revealed to be high, where, in particular, zinc deficiency, which affects the growth adversely, was notable (Süoğlu, 1999; Yaşar, 1999). Among the Turkish children, skipping meal is a major problem for students who are going to state schools, while disliking meals and consuming poor foods are so for the private school students (Yaşar, 1999). Obesity, anemia, and tooth decay are also observed among the Turkish children.

Sample menu for school children between 6 and 10:

Breakfast:	A water glass of milk or fresh fruit juice An egg or cheese sized as a match box 2 dessert spoons of honey or jam or hazelnut paste 5 or 6 pieces of olive 2 thin slices of bread
Mid-Morning:	A medium sized fruit
Midday:	7 or 8 table spoons of meat pasty 3 or 4 table spoons of vegetables with olive oil A thin slice of bread (if a slice eaten at breakfast)
Mid-Afternoon:	A bowl of ice-cream
Evening:	A bowl of lentil soup A bowl of chicken with vegetables A thin slice of bread
Postprandial:	10 or 12 pieces of nut, hickory nut A medium sized fruit

2.5 Nutrition of adolescent

Adolescence can be a term in which unhealthy nutrition habits are earned. Skipping meals (especially breakfast), excessive eating, getting on a diet, consuming poor or food with high calories are so common. Consuming excessive sugar because of some drinks like soda water fruit juices, coffees and teas can cause excessive increases in weight and tooth decay. Also these drinks replace with the foods necessary for body. Inadequate calcium taken at his term can trigger osteoporotic hip fractures in adult term. Diet poor in calcium, inadequate calcium taken or osteopenia improved after calcium absorption destructions, is seen in child and adolescent more often and treated (UNICEF, 1994).

It is the parents who usually consult to the healthcare staff in eating disorders. These disorders are *anorexia nervosa* (significant weight-loss due to causing to vomit deliberately) and *bulimia nervosa* (stable weight by deliberate vomiting despite excessive eating). Prolonged diarrhea, repeating vomits, weight-loss, and inexplicable physical discomfort like amenorrhea are among the symptoms that will expose these illnesses. Adolescents who cause these symptoms deliberately are overly-concerned with their physical shapes; they keep their intents secret -along with the symptoms- for a long time. Among the ways serving that goal are putting on loose-fitting dresses, starting excessive physical trainings, picking up low-calorie and low-fat foods, complaining from some allergy resulting from tasting or smelling the foods, and dumping off what they got sneakily (either through vomiting or intentional diarrhea). Determining the risk of death due to the disguising frequency is a diagnostic difficulty (Swift & Johston, 2007).

Food Group	Nutritional Value	Required Daily Portion
Breads, cereals Other grainy goods (whole grain, enriched)	Carbohydrate, thiamine, niacin and rich than iron	At least 6 portions (1 portion: 1 thin slice of bread, 3 or 4 small or 2 big crackers, 30 g ready cereal for breakfast)
Fruits (Citrus, melon, strawberry and others)	Carbohydrate, A & C Vitamins	At least 2 portions (1 portion: middle sized apple, banana or mandarin, a half grapefruit, a slice of melon, a half bowl of strawberry, ¼ bowl of dried fruits)
Vegetables (dark green-leafy vegetables, legume, pea, other vegetables which contains high amylum)	Carbohydrate, A and C vitamins (different types must be consumed a few times a week)	At least 3 portions (1 portion: a half bowl of cooked vegetables, a half bowl of fresh-cut uncooked vegetables, a bowl of leafy uncooked vegetable like spinach)
Meat, barnyard fowl, fish and equivalents (egg, legume, crusty nutshells)	Protein, thiamine, niacin, iron	2 or 3 portions (Total daily intake 150-200 g lean meat, must be same as barnyard fowl or fish; 1 egg, a half bowl of cooked legume or 2 table spoons of peanut butter that is equal to 30 g meat)
Milk, cheese, yoghurt	Protein, Calcium, Riboflavin	2 portions (for adolescences, 3 portions) (1 portion: 1 bowl of milk, 250 cc yoghurt, 45g natural cheese, 60 g processed cheese)
Butter & desserts	Energy	The incomplete energy requirements following the consumption of the amounts from other nutrition groups

Table 5. Healthy Food Alternatives for School Children (Yaşar, 1999)

Sample menu for girls at adolescence:

Breakfast:	A water glass of milk or fresh fruit juice An egg or cheese sized as match box A table spoon of honey or jam pr hazelnut paste 5 or 6 pieced of olive 3 thin slices of bread Few slices of tomatoes or orange (for milk drinkers)
Midday:	2 pieces of grilled meatballs (cold cuts vegetable) 3 or 4 table spoons of borlotti beans in olive oil A bowl of milk puddings 1 or 2 thin sliced of bread
Mid-afternoon:	4 or 5 table spoons of burghul salad A water glass of ayran
Evening:	A portion meat and vegetable stew 4 or 5 table spoons of macaroni
After the meal	A medium sized fruit 10 or 12 pieces of nut or hickory nut, 2 or 3 pieces of dried apricots or fig

Sample menu for boys at adolescence:

Breakfast	A water glass of milk Cheese sized as 1 or 2 match boxes 1 or 2 table spoons of honey or jam or hazelnut paste 6 or 7 pieces of olive 4 or 5 thin slices of bread Few slices of tomatoes or orange
Midday:	7 or 8 table spoons of vegetable meal with meat 3 medium slices of pastry with potatoes 1 or 2 water glasses of ayran
Mid-afternoon	A toast with yellow cheese A water glass of fruit juice or 1 medium sized boiled corn, a tin of ayran
Evening:	1 or 2 bowls of tarhana soup Grilled fish sized as 2 meatloaves, salad Tahina halva sized as 2 match boxes
After the meal:	1 or 2 medium sized fruits 1 water glass of milk

2.6 Obesity

Obesity is a medical condition and an illness in which excess body fat has accumulated to such extent that it may give rise to various other illnesses, and lead to reduced life expectancy, besides an apparent deformation very notable at the first glance. Observations and statistics indicate a gradual increase in obesity among children and adolescents. The concern here is that while obesity adversely affects mental and physical health of the individual, it also brings economic burden to the society (Arslanoğlu, 2009).

Pathology -- constitutes a significant portion in the increase of adiposity mass among the normal-weight infants. The total adiposity number gradually increases between the month 6 and age 2, and stays stable until the ages of 8 and 10. Associated with puberty, a leap may occur in this number and in the height. In obese children, the fat cells are larger and more in comparison with those who have normal weight (Tershakovec, & Stallings, 1996).

Epidemiology -- despite the familial tendencies toward obesity, the key point here is how much the genetic and environmental factors contribute to these tendencies. Comparing the twins adopted together, the 80% of the changes in weight/height or skin thickness can be explained on genetic basis (Tershakovec, & Stallings, 1996).

The obesity at mother is founded related with increase in adipose tissue at newborn. The children of one or two of obese parents are inclined of being obese in adulthood. (If one of the parents is obese, the risk is nearly 40%; if both of them are obese the risk is 80%) In the first year of life, there is a moderate correlation between putting on excessive weight or the rate of being obese and getting obese later. But infants with excessive weights do not be obese child. Most of obese babies and children do not be obese adults. The risk of being obese that continues in adulthood, increases with the increase in the starting age for obesity (adolescence across infanthood) and severity of obesity (If the ideal body is more at its 180%, the possibility of being obese in adulthood is 100%)(Tershakovec, & Stallings, 1996).

Obesity diagnosis which is age-adjusted is putted with determining ideal percentage deviations at weight of the body according to height. The real weight more than 120% of ideal weight, accepted as obese. But weight deviations related with height can cause defining as wrongly obese of a muscular person. For this reason, measurement of triceps skin thickness by compasses is more certain, useful method at evaluating adiposity; values above 85% at improvement curve are accepted in favor of obesity. (Tershakovec, & Stallings, 1996).

The main problems must be solved of a child determined as obesity; whether being a syndromic or endocrine reason of this issue or not, if there is an external (exogenous) obesity, being expected complications for the moment whether or not or in which the risk is more, if there is no complications, in which conditions the external obesity improves and determining the ones that can be changeable and making appropriate suggestions (Arslanoğlu, 2009).

Being useful of protection, increasing exercise and reducing fat intake, there is no protection method defined. Although energy taking /brim weight is stable, there exist big differences in rate of fat accumulation among normal children. For this reason, it can be difficult to determine the appropriate calorie level for any children. Dietary recommendations accepted as more than a fixed number of calories per kilogram of body weight must be made according to the speed of growth (Tershakovec, & Stallings, 1996).

Beating with the obesity problem, carries two versatility as in the example of social-individual and preventing- nursing. For giving an example of societal preventions, in England at school canteens, being forbidden of food and beverages (with sugar) advertising on TV at the hours of children program published. Nutritional education for groups and physical activities can be an example of social therapeutic approach. Individual preventing approach is as arranging nutrition at pregnancy, being fed with breast milk, planning nutrition habits will be earned later, educating for defected behavior of the child within an obese family or group of friends. Individual therapeutic approach is being followed of obesity child by appropriate nutritionist (Arslanoğlu, 2009).

2.7 Nutritional education

A good nutrition is not only an important factor for the healthy development of individuals, families, and societies, but it helps us overcome the global issues like development of dietary levels of mother and infants, chronic diseases, mother deaths, malaria, AIDS, and other health concerns world is facing (Bellamy, 1998).

Nutritional education aims to gain society balanced nutritional habits by helping the individuals rid of incorrect and unfavorable practices. Such programs prevent nutrients from becoming health-risks, and teach the way of using food resources more efficiently. Nutritional teaching is an academic and practical concept regarding nutrition, dietetics, and nutrition science, including various scientific, economic and social aspects (Baysal, 1993).

The goal of nutritional education is to teach individuals how to use their foods in the best way with respect to the nutrition principles (Ozgur & Ozgur, 1994).

Most of the nutritional problems on national scale can be solved if the children are provided their food and bad nutritional habits are replaced by correct ones (Özgür & Özgür, 1994).

Nutritional education programs realize in two steps:

a. Raising the personnel needed to carry out these programs
b. Preparation of a program and its performance according to relevant analysis reports (Özgür & Özgür, 1994).

It is not necessary to include qualified nutritionists into these programs. As a matter of fact, these specialists are not in enough numbers at developing countries. Instead, those who have developed close relationships within the community should be placed. Of the good examples are nurses and midwives, health officials, the alumni of vocational high school for girls, and the primary school teachers. Should they have education on food production and consumption, by the help of the available specialists, such as agriculturalists, environmental health technicians, etc, they can be beneficial at the rural areas by aiming to educate teachers and the women of villages. Although our country has this potential our educating personnel should be made aware of this (Özgür & Özgür, 1994).

For instance giving up nursing early, is often based on the medical staff's apathy. If the nurses become conscious enough during their educations, nutritional education would be the main concerns. The programs of schools that train medical staff must aimed to think about this subject, seek solution ways, develop a creative talent (Özgür & Özgür, 1994).

Today, problems at nutrition area are; negativeness come from not being able to feed enough and balanced, deficiency of nourishment health applications, problems come with ignorance and inadequacies. Solutions will be brought for enough-balanced feeding and healthy nutrition problems must be handled together and a comprehensive point of view must be created (Perk, 1992).

These are the factors in the Assessment of Nutrition and Metabolism:

- The outlook
- model for food and liquid intake
- understanding of a balanced diet

- cultural and psychosocial factors affecting diet
- metabolic condition
- physiologic changes upon nutritional disorder
- Physical identifiers of malnutrition (Fuller & Schaller-Ayers, 1990).

In the study of Varol and Kocoglu (1997) with the purpose of examining education effect given to the mother, at growth and improvement conditions of low birth weight babies with following response group regularly and control group only 1st, 3rd, 6th, 9th and 12th months within the scope of education program, weight and height measurements are compared, improvement and starting months to additional supplement are evaluated. According to the study results, 90% of the babies in response group recover from malnutrition at 3rd month, this condition creates a statistically thoughtful difference between two groups ($p<0.05$). Activity attributed to education at this month is found 24.2%in weights, 34.5% in height. 70% of babies in response group have been breastfed during 8 months and 1 year, 75-80% of them timely started to additional supplements (Varol & Koçoğlu, 1997).

2.8 The role of nurse at the infant nutrition

- Nutrition is the first duty a family has to learn. Parents are, therefore, given information about nutrition methods (breast-feeding or formula feeding).
- Mothers are assisted with knowledge and awareness in such a way that they give better nutrition to their infants.
- In prenatal term, the parental attitudes on breast-feeding and other nutrition methods are examined. Those who have interest in breastfeeding are shown breast anatomy and its physiology, and taught how to prepare breast tissue (Çavuşoğlu, 2000).
- The infant may be restless due to the need of touching her mom or because of hunger. The nurse teaches hunger symptoms to the parents (ex: uneasiness, crying, suckling gestures, activities in hand and mouth, tenseness and no sleeping, etc.) (Kilegman & Marcdante, 2008).
- Teaching how to feed and wind, more satisfying nutrition time is provided for both mother and infant.
- Mothers are taught about the importance of 'breast-milking-only' that is during the first six months.
- Starting to additional supplements which consists of purees and liquid foods following the sixth month is told to parents. Mothers are further informed about the ingredients of these supplements and their methods.
- For game children, the child can stay with the game and ignore nutrition. In this case, the child shouldn't be forced to have its meal no matter how resistant it can get against eating (Baysal, 2002).
- Monitoring of height and weight of the children is recommended in order to make a nutritional assessment.
- The nutrition and physical activity habits of the children should be arranged to maintain their nominal body-mass (Baysal, 2002; Turkish Republic Ministry of Health, 2004)
- If the infant or child has over-weight problem, the family and child should be encouraged for increased physical activities and directed to a dietician if necessary (Baysal, 2002).

- For school children, the families should be informed about how to overcome unwillingness about breakfasts, which might be related to having snacks at school or developing the habit of meal skipping. For this sense, the children should never be allowed to leave their home without having breakfast, and they should be supported with a lunch-box if necessary (Turkish Republic Ministry of Health, 2004).
- It is crucial for balanced and efficient nutrition not to skip a meal, and not a single breakfast. Besides with the three-times a day main meals, extra nutrient consumption should be encouraged in between them (Turkish Republic Ministry of Health, 2004)
- The weight-reducing diets in adolescence which are carried out incorrectly cause malnutrition and further health problems may arise afterwards. The family and child should be confronted, and directed to a dietician where necessary. If desire to lose weight is found to be overwhelming, a psychiatric intervention is therefore required (American Heart Association, 2006).

Nutrition of a child is very important with respect to its development; its nourishment should not be overlooked beginning from the infancy.

Upon the delivery, the pediatric nurse should support establishing the mother-and-child bond, support and monitor the early-term breastfeeding, support and encourage the breast-milk-only period, help mother and infant stay in the same room, and help mother be supported by the father and the entire family. Moreover, mothers should be given information about mother milk and lactation mechanisms, suckling methods, infant care, practical solutions to frequent problems, nipple care, mother's self-care, nutrition and exercise. Any missing points should be identified by observing the mother's breastfeeding and they should be assisted to make sure they become self-sufficient (İnce, 2001; Pilleteri, 1999; Yıldız, 2001).

Special diagnosis instruments can be used to help determine an objective breastfeeding plan in the shortest time (Hamelin & McLeman, 2000; Yenal & Okumuş, 2003).

Regarding the prevention of emerging problems, nurses should play a very active role as instructors and advisors for mothers beginning from the delivery, in order to start and maintain a healthy breastfeeding period.

3. References

Adams, D. & Hewell, S. (1997). Maternal and Professional Assesment of Breast Feeding. Journal of Human Lactation. 13(4):279-83.

Allen, L. & Gillespie, S. (2001). What Works? A review of the Efficacy and Effectiveness of Nutrition Interventions, United Nations Administrative Committee on Coordination Sub-Committee on Nutrition, Asian Development Bank, September, ACC/SCN Nutrition Policy Paper No.19.

American Academy of Pediatrics (2003). American Academy of Pediatrics: Pediatric Nutrition Handbook. Committee on Nutrition, 3rd ed. Elk Grove Village, IL, American Academy of Pediatrics.

American Heart Association, Gidding, S.S., Dennison, C.B.A., Birch, C.L.L., Daniels, S.R., Gilman, M.W., Lichtenstein, A.H., Rattay, K.T., Steinberger, J., Stettler, N. &Van

Horn, L. (2006). Dietary Recommendations for Children and Adolescents: A Guide for Practitioners. Pediatrics. 117(2):544–559.

Arcasoy, M., Keskinoglu, A., Mir, S., & Taneli, B. (1994). Physical care and nutrition of infants, 1st edition. İzmir: Saray Medikal Yayıncılık San. ve Tic Ltd. Şti., Kanyılmaz Matb, ss. 269-273. ISBN: 975-7816-55-8.

Arslanoğlu, İ. (2009). Adiposity in infants and adolescents, an approach to this problem. Turk Arch Ped 44:115-119.

Aslan, D. (2007). The journal of maternal care and nutrition problems. 16 (6), VIII-XI

Baysal, A. (1993). General nutrition. 8. Baskı. Ankara: Feryal Matbaacılık San. ve Limited Şti. 9-11,103-41.

Baysal A. (2002). Nourishment. Ankara: Hatipoğlu Yayınevi.

Baysan, N., Dündar, P., Özgür, A., Aslan, M. & Marisal, S. (2009). The knowledge - behaviour - attitudes of the mothers of 0-24 months-old infants about breastfeeding and infant nutrition around a healthcare centre in the city of Manisa, STED. 18(1):1-7.

Beaudry, M., Dufour, R. & Marcoux, S. (1995). Relation between infant feeding and infections during the first six months of life. J Pediatri. 126:191-7.

Bellamy, C. (1998). Condition of infants in the world 1998. UNICEF. Ankara: Barok Ofset Matb.

Bertan, M. & Güler, Ç. (1995). Rudiments on public health. Ankara: Özışık ofset. ss. 294-302.

Bertan, M. & Özcebe, H. (1995). BObserving the growth". In: Yurdakök, M., Çoşkun T. (Edt). Pediatri. Ankara: Özışık Ofset. ss. 840-847.

Bilgel, N. (1997). Maternal and infant health from the viewpoint of public health. İstanbul: Hünkar Ofset Matb. ss. 233-36, 342-50.

Birol,L. (1997). Nursing Period, a systematic approach in nursing care. İzmir: Etki Matb. ss. 13-4.

Çavuşoğlu H. (2000). Paediatric nursing. 5. Baskı. Cilt: 1. Ankara: Bizim Büro Basımevi. ISBN: 975-94996-3-0, 975-94996-5-7.

Coşkun, T. (1996). Principles on infant nourishment. Katkı Pediatri Dergisi. Beslenme-I Özel Sayısı. Hacettepe Üniversitesi Tıp Fakültesi Çocuk Sağlığı ve Hastalıkları Ana Bilim Dalı ve Çocuk Sağlığı Enstitüsü Yayını, Ankara. 17(1):7-36.

Çetin, M. (2011). Anaemia in children. http://www.hamilebilgi.com/cocuklarda_kansizlik.html.

Çivi, S., Güler, S. & Tanrıkulu, Z. (1997). Diarrheic and URTI prevalence of the infants of 0-59 months old at Konya Cimenlik region, and their growth levels. V. Halk Sağlığı Günleri (Beslenme ve Yasal Durum) Bildiri Özet Kitabı. Süleyman Demirel Üniversitesi Tıp Fakültesi Halk Sağlığı Anabilim Dalı, Isparta. 8-10 Eylül. ss. 120.

Coşkun, T. (1991). Nutrition at the weaning term. Katkı Pediatri Dergisi. Anne Sütü Özel Sayısı. Hacettepe Üniversitesi Tıp Fakültesi Çocuk Sağlığı ve Hastalıkları Anabilim Dalı ve Çocuk Sağlığı Enstitüsü Yayını, Ankara.12 (5-6):630-636.

Dallar, Y., Tıraş, Ü., Ünsal, R., Gökay, S. & Bıyıklı, Z. (2007). Development of dehydration connected with breastfeeding problems at the newborn period, Türkiye Klinikleri J. Pediatr. 16: 238-44.

Demirçeken, F. G. (2011). Gluten enteropathy (celiac disease): a classical story and recent developments. Güncel Gastroenteroloji 15/1. Mart. ss. 58-72. http://guncel.tgv.org.tr/journal/ 36/pdf/100006.pdf

Egemen, A., Akşit, S. & Kusin, N. (1997). A danger often overlooked about newborn nutrition: incorrect watering of the infant formulations. V. Halk Sağlığı Günleri (Beslenme ve Yasal Durum) Bildiri Özet Kitabı. Süleyman Demirel Üniversitesi Tıp Fakültesi Halk Sağlığı Anabilim Dalı-Isparta. 8-10 Eylül 31.

Fuller, J. & Schaller-Ayers,J. (1990). Health Assesment A Nursing Approach. Philadelphia: J.B. Lippincott-Company. ss. 79-89.

Gökçay, G. & Garibağaoğlu, M. (2002). Nutrition of a healthy children, Neyzi O, Ertuğrul T (Editörler), İstanbul, Nobel Kitabevi, 183-203.

Hacettepe Üniversitesi Nüfus Etütleri Enstitüsü (2003). 2003 Turkey demographic and health survey. http://www.hips.hacettepe.edu.tr/tnsa2003.index.html

Hamelin, K. &McLeman, J. (2000). An Examination of the Use of an in Hospital Breastfeeding Assesment Tool, http://www.umanitobaca/womens-health/br-latch.htm.

http://www.scribd.com/doc/21717405/TNSA-2008-ana-Rapor-tr,172.

İnanç, N. & Hatipoğlu,S. (1995). Healthy family for healthy societies. Ankara.

İnce, Z. (2001). Nutrition with mother milk: concerns and solution approaches, 23. Pediatri Günleri ve 3. Pediatri Hemşireliği Günleri Özet Kitabı, İstanbul. ss. 126-7.

İnce, Z. (2001). Nutrition with mother milk: concerns and solution approaches, 23. Pediatri Günleri ve 3. Pediatri Hemşireliği Günleri Özet Kitabı, İstanbul 126-127.

Jensen, D., Wallace, S. & Kelsay, D. (1994). LATCH: Breastfeeding Charting System and Documentation Tool. Journal of Obstetric Gynecology Neonatal Nursing, 23(1): 27-32.

Jinabhai, C.C., Tay lor, M. & Sullivan, K.R. (2003). Implications of the prevalence of stunting, over weight and obesity amongst South African primary school children: a possible nutritional transition. Eur J Clin Nutr 57: 358-65.

Kavaklı, A. (1992). Growth and development at the infancy. İstanbul: Hilal Matb. 61-71.

Kilegman, M. R., Marcdante, J. K, Jenson, B.H. & Berhman E.R. (2008). Basic of pediatric. ss. 138-139

Köksal, G. (2007). Complementary foods and their significance in newborn feeding, Türkiye Klinikleri Pediatrik Bilimler Beslenme ve Metabolizma Hastalıkları Özel Sayısı. (3):6.

Lytle, L.A. & Ful ker son J.A. (2002). Assessing the dietary environment: examples from school based nutrition interventions. Public Health Nutrition. 5. 893-9.

Netsel, P., Briend, A, Benoist, B., Decker E., Ferguson, E., Fontaine, O. Micardi, A. & Nalubola, R. (2003). Complementary food supplements to achieve micronutrient adequacy for infants and young children. J Ped Gastr Nutr 36: 316-328.

Nielsen, G.A., Thomsen, B.L. & Michaelsen, K.F. (1998). Influence of Breastfeeding and Complementary Food on Growth Between 5 and 10 Months. Acta Paediatr. 87: 911-7.

Ok, Ş. (1991). The tendency of mothers applied to healthy child clinics to breastfeed, and determination of the underlying factors. Ege Üniversitesi Sağlık Bilimleri Enstitüsü. Yüksek Lisans Tezi. İzmir.

Oran, O. & Yurdakök, M. (1996). Feeding newborn infants, Ankara: Güneş Yayınları. ss. 32-9.

Özalp, İ. (1991). Mother milk as a nutritive. Katkı Pediatri Dergisi. Anne Sütü Özel Sayısı. Hacettepe Üniversitesi Tıp Fakültesi Çocuk Sağlığı ve Hastalıkları Anabilim Dalı ve Çocuk Sağlığı Enstitüsü Yayını, Ankara.12 (5-6): 510-20.

Özalp, İ. (1996). Mother milk and nutrition with mother milk. Katkı Pediatri Dergisi. Beslenme-I Özel Sayısı. Hacettepe Üniversitesi Tıp Fakültesi Çocuk Sağlığı ve Hastalıkları Ana Bilim Dalı ve Çocuk Sağlığı Enstitüsü Yayını, Ankara. 17 (1): 37-52.

Özgür, S. & Özgür, T (1994). Sosyal Pediatri. İzmir: Ege Ünv. Basımevi. pp. 209-228. ISBN: 975-483-235-8.

Pehlivanoğlu, E. (2007). Prebiotics and probiotics. Clinic Pediatri. 2 (2): 12-12. http://www.scribd.com/doc/60176255/3/Prebiyotik-ve-Probiyotikler. SSN: 1306-2131.

Perk, M. (1992). Nutrition healthı. In. Güçhan, N. Anadolu Üniversitesi Açık Öğretim Fakültesi Hemşirelik Önlisans Eğitimi. Halk Sağlığı Hemşireliği. Açık Öğretim Fakültesi Yayınları No:266. ETAM A.Ş. Web-Obset, Eskişehir. 250-70.

Pilleteri, A. (1999). The Nursing Role in Caring Fort the Family During the Postportal Period. Maternal and Child Health Nursing. Third Edition, New York.

Richard, J.S. (2001). Breastfeeding 2001, Part II. Pediatric Clinics of North America. 48:273 - 537.

Savino, F., Stefonia, A.L., Maria, F.F. & Roberto, O. (2009). Breast Milk Hormones and Their Protect Effect on Obezity. International Journal of Pediatric Endocrinology, November 4.

Schack, N.L. & Michaelsen, K.F. (2006). Breastfeeding and Future Health. Current Opinion in Clinical Nutrition and Metabolic Care. 9:289-96.

Stitzel F. (2004). Child Nutrition Programs Legislation. Top Clin Nutr. 19: 9-19.

Süoğlu, Ö.D., Fırat, A., Saner, G., Sökücü, S. & El kabes, B. (1999). ÇEffect of zinc supplementation during infancy to the growth. V. Ulusal Metabolik Hastalıklar ve Beslenme Kongresi Özet Kitabı. 15-18 Eylül, Balcalı-Adana. ss. 204.

Swift, W. J & Johston, H. F. (2007). (Çeviren: Evliyaoğlu N, Tahiroğlu A. Y.). Unusual behaviours, In: Robert M. Kliegman, Larry A. Greenbaum, Patricia S. Lye, (Ed), (Çeviri Editörü: Narlı N.) Pediatrik Tanı ve Tedavide Pratik Yaklaşımlar (Practical Strategies in Pediatric Diagnosis and Therapy), 2th Edition, İstanbul: Nobel Kitapevi, pp. 585-610. ISBN 978-9944-73-024-2 (Orijinal ISBN: 0-7216-9131-5).

Taşkın, L. (1997). Obstetrical and maternal nursing - extended 2nd edition. Ankara: Sistem Ofset Matb. ss. 381-97.

TC. Sağlık Bakanlığı, Ana Çocuk Sağlığı ve Aile Planlaması Genel Müdürlüğü, (1996). Booklet for the consultancy course about (nutrition with) breastfeeding, Ankara.

TC. Sağlık Bakanlığı Sağlık Projesi Genel Koordinatörlüğü, Temel Sağlık Hizmetleri Genel Müdürlüğü & Ankara Üniversitesi Tıp Fakültesi Çocuk Psikiyatrisi Bilim Dalı. (1996). A primer for mothers and fathers. Ankara: Aydoğdu Ofset. Mayıs.

TC Sağlık Bakanlığı Temel Sağlık Hizmetleri Genel Müdürlüğü, Hacettepe Üniversitesi Beslenme ve Diyetetik Bölümü. (2004). Nutrition guide peculiar to Turkey, Ankara.

Tershakovec, A. M. & Stallings, V. A. (Çeviren: Aydın, A.) (1996). Infant nutrition and nutrition disorders. In: Richard E. Behrmann, Robert M. Kliegman, (Ed), (Çeviri Editörü: Tuzcu M.) Nelson Essentials of Pediatrics Türkçesi, 2th Edition, İstanbul: Yüce Yayım, Alemdar Ofset, pp. 55-89. ISBN: 975-411-275-4

Tokatlı, A. (1996). Transition to nutritional supplements: nutrition at the weaning. Katkı Pediatri Dergisi. Beslenme-I Özel Sayısı. Hacettepe Üniversitesi Tıp Fakültesi Çocuk Sağlığı ve Hastalıkları Anabilim Dalı ve Çocuk Sağlığı Enstitüsü Yayını, Ankara. 17 (1): 64-72.

TUIK, Results of 2006 Poverty survey, http://www.tuik.gov.tr, Erişim tarihi: : 10 Aralık 2010

Tuncel EK, Dündar C, Pekşen Y (2005). Assessing the midwives' knowledge and applications regarding breast milk, Kocatepe Tıp Dergisi, 6: 43-8.

Tunçdoğan, İ. &Tunçdoğan, A. (2005). Çocuğumuz ve Sağlıklı Beslenmesi. Ankara ss. 257-258

United Nations Children's Fund UNICEF. (1994). The Basics of Maternal and Children Health. Ankara. ISBN: 92-806-3136-5.

Varol, N. & Koçoğlu,G. (1997). Effect of maternal education on the growth and development of the infants with low birth-weight. V.Halk Sağlığı Günleri (Beslenme ve Yasal Durum) Bildiri Özet Kitabı. Süleyman Demirel Üniversitesi Tıp Fakültesi Halk Sağlığı Anabilim Dalı-Isparta. 8-10 Eylül. ss. 93.

Weisstaub, G., Ara ya M. & Uauy, R. (2003). Community Nutrition and Its Impact on Developing Countries (The Chile an Experience). In: Walker, Watkins, Duggan. (Eds) Nutrition in Pediatrics. BC Decker Inc, Ontario. Third Edition, pp. 161-73.

Wilson, A.C., Forsyth, J.S., Greene, S. A., Irvine, L., Hau, C. & Howie P. W. (1998). Relation of Infant Diet to Childhood Health: Seven Year Follow Up of Cohort of Children In Dundee Infant Feeding Study. BMJ. 3, 316 (7124), Jan. ss. 21-25.

World Health Organization Report, (2010). www.who.int/whosis/whostat/EN_WHS10_full.pdf. sf: 45.

Yapıcıoğlu, H., Tutak, E., Yıldızdaş, D., Narlı, N., Evliyaoğlu, N. & Satar, M. (2002). Knowledge of nurses about breast milk, Attitudes of the Nurses on breastfeeding who are mothers themselves, Medical Network Klinik Bilimler, 8(1): 71-5.

Yaşar, A., Ilıca, B. & Rakıcıoğlu, N. (1999). A study with regards to the nutritional condition of the children attending to either private or state elementary schools in Ankara. Beslenme ve Diyet Dergisi. 28 (1): 28.

Yenal, K. & Okumuş, H. (2003). A study to analyze the reliability of LATCH breastfeeding characterization instrument, Hemşirelikte Araştırma Geliştirme Dergisi. 1: 38-44.

Yıldız, S. (2001). Responsibility of the nurse in breastfeeding, 11. Ulusal Neonatoloji Kongre Kitabı, Samsun. ss. 247-52.

Yurdakök, M. (1991). Breastfeeding and fathers. Katkı Pediatri Dergisi. Anne Sütü Özel Sayısı. Hacettepe Üniversitesi Tıp Fakültesi Çocuk Sağlığı ve Hastalıkları Anabilim Dalı ve Çocuk Sağlığı Enstitüsü Yayını, Ankara. 12 (5-6): 628-29.

Yurdakök, K. (1996). Breastfeeding. Katkı Pediatri Dergisi. Beslenme-I Özel Sayısı. Hacettepe Üniversitesi Tıp Fakültesi Çocuk Sağlığı ve Hastalıkları Anabilim Dalı ve Çocuk Sağlığı Enstitüsü Yayını, Ankara. 17(1):53-63.

6

The Growth and Development in Healthy Child

Şenay Çetinkaya
Pediatric Nursing,
Adana School of Health,
Çukurova University,
Turkey

1. Introduction

Child - our assurance for the future...

A healthy society consists of healthy families and healthy children. Therefore, healthy growth of children is important for society and for families. A healthy child is defined as the one who does not show any illness syndromes, but a steady body growth, physiological maturity and cognitive development (Çetinkaya & Conk, 2009; Kavaklı, 1992; Neyzi & Koc, 1983).

The term "growth" is used for defining a quantitative increase in the body or in some of its parts, whereas the "development" is used for functional changes including those which arouse from emotional and social interactions (Behrman & Kliegman, 1996; Beyazova, 1996).

Growth is product of various factors, thus, a complex situation. In this complex, the answers to genetic factors, nutrition, metabolism, endocrine system, and peripheral tissue are of great significance, and required for such a sensitive coordination (Arcasoy et al, 1994; Kandemir & Yordam, 1995). Starvation and inadequate nutrition cause resistance against the growth hormone (Kandemir & Yordam, 1995). In small children, malnutrition has a dampening effect for motivation and curiosity, limiting their desire to play games and make observations. Due to the decreased level of interactions with surroundings, mental and cognitive development of children are adversely affected (Bellamy, 1998).

The growth of head and brain tissues is closely associated with nutrition. This growth is accelerated particularly at the intrauterine period and within the 4 -5 years after delivery. At the age of 5, the brain tissiues are grown up to the 90–95% of an adult person's brain tissue. This period is important for the development of brain, intelligence, and mental state. The remaining 5 - 10% of development is achieved by the ages of 18 - 20 (Bertan & Guler, 1995).

For healthy and desired growth energy is required (Kandemir & Yordam, 1995). Hypothyroidism and hypopituitarism are of the most notable examples. Monitoring child's growth is essential for bringing up healthy generations.

To this end, regular checkups of infants and their measure analysis should be made carefully, while problematic situations that might arise from environmental factors should be resolved (Arcasoy et al, 1994).

A child requires emotional support and cognitive stimulation for an ideal growth. Parents and / or other caretakers have a profound significance in terms of responding to infant behavior and needs (Bégin et al, 1997). Today, it is commonly recognized that the distinction between growth and developments of the children who are lacking or away from parental love, and their peers who are having is notable, thus, significant (Arcasoy et al, 1994).

Monitoring of growth and development is not only meant for determining sick children, but it is a period in which the health officers are put into face-to-face situations with the infants and their families. During these interactions, a unique opportunity for parents is gained to resolve other health issues following a guidance in nutrition, vaccination, and topics alike. Maintaining continuity is important during healthy growth and development (Darendeliler, 2001).

Besides, parents need to be well-educated and well-aware to provide efficient support to their children, in the first place. Nurses, inevitably, play vital role in delivering a thorough, practical, and continuous training program for maintaining the infant development and health (Çetinkaya & Conk, 2009).

Pediatric nursing has holistic approach in nursing-care as it involves studying development and growth characteristics from delivery to adolescence, as well as observing deviation from health-norms according to systems (Cavusoglu, 2000).

2. Assessment of growth and development

The technique which is used for measuring body sizes is called anthropometric measurement. These anthropometric measurements are used to determine whether a child is underdeveloped or not compared to his peers.

a. Measurements used for assessing growth (gaining size)
1. Body scale
2. Stature
3. Head circumference, sutures, fontanels
4. Ratio of the body parts
5. Chest circumference
6. Stomach circumference
7. Pelvis circumference
8. The height of sitting
9. Sub-dermal thickness
10. Arm circumference
11. Calf circumference
b. Measurements used for assessing development (maturation)
1. The maturation degree of the bones
2. The age of tooth eruption and alteration
3. The degree of neuromotor development
4. Psychological development
a. Mental
b. Emotional
c. Social development
5. Sexual development

In the absence of precise definition of normal, the efficiency of child growth is determined by the comparison with others at the similar age and sex and whether there are harmony between growth parameters and the consistency of the growth parameters over time (Overby, 2003).

Body parts, head and chest circumference are more importantly clinical measurements (Bertan & Özcebe, 1995; Beyazova, 1996). These anthropometric measurements can be used in monitoring growth of children. However, it is usually a measurement of weight for the target age. It is a preferred method of assessment, because it is the first affected parameter of discontinuation of weight growing especially in the first two years of growth (Bertan &Özcebe, 1995).

We also need norms to interpret the values determined by measurements (Arcasoy et al, 1994). Weight, height, and head circumference parameters should be drawn on the National Center for Health Statistics (NCHS) growth chart and should be monitored according to standard growth rate (Keane&Fiegelman, 2007; Overby, 2003). Standard growth curve, primarily white, is formed by measuring different groups of middle-class children of all ages. When it is applied to children of different ethnic or racial origin these data can incorrectly identify their growth as abnormal (Overby, 2003). On this subject there are growth percentile curves developed by Olcay Neyzi and his friends for the children of our country (Neyzi et al, 1985; Neyzi et al, 1978). Measurements are compared to the norms taken from the general population to determine whether the infant is within the normal limit or not (Kavaklı, 1992). The research Çetinkaya and Conk did to determine the relation between mothers and growth-development knowledge on development statuses of the infants of 12 months in Malatya city center Turkey has shown that: With respect to weight, 3 % of the girls were under the 3 % percentile while 0.7 % of the boys were under the 3 % percentile. Length measurements indicated that 1.5 % of the girls were under the 3 percentile and 1.6 % of them were under the 3 % percentile. Mothers who were informed about infant growth and development were compared to mothers who were not. Results showed that 58% of mothers who were informed about infant care and 40% of non-informed ones took their infants to routine health checks ($p<0.05$). Due to the fact that mothers' level of information on growth and development of infants has a direct link with their taking infants to health checks, mothers must be informed on the subject (Cetinkaya & Conk, 2009).

2.1 Childhood periods

a. Prenatal Period

Embryonic Period (0 - 10 weeks)

Fetal Period (10 weeks-Until the birth=

b. Postnatal Period

Infanthood period (0 - 1 year)

Pre-play period (1 - 3 years)

Preschool period (3 - 6 years)

School period (6 - 12 years)

Preadolescence

10-12 years
12-14 years

Adolescence

12-18 years
14-20 years (Kavaklı, 1992).

2.1.1 0 – 1 year old child's physical motor and emotional

2.1.1.1 Intrauterine life to extra-uterine life transition

Massiveness and weight of the infant changes according to mother's body structure, the size of the uterus, birth order (2 or 3 children's birth weight is more than the first one. The body weight of a infant filled his gestation age and born mature changes according to racial and regional differences. In our country at Marmora region it is noted as 3,3 kg. Within 3-4 days of birth %5-6 of body weight of the child is lost. 10 days after birth, child replaces this loss and continues to gain weight on a regular basis (Kavaklı, 1992). Newborns gain 20-30 grams for the first 3 months and there will be ½-2/3 times more increase in weight for the next 3 months and ½-2/3 times more increase in weight for the next 6 months. The infant doubles its birth weight in 4-6 months and triples it before 12 months (Keane&Feigelman, 2007). It is proposed that a child's height is affected by two groups of independent genes each coming from mother and father. The first group determines the potential of child's growth. If the other factors are adequate after the child is 2 years old, there is an important degree of correlation between the child's height and the potential adult height. The second group determines the maturation speed of the organism, in other words the start of puberty and the termination age of growth (Kandemir & Yordam, 1995).

The height of the child is adjusted by the interaction between skeletal system and endocrine glands. The height of the mature-born infants is generally 50-52 cm. At birth a male child is longer than a female child because in the first 6 months of intrauterine life male children grow faster. Head growth reflects brain growth and development. The head is the fastest growing part of the body towards the end of fetal life and after birth. At birth the head and the chest circumference of a newborn are almost equal. At birth, chest circumference is 30.5-33 usually 33 cm (Kavaklı, 1992).

The birth of the first infant starts a transition to a new life for the family. This transition period is expected to be a joy by the parent. However they are not prepared for the stress that comes with the infant. They immediately recognize that they are sensitive and fragile in this period. The main task of the child and the family is the integration of a new healthy one to an existing family. In this process; the family has to accept the existence of the child, should provide the child's needs, should keep up the morale and should adopt the available resources. In a union each one of these values are usually a stress creator. The new pediatric nurse working with the family should keep in mind the causes of stress and should counsel to the family to solve their own problems. Nurse's relaxing the mother, helping her to overcome the causes of stress will help the mother to build up confidence and solve her problems. A healthy mother-child relationship does not occur spontaneously at birth, but mother and child from birth with the help of the nurse responded to each other by learning to develop over time.

A healthy mother-child relationship does not occur spontaneously at birth, but it is developed over time, with the help of the nurse, from the birth by mother and child responding each other. The early bound between the father and the child is also important. Father's and the other family members' positive contribution to the process will affect the mother and the infant in a positive way. Nurses can do a lot to create the atmosphere in which the family members and the child mutually affect one another (Foster&Anderson, 1989).

2.1.1.2 Infant (birth through 12 months)

2.1.1.2.1 Neonate (birth to 1 month)

Physical tasks

- Weight: 6-8 Ib (2750-3629 g) ; gains 5-7 oz (142-198 g) weekly for first 6 months.
- Height: 20 inches (50 cm); grows 1 inch (2.5 cm) monthly for first 6 months.
- Head growth
    - head circumference 33-35.5 cm (13-14 inch)
    - head circumference equal to or slightly larger than chest
    - increases by ½ inch (1.25 cm) monthly for first 6 months
    - brain growth related to myelination of nerve fibers; increases in size of brain reflects this process, reaches 2/3 adult size at 1 year; 90% adult size at 2 years
    - no control of muscles of the head
- Vital signs
    - pulse: 110-160 and irregular; count for a full minute apically
    - respirations: 32-60 and irregular; neonates are abdominal
    - blood pressure: 75/49 mmHg
    - poor development of sweating and shivering mechanisms; impaired temperature control
- Motor development
    - behavior is reflex controlled
    - flexed extremities
    - can lift head slightly off bed when prone
- Sensory development
    - hearing and touch well developed at birth
    - sight not fully developed until 6 years
    - differentiates light and dark at birth
    - rapidly develops clarity of vision within 1 foot
    - fixates on moving objects strabismus due to lack of binocular vision (Stein & Miller, 1997).

Utterance and Language Development: Newborn cries when it is restless and hungry. He responds to the strong sounds like doorbell, phone ring by stopping his own movement (Fenwick, 1993; Kavaklı, 1992; Mott et al, 1990).

Emotional Development: Each infant has a unique development. There are strong and weak sides of hereditary features. These features affect the child's relationships and his adaptability to environment. Parents' own childhood experiences, life challenges, intense pace of work, adaptation to the social and cultural changes and economic difficulties affect mother-father and child relationships. The parents taken care of the infant carefully, showing adequate interest and affection to the infant is due to parents' loving each other and being healthy and happy. The interaction of all these factors affects the infant's psychological development and forms individualism (T.C. Ministry of Health et al, 1996).

Psychosocial Development: At first, the infant's relationship with the environment is seldom. External stimuli are not much of a concern. He looks into the human face speaking to him especially the mother's face. He likes to be fed, taken on the lap, to be shaken on a crib. Following breastfeeding and the satisfaction of basic needs the infant feels satisfied.

Game: Position diversity. The mother should talk to the infant and should hold big and bright objects.

2.1.1.2.2 0-2 Months

The infant gains 20-30 grams in a day, 150- 250 in a week, 200 grams on average.

Nutrition: Breast-feeding or formula reinforcement.

Emotional- Social Ability: After breastfeeding and satisfaction of basic needs, the infant laughs.

Mental Ability: Reflex is active and the infant can produce the sounds of the vowels.

Psychosocial Development: Crying has a purpose. He responds to different stimuli by laugh of body movements. He starts to recognize the environment. Human faces, especially the mother's face, attract the infant and the infant starts to recognize the mother's face.

Producing Sound and Language Development: He makes sounds, listens to the sounds and produces his own sounds. His sounds are different from weeping. The infant responds to familiar sounds by producing sounds.

Security: Car carrier should be proper for the infant's use and sit.

Mother and Father-Related Activities: He recognizes the parents. He starts to produce sounds and Laughs spontaneously (Fenwick, 1993; Kavaklı, 1992; Mott et al, 1990).

2.1.1.2.3 2-4 Months

The infant continues to gain 20-30 grams in a day, 150-250 grams a week. The infant lengthens 8 cm in the first 3 months. The head circumference being 35 cm approximately at birth becomes approximately 40,5 cm in a three months infant.

Nutrition: Breastfeeding or formula reinforcement.

Physical Ability: Rolls back and wide, head and chest rises out of bed 45-90 degrees and the weight is supported in the arms, extends for the objects, follows the objects in mid-line, says meaningless words, and starts to localize sounds. Distinguishes the people.

Mental Ability: The imitation of the behaviors acquired by the ordinary activities. Localizing the sounds making sounds by shouting. Does not follow the moving away objects.

Cognitive Development: Provides an optical attention to somewhat complex stimuli.

Producing Sound and Language Development: Turns toward the sound of adults talking and reacts. When enjoyes it, makes sounds (like agu agu). Starts to differentiate the sounds. Cries less when he's awake.

Emotional-Social Skills: Laughs at familiar people, recognizes the non-primer caretakers.

Psychosocial Development: Very interested in environment. Quits crying when the mother comes in if he was crying. Identifies the familiar faces and items (mother's face, feeding bottle) Refuses the food he dislikes. Make sounds when rejoices (babbling). Likes breastfeeding, puts everything in his mouth. Likes music. Does not like being alone.

Game: Holding and speaking. Musical toys, polyphonic mobile. Color differences of the objects, the size and the structure; mirror, children's cot toys, the diversity of the environment.

Security: Not to be left alone in places such as bed, sofa. All small toys accessible should be removed (Fenwick, 1993; Kavaklı, 1992; Mott et al, 1990).

2.1.1.2.4 4-6 Months

Infant continues to gain 20- 30 grams per day. Gets 8 cm taller. His 50 cm height at birth becomes 66 cm at the end of 6 months gaining 8 cm for each 3 months. Head circumference is 43 cm.

Nutrition: Presentation of solid foods, first iron stock is used up.

Physical Ability: Birth weight is doubled, the teeth begin to appear slowly, with constant head and neck control the infant can sit, can roll back from belly, and can hold objects with a movement of grasp.

Mental Ability: Some conscious movements, some sensations, searching for the missing objects that are within sight, recognizing the objects that half parts are hidden, more systematical mimics, producing incomprehensible sounds.

Producing Sound and Language Development: Turns his head towards the sound to the ringing, or the familiar sounds. Reacts to sounds by producing sounds. Laughs out loud. The sounds vary according to whether the infant is happy or not. Listens to the conversation. Makes exciting sounds when sees the mother.

Emotional-Social Ability: Prefers primary care takers. The need for the breastfeeding is reduced. Laughs when it is appropriate. Takes pleasure in laughter.

Psychosocial Development: Doesn't like to be alone, like to be accompanied by people, wants constant affection. When sees the foot or hears the spoon rattle the infant rejoices. Shows excitement with his whole by curling, taking deep breaths or holding his breath

Game: Holding and speaking, game place should be provided for grasping and holding objects.

Security: Protected from safety hazards and environment; Toys should be checked for fragile parts.

2.1.1.2.5 6-8 Months

After the first 6 months the infant's putting on weight reduces a bit, 15- 20 grams per day, 100-200 grams per week it reduces approximately 150 grams. After the 3rd month the average weight increase appropriate for the age can be evaluated by this formula: Age (*months*) +9: 2 = kg. *E.g.* body weight of an 8 month infant:

(8 +9) / 2 = 8.5 kg.

Nutrition: Additional foods begin. A diet containing 4 basic nutrients are applied. After starting the additional foods, unseasoned meatballs can be served.

Physical Ability: Can sit solo, crawl, passes objects from hand to hand, and returns to the sounds coming from his back.

Mental Ability: Developments between 4-6 months continue.

Cognitive Development: The perception of consecutive relationships. Editing the right, accidental goals by using hand-eye.

Emotional-Social Ability: Distinguishes the non-primary responds. Stranger situation or breaking up anxiety.

Psychosocial Development: Look to his reflection in the mirror. Can feed himself by holding the infant bottle with both hands. Enjoys games. Makes unhappy sounds when his toys are taken from him. Likes to play with toy and the body parts like arms and legs of the people especially his mother's. Can distinguish foreigners from family members. Laughs out laud. Can sleep all night without any food. Emotional status is very variable. Can identify family members especially mother even if she is dressed differently. Begins to fear from strangers. Extends his arms to be cuddled. Can imitate sticking out the tongue and coughing. Footsteps of an upcoming person excites him. when his head is covered, he understands it is a joke and he laughs. Looks for a missing or thrown away toy for a while.

Producing Sound and Language Development: Likes to make sounds. Makes incomprehensible sounds. Chirps, chuckles. Responds to sounds and music by producing sounds. starts to imitate the sounds. Turns his head to the sounds coming from a horizontal position within 60 cm. Starts to imitate the rhythm of the sounds. Pretends to be talking while someone else is talking.

Game: Provides space for research . Hoards the toys.

Security: Infant's expanding environment needs to be controlled for dangers (Fenwick, 1993; Kavaklı, 1992; Mott et al, 1990).

2.1.1.2.6 8-10 Months

Nutrition: Liver or brain paste, spleen, pasta, stuffed with minced meat inside, rice can be started. 8-9 months of age, fish, and poultry can be started.

Physical Ability: Crawls, positions, makes forceps movement with his hands.

Mental Ability: Movements are intended for a goal, starts to solve basic problems with previously learned answers, searches for the actively lost object.

Cognitive Development: Target orders, the imitation of facial movements.

Producing Sound and Language Development: Listens carefully to the familiar words. Can produce syllables like "father", "ma-ma" and can associate them. Starts to produce consonants. Repeats sounds. Pretends to be talking with the toys.

Shouts to draw attention. Responds to simple commands. Understands the meaning of the word "No". Can recognize voice sources from 1 meter away even if it is diagonal. Makes incomprehensible sounds but understands a lot of words. Imitates the sounds. Starts to say "Father".

Emotional-Social Ability: Commitment completes the process of love.

Psychosocial Development: There is an increase in the fear of strangers. Shows signs of restlessness when his mother is out of sight. Imitates basic sounds and movements. Can repeat the movements that he likes. Starts to get attention by making sounds. Reacts to food that he dislike by closing his lips. Reacts when he is shown affection or he is rebuked. Knows the meaning of the word "No". Does not like his clothes to be changed. Can find the hidden toys. Likes to eat by his own hands. Can perform a simple verbal request. Starts to cry when his request is not fulfilled. For him the family especially the mother is very important. The desire to satisfy the mother is increased. Shows signs of fear when he is left alone or put into bed. Turns his arms into his face to not to shower.

Game: Storage and search, secretly looking, yelling like Boo, looking at pictures in a book.

Mother and Father-Related Activities: Can roll facedown while he is lying on his back. The word no inhibits him. Can walk aided by holding the furniture's. Carries out single-digit verbal orders like "come here", "give it to me".

Security: Needs to be protected. Electrical outlets, cords should be kept out of reach, stairs needs to be blocked, and tables should be arranged considering their potential dangers.

2.1.1.2.7 10-12 Months

In the first 6 months the infant gains 16 cm, in the second 6 months infant gains (4+4) 8 cm so a 12 months old infant, with the addition of the height at birth (50 cm), will be 16+8 = 24 cm. 50+24 = 74 cm (approximately)

After 3-6 months, children usually fit into their own growing pace and they grow by following their curve percentile of proper age.

At the end of the first year, the infant triples the birth weight and is 1.5 times taller than the birth height. Head circumference is approximately 46 cm when the infant is 12 months old.

Nutrition: Liquids more than solid foods, the use of cup increases, breast-feeding may start to wean.

Physical Ability: Weight birth triples. Stands on his own. Can use a spoon. Can walk around.

Mental Ability: Copycat behavior starts, but these behaviors are never seen before. Understands the words, can say 1 to 4 words, there is willingness and intent.

Cognitive Development: Problem-solving and experience for new information and searching for the mistake.

Producing Sound and Language Development: Responds on his behalf. Knows his parents by their names. Tries to produce familiar sounds by imitation. Understanding of the spoken words are developed. Establishes a link between the words he know and his actions. E.g. can perform the commands like stand, sit, walk. Knows the meaning of 3 words. Forms a sentence without using any real word.

Emotional-Social Ability: Starts to research, differentiates his family from the others.

Psychosocial Development:

10 Months: Understands the word don't and his own name. Imitates facial mimics. Understands games like "see ya" and performs it. Stands over his toy but does not give it away. Looks for a toy under the pillow or in another corner of the house. Repeats the movements that draw attention or make people laugh. Pulls someone's dress to draw attention. Play games such as hand flapping. Cries when he is rebuked by a grown up. Starts to show independent behaviors when it comes to dressing, feeding and motor skills. Can look at the pictures in a book carefully by turning over a few pages together.

11 Months: Shows signs of joy when a behavior is confirmed. Can roll the ball to someone else when it is asked. When hears a familiar music, tries to join it by body movements. Nods his head for no.

12 Months: Shows emotional behaviors like Jealousy, love, anger, fear. Can perform behaviors such as hugging, kissing when it is asked. Fears from foreign environment and immediately hugs her mother. An addiction to any toy or blanket may start (something reassure him) Knows a few words. Likes to say words or to pretend like talking even if it is not true. Learning and developing his abilities cover most of the day.

Game: Speech is increased; a book should be read for the infant. Name and body parts should be pointed out. Likes water, sand and ball games.

Mother and Father-Related Activities: Points out the objects he wants. Says one or two different words.

Security: Should not be left alone in bath tub. The use of the safety seat in the car is important. Should be kept locked and away from the doors.

2.1.2 1-3 Years old (toddlers) child's physical emotional and motor development

Toddler (just stated to walk) phase is approximately between 1 and 3 years. Toddler phase is identified as an independence gained by physical variability and increasing cognitive developments. Child rejoices by his success over his new motor abilities. Repeating movements can helps him master the new abilities. Unsuccessful behaviors can cause negative behaviors and moodiness. If these behaviors are blocked by parents', child's opposition is very common. Parents speak of this kind of restive behaviors during toddler years and at the same time when they develop independence in their child's behaviors; the child test his parents' nerves (Potter & Perry, 1993).

2.1.2.1 12-18 Months

Physical Development: In the early toddler years, child walks his belly up front; arms are spread for balance, in a vertical position. Walking up and down the stairs, kicking a ball and standing on one foot for a few seconds is evidence and gross motor skills continue to develop (Potter & Perry, 1993).

[Height (cm):2 + 9.5] ± 2.5 = cm

Height of a 12 months old infant is approximately 74 - 75 cm. According to that:

[(74/2 + 2) + 9.5] = 46.5 cm ± 2.5

Chest circumference, equal to hear circumference at birth, increases after the infant is 1 year old and gets bigger than the head circumference. Chest circumference is 47 cm at the first year. The belly is big in infancy because the liver is big and the pelvis is small. Abdominal circumference is larger until 2 years and bigger than both head and chest circumference. The bladder is an Intra-abdominal organ in infancy. With the expansion of the pelvis, abdominal organs get down and child's tummy starts to disappear. In infancy lower extremity development is very slow. It gets faster after the 1 year (Kavaklı, 1992).

The development of the skeletal system and healthy bone growth is not only important for the evaluation of development but also important to determine the child's health. Because bone maturation reflects the maturation of somatic tissue; the assessment of bone maturation degree is one of the best criteria to determine child's growth. It is also important to diagnose and to treat the diseases and deficiencies of child development and growth (Hathaway et al, 1993; Kavaklı, 1992).

Number of the infant teeth in the first two years is estimated by this formula:

The child's age (month) - 6 = Number of teeth

In 12-18 months sub-top-1st premolars, it is the time of the eruption of upper and lower canine teeth. Even if no bounds between the child's diet and tooth eruption are found, adequate and balanced nutrition for healthy teeth is important. Fattening of protein, calcium, phosphorus, vitamins C and E are also reported to be important for health teeth. Dental care for children less than 2 years old is done by parents with a toothbrush or gauze. Cardiopulmonary system is stable during toddler years. Hearth and respiratory rates are 24 respiration and 110 beats per minute. Both weight and height development speed is slow. Child's weight is 4 times more than his birth weight. Increase in height continues like a result of the length of the main leg during toddler years (Potter & Perry, 1993).

Language Development: Says 2-3 words knowing their meanings. Imitates the animal sounds. Infant calls items with their names. Points out them if he wants - can link up with 2 words. Infant knows approximately 50 words. Less than %25 of the speech is wise and makes sense (Kavaklı, 1992).

The family should talk to the child in a simple, understandable way in the process of learning how to speak. Small children sometimes try to explain what they want by crying instead of talking. This is because of their limited knowledge of vocabulary. Family and environment should be aware of child's inefficiency. Not to understand this situation, forcing the child to speak can create different emotional problems.

Sensory Motor: It is a trial and research phase between 12- 18 months.

Short stage: the indirect reactions of the third degree. Innovations are characterized by interests. He is creative, discovers new meanings by active attempts.

The objective continuity: Follows the translocation of observed objects.

Meaning-Result relationship: Uses trial and error learning method for learning. Discovery of new meaning by trying; uses systematic variations to create a new way to learn.

Plans (Behavioral reflex = scheme): Makes new social plan to show systematic creation with the new plan in special cases.

Game: Meaningful function, repetition of previously learned behavior to satisfy himself; works for amusement (Mott et al, 1990).

Expected Activities in the 12th Month: Walks independently. Says food and dadda meaningfully. Can use forceps to hold an object. Can fill the cubes into a cup after demonstration. Tries to make a tower from 2 cubes (Hathaway et al, 1993).

Mother and Father-Related Activities in the 12th Month: Points out the objects he want. Says one or two different words. Can walk with or without holding the furniture. Can play flapping or wave a hand. Can drink something out of a cup by himself. Can stand with or without support. Can say mum and dad even a few more words. Speaks in his own strange language. Can play ball, rolls the ball back to you. Can understand verbal commands without signs and adapt (Hathaway et al, 1993).

Expected Activities in the 18th Month: Can make towers consist of 3-4 cubes. Can throw the ball. Make spontaneous scribbles. Self-chair and sit. Can empty small objects from the bottle (Hathaway et al, 1993).

Mother and Father-Related Activities in the 18th Month: Can move up and down the stairs by assistance. Can say 4-20 words. Can understand 2 step commands. Hugs and carries the toy (Hathaway et al, 1993).

Child's fear of separation: Understands the difference between presence-absence of mother by remembering the presence. Child feels insecure, excited and scared. These fears begin at the age of 8 months, and reaches to peak at the month 15; the development of new capabilities facilitate the maturation of the central nervous system in an orderly manner toward the end of age 2, when this fear will be lost. Parents can provide objective continuity by putting a picture of the mother so that infant can see easily. This kind of object relaxes him (Hathaway et al, 1993; Kavaklı, 1992; Mott et al, 1990; Ozgur & Ozgur, 1994).

2.1.2.2 18-24 Months

Short stage: Innovations of new meanings. Although the basis of the ideas is mental composition; problem solving is the result of trial and error (Mott et al, 1990).

The objective continuity: Becoming aware of the continuity of objects; mental image of the lost object does not disappear (Mott et al, 1990).

Meaning-result relationship: The discovery of new meanings with being internalized. Agreement on understanding the inside story; foreseeing with the help of mental manipulation (Mott et al, 1990).

Plans: Even if the symbols have mental expressions, makes up new plan, combines them, his capacity for the use of mental symbols increases; names them.

Game: Increases the possibilities of game activities even if there are mental expressions. Game starts (Mott et al, 1990).

Nutrition: The decreased rate of calorie due to the slowing growth rate is accompanied by less food intake which makes parents worry about their child's food intake. Nurse can reassure parents by keeping the records of their child's growing rate on cards (Mott et al, 1990).

Toddler consumes 3-4 glass of milk apart from her mother's milk. Nutrition needs consist of 3 basic food group come together with solid foods. Taking 1 quart milk every day can create a loss of appetite for solid foods so nurses should limit parents for 28 ounce per day. That may reduce parents' anxiety (Mott et al, 1990).

Mealtime is not only important physically but also important psychosocially. If the parents dominate the toddler's food intake, problems may occur. Nurse should encourage parents to serve a mixture of solid foods. Toddler's taking his food between his fingers supports independence and his ability to eat on his own (Mott et al, 1990).

Cognitive Development: Toddler progresses from sensorimotor for pre- conception period of cognitive phase. In this situation child learns the objective continuity, starts to understand the progress and the effects of events in his memory. Thinks egocentric based and does not accept others' thoughts. Toddler often thinks about the dream and magic, and this is certain from the facial gestures (Özgür & Özgür, 1994).

Language Development (2 years): Says the words about his own needs (water, food, etc.). Makes 2-3 words of simple sentence. Vocabulary is increased. Knows about 300 words. Increased attention. Says about 10 words by understanding. Uses the pronouns "I", "You". There is a talk of Telegraph. Starts to learn the concept of time. Says the names of body parts such as eye, ear, and nose. %65 of his speech wise (Kavaklı, 1992).

Psychosocial Development: In toddler phase the child starts to gain identity. In this phase, also known as autonomy, the child gets independence from mother and likes to be with his peers.

Neuromotor development and manipulation ability is highly developed. Child is active and do thing on his own but family trust and intimacy is still important. Family, especially the mother does not support the child in a stressful environment, the resistance of child to stress and his curiosity to explore the environment decreases.

Children assisted to develop trust and autonomy are known to be socialized better. If the child's autonomy is not respected, we do not understand his emotional needs and cannot help him. The child develops emotions like "dependency, shame, doubt". In this situation child never trusts himself and becomes a problematic adult. Games and toys are literally his world and his most important development tool. He best likes the toys that he can do anything with it (bite, hit) (Mott et al, 1990).

Expected Activities in 24th Month: Forms small sentences, 2 or more words. Kick the ball when asked. Can make 6-7 small towers. Can tell the names and point out the objects. Can jump on both feet. Stand on one foot. Use pronouns.

Mother and Father-Related Activities: Can wear simple clothes. Turn the pages of a book. Play games by imitation (Hathaway et al, 1993; Kavaklı, 1992; Mott et al, 1990; Özgür & Özgür, 1994).

2.1.2.3 24-36 Months

Towards the end of the second year the growth rate gets stabilized at the rate of mid-childhood. Weight increase 2-3 kg/year, height increase 5-7.5 cm/year. The child reaches the half height of his or her adolescence at the second birthday.

Towards the middle of childhood after two years of age the head perimeter increases by 2 cm/year (Mott et al, 1990).

Most of the toddlers can run well at the end of 3. year and ride tricycle. Provided that their amazing motor abilities are encouraged they can do crossing and draw circles on their own. At third year children draw stick-shaped men and build castles from little blocks. Corrected (progressing) habit, the ability of taking off and the development of sphincter control are provided. Provided the child's required cognitive ability has developed the development sphincter control enables toilet training. Mother and fathers frequently consult with the nurses for evaluating the readiness (willing) of their children for toilet training. And nurses always remind mother and parents that patience, harmonization and a non-judging manner are important factors in toiler training as well as successful education (Mott et al, 1990).

Many healthcare professionals start the blood measurement routine at the age of 3 with baseline values which are only accepted for children. Standardized values for toddlers are still a matter of discussion; however normal measurements are 100/60 mmHG (Potter & Perry, 1993).

Piaget defines the period of 2-6 age as preoperational. This period starts with the easiness of mental image creating by language in symbolic context. Child learns how to manipulate the symbolic world. Child cannot distinguish between fantasy and real in definite terms. Dreams, desires and meaningless fears may make his or her blood run cold. World recognition is egocentric or gets interpreted through desires, needs and effects. Cause and effect relationship may be mistaken for temporal relationships or can be interpreted as egocentric.

Disease and medical care implications are interpreted in a different way in this period as well. Child relates one of his brothers' or sisters' getting sick to a recent discussion or a negative comment or may raise concern within himself or herself that he or she has wanted one of his brothers or sisters to get sick. And child feels guilty unless mother and fathers recognize that kind of interpretations and spend time to tell the truths (Potter & Perry, 1993).

Child bears humanistic feelings against material objects in this period as well. He or she thinks that human beings are also the reason and creators of natural events.

Also in this period, "sexual identity" starts to appear. Family image is gained with mother and father. The presence of both sexes is essential for child. This is the first reason which leads to objection issues between child and mother and father. Jealousness, rivalry and getting favored either by mother or father awaken guilt feelings in child. The concept of sexual feature, namely penis problem (penis desire in female children; the fear of penis loss in male children), appears as internal conflict. There is oedipal conflict in this period. Jealousnesses, aggressive urges, demand for punishment and the fear of castration appear. Overblaming and punishing child or preventing the child from engaging in his penis lead to sexual problems in the future (Mott et al, 1990).

Expected Activities: He can walk backwards. He can bounce on one leg. He can use prepositions in a sentence. He can imitate a rough circle. He can point to the objects which he learned by using. He can define himself as "I". He can hold crayons in his palm (Mott et al, 1990).

Mother and Father-Related Activities: Child helps with repositioning of goods. And he can maintain a mutual conversation (Hathaway et al, 1993).

Language Development: He makes sentences of 4-5 words. He roughly knows 900-1000 words and uses plural forms. He asks such questions as "who", "what" and "where". He still makes mistakes in grammar; but in a less proportion. Around 70-80% of his conversation is wisely made up (Kavakli, 1992).

Toilet training is almost finished towards the end of this period. The sleep duration (10-14 hours) decreases. He can slightly tolerate getting apart from mother. Motion and environment discovery has a critical importance. Any restriction in child's behaviors (disease etc.) for any reason is the worst thing that can possibly happen. Autism may increase the tendency of child for a depressive character. So unless really necessary preserving the child of this period in family environment, home treatment if possible or in case of an inevitable hospitalization accompany of mother in bed are really important in terms of emotional development and social harmonization (Mott et al, 1990).

2.1.3 Physical, motor and emotional development in the children of age 3-6

It is a transitional period between pre-school years, toddler period and school-age years. This period lasts from the age of 3 to 5-6. Many people consider this period as the most comfortable years of parents because child is less negative and shares more of his or her thoughts. While physical development progresses slowly cognitive and psychosocial developments progress fast (Potter & Perry, 1993).

Pre-school period is the one where basis habits are gained.

The value attached to child in this period helps him or her to form a good basis for personality development in further ages. Because even in the most appropriate environment, personality can develop after overcoming many problems and obstacles.

While a child of this age group tries to harmonize better, adapt to, his environment by developing new abilities he or she also confronts with new problems unique to his or her development period. In shirt, that is what we call getting mature (Kavaklı, 1992).

2.1.3.1 Age of 3-4

Physical Development: Some aspects of physical development keep becoming stabilized in pre-school period. Heart and breathing rate slowly decreases and respectively becomes as follows: 90 pulse/min and 24 breath/min. Blood pressure gets stabilized at 90/60 mmHg. Approximately weight increases by 2.7 kg and height increases by 2.5 cm annually.

Muscular coordination improves. A child of pre-school age runs well and can easily run up and down the stairs and learns how to bounce.

Child needs opportunities to learn and apply these skills. Nursing in healthy and diseased children enables includes creating that kind of opportunities and evaluation. In spite of the fact that children with acute disease benefit from resting and getting away from daily routine activities children who have chronicle conditions or stay in hospital are in continuous need of developmental opportunities. Parents and nurses can alter these opportunities in accordance with the talent, energy, requirement level and daily routine of child (Potter & Perry, 1993).

Language Development: He knows 1500-2100 words. He has better command of grammar. He sets up sentences with any kind of grammar. He uses past tense. He asks many questions. He recognizes types of money. Mostly all of his or her conversation is widely made up (Kavaklı, 1992).

The Concept of Place and Location: He can tell the locations of goods and whether or not they are in their place. He commands by orders. He knows the location of goods: above, below, near. He can tell the name of his home street. He knows where to direct upon entering street. He can recognize whether something is cut in halves or not (Özgür & Özgür, 1994).

The Development of Balance and Motion Functions: He walks and climbs up stairs really confident in himself. He can easily walk backwards, stand on one leg, walk along one line and turn upper part of his body while seated or standing. He better commands his body and is skilled at his hands.

He can throw and catch the ball, ride tricycle, add up building woods, unbutton, play with a infant, eat well with spoon without dirtying his clothes and take off his shoes. He can also copy such simple shapes as circle and triangle (Wechselberg & Puyn, 1993).

Psychosocial Development: He wants to be independent. He is inpatient. He is aggressive in the way he speaks and behaves, envies his sisters or brothers, get angry to his mother and father. He has a quite variable emotional condition. He likes getting praised, making people laugh and cheering them up. He likes to tell inter-family issues to outsiders by exaggerating them. Games have a really important place in this period. He plays imaginary games: he indicates sex difference in such games as "Doctorship", "Nursing" or being "Father", "Mother". Sexual interest and showing their genital organs are frequently seen in this period (Kavaklı, 1992).

Game: Game teaches children how to act charitably with no thought of personal gain and get pleasure from it.

A child conscious of it will also learn to put up with many self-devotions with no thought of personal gain.

Child learns to come to the forefront or to get drawn to background from time to time. So the tolerance, self-devotion and friendship with his friends that he shows in this age form the basis of commitment, self-devotion that he will make to his friends or spouse within family in the future.

They are best at role playing games. They adjust the environment at their pleasure. He acts the roles of things that he observes around his environment such as people, animals, goods, mother, doctor, grocery etc.

He operates his observation and recalling skills in these games and his imagination and thought horizon are broadened. He puts the things he visualizes by various roles in an order and forms them. And by this way he gets more experienced and does not only imitate people; but also put himself in their place.

This role playing game assists children with overcoming his problems on his own. He tries to pleasure his desires which are kept under pressure in reality via games.

He also re-experiences some of the events in which he has been involved but not able to figure out in games. Child needs not to be disturbed especially during these times. Because child manages to overcome his sufferings and his troubles during the game (Wechselberg & Puyn, 1993).

Expected Activities: He can climb up the stairs by switching his legs. He starts to button and unbutton. "What would you like to do as something fun?" (He responses to questions with plural verbs and personal pronouns). He responds to such commands as putting a toy into a container, on the table or under the table. He draws a circle when he is asked for drawing a human being (male, female). He knows his own sex ("Are you a boy or a girl?"). He can tell his name properly. And he can copy the ready drawings ("Can you draw one like this?").

Mother and Father-Related Activities: He can eat his meals on his own at meal times. He can take his shoes and jacket off (Hathaway et al, 1993).

2.1.3.2 Age of 4-5

Physical Development: Approximately weight increases by 2.7 kg yearly. And he gets 24.3 kg until the age of 5. His height increases by less than 2.5 cm. Height increase is up to the increase in legs. Their chest girth is 55 cm at the age of 5 (Kavaklı, 1992; Potter & Perry, 1993).

Language Development: Child cannot find the required words when he tries to explain an event which has excited him or a dangerous event or a demand to his father and mother and he starts spelling them over and over. This spelling over and over cannot be considered as stammering. The child's speaking abilities are not as fast as thinking abilities in such conditions.

Stammering is mostly mistaken for lisping or clipped speech. Being unable to pronounce correctly and pronouncing certain syllables incorrectly cannot be accepted as stammering. And besides, most of the children cannot pronounce some words correctly; e.g. "I'm taking a baf" instead of "I'm taking a bath" or "The wion wawed" instead of "The lion roared".

That the child cannot pronounce a single syllable correctly does not necessarily mean that the case will be the same in the future. After a certain time the child will correct this mispronounced letters on his own.

While lisp speech is not something which is frequently seen it can also not be regarded as something very important. It is not an indication of any failure. All malfunctions generally disappear by themselves towards the end of fifth year.

Father and mother should not emphasize on psychological stammering and lisping. In case that the child's attention is attracted to this situation or that if he or she is tried to get corrected by getting criticized the harmless stammering may turn into a real speech disorder, which means that the child may become stammerer (Wechselberg & Puyn, 1993).

The Concept of Place and Location: Age of 4: He or she gets better at defining adverbs of location and quality (deep, below etc.). He plays hide and seek. He runs in front of an adult. If a place is described he can tell its direction from house. He can play construction games in up and side directions.

Age of 5: He gets interested in distant places. He can describe the way and nearby locations. He obeys to such commands as forward and backward. He can distinguish between such things as thin, fat and slightly deep (Özgür & Özgür, 1994).

The Development of Balance and Motion Functions: From now on child can practically imitate any motion in a game and runs confident and with no fear. He also competes with his friends and can keep himself balanced at height. He hides, climbs and can easily ride a tricycle and drive a car. He gradually gets better at gripping, holding, throwing, playing, drawing, putting on and off (Wechselberg & Puyn, 1993).

Psychosocial Development: Discussion and objections starts to decrease. He is too busy with doing his own works and playing game. His fears partially decrease. The independence begins. But he still needs assistance in putting on and cleanup. He starts to act either as a man or a woman and to learn the codes of society. He wants to obey the rules of game; but can also trick when he realizes that he will lose. He may complain in small injuries. And in serious cases he tries to appear brave and mature. He likes watching television. He gets better at understanding television programs. As his eye-hand coordination is not at required level he cannot concentrate on close studies or small pictures. He wants to utilize real things in games. He likes using real plate instead of paper or real flour instead of mud and sand and etc (Kavaklı, 1992).

Game: He generally starts playing games which we can name as social plays which are played as groups and reflect the behaviors of grown-ups. He finds speaking opportunities. These speaking activities assist child with stimulating and training qualities and abilities which lead to social maturity (Wechselberg & Puyn, 1993).

Cognitive Development: A child of pre-school age proceeds in preoperational period (gets mature in that period). The continued egocentrism (self-centeredness) of early thinking makes difficult for child to present acceptable alternatives. With the increased use of maturation, experience and symbolic way of thinking he starts to take others' opinion and gets less egocentric (Potter & Perry, 1993).

Mental and Psychological Development: Stubbornness period gradually loses its pace. And the second phase of question asking starts this time. He asks such questions as "why is this like this?", "how is it done?" and "why do I have to do this?". His intelligence also improves in parallel with the advancement in speaking. He wants to create his own early by constantly asking question and to organize it. This period can also be called as "fantasy" period and may last until the launch of school. The requests of children are under the effect of some things. In their way of thinking, goods have such a power that it affects people. Children see the events in the way they want to see them and proceed in their own worlds as very confident of themselves. And the world of fables makes a match of these childish beliefs and thought. The child's ability of fantasy reaches its peak in this period. The child learns how to act independently and to adapt with the environment in this period as well.

The strong interest in environment and the education need are the most distinct features of this period. Child learns to recognize the reality better. In spite of that there happens unexpected and surprising changes in child's views. Child may give his mother a piece of wood which he earlier accepted as a ship for burning in oven (Wechselberg & Puyn, 1993).

Expected Activities: He can run and spin without any imbalance. He can stay on one leg for like 10 seconds. He can fasten and tie his shoes (but cannot button). He can count up to 4 by heart. "Give me 2 of them". (He can choose and then give 2 of 4 breads). He can draw a man (it usually consists of a head, two bumps and probably two eyes; yet no body). He knows the days of a week ("Which day is after Tuesday?"). He can give proper answers to the following questions: ("What do you do when you get sleepy, hungry and feel cold?"). He can make + sign by imitating.

Mother and Father-Related Activities: He can meet his toilet need on his own (may need assistance for wiping). He can play for at least 30 minutes outside. He can put on his own except for buttoning process (Hathaway et al, 1993).

Concept of Time: Being not that conscious, he can talk about past, future and present at the age of 4. He knows that sun rises in the morning; and moon at night. He has no concept of season. He relates hot and cold with the concept of season.

He knows to direct himself within time and location in order to live in a reasonably stabilized world at the age of 5. He can tell his age and the days of a week. He cannot recognize the concept of death. Talks about earlier people do not make an impression on him. He wants to finish what he starts and dramatizes natural events. He adds sun, moon, cloud etc. to his stories (Potter & Perry, 1993).

2.1.3.3 Age of 5-6

Physical Development: His birth height usually doubles at the age of 6. The average height is 105 cm. As a result of this slow downed growth nutritional needs get relatively stabilized.

When he reaches 6 he can catch, throw or bounce the ball. His improved subtle motor abilities enable him to accomplish delicate manipulations. Child can make circles, X signs and copy square or triangles. These abilities enable him to write letter and numbers (Potter & Perry, 1993).

Language Development: He roughly knows 3000 words. He can clearly explain his thoughts. He uses such words as: "in case", "because", "why" and "the reason". Such concepts as size, weight and distance improve (Kavaklı, 1992).

In this period the child speaks so fast and urgently that he may speak swallowing some syllables and even some part of sentence apart from syllables. This condition can be overcome provided that required emphasis is addressed (Wechselberg & Puyn, 1993).

The Concept of Place and Location: While home is his focal point he also pays attention to moon, sun and sphere. He recognized right and left in his way. He can tell the names of his favorite and nearby locations. He gets afraid of getting lost when he does not use the regular route. He can draw a small labyrinth with his finger (Özgür & Özgür, 1994).

The Development of Balance and Motion Functions: Child is as command of his motions as grown-ups. He learns such difficult tasks as threading a needle, putting on, bathing, drying, teeth brushing and eating on a table on his own. He also goes to toilet on his own. And it is not difficult for him to learn to ride a bicycle. He can draw simple shapes in detail and paint human being, animal, house, three and automobile.

He can now tie his own shoes. His working abilities do also improve with the muscle strength required for heavy efforts and patience in short time.

Psychosocial Development: He changes his attitudes towards his mother. He really loves her; but he always blames her for anything wrong and hates her in a minute. He envies his sisters or brothers. However he really likes to listen to his infanthood stories. He still needs assistance with bathing. He likes to play in a bathtub; but does not really like his face and neck to get washed. He must be reminded of washing his hands and face before meals. Such accidents as spilling on his clothes or table cloth can frequently be observed. He is more rapacious than he is hungry for foods. Where his playmates or regular friends are from or at which class they are studying does really not concern him. He plays better with counter sex; but slowly starts to choose friends of the same sex (Kavaklı, 1992). The fables that he takes pleasure show variety. While male children like legendary and heroic fables; female ones like fairy and queen fables (Özgür & Özgür, 1994). The biggest problem at this age is that children do not know where to stop while playing games without any physical and emotional damage. A child of 6 can generally be described as a sweet, explorer and investigator kid.

The parents and the people around should give almost real-like answers to the questions that children are asking about their bodies. The processes should be explained in a simple and short form. The effects of parents, teachers, friends and the other people around are really important in creating these concepts on children either in a good or bad way.

That something is cut or removed from their body do really frighten children. So it will be more appropriate to tell a child who is to be circumcised or to have tonsillectomy that these parts will not be removed; but rather be cleaned up and corrected. Children of this age get aggressive against outflow of their blood even in unimportant scratches and injuries and cries "I will run out of all my blood, it flows". Children of this age group are really afraid of blood-drawing and get panicked in such cases. Particularly nurses should be well aware of their approaches against the children of this age group staying in hospital and sympathize with their fears and know the issues of their development period and contact them considering all these facts (Kavaklı, 1992).

Game: An interest in collection, collecting something special, appears in children during this period (Wechselberg & Puyn, 1993).

Cognitive Development: Intuitive thinking replaces egocentrism until the ages of 5 and 6. Pre-school child can solve the problems at an increasing rate by thinking one sided.

The world knowledge of a pre-school child is closely related to structural experiences. Pre-school period is based on the child's recognition of real world via his or her imaginary rich world. In case that two of them are confused by a child it mostly leads to childhood fears. In fact when a child reflects the truth from his own perspective it is generally interpreted as a lie by grown-ups. Early instant thinking improves in pre-school years. Thinking is transductive process, which means that cause and effect relationships interact within each other. If two events are related with each other in terms of time and place child (in terms of cause) relates one to another. For example a child staying in hospital may come up with such a result: "I cried last night and that's why nurse gave me injection." Children around the age 5 start to learn the rules to understand the causes. And then the child starts to draw a conclusion from the general to the specific. That is what forms the basis of logical thinking. Now the child thinks like that: "I daily get two injections. That is why I got another shot last night."

The moral development of a pre-school child also includes a social understanding of proper and improper behaviors. At the same time the child keeps getting motivated by the desire of avoiding from punishment and the wish of a reward. The basic distinction between this phase of moral development and the children of 1-3 age is that pre-school children are better at recognizing which behavior deserves punishment and which behavior deserver reward and start tagging these behaviors as proper and improper.

When a nurse makes preparation for a treatment of a pre-school aged child he or she should consider the fact that whether the child comprehends what is being told (Potter, & Perry, 1993).

Mental and Psychological Development: He establishes better relationships with his environment. His world gets enlarged and he feels in safety around home. The child interacts with other children and makes new playmates this way.

He learns the concept of discipline and to adapt to environment. Child gets away from egocentrism and starts to compare himself or herself to other children. He learns to praise the works of others.

The emotional connection of child to his father and mother gradually decreases as result of joining to new groups and to the society. The child established his own measurement independent of his or her trainer's measurement for good and bad.

He recognizes the worth of money and starts to lose his belief in wonderland or something like that. He can distinguish sexes easily. They show interest to their sex roles. It is very important that boys act as a father or girls act as a mother in terms of healthy development of personality and especially accepting duties necessitated by their sex in the future.

Expected activities: He can catch a ball. He can jump smoothly. He can copy a drawn + sign. He can say his age. His concept of '10' improves (he can count 10 sticks). He can count large numbers by heart. He knows which one of his hands is at right or left. He can draw a human being with at least eight details of him. He can describe his favorite TV program with some details.

Mother and Father-Related Activities: He can do trivial housework (like dumping, wiping up). He can go to school alone or can get in school bus. He is good at motor abilities; but not good enough to be aware of dangers (Hathaway et al, 1993).

Advices to Parents for the Development of Sense of Personality: Encourage children to be independent. Make things easier for them. Want them to help you. Let them decide themselves. Make your children feel special. Often indicate that you love them. Respect their feelings and supply with their needs. Show interest and praise them for their each success. They should learn scolding as well as appreciating. Listen to them curiously while they're talking to you.

2.1.4 Physical, motor and emotional development of school-age child

It should not be forgotten that growing to school maturity requires not only the development of intelligence but also internal, emotional and social maturation. Merely developing the intelligence and underestimating the psychological, emotional and social development mean preventing development of the child's personality and perhaps, the necessary development for school. The child should not be interfered while playing various games, he/she should be prepared to be together with his/her peers and the child should be assisted to enter a new period of life, in other words the school age, without dreading on his/her own (Wechselberg & Puyn, 1993).

It is unfavorable to school the children who develop slower than their peers and are not able to conduct the study that school requires yet, before developing needfully. Otherwise, the child encounters with the problem of failing the class even in the first years. The failure of this type of child does not only cause him/her to be a nervous wreck but also affects his/her behaviors, and it is observed that the child becomes coward, angry, bad-tempered and aggressive (Wechselberg & Puyn, 1993).

Through starting the school, the child leaves the confident environment where he/she recognizes as home and family, and starts to live in a totally new world , full of friends, learning and adventure, for the first time. The world of school is a world that the child cannot entirely share with his/her parents. It is required to support him/her affectionately and try to understand him/her (Platin, 1991).

2.1.4.1 In general at 6-12 years old

Their pulse and breathing rate decrease generally and the blood pressure increases (Newman, 1995). The respiration rate is 19-21. /min. On the other hand the blood pressure is 120/75 mmHg at 6-9 years old (Yigit, 1992). The pulse is 75-115/min (Newman,1995).

Physical Development: The 6-year-old child is different from the pre-school period. The schoolchild is taller and more slightly built than he/she is in pre-school period (Foster et al, 1989).

The child gains 2.5-3.2 kg/year at 6-12 years old which is the schoolchild period (Kavaklı, 1992).

6-12 year olds= Age (Year) X 7 /2 = kg. A 6-year-old child is 20-21 kg (Kavaklı, 1992).

Along with the body and limbs, he/she gets longer by 5.5 cm per year. While he/she loses his/her milk teeth, he/she grows teeth continuously. The skills of coordinated movement and fine motor keep developing. The continuance of growth raises calorie requirement (Foster et al, 1989).

Mental Development: He/she manages definite tasks. The girl or boy behaves egocentrically although he/she is not always right. He/she learns to express his/her emotions and opinions verbally and in written. His/her vocabulary is 3000 and more, he/she makes complex sentence (Foster et al, 1989).

Emotional and Social Development: The child after 6 years old begins to side against the social groups. He/she opposes firstly his/her home, then the society. He/she defends the opposite opinions of the people around. .from now on "the second age of opposing" has begun. At the same time, this is a dangerous age in which this child who goes to school, is not able to know what to do. Also, the precise settlement of truths within the psychism of the child begins in this period (Ozgur & Ozgur, 1994).

He/she lives some crises such as inferiority complex regarding the things that he/she's done and he/she wants to do. The requirement of sex education continues. He/she likes to be with his/her friends, competition is important. He/she is afraid of that his/her body will become permanently disabled and his/her body image will change; he/she may have a phobia and have nightmare. Neurotic behaviors are common (Foster et al, 1989).

Nutrition: His/her appetite fluctuates because of the variability in the activities and the modification of the growth process. There is a tendency of disregarding breakfast due to the hurry of getting to school. Although lunch is provided in many schools, the children do not eat those foods (Foster et al, 1989).

The preferences of child regarding the foods may change frequently. Moreover, the children's food habits begin in the periods of pre-school and school age. The children in this period are curious about buying foods out and trying new different foods. It is required for the family to be sensitive about teaching positive behaviors (Yigit, 1992).

Game: He/she plays group games with his/her fellows and team activities are dominant. They read books at all ages. They like cycling. They are fond of sports equipment. They play card games, board games and table games. Most of the games are active games that do not require equipment or less equipment (Foster et al, 1989).

Safety: It should be kept using safety belt during the travel on the car. Cycling can be taught to him/her and applied. Handicrafts and hobbies with the mechanical tools are taught by providing safety (Foster et al, 1989).

2.1.4.2 Age of 6-7

Physical Development: The excellent development of motor coordination is better than the motor skills. He/she is better good at balance and rhythm, running, jumping, climbing, leaping and speeding. He/she catches and hurtles the ball. He/she wears clothes without help or a little help by his/her own (Foster et al, 1989).

Mental Development: He/she has a vocabulary of 2500 words. He/she learns reading and writing, and begins to be familiar with certain concepts and numbers. He/she knows right-left, morning-noon-evening and money. His/her intuition power improves. He/she likes simple games with simple rules. He/she is verbally aggressive, hectoring, quarrelsome and self-opinionated (Foster et al, 1989).

Emotional and Social Development: He/she is jovial and sympathetic; he/she avoids conflicting with mother and father due to his/her choices. At the age of 7, he/she is silent and thoughtful, and very sensitive. He/she uses telephone. He/she likes to do something, starts to do many things and finishes only some of them. He/she fulfills some responsibilities that the household gives (Foster et al, 1989).

Nutrition: The pre-school child does not like persistence on foods. His/her nutrition has a tendency of showing the deficiencies of riboflavin, vitamin A and iron. The daily water requirement is 100 ml/kg and the daily protein requirement is 3 g/kg (Foster et al, 1989).

Game: They like infant doll, toy car and toy truck. In the games, they prefer to play with both genders in small groups. At about age of 7, they prefer the same gender. They learn cycling. They prefer to pretend with real costumes and dream. They collect for the quantity by not caring the quality. They play active games such as ice-skating, martial arts and hide-and-seek. They are ready to learn music, dance and gymnastics. Their television hour should be restricted to 1-2 hour/day (Foster et al, 1989).

Safety: Safety in traffic should be taught and supported. There is still a need for adult supervision in the games. Staying away from the strangers and avoiding getting something from them should be taught. Prevention and curing of the diseases and other habits for healthy life should be taught. Cycling at home should be restricted, should not be allowed in traffic and cycling safely should be taught. The harms of drug use, alcohol and cigarette should be taught (Foster et al, 1989).

Expected Activities: He/she can copy a triangle. He/she can define the words according to their uses (What is an orange? "It is for eating"). He/she knows that it is morning or afternoon. He/she can draw a human picture with its 12 details. He/she can read the words containing monosyllable. He/she uses pencil to write his/her name (Hathaway et al, 1993).

2.1.4.3 Age of 7-8

Physical Development: His/her weight increases by 1.4 - 2.7 kg (each year). His/her height increases by 2.5 - 5 cm (each year) (Newman, 1995).

Social Development: The rule of pleasure weakens over against the rule of truth, and the sign of a more realist tendency is observed on the child. The child tries to make classification, multiplication and summation in series (Ozgur & Ozgur, 1994).

Psychosocial Development: The age of 7 is a more serious, self-aware, less negative, less problematic, self-enclosed, gentle, dutiful and emotional age. He/she is fond of speaking, speaking bitingly and discussing. The child is sometimes fond of staying alone and having a his/her own room. In addition to not liking bathing so much, he/she can bath on his/her own. He/she likes to wear his/her old clothes. He/she does not have a preference. He/she wears everything that is purchased for him/her, he/she sheds the clothes that he/she took off on the ground or couch, he/she is messy. He/she should be reminded to go to bed. He/she may take along a toy or object which he/she likes or thinks that it assures him/her. He/she sometimes thinks that everybody opposes him/her. He/she complains about his/her family. He/she thinks that he/she is misbehaved and his/her family adopted him/her. He/she wants to escape from his/her family and house. In essence, he/she desires the intimacy and interest of his/her family very much. He/she is admires his/her elderly brother/sister. If he/she has a younger sister, he/she looks after and protects her, but he/she frequently quarrels with her and he/she is mostly jealous of her very much. His/her relations with mother are better, compared to the age of 6. However, the child at this age is closer to father. The games with friends and group games are very important. The consent of the friend interests him/her very much. His/her place in the group and his/her popularity is important for him/her. Female-male discrimination has started to differentiate also in the games. In this period, the child may attach to the opposite sex emotionally. He/she likes his/her school, teacher and reading very much. He/she is fond of reading books and magazines, particularly adventure books. The thoughts of his/her teacher interest him very much. The child at this age is shy. He/she is embarrassed of the changes in his/her body and does not like being touched. Since other people's thoughts and behaviors interest him/her very much, he/she is very sensitive to criticism and jeering (Kavaklı, 1992).

Expected Activities: He/she can count in 2's and in 5's. He/she can do up his/her shoelace. He/she can copy rhombus. He/she knows which week day it is (does not know the date and the year). He/she can sum and subtract the one digit. He/she can draw the picture of a man with 16 details (Hathaway et al, 1993).

2.1.4.4 Age of 8-9

Physical Development: He/she may not see the close. The girls begin to show interest to opposite sex. Hand-eye coordination and fine motor skills have developed. He/she is active and easy going. He/she meets his/her all physical needs. He/she is busy with constant movements, games and hard work. It is difficult to poise the balance between resting and motion (Foster et al, 1989).

The changes in the body ratio are clearer through the gradual loss of the body fat and the longer growing of the crotch line (Newman, 1995).

His/her weight increases by 1.4 to 2.7 kg (each year). His/her height increases by 2.5 to 5 cm (each year) (Newman, 1995).

Mental Development: He/she knows the meanings of the words and learns grammar according to its rules. He/she reads the books that he/she likes alone, examines the newspapers and reads funny texts. He/she draws the things that he/she likes in detail. He/she makes numerical, serial, physical and central classifications. He/she uses the language as word games, slogan, joke, riddle etc. He/she sets up the rules in his/her life. Everything including the rules in work life, how and what is weather, seasons etc. are very interesting (Foster et al, 1989).

Emotional and Social Development: He/she has a good communication with fellows, but he/she is negative against the opposite sex. He/she is self-confident and practical at home; he/she questions the opinions and values of his/her mother and father. He/she likes camping, being out with large groups, group activities and climbing. He/she is modest regarding his/her body; he/she is aware of gender. While working, he/she is careful and shows his/her best skill. He/she is happy, collaborative and he/she is active and easy in family relations. He/she uses the manner of adults and he/she is gentle. The team spirit is at upper level; secret rules and rituals have become prominent. It is better to give suggestions rather than dictatorial approach (Foster et al, 1989).

Psychosocial Development: It is an age in which he/she has opinions about everything, advises everybody and defends himself/herself against the critics of his/her teacher, family and siblings. He/she wants to learn the reason of the events happening in the world and in his/her environment. He/she is ready for everything. He/she is curious and always has hurry. He/she is very busy and active. His/her interest for collection is extreme. He/she collects everything. He/she is willing to establish relationship with the other people in his/her environment. He/she likes to observe and watch the conversations and social activities of the adults very much. He/she likes to play with his/her fellows. He/she feels both love and hate for the opposite gender. He/she begins to a game or work in an ambitious and zippy manner. On consequence, he/she may fail, and abandon himself/herself to despair and cry. He/she likes travelling, seeing new places, having new experiences and new friendships. In general, he/she is loyal to his/her engagements. He/she is at that place in time. He/she can totally wear his/her clothes by himself/herself and likes to choose his/her clothes. He/she is careless, untidy and impatient. His/her sleep is qualified. However the time for going bed should be reminded. He/she is social. His/her behaviors are more positive compared to the age of 7. But it is required to develop them more. He/she is curious about helping the people and being approved and praised by them. 8-year-old child writes texts about sex, and whispering, giggling and laughing regarding this subject are very frequently observed at this age. He/she does not like to be alone and always wants to be with his/her friends and other adults. He/she is the first person who has finished the meal, he/she is precipitant. He/she does not chew the food, in fact swallows. He/she gets on with everybody at home. Especially, he/she needs the close interest and understanding of his/her mother. In addition to preferring mother, his/her love for father has increased. He/she gets on with his/her siblings and loves them. He/she is sensitive to the problems of the family. In case of any stress, he/she shows the behaviors from infanthood such as rubbing his/her eyes nail-biting and eating with hands. He/she is fond of working with father like repairing and helping him. This age is an age in which the friend is more important than the family and he/she is willing for learning and contacting with the people around him/her (Kavaklı, 1992).

Nutrition: His/her nutrient requirement is 2100 cal/day. He/she tends to slur over both meals and thiamin, calcium and iron may be deficient. Adiposity problem starts in this period. He/she can help to prepare food (Foster et al, 1989).

Game: He/she likes walking sports. He/she is attracted by cooking, woodworks and handicrafts. He/she likes card and table games. He/she likes listening to radio and cassette. He/she begins to collect qualitatively. The restriction of TV should be kept (Foster et al, 1989).

Safety: Safety in firearms should be taught, they can be allowed to search and see them only under the control of the adults. Mother and father should be aware of who their child's friends are, and the family should eliminate few bad friends. Swimming should be taught safely under the control of the adults (Foster et al, 1989).

Expected Activities: He/she can define the words better than their usage form (What is an orange? "It is a fruit"). He/she can give proper answers for the questions. He/she improves his/her reading. He/she learns operations in summing and subtracting such as "carry…" and "we take 1 from…" (Hathaway et al, 1993).

2.1.4.5 Age of 9-10

Physical Development: .A 9-year-old-child weighs 30-32 kg. Furthermore, his/her height increases 6 cm (Ozgur & Ozgur, 1994).

Social Development: Self-criticism begins indefinitely in a 9-year-old-child. At the age of 10, he/she can criticize his/her mistakes (Ozgur & Ozgur, 1994).

Psychosocial Development: The girls at the age of around 9 are more portly and mature. This makes the child restless. Hereafter the gender difference is clear. She is aware of the changes in her body. They do not want to show their bodies even to their mothers. Most of the girls know menstruation and discuss this issue with their friends. The child wants to recognize its body better and know the functions of his/her sexual organ better. Both genders have begun to keep their rooms and clothes tidier. The child of this age generally finishes the work that he/she started. He/she can give decision more quickly and easily. He/she generally does what he/she wants rather than what he/she should do. He/she is rebellious against the authority. He/she thinks that his/her family is less important than friends. He/she strictly opposes against their behaviors. He/she is not so much interested in the family, but he/she likes being together and travelling with them very much. He/she wants to have role in family's decisions. He/she becomes very happy by helping his/her mother while she is very busy. In general, he/she is on very good terms with his/her siblings. Going to bed should be still reminded to him/her. He/she understands the things, being told very well. He/she understands the subjects like pray, religion well and can apply them. He/she wants to do the work ideally. He/she likes complicated table games and organized games much more. His/her hobbies have started. He/she likes listening to historical events. It is the age of listening story, tale and adventure. He/she is fond of reading these kinds of books. He/she is social. He/she can be disciplined easily. His/her feelings of empathy and sympathy have developed. He/she may have somatic complaints in case of stress (Kavakli, 1992).

Expected Activities: He/she knows the month, day and year. He/she counts the months respectively. He/she learns simple multiplication operations (Hathaway et al, 1993).

2.1.4.6 Age of 10-11

Physical Development: Gaining weight and development-growth are observed in both genders. Especially, the development and gaining weight are more distinctive in girls compared to boys. It is observed that the girls show more progress than boys in terms of both gaining weight and maturation. This situation may lead anxiety in both genders in terms of many things (Kavakli, 1992).

The pulse is between 70 and 110/min at the age of 10. Breathing rate is 19/min. The blood pressure is 112/64 mmHg (Newman, 1995).

Psychosocial Development: The child indicates a slight transition from the age of 9 to the age of 10. The child at this age is cheerful and happy, it is the age in which he/she likes the physical activities like running, jumping. He/she is excited. He/she likes reading exciting adventurous books such as detective stories, and likes watching these types of films. He/she is closer to family compared to the age of 9. He/she gets on with his/her parents. He/she shows respect to his/her family and their roles. His/her relation with his/her siblings between 6-9 year-old is not so good, but he/she likes his/her younger sibling, if any, younger children and animals very much and protects them. The role in the group games and activities is given according to the gender difference. It is an age in which long lasting, special and intimate friendships are established. He/she cannot know that he/she is tired and when he/she should go to bed. His/her body position while sitting at the table and studying is not good. Continuous reminding may be required. He/she expresses his/her happiness and love explicitly. He/she gets angry and blazes quickly, but this continues very shortly. When he/she gets angry, he/she cries, but he/she never likes being consoled. His/her appetite and health are pretty good. He/she can tolerate stress better. He/she does not want to be alone. He/she argues with the family for everything. His/her relation with his/her father is better. He/she is not on good terms with his/her siblings. However he/she is attentive to choosing friends and getting on with them. He/she is frequently jealous of his/her friend. The sense of shame is considerably high in the child at this age. The boys are annoyed very much and become embarrassed when their mothers kiss them in the presence of their friends or guests. The gender difference is clear. Since the physical growth is not most often parallel with the social and emotional maturation, dumps exist for the children who appear older than their age. Because the child cannot display the behaviors that an adult and the society expect from him/her. His/her interest in money has formed. The desire for being financially independent from the family has begun. In case of stress, he/she turns in on himself/herself, he/she only holds his/her mother. In this period, it is essential to guide the child, establish a clear and understandable relation, help him/her to accept his/her role peculiar to his/her gender, encourage and guide him/her regarding the skill-oriented games and works. Hence the school and the family should be in good relations (Kavakli, 1992).

2.1.4.7 Age of 11-12

Physical Development: Their life symptoms have gotten close to the adults'. For girls, growth has increased; the inequality between the genders, particularly physical power in boys has increased much more (Foster et al, 1989). The girls tend to grow more rapidly than the boys and this comes clearly before two years. The child who feels his/her difference from his/her peers negatively, feels the need to be relieved about that loneliness (singularity) is normal in the growth period (Newman, 1995). Except 3rd molar teeth, all the teeth have been grown. The interest to the opposite gender has begun among boys. The girls may menstruate (Foster et al, 1989).

Mental Development: He/she can have opinions and prejudices about the social problems; this is understood from the others' standpoint. He/she likes strange stories and love tales. He/she begins to be interested in the abstract of opinions. Human health and reproduction are very interesting for him. He/she is more ethical, faithful and responsible in this period (Foster et al, 1989).

Emotional and Social Development: The loyalty to a group is strong; the boys begin to tease the girls and the girls flirt with the boys in order to take attention with their best friends. They want independency. They are rebellious in routine works; their state of mind is fluctuating; they sometimes prefer loneliness in a day. They criticize the works very much. They chat with their friends about the realities of life. Masturbation increases (Foster et al, 1989).

At the age of 11, the limits of criticism broaden and also they begin to criticize the tasks that others gave him. He/she considers about the applications that he/she had and ranks them according to their values. The logical tendency begins to be dominant over thought, judgment and decision. Girls and boys form groups among themselves and they are alienated from common games. While the boys like sport and cycling, the girls like meeting with her friends. The girls at this age enjoy some behaviors such as wearing the same clothes and acting similarly (Ozgur & Ozgur, 1994).

Psychosocial Development: He/she is easy going and relaxed. He/she can control himself/herself, his/her attitude toward the events is more positive. He/she likes himself/herself and the world. He/she is happy. He/she likes making jokes. The child likes difference and variety. Although they do not keen on money so much, they want to earn. They keep their money well. They like talking and try to talk to an adult about any subject. They are good friends for talking. Their interest in the opposite gender has increased. They like to talk about this subject. In particular, the boys are fond of the games and social activities (dance, party etc.) where both genders participate. It may be necessary for the families to control the parties. Their relations with family are pretty good. Their arguments with the family and their requests from them have decreased. They expect their family to show respect to their privacy. He/she less often quarrels with his/her siblings at the age that is close to him/her age. A very young sibling bothers him/her. He/she quietly gets on with his/her siblings at pre-school period and gets along well with them. He/she has a special respect and sympathy for his/her elderly sister/brother. His/her relations with friends are very good. He/she can change his/her friends. For example, while he/she is interested in his/her friend, he/she can have another friend. Although they like groups, they sometimes want to be alone. Their interest in reading has lessened a little. Their interest in outdoor activities and sport has increased. Collecting occupies significantly for the child at this age. If he/she is tired in case of stress, he/she displays extremely nervous behaviors (Kavakli, 1992).

Nutrition: While the daily calorie requirement is 2500 cal/day for boys, this is 2250 cal/day for girls. The daily requirement for water is 75 ml/kg and the daily requirement for protein is 2 g/kg (Foster et al, 1989).

Game: They like the works conducted manually. They like working and running errands in order to learn about money. They want to play sports, dance and call. They like plays and any active things (Foster et al, 1989).

Safety: He/she continues to observe his/her friends; the safe cycling in the streets and traffic should be emphasized (Foster et al, 1989).

3. Conclusion

The challenges today's pediatric nursing faces in providing care for children and their families require skills from a wide spectrum of both technologic and psychosocial arenas. To meet the needs of the child and the family in a variety of settings, the nurse must have a thorough understanding of disease processes, as well as knowledge of emotional, social, cultural, and developmental needs.

To provide this essential knowledge base, this unit begins with a review of growth and development, which is basic to understanding the behavior of children and the influences of illness.

The pediatric nursing includes a holistic approach in terms of nursing criteria by studying the normal growth- development and health problems in a child, from the birth to adolescence (ages of 0-18) according to the systems which are used.

The medical officers who deal with children must know the stages of child growth and development, the theories which are related to the growth and development and to identify and evaluate the factors that affect this process positively or negatively.

It is important to evaluate the growth and development in a healthy child. In order to do that, the medical officers who are responsible for the child health, should at least know the growth and development features according to critical periods in childhood.

4. References

Arcasoy, M., Keskinoğlu, A., Mir, S., & Taneli, B. (1994). Physical care and nutrition for infants. 1. Baskı. İzmir: Saray Medikal Yayıncılık San. ve Tic Ltd. Şti., Kanyılmaz Matb, 228-268. ISBN: 975-7816-55-8.

Bégin, F., Habicht, J.P., Frongillo E.A, & Delisle, H. (1997). The Deterioration In Children's Nutritional Status In Rural Chad: The Effect of Mother's Influence on Feeding. Am. J. Public Health. 87 (8) Aug. 1356-1359.

Behrman, R.E. & Kliegman, R.M. (1996). Essentials of Pediatrics, 7th. Ed., America: W.B. Sounders Company, pp. 1-34.

Behrman, R.E., Kliegman, R.M. & Jenson, H.B. (2000). Textbook of Pediatrics, 16th. Ed., America: W.B. Sounders Company, pp.23-61. ISBN-10: 0721677673, ISBN-13: 978-0721677675

Bellamy, C. (1998). Condition of children in the world 1998. UNICEF. Ankara: Barok Ofset Matb.

Bertan, M. & Güler, Ç., (1995). Public Health Basicsr. Ankara: Özışık ofset. ss. 294-302. ISBN: 975-7467-26-X

Bertan, M. & Özcebe, H. (1995). Monitoring the growth. In Yurdakök, M., Çoşkun T., Pediatri. Ankara: Özışık Ofset. ss. 840-847. ISBN: 975-7467-25-1.

Beyazova, U. (1996). (Çeviren). Development and behaviour at infancy. In: Behrman R. E., Kliegmen R. M., Nelson Essentials of Pediatrics. Second Edition Türkçesi. ss. 1-55. ISBN: 975-411-275-4.

Curry, D.M. & Duby J.C. (1994). Developmental Surveillance by Pediatric Nurses. Pediatric Nursing. 20 (1) Jan/Feb. ss. 40-44.

Conk, Z. (1992). Development and adaptation in the families having adolescents. Ege Üniversitesi Hemşirelik Yüksekokulu Dergisi, 8(1):41-48.

Çavuşoğlu H. (2000). Paediatric nursing. 5. Baskı. Cilt: 1. Ss. 18-27. Ankara: Bizim Büro Basımevi. ISBN: 975-94996-3-0, 975-94996-5-7.

Çetinkaya, Ş. & Conk, Z. (2009). Growth and development of twelve-month infants in central Malatya. Turkey, İnönü Üniversitesi Tıp Fakültesi Dergisi. 16(2):95-100.

Darendeliler, F. (2001). Inspection of Growth - Booklet of the 1st National Congress on the Maternal-Infant Health. Ankara Üniversitesi, Tıp Fakültesi Çocuk Sağlığı ve

Hastalıkları Anabilim Dalı, Halk Sağlığı Anabilim Dalı, Kadın Sağlığı ve Hastalıkları ve Doğum Anabilim Dalı, T.C. Sağlık Bakanlığı Türk Tabipleri Birliği. ss. 150-161.

Ersoy, B. (2006). Vitamin & Mineral requirement and use at the adolescence. Türkiye Klinikleri Dergisi, 2(11):121-126.

Fenwick, E. (1993). Maternal and infant care. ABC kitabevi A.Ş., İstanbul, Ankara, İzmir.

Foster, R.L.R., Hunsberger, M.M. & Anderson, J.J. (1989). Family-Centered Nursing Care of Children. W.B. Saunders Comp. ss: 167-246. ISBN-10: 0721612229, ISBN-13: 978-0721612225.

Hathaway, W.E., Groothuis J.E. & Paisley J. W. (1993) (Çeviren: Sarialioğlu F, Yurdakök M, Kutluk T, Çalıkoğlu AS). (Current Pediatric Diagnosis and Treatment), 1. Baskı. Cilt: 2. Ankara: Barış Kitapevi. ISBN/ISSN: 975-95331-0-3 (Orijinal ISBN-10: 0838514294, ISBN-13: 978-0838514290).

Kandemir, N. & Yordam, N. (1995). "Growth and affecting factors". In Yurdakök, M., ÇoşkunT., Pediatri. Ankara: Özışık Ofset. 90-97.

Kavaklı, A. (1992). Growth and development during adolescence. İstanbul: Hilal Matb., pp. 61-71, 226-229.

Keane, V. & Fiegelman, S. (2007). (Çeviren: Taşkın E, Kılıç M). Growth Retardation and Malnutrition, In: Robert M. Kliegman, Larry A. Greenbaum, Patricia S. Lye, (Ed), (Çeviri Editörü: Narlı N.) Pediatrik Tanı ve Tedavide Pratik Yaklaşımlar (Practical Strategies in Pediatric Diagnosis and Therapy), 2th Edition, İstanbul: Nobel Kitapevi, pp. 233-247. ISBN 978-9944-73-024-2 (Orijinal ISBN: 0-7216-9131-5).

Kliegman, R.M., Marcdante,K., Jenson, H.B. & Behrman, R.E. (2006). (Çeviri) Ovalı F. Nelson Pediatrinin Temelleri. 17. Baskı, İstanbul: Nobel Tıp Kitapevi, ss.15-33.

Mott, S. R. , James, S. R., & Sperhec, A. M. (1990). Nursing Care of Children and Families. Second Edition. Addison-Wesley California New York. pp. 180-181. ISBN-10: 020112923X, ISBN-13: 978-0201129236.

Newman, J.T. (1995) Pediatric Nursing (Clinical Rotation Guides), Springhouse Clinical Rotation Guides. Springhouse Pub Co. pp 20-24. ISBN: 0874347378/0-87434-737-8.

Neyzi, O. (1995). Relations between the nutrition of 0-5 year old infants and the period of growth. Sürekli Tıp Eğitim Dergisi. 4 (10) Ekim : 334-37.

Neyzi, O., Binyıldız, P., Alp, H., (1978). Percentile growth curves of the Turkish children (0-36 months) Tartı-Boy. İstanbul Tıp Fakültesi Mecm., 41: Suppl. 74.

Neyzi, O., Günoz, H., Percentile growth curves of the Turkish children (0-18 months). Baş Çevresi. (Basılmamış).

Neyzi, O. & Koç, L., (1983). Paediatric health and illnesses. İstanbul Üniversitesi Tıp Fak. Yayınları. İstanbul: Bayda Yayını. ss. 232-243.

Overby, J. (2003). Çocuk Sağlığı İzlemi, In: Abraham M. Rudolph, Robert K. Kamei, Kim J. Overby, (Ed), (Çeviri Editörü: Yurdakök M.).Rudolph's Fundamentals of Pediatrics Türkçe, 3th Edition, Ankara: Güneş Kitapevi, pp. 1-69. ISBN: 975-8531-56-5.

Özcebe H. (2002). Attitudes toward the problems of adolescents at the primary healthcare. STED, 11(10): 374-377.

Özgür, S. & Özgür, T (1994). Sosyal Pediatri. İzmir: Ege Ünv. Basımevi. pp. 234-246. ISBN: 975-483-235-8.

Özmert, E.N. (2005). Supporting the early-infant development-I: Nutrition. Çocuk Sağlığı ve Hastalıkları Dergisi,48(2):179-195.

Öztürk, O. (1989). Mental health and disorders. 2. Basım. Bayrak Matb. İstanbul. 79-84.

Platin, N. (1991). Some important highlights when your child begins the school. THD. Cilt: 40, Sayı: 1-2. Ocak-Temmuz, ss. 55.

Potter P. A. & Perry A. G. (1993). Fundamentals of Nursing Concepts, Process and Practice, Infant. St. Louis, MO: Mosby YearBook, pp. 489-490.

Savaşer, S. & Yıldız, S. (2009). The guide of paediatric health and illnesses for nurses, 1. Baskı, İstanbul: İstanbul Medikal Yayıncılık Ltd. Şti. ss. 186-190. ISBN: 978-9944-211-76-5.

Stein, A.M. & Miller, J.C. (1997). NCLEX-RN REVİEW. Third Edition. National Student Nurse's Association. A division of International Thomson Publishing Inc. 351-65.

TC. Sağlık Bakanlığı, Çapa Çocuk Sağlığı Enstitüsü, UNICEF WORKSHOP'u. 27-31 Ocak 1992.

Türkiye İstatistik Enstitüsü (2009). General census of Turkey: population with respect to age and gender, population size of the administrative regions according to age group and gender. Access: http://www.tuik.gov.tr/VeriBilgi.do? tb_id=39&ust_id=11. Erişim tarihi:1.03.2010.

Üstün, B. (1990). Family affairs at the adolescence. THD. Cilt: 39, Sayı: 2, Mayıs-Eylül 1990, ss. 29-30.

Wechselberg, K. & Puyn, U. (1993). Mother and child at the prenatal - delivery - postpartum period. 6. Baskı. Remzi Kitapevi.

Whaley L.C. & Wong D. L., (1987). Nursing Care of Infants and Children. Third Edition. The C.V. Mosby Company. St. Louis Washington D.C. pp. 541, 563-65.

World Health Organization. (2010). Child and Adolescent Health and Development, Erişim:http://www.who.int/child_adolescent_health/topics/prevention_care/adolescent/en/index.html. Erişim tarihi: 01.03.2010.

Yiğit, R. (1992). Growth and development of the children at the age of elementary school. THD. Cilt: 42, Sayı:4. Ekim-Kasım-Aralık. ss. 37-40.

7

Probiotics for Autoimmune Diseases: Is There a Benefit?

Öner Özdemir[1] and Azize Yasemin Göksu-Erol[2,3]
[1]*Department of Pediatrics, Division of Allergy / Immunology, İstanbul Medeniyet University, Göztepe Research and Training Hospital, Istanbul*
[2]*Suleyman Demirel University Medical School, Dept. of Medical Genetics; Isparta*
[3]*Afyonkocatepe University Medical School, Dept. of Histology&Embryology; Afyonkarahisar, Turkey*

1. Introduction

Experimental and clinical trials of probiotic use as capable preventive and therapeutic strategy in different diseases varying from allergic to autoimmune disease have recently reported. Probiotics are used in allergic disease, which have shown to be beneficial in some patients with atopic dermatitis and allergic rhinitis [1]. Based on the hygiene hypothesis, it has been theorized that changes in human intestinal microflora in developed societies cause an increase in the prevalence of autoimmune disease (AD) besides allergies [2]. Regulation of intestinal microflora composition by probiotics may offer the possibility to influence the development of mucosal/systemic immunity as well as ADs. In this article we will consider the etiology of AD and its relation to gut and environmental microbiota (hygiene) before discussing the mechanisms of probiotic effect and the beneficial effects that they may confer to individuals with AD.

2. Brief pathophysiology of AD: What causes an AD?

The immune system normally acts to ensure tolerance to 'self', but a breakdown in the tolerogenic pathways has been hypothesized to lead to AD that may result from loss of tolerance to self antigens in general. A breakdown in the tolerogenic pathways can also lead to other so-called inflammatory diseases e.g. atopic and inflammatory bowel disease (IBD). Allergic disease may result from loss of tolerance to food and environmental antigens; IBD may result from loss of tolerance to commensal bacteria within the intestinal tract. The main characteristics of IBD and AD are tissue destruction and functional impairment as a consequence of immunologically mediated mechanisms which are principally the same as those functioning against dangerous (pathogenic) infections. In case of ADs, a major effort was done in understanding pathogenetic mechanisms leading to the loss of tolerance to self components (autoantigens). Despite the fact that target antigens and the genetic basis of several ADs are now better understood, the initial events leading to a loss of tolerance towards self components remain unknown. One of the most attractive explanations for autoimmune phenomena has always centered on various infections as possible natural events capable of initiating the process in genetically predisposed individuals.

The most accepted conventional hypothesis explaining how infectious components cause autoimmunity is based on the concept of cross-reactivity, "molecular mimicry". This hypothesis assumes a similarity between the epitopes of an autoantigen present in the afflicted organism and the epitopes in the environmental antigen. The latter may consist of a microorganism or another external antigen that causes the autoimmune response. The other hypotheses in the AD pathogenesis such as hygiene-old friends- hypothesis, bystander immunoregulation and T regulatory cell (Treg) defects are briefly discussed below as well.

Because of our long association with environmental organisms (old friends), they are recognized by the innate immune system as harmless or, in the case of some helminths, treated as "friends" because a response would merely lead to immunopathology [2]. Therefore, rather than priming aggressive immune responses, these organisms prime immunoregulation. They do it by inducing an unusual pattern of maturation of dendritic cells (DC) such that these retain the ability to drive Treg. Toll-like receptor 2 (TLR2) may be involved for helminths and TLR9 for lactobacilli. It is interesting that polymorphisms of NOD2 (an intracellular receptor for bacterial peptidoglycan) are linked to increased susceptibility to both Crohn's disease and asthma [3]. Thus an extension of the "hygiene" mechanism suggests that in an environment that less actively primes Treg activity, immunoregulatory disorders will occur first in those individuals whose innate immune systems are least efficient at driving Treg.

The increased regulatory dendritic cells (DCreg) and Treg induced by "old friends" then lead to two immunoregulatory mechanisms mediated in part by release of IL-10 and TGF-β. Firstly, continuing exposure to "old friends" will cause continuous background activation of Treg specific for the "old friends" themselves, resulting in a constant background of "bystander suppression" [4]. This mechanism has been demonstrated in a model of colitis. Secondly, DCreg inevitably sample self and gut contents and so induce Treg specific for the target antigens of the groups of chronic inflammatory disorder. These mechanisms may be aborted when there are legitimate "danger" signals. For example, Treg function can be turned off by appropriate "danger signals" in vitro [5].

The unifying hypothesis explaining the simultaneous increase in T helper type 2 (Th2)-mediated allergies and Th1-mediated autoimmunity is that modern living conditions can lead to defective maturation of Treg and regulatory antigen presenting cell or DCreg [6]. Therefore, rather than Th1/Th2 balance, the crucial factor is likely to be the effector T cells/Treg balance. Thus diminished immunoregulation can lead to inappropriate immune responses to allergens, gut contents, or self. In the absence of optimal levels of immunoregulation, the individual may develop a Th1-/Th2-mediated inflammatory disorder, depending on his/her own particular Th1/Th2 bias, immunological history, and genetic background. Evidence to confirm this hypothesis has come from studies of allergic disorders, MS and autoimmune polyglandular syndromes [6].

3. Any role for hygiene (environmental microbiota) in AD development?

According to the old 'hygiene (old friends) hypothesis', the decreasing incidence of infections in developed and developing countries is at the origin of the increasing incidence of allergic diseases [7]. New practices, introduced as a result of industrialization, such as childbirth by surgical delivery, ingestion of pasteurized food, cleaner homes, and indiscriminate use of antibiotics and so on, have led in recent years to the replacement of probiotics by other microorganisms that are not as well adapted to the microenvironments of the human body. The hygiene hypothesis is based upon epidemiological data, particularly migration studies, showing that subjects migrating from a low-incidence of infections to a high-incidence country acquire the allergic and immune disorders with a high incidence at the first generation as well. Therefore, it was possible to extend the old hypothesis from the field of allergy, where it was formulated, to those of ADs such as T1D or multiple sclerosis (MS) [7,8]. However, some data and others showing a correlation between high AD incidence and high socio-economic level do not prove a causal link between infections and immune disorders. Part of the increased incidence of these diseases may be somewhat attributed to better diagnosis or improved access to medical facilities in economically developed countries. However, this cannot explain the marked increase in immunological disorder prevalence that has occurred over such a short period of time in those countries, particularly for diseases which can be diagnosed easily, such as T1D or MS.

Proof of principle of the hygiene hypothesis is suported by animal models and to a lesser degree by intervention trials in humans. The incidence of spontaneous T1D is directly correlated with the sanitary conditions of the animal facilities, for both the non-obese diabetic (NOD) mouse and the bio-breeding diabetes-prone (BBDP) rat: the lower the infectious burden, the higher the disease incidence [8,9,10]. Diabetes has a very low incidence and may even be absent in NOD mice bred in 'conventional' facilities, whereas the incidence is close to 100% in female mice bred in specific pathogen-free conditions [11]. Furthermore, BBDP rats subject to Cesarean derivation have been noted to develop accelerated disease due to lack of contamination with microbiota in birth canal [12]. Taken together, these data open new therapeutic perspectives in the prevention of allergic and ADs.

4 Intestinal microbiota and their role in ADs?

Based on hygiene hypothesis, the sudden change in human intestinal microflora may importantly contribute to the rise in the incidence of ADs, observed in the last half a 20th century [7]. More than 17 bacterial families encompassing 500 different microbial species can be found in human adults. These commensal bacteria regulate a myriad of host processes and provide several nutrients to their host and their symbionts within the microbial community. In healthy individuals these relationships are thought to occur in equilibrium. However, disruption of this equilibrium may contribute to a variety of conditions including AD, IBD and atopic disease [13]. This connection is gaining credibility as associations between gut microbiota and either the risk for or presence of a variety of specific human diseases is demonstrated.

Accordingly, the pathogenesis of ADs has been recently thought to involve an interaction between genetically determined host susceptibility, the enteric microbiota and dysregulated immune response. Interactions between the intestinal environment, barrier function, and immune system have been shown to have a major impact in the rate of autoimmunity development. Disruption of intestinal barrier function and aberrant mucosal immune activation has been implicated in a variety of diseases within and outside of the gastrointestinal tract [2,9]. The penetration of gut bacterial antigens into lymphoid tissues is one of the suggested initial factors leading to a loss of tolerance towards self components in genetically predisposed individuals. With this model in mind, recent studies have shown a link between diet, composition of intestinal microbiota, and pathogenesis of ADs. Furthermore, this new paradigm subverts traditional theories underlying autoimmunity development, which are mainly based on molecular mimicry, and suggests that the autoimmune process can be arrested if the interplay between genes and environmental triggers is prevented by re-establishing intestinal barrier function [14].

A hypothesis previously has been proposed involving a trio of interacting factors that may create a "perfect environment " for ADs such as type 1 diabetes (T1D) development. These factors include (i) an aberrant intestinal microbiota, (ii) a 'leaky' intestinal mucosal barrier, and (iii) altered intestinal immune responsiveness [15]. In support of this model, modulation of T1D pathogenesis in animal models has proved successful through early intervention with a variety of dietary alterations. Indeed, the administration of a hydrolyzed casein diet or the administration of antibiotics has strengthened the hypothesis that an aberrant microbiota could accelerate disease development. More importantly, this is not a phenomenon that occurs only in rodent models of diabetes, as very recent studies have noted that humans with a propensity to develop T1D as well as other ADs possess an abnormal intestinal barrier; the so called "leaky gut" [8,14]. Together with the gut-associated lymphoid tissue and the neuroendocrine network, the intestinal epithelial barrier, with its intercellular tight junctions, controls the equilibrium between tolerance and immunity to nonself-antigens. Other modulators of tight junction proteins such as certain probiotics may also play a role in modulation of "intestinal leakiness" [8,9,13,15].

5. What are probiotics?

Probiotics are usually isolated from the commensal microflora that inhabits the skin and mucosas. And they represent the species of viable microorganisms (bacteria or yeasts) that have a clear beneficial effect on the health of the host thru establishing a true symbiotic relationship with humans for the longest time. Probiotic is derived from the Greek word meaning "supporting or favoring life". The works of Metchnikoff and Tissier were the first to make scientific suggestions about the probiotic use of bacteria, even if the word "probiotic" was not coined until 1960, to name substances produced by microorganisms which promoted the growth of other microorganisms [16].

Probiotics are first described as selective nonpathogenic living microorganisms or components of bacteria in food supplements, including some commensal bacterial flora, which have beneficial effects on host health and disease prevention and/or treatment [17]. However, experts have debated how to define probiotics. One widely used definition, developed by the World Health Organization and the Food and Agriculture Organization of the United Nations, is that probiotics are "live microorganisms, which, when administered in adequate amounts, confer a health benefit on the host." Probiotics are also defined as 'mono- or mixed cultures of live microorganisms which, when applied to animal or man, beneficially affect the host by improving the properties of the indigenous microflora' [16].

A probiotic bacterium is required to fulfill certain criteria to be of benefit [1]. These include being of human origin and having generally regarded as safe status, acid and bile stability, adherence to intestinal cells, persistence for some time in the gut, ability to produce antimicrobial substances, antagonism against pathogenic bacteria, and ability to modulate the immune response. Probiotic activity has been found to be associated with Lactobacilli, Lactococci, Bifidobacteria (longum, infantis), Streptococcus (thermophilus), Enterococcus (faecium), nonpathogenic E. coli (Nissle 1917), Bacillus coagulans and Saccharomyces strains (boulardii and cerevisiae) [1,17]. The most popular lactic acid bacteria are members of the genera Lactobacilli and Lactococci, which have a long history of safe use. Lctb acidophilus is the most well-known probiotic and one of the most important for the health of the small intestine. Other examples of probiotics are Lctb rhamnosus GG (LGG), Lctb gasseri, Lctb fermentum, Lctb salivarius, Bfdbm bifidum and Streptococcus strains include cremoris, faecium and infantis.

The number of commercially available products that are supplemented with probiotics is rising. Dairy products that contain probiotics are sold in every supermarket and probiotic food supplements (for example; capsules, tablets, and powders) can be purchased in pharmacies or via the internet. For infants, infant formulas containing probiotics are also currently available. Live probiotic cultures are available in fermented dairy products and probiotic fortified foods. Examples of foods containing live probiotics are yoğurt, fermented and unfermented milk, miso, tempeh, and some juices and soy beverages. However, tablets, capsules, powders and sachets containing the bacteria in freeze dried form are also available.

6. A cultural product related to probiotics: Yogurt (Yoğurt)

Increasing interest has also been paid to the beneficial functions of Lactobacilli in addition to their importance in the preparation process of fermented foods such as yoğurt and cheese. Here, the reason for selecting yoğurt as a probiotic food was several-fold. It can be produced in a sustainable manner locally and therefore doesn't rely on importation, and it provides nutrition and is an excellent carrier for probiotic organisms.

Fermented foods, particularly dairy products like yoğurt, have been consumed for centuries in some cultures including Turkish. A similar health effect is also observed for lactose fermenting starter bacteria such as Lctb delbrueckii ssp. bulgaricus and Streptococcus thermophilus in fermented milk products like yoğurt. However, these traditional starters are not considered probiotics by some researchers since they lack the ability to proliferate in the intestine [16]. Therefore probiotic yoğurt including different probiotic strains (lactobacilli and/or bifidobacteria) than standard one has been produced and become popular in recent literature. Probiotic yoğurt includes a probiotic strain or multistrain probiotics that has been shown to have beneficial effects on the health of the host with HIV/AIDS and diarrhea [18]. Traditional yoğurt was compared in a study with probiotic yoğurt in non-inflammatory acute gastroenteritis. Acute non-inflammatory gastroenteritis improvement is accelerated by probiotic yoğurt consumption [19]. Probiotic yoğurt intake was associated with significant anti-inflammatory effects that paralleled the expansion of peripheral pool of putative T(reg) cells in IBD patients and with few effects in controls [20].

Yoğurt contains viable bacteria culture including Streptococcus thermophilus and Lctb delbrueckii sp. bulgaricus [1]. Although these cultures clearly fulfill the current concept of probiotics, only a small number of these bacteria have been studied. Yet some specifically have been shown to have a probiotic effect [1,21,22]. Health effects of traditional (standard) yoğurt will not be reviewed in detail here; several reviews have already been published on this topic [1,16,21]. Yoğurt has been shown to be successful for reducing the duration of symptoms in acute non-bloody diarrhea in 6-24-month-old hospitalized infants [23]. Yoğurt feeding was associated with a clinically relevant decrease in stool frequency and duration of diarrhea in children who have reducing sugars in stools [24]. Positive changes in lipid profile were observed in both yoğurt groups [25].

Although there is well-known assumption of longer human life in the cultures consuming frequently yoğurt, the neat probiotic effect of yoğurt on the frequency of ADs is unknown.

7. Can probiotics really prevent and/or treat any type of ADs?

The new version of 'hygiene hypothesis' proposes that reduced exposure to environmental and/or enteric stimuli, including microbes, underlies the rising incidence of childhood ADs [7,15,26]. This hypothesis is supported by data that highlight the importance of infant exposure to environmental microbes for appropriate development of the immune system. This might explain the observation that administration of microbes or their components inhibits AD in animals such as T1D, as mentioned above [2,13-15]. These findings raise the possibility of using live, nonpathogenic microbes (for example, probiotics) or microbial components to modulate or're-educate' the immune system.

For some time now, microbial agents have been implicated in the etiology of ADs, including insulin dependent diabetes mellitus (T1D). Recent studies, however, have revealed that exposure of genetically diabetes-susceptible animals to certain microbes or microbial agents at an early age prevent the induction and progression of disease. This suggests that microbes may act to modulate the immunological status or immune repertoire of an individual genetically programmed for T1D away from an autoimmune response [27]. Immunization with microbial agents at an early age may offer an important new direction for the immunotherapy of T1D [10,28]. The protective effect of a probiotic and a bacterial extract was reported on the onset of diabetes in NOD mice.

Similarly, there is an increasing amount of data showing that intestinal microbiota changes could contribute to the modulation of immune disorders but evidence is still slim, except in IBD. The case of probiotics in IBD is more complex because of the possible local anti-inflammatory effect, which could explain the relief of symptoms without changes in disease progression, as implicated in the hygiene hypothesis. Following a number of uncontrolled studies in a small cohort of 14 pediatric patients with newly diagnosed ulcerative colitis (UC), probiotic treatment induced a significant rate of remission compared to the control group and a lower relapse rate [29].

Supposed Mechanisms of Probiotics` Effects in the Prevention/Treatment of ADs

Some supposed mechanisms of probiotics` effects in the development of autoimmunity defined in the recent literature are discussed below (as summarized and shown in figure 1).

1. Immunoregulation by TGF-β-bearing Treg cells

CD4+/CD25+ - Tregs have shown to be pivotal players in the maintenance of immune tolerance. Their role in the prevention of autoimmunity in animal models and evidence for disturbed or dysfunction of Tregs have also been observed in patients with different ADs, including MS [6]. Recent studies provided evidence that one effect of probiotics may involve induction of differentiation of IL-10-dependent, TGF-β-bearing Tregs [6]. They also can suppress immune responses distinct from responses against the antigen in question, here antigens expressed by infectious agents (a phenomenon called bystander suppression).

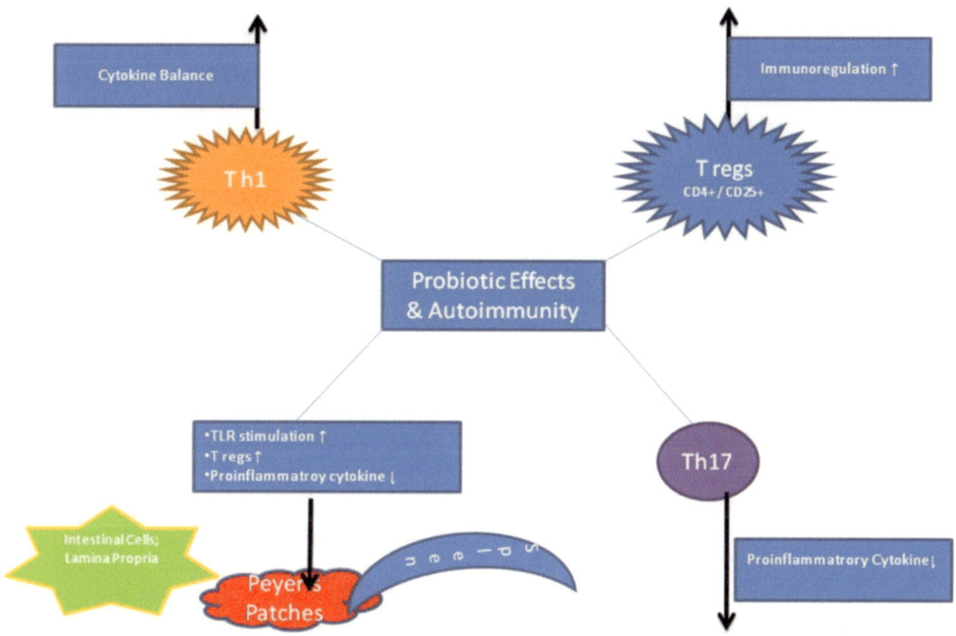

Fig. 1. This figure illustrates some supposed mechanism of probiotic effects on the development of autoimmunity and autoimmune diseases. Probiotics seem to have a regulatory effect on Treg, Th1, Th17, intestinal cells and splenocytes.

2. Development of tolerogenic DCs

Lctb reuteri / casei have been also shown to prime monocyte-derived DCs through the C-type lectin DC-specific intercellular adhesion molecule 3-grabbing non-integrin (DC-SIGN) to drive the development of Tregs [30]. These Tregs produce increased levels of IL-10 and are capable of inhibiting the proliferation of bystander T-cells. This study suggests that the targeting of DC-SIGN by certain probiotic bacteria might explain their beneficial effect in the treatment of a number of inflammatory diseases, including AD [1].

3. Reducing proinflammatory cytokines through Th17 cells

Th17 has been also shown as pathogenic cells in some ADs such as experimental autoimmune encephalomyelitis (EAE) and arthritis [31]. Suppression of this newly discovered subset of T cells by probiotics might explain effects observed in different experimental models that all involve inflammatory responses, i.e. colitis. For instance; Lctb casei suppressed experimental arthritis by reducing proinflammatory cytokines released from Th17 cells.

4. Stimulating Th1 cells

Although there are still some studies showing no significant effects of probiotics on either Th1/Th2 cell responses, certain strains of Lctb and Bfdbm modulate the production of cytokines, and may divert the immune system in a regulatory or tolerant mode. Changes in cytokine profile induced by probiotics may be probiotic strain- or site-specific and dependent on the experimental system used. For instance, Lctb reuteri induced proinflammatory and Th1 cytokines; and Bfdbm bifidum/infantis and Lctb lactis reduced Th2 cytokines and acted as potent inducers of IL-10 production [32].

5. Probiotic regulation in intestinal epithelium and upregulation of host immune responses to defend against infection

Probiotics compete with non-commensal bacteria and eliminate them by secreting antimicrobial products, increase the production of antibodies and macrophage activity and contribute to the appropriate host nutrition by producing some vitamins and by breaking down undigested molecules. These characteristics argue in favor of a symbiotic relationship between humans and probiotics [1]. Probiotic administration in humans and animals has also been shown to be beneficial in the treatment and prevention of intestinal infections and to reduce mucosal inflammation. Their ability to deviate tissue cytokine secretion from a pro-inflammatory to an anti-inflammatory profile has been specifically described. This effect probably results from the ability of probiotics to adhere to mucosal surfaces and inhibit the attachment of other pathogenic bacteria, to secrete factors that enhance barrier integrity, and to modulate cells of the immune system [33].

6. Anti-inflammatory effect of probiotics

The anti-inflammatory effect of probiotics has been attributed to increased production of IL-10 by immune cells in the lamina propria, Peyer's patches and the spleen of treated animals [34]. Moreover, a decrease in the secretion of pro-inflammatory cytokines, IFN-γ, TNF-α and IL-12 has been demonstrated [33].

7. Maturing gut barrier

Recent data indicate that commensal intestinal microbiota represents a major modulator of intestinal homeostasis. Dysregulation of the symbiotic interaction between intestinal microbiota and the mucosa may result in a pathological condition with potential clinical repercussions. For instance, it is shown that mice reared in germ-free conditions have an underdeveloped immune system and have no oral tolerance. In contrast, pathogen-free mice are capable of reconstituting the bacterial flora with Bfdbm and tolerance development. In addition to providing maturational signals for the gut-associated lymphoid tissue, probiotics balance the generation of pro- and anti-inflammatory cytokines in the gut. After probiotic consumption, decrease in fecal α-1 antitrypsin, serum TNF-α, and changes in TGF-β and other cytokines point to down-regulation of inflammatory mediators [33]. Furthermore, probiotic bacteria may counteract the inflammatory process by stabilizing the gut microbial environment and the permeability barrier of the intestine, and by enhancing the degradation of enteral antigens and altering their immunogenicity. This gut-stabilizing effect of probiotics could be explained by the improvement by probiotics of the immunological barrier of the intestine through intestinal IgA responses, specifically [1,35].

8. Systemic TLR stimulation via non-antigenic ligands

A number of experiments indicate that infectious agents can promote protection from ADs through mechanisms independent of their constitutive antigens, leading to stimulation of non-antigen specific receptors such as TLRs. A family of pattern recognition receptors such as TLRs on gut lymphoid and epithelial cells mediates innate immune responses to bacterial molecular patterns and, thereby, orchestrates acquired immunity. An observation made for TLR-2/-3/-4/-7 and -9 that TLR stimulation could prevent the onset of T1D in NOD mice [9,10,36].

Although the beneficial effects of probiotics on wide variety of diseases have been shown, little is known about how probiotics modulate the immune system and autoimmunity development. Currently, only limited publications are available mentioning the effects of probiotics on ADs in rodent models or human. Therefore, it was important to explore the effect of human probiotics in various autoimmune experimental and clinical disease models. Here, firstly experimental and later clinical studies of probiotics in different ADs under the recent literature gathered from Medline and Pubmed are discussed.

8. Animal experimental models and human clinical trials describing supposed effects of probiotics in ADs

Benefits of probiotic use in firstly animal experimental and later human clinical models of ADs including arthritis, T1D, EAE and IBD will be mentioned correspondingly in this assessment. Presumed favorable effects of probiotics in various ADs reviewed in this article are also shown in table 1 and 2.

Disease model	Probiotics	Assessment	Outcome	Ref.
		Animal Experimental Autoimmune Encephalomyelitis Models		
EAE	LcS	↑IL-10, ↑TGF-β	↓disease activity	55,56
EAE	LcS	↑ Th1 cytokines	↑ disease activity	55,56
EAE	Lctb reuteri	↑ proinflammatory cytokines	↑ disease activity	32,54
EAE	LcS, BbY	myelin basic protein	Ø disease activity	56
EAE	Lctb casei 393	↑ IL-10, ↑TGF-β	↓disease activity	55,56
EAE	Bfdbm animalis	↑Tregs, ↓ immune parameters, ↑ body weight gain,	↓disease activity	57
EAE	Lctb casei	↑ immunoregulatory cytokines	↓disease activity	55,56
EAE	Lctb paracasei	↓ proinflammatory cytokines, ↑ Tregs dependent on IL-10	↓disease activity	55,58
EAE	Lacto-mix	↑ Tregs, ↑IL-4, ↑IL-10, ↑TGF- β1	↓disease activity	55,58
		Animal Experimental Inflammatory Bowel Disease Models		
DSS colitis	VSL#3	inflammation	↓disease activity	66
DSS colitis	E. coli Nissle 1917	inflammation	↓disease activity	66

Disease model	Probiotics	Assessment	Outcome	Ref.
IL-10-/- mice colitis	Lctb salivarius	↓IFN-γ	↓disease activity	62,63
IL-10-/- mice colitis	Bfdbm infantis	↓IFN-γ	↓disease activity	62,64
IL-10-/- mice colitis	Lctb reuteri	inflammation	↓disease activity	61
IL-10-/- mice colitis	Lctb plantarum	↓IL-12, ↓IFN-γ	↓disease activity	60
Animal Experimental Diabetes Mellitus Models				
T1D	Lctb casei	↓ β-cell destruction, ↓IFN-γ, ↑IL-2	↓ disease activity	51,52
T1D	LcS	↓ β-cell destruction, ↓autoreactive CD8+ T-cells	↓ disease activity	51,52
T1D	VSL#3	↓ insulitis and β-cell destruction, ↑IL-10, ↑IFN-γ	↓ disease activity	50
T1D	Lctb johnsonii	modify gut microbiota:↓ pro-inflammatory cytokine , ↓IFN-γ, ↓ iNOS and ↑Cox2, ↑claudin (the tight junction protein)	↓ disease activity	48,49
T1D	Lctb reuteri	modify gut microbiota	↓ disease activity	51,52
Animal Experimental Arthritis Models				
CIA	LcS	↓CII-induced IgG2a/2b, ↓IFN-γ production by spleen cells	↓ disease activity	41
CIA	Lctb casei	↓proinflammatory cytokines, ↓T-cell proliferation, ↑IL-10, ↓CII-induced IgG2a/2b, ↑Foxp3+/CD4+-T cells	↓paw swelling, ↓disease activity, ↓cartilage degradation	40
CIA	Lctb fermentum	↓proinflammatory cytokines, ↓T -cell proliferation, ↓ IL-10	↓disease activity, ↓cartilage degradation	42
CIA	Lctb delbrueckii	↓proinflammatory cytokines, ↓T-cell proliferation, ↓ IL-10	↓disease activity, ↓cartilage degradation	42
AA	LGG	inflammation	↓ disease activity	55
AA	Enterococcus faecium	disease intensity	↓ disease activity	38
CIA	Lctb bulgaricus	inflammation	↓ disease activity	42

Abbreviations: Lctb: lactobacillus; Bfdbm: bifidobacterium; LcS: Lctb casei Shirota; BbY: Bfdbm breve strain Yakult; Lacto-mix: Lctb paracasei, Lctb plantarum, Lctb delbrueckii; LGG: Lctb GG; VSL#3: a mixture of four species of lactobacilli, three species of bifidobacteria and Streptococcus thermophilus; DSS: dextran sulfate sodium colitis; EAE: experimental autoimmune encephalomyelitis; CIA: collagen induced arthritis; AA: adjuvant arthritis; T1D: insulin-dependent Diabetes Mellitus; CII: Type II collagen; ↓: decreased in severity of disease; ↑: increased in severity of disease; Ø: no effect on severity of disease.

Table 1. Probiotic effects in animal experimental autoimmune disease models are shown.

Disease	Probiotics	Assessment	Outcome	Ref.
Human Clinical Arthritis Trials				
RA	LGG	clinical/biochemical parameters, ↓proinflammatory cytokines	↓ disease activity	43,44
RA	Bacillus coagulans	inflammation	↓ disease activity	45
RA	Living / vegan food	health assessment questionnaire	↓ disease activity	46
Spondyloarthritis	Combination	clinical/biochemical parameters	Ø disease activity	47
Human Clinical T1D Trials				
T1D	Various	autoantibodies	Ø disease activity	53
Human Clinical Inflammatory Bowel Disease Trials				
Pouchitis	VSL#3	inflammation	↓ disease activity	68,70,71
Pouchitis	LGG	inflammation	↓ disease activity	69,72,73
Active UC	E. coli Nissle 1917	inflammation, induction of remission	↓ disease activity	75,76
Active UC	VSL#3	inflammation, induction of remission	↓ disease activity	68,70,71
Active UC	BbY	endoscopic and histological scores	↓ disease activity	77,78
Active UC	LGG	induction of remission	Ø disease activity	69,72,73
UC remission	VSL#3	maintenance of remission	↓ disease activity	79
UC remission	LGG	maintenance of remission	Ø disease activity	76,80
UC remission	Bfdbm breve / bifidum Lctb acidophilus	maintenance of remission	↓ disease activity	78
Active CD	LGG	inducing remission	Ø disease activity	81,82
Active CD	E. coli Nissle 1917	inducing remission	Ø disease activity	81
CD remission	S. boulardii	maintenance of remission	↓ disease activity	83
CD remission	LGG	maintenance of remission	Ø disease activity	82,84,85
CD remission	Lctb johnsonii	maintaining surgically induced remission	↓ disease activity	86,87
CD remission	VSL#3	maintaining surgically induced remission	↓ disease activity	88

Celiac disease	Lctb sanfranciscensis	proteolytic activity	↓ disease activity	89
Celiac disease	Lctb plantarum	proteolytic activity	↓ disease activity	89
Celiac disease	VSL#3	proteolytic activity	↓ disease activity	90
Celiac disease	Bfdbm lactis	proteolytic activity	↓ disease activity	91
Human Clinical Multiple Sclerosis Trials				
Multiple Sclerosis	Various	dysbiosis	↓ disease activity	59

Abbreviations: Bfdbm: bifidobacterium; Lctb: lactobacillus; BbY: Bfdbm breve strain Yakult; LGG: Lctb GG; VSL#3: a mixture of four species of lactobacilli, three species of bifidobacteria and Streptococcus thermophilus; CD: Crohn`s disease; UC: ulcerative colitis; RA: rheumatoid arthritis; T1D: insulin-dependent diabetes mellitus; ↓: decreased in severity of disease; ↑: increased in severity of disease; Ø: no effect on severity of disease.

Table 2. Probiotic effects in human clinical autoimmune disease trials are shown.

8.1 Ia-probiotic effect in animal experimental arthritis models

Changes in the normal gastrointestinal microflora and dysregulation of the mucosal immune response to these pathogens may contribute to the development of ADs such as rheumatoid arthritis (RA). This possibility has led investigators to evaluate the efficacy of probiotics for alleviating RA symptoms through modulation of the aberrant inflammatory autoimmune response. Of particular interest are LAB probiotics and their immunomodulating and anti-inflammatory effects, which have been shown to lessen the symptoms of arthritis. LAB have been shown to significantly downregulate proinflammatory cytokines (eg, IFN-γ, IL-12, TNF-α) without altering regulatory cytokines (eg, IL-10, TGF-β) to cause anti-inflammatory effects alleviating RA symptoms [37].

Adjuvant arthritis (AA) is a classic murine model for RA, which has been considered a prototype of Th1 disorders. Feeding dairy products fermented with lactobacilli, especially LGG, to rats with AA had a noticeable beneficial effect, surpassing even the effect of oral *Lctb GG* (LGG) alone. There was a statistically significant decrease in inflammation histologically over one month in rats fed yoğurt containing LGG compared with rats fed plain yoğurt or milk. Ingestion of live or heat-killed human LGG had the same clinical beneficial effect. The authors concluded that the LGG, especially in the form of fermented yoğurt, apparently exert both preventive and therapeutic effects on the T-cell-dependent experimental arthritis [37]. Accordingly, AA rats treated in combination with methotrexate and lyophilized probiotic bacteria *Enterococcus faecium*, enriched with organic selenium, had a significantly greater reduction in disease intensity than the methotrexate group [38].

Type II collagen (CII)- induced arthritis (CIA) is considered to be a good model of RA in humans and is often used as a system to evaluate antiinflammatory drugs. An earlier study found that *Lctb casei* reduced the incidence and development of CIA in mice in a dose dependent manner. Oral administration of Lctb casei for 12 weeks reduced signs of CIA including paw swelling, lymphocyte infiltration into the joint, and degradation of cartilage when compared with control animals. Lctb casei administration reduced CII-reactive proinflammatory molecules by CD4+-T cells. Lctb casei administration also reduced CII-reactive Th1-type IgG isotypes IgG2a and IgG2b, while up-regulating immunoregulatory IL-10 levels. These results suggest that oral administration of Lctb casei suppresses the CII - reactive effector function of Th1-type cellular and humoral immune responses in arthritic inflammation [39]. Furthermore; in another study CII alone or together with Lctb casei was orally administered into rats with CIA, and its effects on the clinical and histopathological aspects of arthritis were investigated. Coadministration of Lctb casei with CII more effectively suppressed clinical symptoms, paw swelling, lymphocyte infiltration and destruction of cartilage tissues of experimental arthritis than the rats treated with CII alone. The enhanced therapeutic efficacy was associated with an increase in anti-inflammatory cytokines while decreasing proinflammatory cytokines. Coadministration of Lctb casei with CII more effectively suppressed CII-reactive T cell proliferation and the levels of Th1-type IgG isotypes (IgG2a and IgG2b), while up-regulating Foxp3 expression levels and the population of Foxp3+/CD4+ -T cells. This study indicates that Lctb casei could potentiate antigen-specific oral tolerance and suppress Th1-type immune responses of arthritic inflammation [40].

Also, oral administration of *Lctb casei Shirota (LcS)* into CII-sensitized DBA/1 mice reduced CII-induced IgG2a/2b antibodies in serum and suppressed the CII-induced secretion of IFN-γ from splenocytes ex vivo. It has also been shown that LcS prevented the onset of CIA in DBA/1 mice [41]. Other studies have reported similar improvements in measures of arthritis after administration of *Lctb fermentum* and *Lctb. delbrueckii*. Oral intake of skimmed milk fermented with *Lctb delbrueckii subsp. bulgaricus OLL 1073R-1* prevented CIA in mice. A weaker beneficial effect was noted with fresh skimmed milk and with skimmed milk fermented with another strain of the Lctb. bulgaricus, OLL 1102 [42].

8.2 Ib-probiotic effect in human clinical arthritis trials

A pilot double-blind clinical study evaluated the long-term effects of *LGG* on symptoms of RA. Twenty-one RA patients were randomized to receive 2 capsules of LGG or placebo twice daily for 12 months. RA activity was reduced in 71% of patients in the LGG group vs 30% of patients in the placebo group. Although there were no statistical differences in clinical or biochemical parameters, more patients in the LGG group reported a greater feeling of well-being [43]. Furthermore, the effects of an orally administered probiotic LGG on sulfasalazine metabolism in individuals with RA were studied in a preliminary study. Although there were also no statistical significant differences in the activity of RA, more subjects in the LGG group reported subjective well being [44].

In another pilot study, RA patients who received *Bacillus coagulans* experienced significant improvement in the pain, greater improvement in patient global assessment, patient self-assessed disability, and reduction in total CRP. Bacillus coagulans is a gram-positive, spore-forming, aerobic to microaerophilic LAB bacillus that releases anti-inflammatory molecules or acts indirectly to eradicate organisms in the gut responsible for the inflammatory immune response [45].

A change in the fecal microflora was connected with decreasing activity of RA for one year intervention with living food. 'Living food' is an uncooked vegan diet, which contains no animal products, raffinated substances or added salt. The effects of this diet, *rich in lactobacilli,* in RA patients randomized into diet and control groups were tested. The intervention group experienced subjective relief of rheumatic symptoms during intervention. A return to an omnivorous diet aggravated symptoms. Half of the patients experienced adverse effects (nausea, diarrhoea) during the diet and stopped the experiment prematurely. Nonetheless there was a decrease in the disease activity with lactobacilli-rich and chlorophyll-rich drinks, increase in fibre intake, and no need for gold, methotrexate or steroid medication [46].

In another randomized controlled trial, sixty-three patients with active spondyloarthritis (enteropathic peripheral arthropathies) were randomized to oral probiotic (n = 32) or placebo (n = 31) for 12 weeks. No significant difference was noted between groups in any of the core domains (pain, spinal mobility, patient global, peripheral joint and entheseal scores, stiffness, C-reactive protein, and fatigue) [47].

8.3 IIa-probiotic effect in animal experimental T1D models

The NOD mouse and BBDP rat develop a spontaneous form of human T1D that mimics many features of the human disease, thus representing a model for investigating possible therapeutic approaches. A study reported a culture-independent analysis of the bacteria in fecal samples collected from BBDP and BioBreeding diabetes resistant (BBDR) rats. Two genera of bacteria, Lctb and Bfdbm, emerged as dominant groups negatively correlated with the onset of T1D. Further analysis of the Lctb population within these groups established that Lctb strains with cinnamoyl esterase activity, Lctb johnsonii N6.2 and Lctb reuteri TD1 were negatively correlated with T1D development [48]. Taken collectively, these data suggest that the gut and the gut microbiota are potential agents of influence in T1D development. Consistently, recent accumulating data suggest that the gut immune system plays a role in the development of T1D.

Administration of *Lctb johnsonii N6.2* isolated from BBDR delayed or inhibited the onset of T1D in BBDP rats when administered postweaning. Analysis of the intestinal ileum showed administration of Lctb johnsonii induced changes in the native microbiota, host mucosal proteins, and host oxidative stress response. The administration of Lctb johnsonii also resulted in higher levels of the tight junction protein claudin. In this study, low expression of pro-inflammatory cytokines IFN-γ correlated with the administration of Lctb johnsonii N6.2, whereas low expression of TNF-α correlated with overall healthy status [49]. These results indicate that the mechanisms involved in T1D inhibition in BBDP rats may be different from the effect mediated by the probiotic treatment VSL#3.

Previous reports in the NOD model of diabetes have shown that the administration of the probiotic formulation VSL#3 decreased the incidence of T1D through IL-10 immunomodulation and induction of proinflammatory cytokine IFN-γ. Early orally administered the probiotic compound *VSL#3* induced immunomodulation by a reduction in insulitis severity and a decreased rate of β-cell destruction in NOD mice. Prevention was associated with an increased production of IL-10 from Peyer's patches and the spleen and with increased IL-10 expression in the pancreas, where IL-10-positive islet-infiltrating mononuclear cells were detected [50].

Oral feeding of *Lctb casei* to young NOD mice inhibited the occurrence of T1D, prevented the disappearance of insulin-secreting β -cells, and regulated the host immune system response, as reflected by lower IFN-γ and higher IL-2 production [51]. From the age of 4 wk, female NOD mice were fed a diet containing *LcS,* and the onset of diabetes was recorded thereafter. The incidence of diabetes in the control group was significantly higher than that in the LcS-treated group, and pathological analysis of the LcS-treated group revealed strong inhibition of the disappearance of insulin-secreting β-cells in Langerhans islets. Moreover, the proportion of CD8+-T cells among spleen cells was decreased in the LcS treated group, suggesting the inhibition of autoreactive T cells. It is postulated that LcS may alter the imbalance of Th1/Th2 cytokine production, which is thought to be the cause of the onset of T1D [13,51].

8.4 IIb-probiotic effect in human clinical T1D trials

The feature of immune-mediated T1D is T cell-mediated destruction of the insulin-producing β-cell in the islets, which results from an imbalance between disease promoting factors and protective elements. The particular mechanisms of β-cell destruction leading to diabetes remain still unclear [52]. A pilot study of PRODIA (probiotics for the prevention of β-cell autoimmunity in children at genetic risk of T1D) included 200 children with genetic risk for T1D. This study was planned to show whether the use of probiotics during the first 6 months of life is safe and feasible and to determine whether the use of probiotics during the first 6 months of life decreases the appearance of T1D-associated autoantibodies. However, the prevalence of autoantibodies among the study subjects at 6, 12, and 24 months of age was at levels close to the expected and the clinical follow-up did not either indicate problems in the feasibility of the study [53].

8.5 IIIa-probiotic effect in animal EAE models

EAE, which is an experimental model for MS, is assumed to be induced by activation of autoreactive Th1 cells that recognize myelin basic protein (MBP), which causes inflammatory demyelination in the central nervous system. It has been previously demonstrated that effects of probiotics on EAE in mice were strain-dependent, either stimulating or suppressing the clinical symptoms. In a murine EAE model it was shown that the outcome of EAE was dependent upon the cytokine profile induced by different probiotic strains. Strains that induced proinflammatory cytokines in the gut aggravated the cumulative disease burden, whereas strains that induced regulatory cytokines reduced this burden. For instance, LcS and Bfdbm strains induced immunoregulatory cytokines and improved EAE, while *Lctb reuteri* induced proinflammatory cytokines and aggravated EAE thru release of Th1-associated cytokines [32].

LcS was previously reported to increase the duration of clinical symptoms in a rat EAE model [54]. Because experiments involving LcS detected mainly enhancement of innate immune responses and promotion of Th1-mediated immune reactivity. To confirm and further investigate modulation of Th1 responses and development of AD by LcS, the consequences of oral administration of LcS were assessed in several experiments. And a recent data also showing strain-specific differences on the effect of commercially available probiotic drinks in an EAE rat has been described. In this particular model, these probiotic drinks do not enhance but rather suppress the disease by increasing the production of the regulatory cytokines IL-10 and TGF-β, which is consistent with the indications that Tregs are involved in EAE [55].

Furthermore, to evaluate the effects and safety of two probiotic strains, LcS and *Bfdbm breve strain Yakult* (BbY) were orally administered to Lewis rats with EAE. Three experimental designs were examined by combining different antigen types and probiotic administration periods: (1) EAE was induced with a homogenate of guinea pig spinal cord as the sensitizing antigen, and LcS was orally administered from one week before this sensitization until the end of the experiment; (2) EAE was induced using guinea pig originated MBP as the sensitizing antigen, and LcS was orally administered from one week before this sensitization to the end of the experiment; (3) EAE was induced using guinea pig MBP as the sensitizing antigen, and the probiotic strains (LcS and BbY) were administered starting in infancy (two weeks old) and continued until the end of the experiment. In experiment 1, oral administration of LcS tended to suppress the development of neurological symptoms. Differences in neurological symptoms between the control group and the administration groups did not reach statistical significance in experiments 2 and 3. As a result, these findings support the notion that neither LcS nor BbY exacerbates AD [56].

Effects of *Bfdbm animalis* were evaluated during lactation on autoimmune responses in rodents. In the EAE model, Bfdbm animalis significantly reduced the duration of clinical symptoms and improved the body weight gain compared with the control group. Hence, animals that receive Bfdbm animalis recover faster than controls. The mechanisms by which Bfdbm animalis induced these beneficial effects on EAE are unclear, but do suggest an involvement of Treg cells [57].

The preventive effects of five daily-administered probiotic mixture strains (two strains of *Lctb paracasei*, two strains of Lctb *plantarum* and the traditional yogurt bacterium Lctb delbrueckii *subsp. bulgaricus*) were evaluated comparatively on EAE development in mice. This novel probiotic mixture exerts a therapeutic effect on EAE mediated by Tregs producing IL-10. After a primary screening, three strains, Lctb paracasei DSM 13434, Lctb plantarum DSM 15312 and Lctb plantarum DSM 15313, that efficiently prevented EAE development were chosen for further evaluation. This new mixture of three probiotics is subsequently referred to as "Lacto-mix". The immunosuppressive potential of Lacto-mix strains was associated with induction of Tregs and production of IL-4, IL-10 and TGF-β1 in mesenteric lymph nodes and spleen. Despite a preventive effect on EAE, administration of each individual strain to mice with established EAE was not capable to suppress the disease [55]. In another study, treatment with *Lacto-mix* successfully reversed established EAE and demonstrated a unique synergistic effect of these strains to regulate systemic IL-10 release and induce functional Tregs in, not only intestinal lymph nodes, but also in the periphery and central nervous system of diseased animals [58].

8.6 IIIb-probiotic effect in human clinical MS trials

Much of the epidemiological data in MS is consistent with a role for diet in its initiation, exacerbations, or progression. Some of the dietary factors contributing to the worsening of

MS include a high animal-fat diet; food allergies/intolerances; and digestive malfunctions, including malabsorption and dysbiosis. Gut malabsorption and dysbiosis can be corrected using probiotics. Although there is no known clinical data on the use of probiotics in MS patients, probiotics might have an indirect effect in MS thru correcting dysbiosis [59].

8.7 IVa-probiotic effect in animal experimental IBD models

IBD is a life-long and chronic inflammatory condition of the gastrointestinal tract including the 2 major diseases, Crohn's disease (CD) and UC. A convergence of findings show that intestinal microflora play a central role in the pathogenesis of IBD and thus investigators have pursued studies to seek therapeutic effects of manipulating intestinal microflora. A reduction in microbial burden of gut by public health measures contributes to an immunological imbalance in the intestine, which has been explained by the 'hygiene hypothesis'. The question is posed to determine whether a similar explanation can be proposed for the increased incidence of IBD [9,13-15]. The extension of the hygiene hypothesis to IBD opens new therapeutic perspectives including the revisiting of probiotics and other forms of exposure to bacteria or parasite components.

A number of reports have been published that describe the influence of probiotic consumption on colitis in animal trials. In particular, the IL-10 $^{-/-}$ (knockout) mouse has been extensively studied. IL-10 knockout mice develop colitis when colonized with a conventional flora but remain disease-free when maintained under germ-free conditions. Schultz et al. colonized IL-10$^{-/-}$ mice with *Lctb plantarum 299v* two weeks before transfer from a germ free environment to a specific pathogen-free environment. This resulted in significant attenuation of disease and a significant reduction in mesenteric lymph node IL-12 and IFN-γ production [60].

Madsen et al. demonstrated a role for *Lctb reuteri* in prevention of colitis in IL-10$^{-/-}$ mice. Neonatal IL-10$^{-/-}$ mice were shown to have a decreased concentration of colonic Lctb species and an increased concentration of mucosal adherent bacteria. Oral administration of the prebiotic lactulose (shown to increase the levels of Lctb species) and rectal swabbing with Lctb reuteri restored Lctb levels to normal and reduced the number of adherent bacteria within the colon. These effects were associated with the attenuation of colitis [61].

In another placebo-controlled trial the efficacy of *Lctb salivarius* UCC118 and *Bfdbm infantis* 35624 in attenuation of colitis in the IL-10$^{-/-}$ mouse model was demonstrated. Further studies examined the effect of Bfdbm infantis 35624 on early inflammation in IL-10$^{-/-}$ mice and wild-type mice of the same genetic background. Pronounced changes occurred in the Peyer's patch following probiotic consumption, with IFN-γ reduced in both wild-type and IL-10$^{-/-}$ mice [62].

The oral route of administration may not be required for certain probiotic effects. Reduced inflammatory scores and reduced production of proinflammatory cytokines have been observed in IL-10$^{-/-}$ mice that had been injected subcutaneously with Lctb salivarius UCC118 [63]. Additionally; in order to enhance the probiotic effect in these murine models, investigators have combined probiotic treatment with prebiotics, antibiotics, immunostimulatory DNA sequences or they have genetically engineered the probiotic strain to secrete antiinflammatory mediators. The prebiotic *inulin* and a combination of the probiotic organisms Lctb acidophilus La-5, Lctb delbruckii subsp. bulgaricus, Bfdbm Bb-12, and Streptococcus thermophilus significantly reduced inflammation [64]. The effect was enhanced by combination with metronidazole, suggesting a synergistic effect of the combination of anti- and probiotics in the treatment of experimental colitis [65]. Attenuation of DSS (dextran sulfate sodium) colitis was caused by *VSL#3* DNA mediated through TLR- 9 signaling. Isolated DNA of E. *coli strain Nissle 1917* showed an antiinflammatory effect in the DSS model as well. Interestingly, specific immunostimulatory DNA sequences have also been shown to attenuate the production of proinflammatory cytokines in UC patients [66]. Genetically modified probiotics have been tested for their ability to attenuate colitis in the IL-10 knockout model. *Lactococcus lactis* was engineered to secrete biologically active IL-10. A significant reduction in inflammation was observed in both murine models [67].

8.8 IVb-probiotic effect in human clinical IBD trials

Studies on the use of probiotics in the treatment of noninfectious inflammatory bowel disorders found that 4 strains of Lctb and 1 strain of Streptococcus were effective in maintaining remission of UC and reducing the postop recurrence of CD. In the randomized controlled trials, 12 of 16 UC but only 2 of CD trials of probiotic therapy were successful. No superiority of any probiotic was clearly evident, but a multi-agent mixture, VSL3# may be better suited in UC and pouchitis [68]. And studies of probiotics e.g. LGG in CD have been disappointing, and a recent Cochrane systematic review has concluded that their use could not be recommended on the available evidence [69].

9. Pouchitis

The most compelling evidence for the use of probiotics in IBD comes from randomised double-blind placebo controlled trials with *VSL#3* (a mixture of four species of lactobacilli, three species of bifidobacteria and Streptococcus thermophilus) in patients with pouchitis. The efficacy of *VSL#3* as a maintenance treatment in 40 patients with chronic relapsing pouchitis after antibiotic-induced remission was assessed. After 4 months fewer relapses were found to occur in the intervention group than in the control group. Moreover, all patients were subsequently found to relapse 3 months after cessation of *VSL#3*. Later, the same group assessed *VSL#3* in the primary prevention of pouchitis in 40 patients following surgery. The incidence of pouchitis was found to be reduced and the quality of life improved in the *VSL#3*-treated group compared with the placebo group [68]. Finally, a further study has confirmed the effectiveness of VSL#3 as maintenance therapy in patients with recurrent or chronic pouchitis [70]. In contrast, Shen et al. have reported no significant benefit of *VSL#3* in maintaining antibiotic-induced remission in 31 patients [71].

Trials of other probiotics in the management of pouchitis have yielded mixed results. One observational study of patients receiving *LGG* after pouch formation has reported a lower rate of pouchitis than in historical controls [72]. However, Kuisma et al. have found no difference in mean pouchitis scores between placebo and LGG-treated groups at the end of a 3-month study period [73]. Finally, a reduction in endoscopic and clinical disease activity associated with an increase in faecal probiotic species has been demonstrated in 51 patients with pouchitis after surgery for UC who consumed fermented milk containing lactobacilli and *bifidobacteria* [74].

10. UC

10.1 Probiotics to treat active UC

In a study comparing the effect of probiotic E. coli Nissle 1917 vs. mesalamine on induction of remission in UC, both groups had similar time to remission, demonstrating equal efficacy of treatments. Consistently, several controlled trials have demonstrated that *E. coli Nissle 1917* has similar efficacy to conventional mesalazine treatment with fewer side effects [75]. Efficacy of direct delivery of the probiotic to the colon with E. coli Nissle 1917 enemas in left-sided UC has been demonstrated [76].

In an open-label trial, *VSL#3* was added to current regimen for patients who had failed to respond to conventional therapy for active UC. Addition of VSL#3 for 6 weeks led to either remission or response in 77% of patients as measured by the disease activity index [68].

Active UC was treated with fermented milk including *BbY,* Bfdbm bifidum strain Yakult and an Lctb acidophillus strain [77]. A recent clinical trial demonstrated that treatment of patients with Bfdbm fermented milk compared to placebo leads to a significant decrease in a clinical activity index score, as well as a significant decrease in endoscopic and histological scores after 12 weeks of treatment [78].

10.2 Probiotics as maintenance therapy in UC

Treatment with *VSL#3* to maintain remission in UC was found to be only 4 of 20 patients had experienced relapse at the end of the study [79]. Several studies examining the use of lactobacilli or bifidobacteria as maintenance treatment in UC have demonstrated conflicting results. Ishikawa et al. have demonstrated a reduction in the number of disease exacerbations in a group of Japanese patients receiving fermented milk containing *Bfdbm breve, Bfdbm bifidum and Lctb acidophilus* compared with placebo. However, this clinical benefit was not found to be associated with an increase in steroid-free remission or endoscopic improvement in disease activity [78]. Another open-label trial showed that for maintenance of remission in UC that *LGG* alone, or in combination with mesalamine, demonstrated equal efficacy to mesalamine alone [76,80].

11. CD

11.1 Probiotics to treat active CD

Previous two studies with *E. coli Nissle 1917* and *LGG* had evaluated probiotics in active CD patients, but neither study has demonstrated convincing efficacy, in part because of small numbers of patients [81]. A recent double-blinded placebo controlled trial randomized 11 patients with active CD to receive either LGG or placebo. There was no difference in at the rate of inducing remission for 6 months between the two groups [82].

11.2 Probiotics to maintain remission in CD

Evidence for use of probiotics as maintenance therapy in CD is not persuasive, with only a couple of studies reporting positive results. A study comparing *S. boulardii*+antibiotic+mesalazine with mesalazine alone has shown fewer relapses in the former group in patients with medically-induced remission of CD [83]. A recent double-blinded placebo controlled trial randomized 11 patients with active CD to receive either *LGG* or placebo. There was no difference at the rate of sustaining remission for 6 months between the two groups [82]. Another randomized, double blind study compared *LGG* vs. placebo in addition to standard maintenance therapy in a group of 75 children. These studies did not find any advantage for *LGG* compared with placebo in maintaining medically-induced remission [84].

Several clinical studies have been performed to analyze the effects of probiotics on maintaining surgically-induced remission. Three studies using LGG have not confirmed the effectiveness of this probiotic as a maintenance strategy after surgically-induced remission [84,85]. Another clinical trial utilizing treatment with LGG after surgical resection failed to show prevention of early endoscopic recurrence when compared to placebo. One study suggested modest but not significant improvement in recurrence rates of patients after surgical resection of diseased bowel by *Lctb johnsonii* LA1 [86]. However, two randomised double-blind placebo-controlled studies have reported no effect of Lctb. johnsonii LA1 in preventing recurrence in CD patients in surgically induced remission [86,87]. Lastly; Campieri et al. have shown benefit of *VSL#3* in preventing post-operative recurrence in 40 patients randomised to 3 months of rifaximin followed by 9 months of *VSL#3* or to 12 months of mesalazine [88].

12. Celiac disease

The only effective treatment for Celiac is a strict adherence to a gluten-free diet throughout the patient's lifetime. Otherwise, wheat gliadin induces severe intestinal symptoms and small-bowel mucosal damage in patients. Gluten-free products are not widely available and are usually more expensive than their gluten-containing counterparts. There is, therefore, an urgent need to develop safe and effective therapeutic alternatives, to develop high-quality gluten-free products and to investigate the potential of the bread making biotechnology following ancient protocols, which include long-time fermentation by selected sourdough LAB. There is a necessity for new biotechnologies using probiotics as starters for sourdough fermentation to investigate their potential to decrease the risk of gluten contamination in gluten-free products.

Thus, 46 strains of sourdough LAB were screened for proteolytic activity and acidification rate in gluten-free flours. The sourdough cultures consisted of *Lctb sanfranciscensis* and *plantarum* were selected and used for the manufacture of gluten-free bread [89]. Moreover, proteolytic activity by probiotic *VSL#3* was also found to have an importance during food processing to produce predigested and tolerated gliadins for increasing the palatability of gluten-free products [90]. In addition; *Bfdbm lactis* was found to inhibit the toxic effects of gliadin in intestinal cell culture conditions [91].

13. Conflicting results and reasons of failure in human AD clinical trials

Although human clinical trials for therapeutic probiotic use in AD have been somewhat disappointing, human trials are also performed unsatisfactorily. Firstly, one of the main reasons for this failure is that the topic is becoming currently popular and further studies need to be done. For instance: although arthritis trials both in human and animal are partly successful, there is no still enough clinical data on the use of probiotics in MS and T1D patients.

Secondly; since human is a more complex organism than cell cultures and animals, performing a research in human is very difficult. As expected, most of the hopeful data firstly have come from in vitro cell culture studies and experimental animal models.

Thirdly, there are also difficulties of recognizing mechanisms implicated in ADs. As mentioned upper part of this review; there at least several hypotheses for autoimmunity development and there a lot need to be further clarified. Thus, it is very difficult to decide what kind of probiotic strain would be helpful.

Fourthly, it is very hard to measure net effect of probiotic since the effect of probiotic use is specifically dependent upon strain. Consequently, there is also a large amount of conflicting data on the probiotic use in ADs.

Fifthly, there is also fear from possible side effects of probiotics. As mentioned above, the fact that certain probiotics are known to stimulate Th1 immunity, which might be an additional safety issue. Excessive immunostimulation might aggravate or induce Th1-mediated immune responses, e.g. ADs.

14. Expert commentary (Conclusion)

As mentioned above, there is a large amount of conflicting data on the preventive/therapeutic effects of probiotics in ADs. Results from metaanalyses and systematic reviews that combine results of studies from different types of probiotics to examine the effects in any disease should be interpreted with caution. There are also difficulties of recognizing etiology and pathogenesis of ADs from RA to IBD in which have many mechanisms involved. Similarly, with various strains, especially LcS, stimulation of Th1-mediated immune responses has been described. Additionally, if probiotics are used in patients with ADs for any reason -therapy or prevention- cautionary approach ought to be taken. Thus, probiotics cannot be recommended generally for primary prevention of ADs. Any probiotics should not be used especially in immune-compromised children; even they have at risk for ADs. Finally, there is insufficient but fairly promising evidence to recommend the addition of probiotics to foods for prevention and treatment of ADs.

14.1 Five-year view

Involvement of commensal enteric microflora and its components with strong immunoactivating properties in etiopathogenetic mechanism of multifactorial diseases, including IBD, T1D, RA, and allergy has been recently suggested. Regulation of intestinal microflora composition (e.g. by probiotics) offers the possibility to influence the development of mucosal and systemic immunity as well as it can play a role also in prevention and treatment of some ADs. Progress has been made by the identification of receptors and pathways through which gut microbes influence development of the immune system. Such mechanistic data have moved a field that was once regarded as being on the scientific fringe to the mainstream, and support increased funding to advance this promising area of research in the hope that it might deliver the long awaited answer of how to safely prevent ADs.

Better understanding of the effects of different probiotic strains and a deeper insight into the mechanisms of the heterogeneous manifestations of AD are needed for the validation of specific strains carrying anti-autoimmune potential. Therefore, research activities are currently focusing on identification of specific probiotic strains with immunomodulatory potential and on how dietary content interacts with the most efficacious probiotic strains. Moreover, the selection of the most beneficial probiotic strain, the dose, and the timing of supplementation still need to be determined. Further studies should also clarify if any susceptible groups of ADs exist and how these groups benefit from supplementation with certain probiotic strains.

Some studies in the management of ADs suggest that therapeutic benefit requires a combination of probiotic species (as with VSL#3 or Lacto-mix) or that the component(s) responsible for the anti-inflammatory effect in combination preparations have specific properties that monotherapy probiotics do not. This concept also supports the use of prebiotics that increase concentrations of several commensal immunoregulatory bacteria. Prebiotic use was shown to be associated with a reduction in the faecal concentration of Bacteroides fragilis, but had no effect on lactobacilli or bifidobacteria. Genetically modified probiotics will be tested for their ability to attenuate ADs thru secreting regulatory cytokines in experimental models as well. In near future, the researchers will look for more appropriate combinations of probiotic species or modified probiotics with/without prebiotic and test them in human/rodent AD models.

Additionally, side effects are very low and they might not be nonexistent, as shown in a set of patients with different diseases. However, probiotics should not be considered as totally harmless, particularly in the immunodeficient host, and more safety studies are needed. As imagined, probiotics may have unpredictable behaviour like all microorganisms, such as unanticipated gene expression in nonnative host environment, or acquired mutations occurring spontaneously via bacterial DNA-transfer mechanisms. Certain probiotics are known to stimulate Th1 immunity, which has been suggested as one of the mechanisms by which they can suppress Th2-mediated allergic diseases. However, this presumed excessive immunostimulation might aggravate or induce Th1-mediated immune responses and diseases such as T1D, MS; and it might cause an additional safety issue.

Consequence of over-activation of the immune system by probiotics in hosts with immune dysfunctions, such as individuals genetically predisposed to autoimmunity, has raised some concerns too. With respect to the association between bacterial antigens and autoimmune responses and the adjuvant activity of LAB strains, the involvement of LAB in the pathogenesis of some models of autoimmunity in experimental animals and possibly in humans has been suggested. Thus, from a safety point of view, the potential of probiotic bacteria (especially the immunostimulatory strains), to induce destructive inflammation or autoimmunity needs to be investigated. For instance, it has been experimentally demonstrated that *Lctb casei* cell wall components (given intraperitoneally) are able to induce cardioangitis (an autoimmunity-associated heart disease) in mice [92].

14.2 Key issues

- Since conclusions on probiotics are limited to specific strains and models, they should not be generalized [32,54,55].
- Probiotics should not be considered as completely harmless, particularly in the immunodeficient host, and more safety studies are needed [54,92].
- Physiological use (normal route, normal dose, normal growth phase, specific strain or substrain/species) is studied in all cases, so as not to overwhelm (high dose) or circumvent natural immune processing [54,92].

- Do probiotics really induce/exacerbate ADs? LGG and others have specific dose- and duration- dependent immunomodulatory effects on the proliferation of B-/T-lymphocytes. Some mice orally fed lactobacilli were demonstrated to have an increased Th1 cytokine production. And this type of immunomodulatory mechanism might exacerbate Th1-dependent ADs [32,54,55,92].
- Th1-mediated immune response stimulation also seems to be dependent on type of disease model as well as probiotic strain. In SJL mice with EAE showed that different lactobacilli strains could enhance or inhibit development of ADs [32,54]. And some immunostimulatory probiotics do not always seem to induce autoimmune responses in models that have the genetic potential to develop autoimmunity. Such as Lctb rhamnosus HN001 and Bfdbm lactis HN019 do not induce pathological inflammation in mouse model of experimental autoimmune thyroiditis [93].
- The researchers ought to look for more appropriate and safe combinations of probiotic species (as with VSL#3 or Lacto-mix) or modified probiotics with/without prebiotic and test them in human/rodent AD models [55].
- Research activities are currently focusing on identification of specific probiotic strains with immunomodulatory potential and on how dietary content interacts with the most efficacious probiotic strains. Further studies should be made for the identification of receptors and pathways through which gut microbes influence development of the immune system.

15. References

[1] Özdemir Ö. Various effects of different probiotic strains in allergic disorders: an update from laboratory and clinical data. Clin. Exp. Immunol. 160, 295–304 (2010).

[2] Tlaskalová-Hogenová H, Stepánková R, Hudcovic T et al. Commensal bacteria (normal microflora), mucosal immunity and chronic inflammatory and autoimmune diseases. Immunol. Lett. 93(2-3), 97-108 (2004).

[3] Billmann-Born S, Till A, Arlt A et al. Genome-wide expression profiling identifies an impairment of negative feedback signals in the Crohn's disease-associated NOD2 variant L1007fsinsC. J. Immunol. 186(7), 4027-4038 (2011).

[4] Walsh KP, Brady MT, Finlay CM, et al. Infection with a helminth parasite attenuates autoimmunity through TGF-beta-mediated suppression of Th17 and Th1 responses. J. Immunol. 183(3), 1577-1586 (2009).

[5] Sgouroudis E, Kornete M, Piccirillo CA. IL-2 production by dendritic cells promotes Foxp3(+) regulatory T-cell expansion in autoimmune-resistant NOD congenic mice. Autoimmunity. 44(5), 406-14 (2011). doi: 10.3109/08916934.2010.536795.

[6] Schwartz RH. Natural regulatory T cells and self-tolerance. Nat. Immunol. 6, 327–330 (2005).

[7] Okada H, Kuhn C, Feillet H, Bach JF. The 'hygiene hypothesis' for autoimmune and allergic diseases: an update. Clin. Exp. Immunol. 160 (1), 1–9 (2010).

[8] Bach JF. The effect of infections on susceptibility to autoimmune and allergic diseases. N. Engl. J. Med. 347, 911–920 (2002).

[9] Feillet H, Bach JF. Increased incidence of inflammatory bowel disease: the price of the decline of infectious burden? Curr. Opin. Gastroenterol. 20(6), 560-564 (2004).

[10] Bach JF. Protective role of infections and vaccinations on autoimmune diseases. J. Autoimmun. 16(3), 347-353 (2001).

[11] Singh B, Rabinovitch A. Influence of microbial agents on the development and prevention of autoimmune diabetes. Autoimmunity. 15(3), 209-213 (1993).
[12] Brugman S, Klatter FA, Visser JT et al. Antibiotic treatment partially protects against type 1 diabetes in the Bio-Breeding -prone rat. Is the gut flora involved in the development of type 1diabetes? Diabetologia. 49(9), 2105-2108 (2006).
[13] Matsuzaki T, Takagi A, Ikemura H, Matsuguchi T, Yokokura T. Intestinal microflora: probiotics and autoimmunity. J. Nutr. 137(3 Suppl 2), 798S-802S (2007).
[14] Fasano A, Shea-Donohue T. Mechanisms of disease: the role of intestinal barrier function in the pathogenesis of gastrointestinal autoimmune diseases. Nat. Clin. Pract. Gastroenterol. Hepatol. 2(9), 416-422 (2005).
[15] Vaarala O, Atkinson MA, Neu J. The "Perfect Storm" for type 1 diabetes: The complex interplay between intestinal microbiota, gut permeability, and mucosal immunity. Diabetes. 57, 2555–2562 (2008).
[16] Joint FAO/WHO, author. Evaluation of health and nutritional properties of powder milk and live lactic acid bacteria. Food and Agriculture Organization of the United Nations and World Health Organization Expert Consultation Report. October 2001. http://www.fao.org/ag/agn/Probio/probio.htm.
[17] Lilly DM, Stillwell RH. Probiotics: Growth-promoting factors produced by microorganisms. Science. 147, 747–748 (1965).
[18] Anukam KC, Osazuwa EO, Osadolor HB, Bruce AW, Reid G.Yogurt containing probiotic Lactobacillus rhamnosus GR-1 and L. reuteri RC-14 helps resolve moderate diarrhea and increases CD4 count in HIV/AIDS patients. J. Clin. Gastroenterol. 42(3), 239-243 (2008).
[19] Al-Mendalawi MD, Heydarian F. Comparison between traditional yogurt and probiotic yogurt in non-inflammatory acute gastroenteritis. Saudi Med. J. 31(9), 1071-1072 (2010).
[20] Lorea Baroja M, Kirjavainen PV, Hekmat S, Reid G. Anti-inflammatory effects of probiotic yogurt in inflammatory bowel disease patients. Clin. Exp. Immunol. 149(3), 470-479 (2007).
[21] Guarner F, Perdigon G, Corthier G, Salminen S, Koletzko B, Morelli L. Should yoghurt cultures be considered probiotic? Br. J. Nutr. 93, 783-786 (2005).
[22] Hitchins AD, McDonough FEM. Prophylactic and therapeutic aspects of fermented milk. Am. J. Clin. Nutr. 49, 675–684 (1989)
[23] Pashapour N, Iou SG. Evaluation of yogurt effect on acute diarrhea in 6-24-month-old hospitalized infants. Turk. J. Pediatr. 48(2), 115-118 (2006).
[24] Boudraa G, Benbouabdellah M, Hachelaf W, Boisset M, Desjeux JF, Touhami M.Effect of feeding yogurt versus milk in children with acute diarrhea and carbohydrate malabsorption. J. Pediatr. Gastroenterol. Nutr. 33(3), 307-313 (2001).
[25] Sadrzadeh-Yeganeh H, Elmadfa I, Djazayery A, Jalali M, Heshmat R, Chamary M. The effects of probiotic and conventional yoghurt on lipid profile in women. Br. J. Nutr. 103(12), 1778-1783 (2010).
[26] Canche-Pool EB, Cortez-Gómez R, Flores-Mejía R et al. Probiotics and autoimmunity: an evolutionary perspective. Med. Hypotheses. 70(3), 657-660 (2008).
[27] Akerblom HK, Virtanen SM, Ilonen J et al. Dietary manipulation of beta cell autoimmunity in infants at increased risk of type 1 diabetes: a pilot study. Diabetologia. 48(5), 829-837 (2005).
[28] Petrovsky N. Immunomodulation with microbial vaccines to prevent type 1 diabetes mellitus. Nat. Rev. Endocrinol. 6(3), 131-138 (2010).

[29] Miele E, Pascarella F, Giannetti E et al. Effect of a probiotic preparation (VSL#3) on induction and maintenance of remission in children with ulcerative colitis. Am. J. Gastroenterol. 104(2), 437-43 (2009).
[30] Smits HH, Engering A, van der Kleij D, de Jong EC, Schipper K, van Capel TM, et al. Selective probiotic bacteria induce IL-10-producing regulatory T cells in vitro by modulating dendritic cell function through dendritic cell-specific intercellular adhesion molecule 3-grabbing nonintegrin. J. Allergy Clin. Immunol.115(6), 1260-1267 (2005).
[31] So JS, Kwon HK, Lee CG et al. Lactobacillus casei suppresses experimental arthritis by down-regulating T helper 1 effector functions. Mol. Immunol. 45, 2690–2699 (2008).
[32] Maassen CB, Claassen E. Strain-dependent effects of probiotic lactobacilli on EAE autoimmunity. Vaccine. 26(17), 2056-2057 (2008).
[33] Dotan I, Rachmilewitz D. Probiotics in inflammatory bowel disease: possible mechanisms of action. Curr. Opin. Gastroenterol. 21(4), 426-430 (2005).
[34] Fedorak RN. Understanding why probiotic therapies can be effective in treating IBD. J. Clin. Gastroenterol. 42 Suppl 3 Pt 1, S111-115 (2008).
[35] Isolauri E, Sütas Y, Kankaanpää P, Arvilommi H, Salminen S. Probiotics: effects on immunity. Am. J. Clin. Nutr. 73(2 Suppl), 444S-450S (2001).
[36] Rachmilewitz D, Katakura K, Karmeli F et al. Toll-like receptor 9 signaling mediates the anti-inflammatory effects of probiotics in murine experimental colitis. Gastroenterology. 126, 520–528 (2004).
[37] Baharav E, Mor F, Halpern M, Weinberger A. Lactobacillus GG bacteria ameliorate arthritis in Lewis rats. J. Nutr. 134, 1964-1969 (2004).
[38] Rovensky J, Svik K, Stancikova M, Istok R, Ebringer L, Ferencik M. Treatment of experimental adjuvant arthritis with the combination of methotrexate and lyophilized Enterococcus faecium enriched with organic selenium. Folia Microbiol. 47, 573–578 (2002).
[39] So JS, Kwon HK, Lee CG et al. Lactobacillus casei suppresses experimental arthritis by down-regulating T helper 1 effector functions. Mol. Immunol. 45(9), 2690–2699 (2008).
[40] So JS, Lee CG, Kwon HK et al. Lactobacillus casei potentiates induction of oral tolerance in experimental arthritis. Mol. Immunol. 46(1), 172-180 (2008).
[41] Kato I, Endo-Tanaka K, Yokokura T. Suppressive effects of the oral administration of Lactobacillus casei on type II collagen-induced arthritis in DBA/1 mice. Life Sciences. 63, 635–644 (1998).
[42] Kano H, Kaneko T, Kaminogawa S. Oral intake of Lactobacillus delbrueckii subsp. bulgaricus OLL1073R-1 prevents collagen-induced arthritis in mice. J. Food. Prot. 65, 163–166 (2002).
[43] Hatakka K, Martio J, Korpela M et al. Effects of probiotic therapy on the activity and activation of mild rheumatoid arthritis--a pilot study. Scand. J. Rheumatol. 32(4), 211-215 (2003).
[44] Lee HJ, Waller RD, Stebbings S et al. The effects of an orally administered probiotic on sulfasalazine metabolism in individuals with rheumatoid arthritis: a preliminary study. Int. J. Rheum. Dis. 13(1), 48-54 (2010).
[45] Mandel et al. Bacillus coagulans: a viable adjunct therapy for relieving symptoms of rheumatoid arthritis according to a randomized, controlled trial. BMC Comp. Altern. Medicine 10, 1-7 (2010).
[46] Nenonen MT, Helve TA, Rauma AL, Hanninen OO. Uncooked, lactobacilli-rich, vegan food and rheumatoid arthritis. Br. J. Rheumatol. 37, 274–281 (1998).

[47] Garrett SL, Kennedy LG, Calin A. Patients' perceptions of disease modulation by diet in inflammatory (rheumatoid arthritis/ankylosing spondylitis) and degenerative arthropathies. Br. J. Rheumatol. 32(suppl. 2), 43 (1993).

[48] Scott FW, Cloutier HE, Kleemann R et al. Potential mechanisms by which certain foods promote or inhibit the development of spontaneous diabetes in BB rats: dose, timing, early effect on islet area, and switch in infiltrate from Th1 to Th2 cells. Diabetes. 46(4), 589-598 (1997).

[49] Valladares R, Sankar D, Li N et al. Lactobacillus johnsonii N6.2 Mitigates the development of Type 1 diabetes in BB-DP Rats. PLoS ONE 5 (5), 10507 (2010).

[50] Calcinaro F, Dionisi S, Marinaro M et al. Oral probiotic administration induces interleukin-10 production and prevents spontaneous autoimmune diabetes in the non-obese diabetic mouse. Diabetologia. 48(8), 1565-1575 (2005).

[51] Matsuzaki T, Nagata Y, Kado S et al. Prevention of onset in an insulin-dependent mellitus model, NOD mice, by oral feeding of Lactobacillus casei. Acta Pathol. Microbiol. Immunol. Scand. 105, 643–649 (1997).

[52] Kawasaki E, Abiru N, Eguchi K. Prevention of type 1 diabetes: from the view point of beta cell damage. Diabetes Res. Clin. Pract. 66 Suppl 1, S27-32 (2004).

[53] Ljungberg M, Korpela R, Ilonen J, Ludvigsson J, Vaarala O. Probiotics for the prevention of beta cell autoimmunity in children at genetic risk of type 1 diabetes--the PRODIA study. Ann. N. Y. Acad. Sci. 1079, 360-364 (2006).

[54] Maassen CB, van Holten JC, Balk F et al. Orally administered Lactobacillus strains differentially affect the direction and efficacy of the immune response. Vet. Q. 20 (Suppl. 3), S81–83 (1998).

[55] Lavasani S, Dzhambazov B, Nouri M et al. A novel probiotic mixture exerts a therapeutic effect on experimental autoimmune encephalomyelitis mediated by IL-10 producing regulatory T cells. PLoS ONE 5(2), e9009 (2010).

[56] Kobayashi T, Kato I, Nanno M et al. Oral administration of probiotic bacteria, Lactobacillus casei and Bifidobacterium breve does not exacerbate neurological symptoms in experimental autoimmune encephalomyelitis. Immunopharmacol. Immunotoxicol. 32(1), 116-124 (2010).

[57] Ezendam J, de Klerk A, Gremmer ER, van Loveren H. Effects of Bifidobacterium animalis administered during lactation on allergic and autoimmune responses in rodents. Clin. Exp. Immunol. 154(3), 424-431 (2008).

[58] McGeachy MJ, Stephens LA, Anderton SM. Natural recovery and protection from autoimmune encephalomyelitis: contribution of CD4+CD25+ regulatory cells within the central nervous system. J. Immunol. 175, 3025–3032 (2005).

[59] Kidd PM. Multiple sclerosis, an autoimmune inflammatory disease: prospects for its integrative management. Altern. Med. Rev. 6(6), 540-566 (2001).

[60] Schultz M, Veltkamp C, Dieleman LA et al. Lactobacillus plantarum 299v in the treatment and prevention of spontaneous colitis in interleukin-10- deficient mice. Inflamm. Bowel Dis. 8, 71–80 (2002).

[61] Madsen KL, Doyle JS, Jewell LD, Tavernini MM, Fedorak RN. Lactobacillus species prevents colitis in interleukin 10 gene-deficient mice. Gastroenterology. 116(5), 1107-1111 (1999).

[62] Sheil B, MacSharry J, O'Callaghan L et al. Role of interleukin (IL)-10 in probiotic-mediated immune modulation: an assessment in wild-type and IL-10 knock-out mice. Clin. Exp. Immunol. 144, 273-280 (2006).

[63] Sheil B, McCarthy J, O'Mahony L et al. Is the mucosal route of administration esential for probiotic function? Subcutaneous administration is associated with attenuation of murine colitis and arthritis. Gut. 53, 694-700 (2004).

[64] Welters CF, Heineman E, Thunnissen FB, van den Bogaard AE, Soeters PB, Baeten CG. Effect of dietary inulin supplementation on inflammation of pouch mucosa in patients with an ileal pouch-anal anastomosis. Diseases of the Colon and Rectum 45, 621–627 (2002).

[65] Schultz M, Munro K, Tannock GW et al. Effects of feeding a probiotic preparation (SIM) containing inulin on the severity of colitis and on the composition of the intestinal. microflora in HLA-B27 transgenic rats. Clin. Diagn. Lab. Immunol. 11, 581–587 (2004).

[66] Rachmilewitz D, Kermeli F, Takabayashi K et al. Immunostimulatory DNA ameliorates experimental and spontaneous murine colitis. Gastroenterology. 122, 1428–1441 (2002).

[67] Huibregtse IL, Snoeck V, de Creus A et al. Induction of ovalbumin-specific tolerance by oral administration of Lactococcus lactis secreting ovalbumin. Gastroenterology. 133(2), 517-528 (2007).

[68] Bibiloni R, Fedorak RN, Tannock GW et al. VSL#3 probiotic-mixture induces remission in patients with active ulcerative colitis. Am. J. Gastroenterol. 100, 1539 -1546 (2005).

[69] Rolfe VE, Fortun PJ, Hawkey CJ, Bath-Hextall F. Probiotics for maintenance of remission in Crohn's Disease. The Cochrane Database of Systematic Reviews 2006, issue 4, CD004826. Chichester, West Sussex: John Wiley and Sons Ltd.

[70] Mimura T, Rizzello F, Helwig U et al. Once daily high dose probiotic therapy (VSL#3) for maintaining remission in recurrent or refractory pouchitis. Gut 53, 108–114 (2004).

[71] Shen B, Brzezinski A, Fazio VW et al. Maintenance therapy with a probiotic in antibiotic-dependent pouchitis: experience in clinical practice. Aliment. Pharmacol. Therapeutics 22, 721-728 (2005).

[72] Gosselink MP, Schouten WR, van Lieshout LM, Hop WC, Laman JD, Ruseler-van Embden JG. Delay of the first onset of pouchitis by oral intake of the probiotic strain Lactobacillus rhamnosus GG. Diseases of the Colon and Rectum 47, 876–884 (2004).

[73] Kuisma J, Mentula S, Jarvinen H, Kahri A, Saxelin M, Farkkila M. Effect of Lactobacillus rhamnosus GG on ileal pouch inflammation and microbial flora. Alimentary Pharmacology and Therapeutics 17, 509–515 (2003).

[74] Laake KO, Bjorneklett A, Aamodt G et al. Outcome of four weeks' intervention with probiotics on symptoms and endoscopic appearance after surgical reconstruction with a J-configurated ileal-pouch-anal-anastomosis in ulcerative colitis. Scan. J. Gastroenterol. 40, 43–51 (2005).

[75] Rembacken BJ, Snelling AM, Hawkey PM et al. Non-pathogenic Escherichia coli versus mesalazine for the treatment of ulcerative colitis: a randomised trial. Lancet. 354, 635- 639 (1999).

[76] Matthes H, Krummenerl T, Giensch M, Wolff C, Schulze J. Treatment of mild to moderate acute attacks of distal ulcerative colitis with rectally-administered E. coli Nissle 1917: Dose-dependent efficacy. Gastroenterology 130 (Suppl. 2), A119 (2006).

[77] Kato K, Mizuno S, Umesaki Y et al. Randomized placebo-controlled trial assessing the effect of bifidobacteria-fermented milk on active ulcerative colitis. Aliment. Pharmacol. Ther. 20, 1133–1141 (2004).

[78] Ishikawa H, Akedo I, Umesaki Y, Tanaka R, Imaoka A, Otani T. Randomized controlled trial of the effect of bifidobacteria- fermented milk on ulcerative colitis. J. American College Nutrition 22, 56–63 (2003).

[79] Venturi A, Gionchetti P, Rizzello F et al. Impact on the composition of the faecal flora by a new probiotic preparation: preliminary data on maintenance treatment of patients with ulcerative colitis. Aliment. Pharmacol. Therapeutics 13, 1103–1108 (1999).

[80] Zocco MA, dal Verme LZ, Cremonini F et al. Efficacy of Lactobacillus GG in maintaining remission of ulcerative colitis. Alimentary Pharmacology and Therapeutics 23, 1567–1574 (2006).

[81] Malchow HA. Crohn's disease and Escherichia coli. A new approach in therapy to maintain remission of colonic Crohn's disease? J. Clin. Gastroenterol 25, 653–658 (1997).

[82] Schultz M, Timmer A, Herfarth HH et al. Lactobacillus GG in inducing and maintaining remission of Crohn's disease. BMC Gastroenterol. 4, 5 (2004).

[83] Guslandi M, Mezzi G, Sorghi M, Testoni PA. Saccharomyces boulardii in maintenance treatment of Crohn's disease. Digestive Diseases and Sciences 45, 1462– 1464 (2000).

[84] Bousvaros A, Guandalini S, Baldassano RN et al. A randomized, double-blind trial of Lactobacillus GG versus placebo in addition to standard maintenance therapy for children with Crohn's disease. Inflamm. Bowel Dis. 11, 833– 839 (2005).

[85] Prantera C, Scribano ML, Falasco G, Andreoli A, Luzi C. Ineffectiveness of probiotics in preventing recurrence after curative resection for Crohn's disease: a randomised controlled trial with Lactobacillus GG. Gut. 51, 405–409 (2002).

[86] Van Gossum A, Dewit O, Louis E et al. Multicenter randomized-controlled clinical trial of probiotics (Lactobacillus johnsonii, LA1) on early endoscopic recurrence of Crohn's disease after ileo-caecal resection. Inflamm. Bowel Dis. 13, 135–142 (2007).

[87] Marteau P, Lemann M, Seksik P et al. Ineffectiveness of Lactobacillus johnsonii LA1 for prophylaxis of postoperative recurrence in Crohn's disease: a randomised, double blind, placebo controlled GETAID trial. Gut. 55, 842–847 (2006).

[88] Campieri M, Rizzello F, Venturi A et al. Combination of antibiotic and probiotic treatment is efficacious in prophylaxis of post-operative recurrence of Crohn's disease: A randomized controlled study vs mesalamine. Gastroenterology. 118, G4179 (2000).

[89] Di Cagno R, Rizzello CG, De Angelis M et al. Use of selected sourdough strains of Lactobacillus for removing gluten and enhancing the nutritional properties of gluten-free bread. J. Food Prot. 71(7), 1491-1495 (2008).

[90] De Angelis M, Rizzello CG, Fasano A et al. VSL#3 probiotic preparation has the capacity to hydrolyze gliadin polypeptides responsible for Celiac Sprue. Biochim. Biophys. Acta. 1762(1), 80-93 (2006).

[91] Lindfors K, Blomqvist T, Juuti-Uusitalo K et al. Live probiotic Bifidobacterium lactis bacteria inhibit the toxic effects induced by wheat gliadin in epithelial cell culture. Clin. Exp. Immunol. 152(3), 552-558 (2008).

[92] Okitsu-Negishi S, Nakano I, Suzukim K, Hashira S, Abe T, Yoshino K. The induction of cardioangitis by Lactobacillus casei cell wall in mice: I. The cytokine production from murine macrophages by Lactobacillus casei cell wall extract. Clin. Immunol. Immunopathol. 78, 30-40 (1996).

[93] Zhou JS, Gill HS. Immunostimulatory probiotic Lactobacillus rhamnosus HN001 and Bifidobacterium lactis HN019 do not induce pathological inflammation in mouse model of experimental autoimmune thyroiditis. Int. J. Food Microbiol. 103(1), 97-104 (2005).

Part 3

Pediatric Cardiology

8

Infants Born with Intrauterine Growth Restriction: Renal and Cardiovascular Follow-Up

Silvia Visentin, Martina Bertin,
Michela Rampon, Daniele Trevisanuto,
Vincenzo Zanardo and Erich Cosmi*
Department of Woman and Child Health,
University of Padua School of Medicine, Padua,
Italy

1. Introduction

Intrauterine growth restriction (IUGR) is a abnormal fetal growth pattern, occurrung in 8% of pregnancies (Mandruzzato & al., 2008), but its prevalence changes in different categories of pregnant women, with rates of 3-5% for healthy mothers and 25% or more in some high-risk groups such as hypertensive mothers. This condition is the leading cause of fetal mortality and perinatal morbidity and significantly increased short-and long-term mortality (Froen & al., 2004). The modern purpose of Obstetrics is "To ensure that every baby born with a potential psychological and physical development as much as possible unchanged compared to the one inherited by the two parental gametes at the time of their union" (JP Greenhill, 1976). The identification of intrauterine growth restriction is important not only to choose the timing of delivery, but also, in cooperation with neonatologists, an appropriate follow-up of cardiovascular complications, renal, neurological and endocrinological that may arise in these infants (McIntire & al., 1999). Several factors have contributed to the confusion in terminology associated to IUGR (Battaglia & al., 1967). By definition, 10% of infants in any population, has a birth weight less than or equal to 10 th percentile (Figure 1). Often the distinction between pathological and normal growth cannot be performed reliably in clinical practice, especially before the fetus is born. Furthermore, although define a condition based on the 10th percentile seems to have a statistical significance, may prove to be clinically relevant. Although fetal growth curves for specific ethnic origin and geographical are increasingly used to assess the weight at birth, remains unclear whether or not they are appropriate (Zhang & al., 1995). The correct use of the terms "small for gestational age" (SGA) and "intrauterine growth restriction "(IUGR) is still unclear and often the two words are switched. Given these difficulties, the American College of Obstetricians and Gynecologists (ACOG) Practice Bulletin, in January 2000, advised to apply

* Corresponding Author

the first term to infants and the second to fetuses (American College of Obstetricians and Gynecologists [ACOG] 2001).

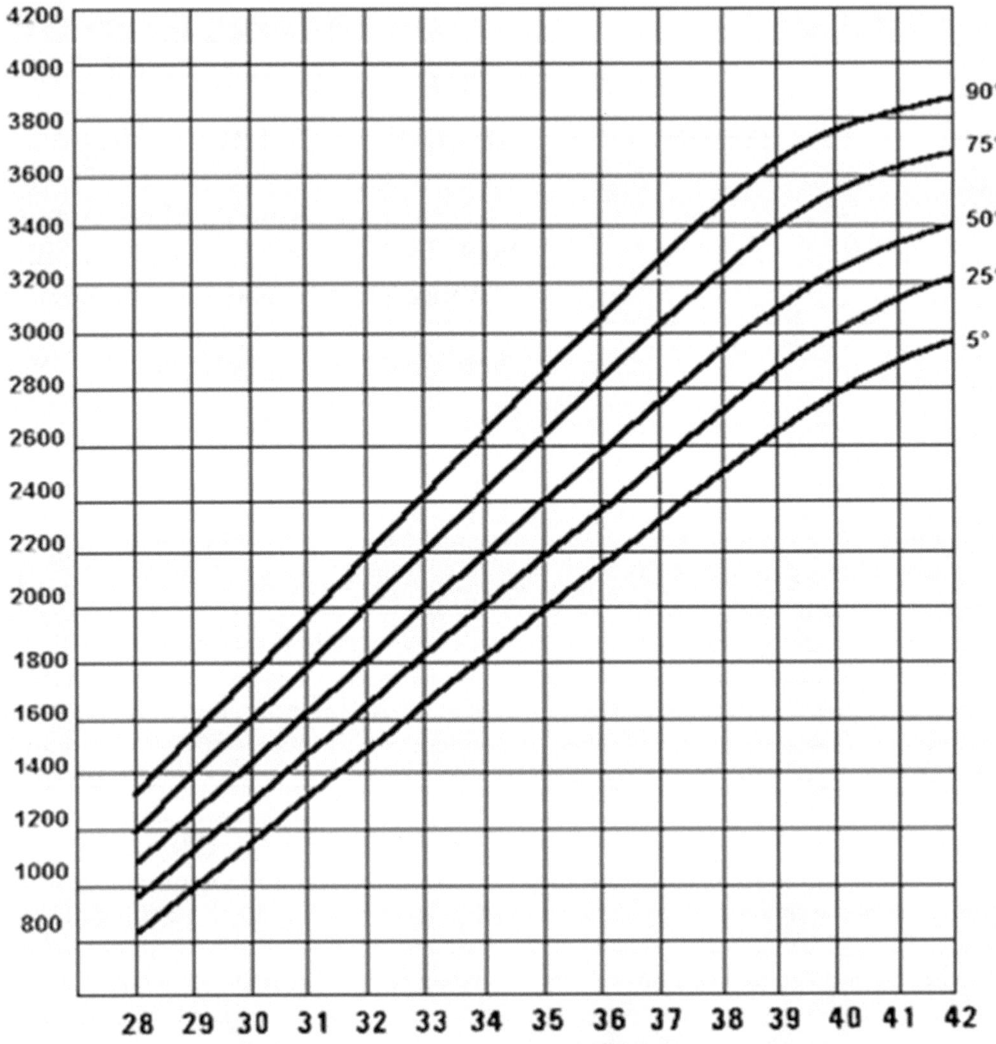

Fig. 1. Curve of fetal weight percentiles throughout the gestation.

The infants defined SGA are fetuses whose birth weight corresponding to lower ends of the curve of normality and, especially in the United States of America, the infants whose weight is below 10th percentile for gestational age, are called SGA. The fetus whose estimated weight is lower than expected, lower than the classically 10th percentile, is classified IUGR, so this definition will include fetuses with normal growth corresponding to lower values of the curves normality, but also those with specific clinical conditions which prevent them from reaching their growth potential. In the second case may be influenced by the extrinsic conditions (eg, mother smoker), or inherent genetic defects (eg aneuploidy).

1.1 Etiology of IUGR

Growth retardation in utero is not a specific disease caused by a single etiology, but the result of the simultaneous presence of multiple and diverse maternal and fetal abnormalities. Among the factors that determine fetal growthdistinguish intrinsic ones, or fetal and extrinsic ones, both maternal and placental (Figure 2). IUGR is not a specific entity but is the result of idiopathic, maternal, fetal and placental disorders. The management and neonatal outcome depends in part on the etiology of delayed fetal growth and thus is always important to try to identify it, but this makes it possible in only 40% of IUGR fetuses. In the remaining 60% of cases the factors etiologic known to date do not appear to be involved: idiopathic IUGR fetuses.

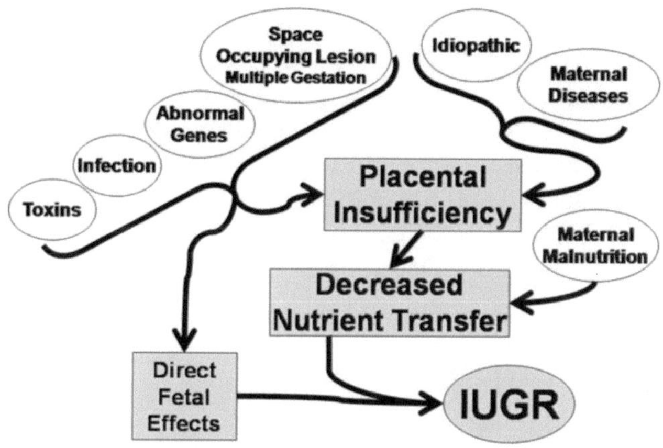

Fig. 2.

Fetal factors may contribute up to 15 to 20% of IUGR (Baschat, 2004). There is a strong correlation between chromosome disorders, congenital malformation and IUGR, which constitutes about 7% of all fetal growth restriction (FGR). Fetuses with aneuploidy such as trisomy 13, 18, 21, as well as with other disorders (multifactorial congenital malformation, X-linked disorders or other autosomal disorders) are usually growth restricted (Snijders & al., 1993) Fetal infection

may be responsible up to 10% of fetal growth restriction. These infections are usually acquired in utero congenital incurred by agents viral infections (rubella, CMV, HSV, HIV), protozoa (Toxoplasma gondii, Plasmodium falciparum) and bacteria (Listeria, Treponema pallidum). In the placenta, the infection can replicate and be transmitted to the fetus, thus causing a delay in organogenesis which will be a direct or an indirect consequence of fetal response to infection. Maternal causes associated with a decrease in uteroplacental perfusion, is responsible to account for 25-30% of all IUGR cases (Lin & Santolaya-Forgas, 1998). The placental factors explain 25-40% of cases of growth retardation and include: inadequate trophoblastic invasion of the endometrium, multiple placental infarcts and abnormalities in size or shape of the placenta. It is observed that the placenta of IUGR fetuses was smaller than the normality and that a ratio of placental weight greater than the value of 10 can be considered an index diagnosis of IUGR, irrespective of fetal weight. Thus chronic vascular disease secondary to hypertension, renal disease, diabetes mellitus, and collagen vascular diseases, especially in combination with superimposed preeclampsia are the most common cause of IUGR. Thrombophylic disorders cause IUGR but it is yet unclear if the effect on fetal growth is mediated by placental thrombosis or is a consequence of maternal hypertension. The antiphospholipid syndrome, an acquired coaugulopathy, is also correlated in determining IUGR. Other maternal causes are represented by nutritional abnormalities such as women with bowel inflammatory disease. Usually twin gestation is associated with IUGR. Maternal substance abuse *i.e.*smoking, alcohol, and drug consumption is also correlated with IUGR. Placental factors, such as abnormality in size and/or function are implied in IUGR. Between the exogenous toxic substances consider firstly smoke because it causes an increase in concentration of carboxyhemoglobin resulting in reduced maternal oxygenation of the fetus. Nicotine also seems to cause arched and spiral artery vasoconstriction, with subsequent reduction of placental flow and indeed the infants of smoking mothers have a birth weight of 150-250 grams less on average than those born to non-smokers mothers. Another environmental factor is alcohol, which determine in the 10-30% of pregnant women who do abuse, the fetal alcohol syndrome, characterized by growth retardation and morphological abnormalities such as deformation of the limbs, cardiac structural abnormalities, abnormal facies, microcephaly, and cognitive delay. Recently it has been shown that IUGR fetuses may be caused by idiopathic factors, in this case the cause determining IUGR is not known (Harkness & Mari, 2004), nevertheless exist placental insufficiency.

1.2 Physiopathology

The said etiologies may lead to fetal pathophysiological three paintings: a abnormal placental function, an inadequate supply of oxygen and / or nutrients maternal and a reduced ability of the fetus to use such substances, with subsequent loss of its ability to adapt. Uteroplacental circulation is characterized by low vascular resistance and a remarkable capacity of vasodilatation. If the phenomenon of placentation, or trophoblastic invasion of the endometrium, is adequately, then the placental blood flow exceeds those that are the fetal metabolic demands, maintaining a safety margin that ensures the well-being of the fetus if occurring conditions of the sudden drop in nutrient supply. In the above occurrence the fetus reacts by introducing a characteristic response, whose mechanisms are well known (Brodsky & Christou, 2004). Redistribution and increase in vascular resistance in the umbilical artery that occur in the event of fetal distress in IUGR seem to be the result of an imbalance between factors acting vasoconstrictor and vasodilator, which are all metabolites of arachidonic acid. In particular, there was a concentration of thromboxane A2 (TXA2) increased compared to that of prostacyclin (PGI2): the first is platelet-derived and/or trophoblastic and has a vasoconstrictor and platelet aggregating effect, while the second is produced by the endothelium and the renal cortex and has a vasodilator and platelet anti-aggregating. In addition to these metabolites, there are high concentrations of endothelin-1 and NO-synthase inhibitors, as well as a reduction of VEGF and placental growth factor (PlGF) (Greiss, eds Masson Publ, 1982). Vasoconstriction and thrombosis of placental vessels cause the reduction of exchange of nutrients and oxygen, with subsequent hypoxia, metabolic acidosis, asphyxiation and activation of compensatory mechanisms of type vasopressor. In fetal circulation there is a massive release of catecholamines, which determines selective vasoconstriction of the territories tributary of descending aorta (especially in the districts splanchnic and skeletal muscle) and vasodilation in brachio-cephalic vessels to facilitate the flow to the brain. The persistence of this compensatory mechanism creates an overload of the ventricle left with a high risk of myocardial ischemia, and contemporary overloading of the right ventricle, due to splanchnic vasoconstriction. One therefore understand the reason for the reduced fetal myocardial contractility, which accompanies the reduction in cardiac output, the peak rate in large vessels and ventricular filling, resulting in increased central venous pressure and subdiaphragmatic venous pulsatility. The increase of indices of resistance in the umbilical artery indicates worsening of placental impairment, while the concomitant reduction of the same in middle cerebral artery and cerebro-placental ratio inversion (ratio umbilical and cerebral resistance) indicates that there began the phenomenon of brain-sparing effect. The caliber of the middle cerebral artery (MCA) continues to increase gradually until it reaches a zenith, before the onset of an abnormal fetal heart rate patterns, a sign of imminent death of the fetus. The ability to protect the brain parenchyma, with vasodilatation of ACM, just before the exitus, is lost, probably because the vessels lose their sensitivity to hypoxia, or due to the reduction of output fetal heart. At this point flow changes and appear similar to those in the umbilical artery also in the peripheral vessels (Krebs & al., 1996).

1.3 Classification

The IUGR fetus is usually divided into two clinical patterns: symmetric and asymmetric. This classification is related to the morphometric ultrasonography measurements of the head circumference (HC) and abdominal circumference (AC). In the moment that exist a reduction in the growth rate of both the above measurements the IUGR fetus is named symmetric; if only the AC is compromised the IUGR is asymmetric. The clinical pattern of IUGR is related to the nature of the causative factor, the stage of gestation in which the insult acts, and its duration. The above patterns are classified on the basis of antepartum and postpartum morphometric measurements of the head and abdomen of the fetus and newborn respectively. Approximately 20 to 30% of IUGR fetuses are symmetric type and 70 to 80% asymmetric. The clinical pattern divided into symmetric and asymmetric IUGR depends on the time the insult on the fetal growth occurs. In fact, during intrauterine life, fetal growth can be classified into three dynamic stages (Winick, 1971) . The first phase is represented by cellular hyperplasia and occurs during the first 16 weeks of gestation determining a rapid increase in cell number; in the second stage a concomitant cellular hyperplasia and hypertrophy involves an increase in both cell number and size occurring during the mid trimester. The last phase is characterized by a rapid increase in cell size as cellular hypertrophy dominates up to 32 weeks of gestation. Thus fetal growth rate in these three different dynamic stages is from 5g/day at 15 weeks, 15 to 20 g/day at 24 weeks, and 30 to 35 g/day at 34 weeks gestation. There have been many controversies surrounding the prognosis of the two patterns of growth-restricted fetuses. Many studies suggested that the symmetrically growth restricted fetuses were at greater risk of adverse outcome. This was particularly correlated to the high incidence of malformation and infections in the symmetric IUGR fetuses. A more recent study reports that the outcome of asymmetric IUGR is poorer if compared to the symmetrical one, also if the abnormalities in the first group were higher. So far, It is unclear if body proportionality (asymmetric / symmetric IUGR) is important with respect to etiology and neonatal outcome.

2. Diagnosis and management of IUGR

The detection of the IUGR fetuses is essential because of the high mortality and morbidity associated with this condition. In a study with a 10 years follow up, it was reported that in IUGR fetuses there is an incidence of 10 % of physical handicap and a 5% of neurodevelopment delay.

2.1 Diagnosis

Accurate pregnancy dating is the first step that should be considered in order to detect accurately IUGR fetuses. In the moment that pregnancy age is accurately dated, the diagnosis of IUGR consists essentially on clinical history, physical examination, ultrasonography and Doppler ultrasonography. The correct dating of the pregnancy (it is considered that the gestational age is uncertain at the 20-40% of pregnancies) is the key point of diagnosis, as only once in possession of this last, we compare the measurements with those obtained by us of reference curves. The determination of gestational age is possible through the date of last menstrual period (Last Menstrual Period - LMP), which is reported by pregnant or with ultrasound evaluation of fetal biometric parameters or during the clinical examination of the newborn immediately after birth. The LMP is often not correct, as reported by pregnant women, and vitiated by any menstrual irregularities. In contrast, the ultrasound parameters almost always show a high accuracy, especially if you use the measurement of the length of the top-sacred (Crown Rump Length - CRL) trans vaginal ultrasound during the first trimester of pregnancy (Soothill & al., 1999). Clinical history is important to find out the cause of IUGR, which is important for the clinical management. In this condition a detailed fetal echo is indicated. Physical examination consists in fundal height measurements of the uterus that can detect the small for gestational age fetus. A single measurement at 32 to 34 weeks of gestation has a sensitivity of 69% to 85% combined with a specificity of up to 96%. The diagnostic accuracy in predicting an IUGR fetus measuring the fundal height is similar if compared to AC measurement. Ultrasonography is able to predict the EFW of a fetus and several morphometric parameters should be used (Shepard & al., 19824). The error in the prediction of EFW may reach up to 25% (Hadlock & al., 1984). The most accurate parameter in the estimation of fetal weight is the AC, which is the most sensitive parameter for the detection of IUGR. In fact the AC measurements fall within 10% of the actual weight. It can be considered affected by intrauterine growth restriction fetus that shows (Cosmi & al., 2005): abdominal stunted controls seriated, CA decline from normal values to values below 10 th percentile and AC <10 th percentile and head circumference in the norm. The slight delay is defined if the AC is <10 °, and severe if <2SD, equal to 2.5 th percentile for the age gestationa. A normal CA excludes the diagnosis of IUGR with a false negative rate of about 40 to 10%. Dudley has completed a review of ultrasonographic fetal weight estimation and concluded that the method is inaccurate, with low sensitivity and predictive value for fetal compromise, but by its method of analysis does not reveal any significantly better (Dudley, 2005). In conclusion, since fetal growth is a dynamic process, the "serial do biometrics in order to obtain a longitudinal analysis of the actual rate of growth of each fetus, improves the sensitivity of diagnosis of IUGR.

2.2 Management

Current management of IUGR fetuses consists of serial ultrasound measurements to assess the growth rate, amniotic fluid, fetal heart rate (FHR) monitoring and Doppler velocimetry.

The fetal non stress test (NST) is used as the primary fetal surveillance method for the assessment of fetal well-being, its interpretation can recognize fetuses compromised or not (Cagnon & al., 1987). In the current practice an abnormal NST is usually followed by the evaluation of the biophysical profile score (BPP). The latter assess 5 parameters being the FHR, fetal tone, fetal gross body movements, fetal breathing movements (FBM), and the AF. To each parameter assessed a numeral scale from 0 to 2 is given. Thus the BPP is considered normal when the score is from 8 to 10, and the test is repeated at weekly interval because the occurrence of fetal death is very rare within 1 week; a score less than 6 is considered abnormal as chronic asphyxia is suspected. In the latter situation the BPP should be repeated in 4-6 hrs. and delivery should be considered if oligohydramnios is present (Dayal & al., 1999). The Non stress test (NST) and BPP are useful screening tool in the evaluation of fetal well being. At present, there is not enough evidence from randomized trials to evaluate the use of biophysical profile score as a test of fetal well being in high-risk pregnancies (Manning & al., 1980). Furthermore, the NST become abnormal too late if compared to the Doppler velocimetry changes. Doppler investigation should be used for the antenatal surveillancein IUGR fetuses, as it select which fetus could benefit from a more intense antenatal surveillance. In fact Doppler velocimetry in IUGR fetuses versus NST is superior in identifying the need of intervention. Doppler investigation is very useful in order to find out the possibility of fetal hypoxia and/or hypercarbia. Doppler meta-analysis has shown the use of the umbilical artery in high-risk pregnancies reduces the number of antenatal admissions (44%), inductions of labor (29%), cesarean sections for fetal distress (52%), and perinatal mortality (38%). The ACOG recommends the use of Doppler investigation in IUGR fetuses. Many studies have focused their attention on the temporal sequence of changes in fetal parameters in the IUGR fetus (ACOG, 1997). Thus an IUGR fetus is considered that with an EFW < 10th percentile, with an abnormal Doppler investigation and oligohydramnios. This group of IUGR fetuses constitute about 35-40% of all IUGR fetus and the antenatal surveillance has to be increased; the remaining IUGR fetuses, those with EFW < 10th percentile, normal Doppler investigation and amniotic fluid could be managed as AGA fetuses as have the same outcome. Fetuses whose weight is less than 10th percentile are usually managed with weekly NST or BPP to search for evidence of fetal distress. Doppler investigation of the umbilical artery (UA) is important to find out abnormalities, such as resistence increase, absent of end diastolic flow, reversed flow, in the UA, which constitutes pathological findings. Fetal growth restriction is a significant factor for increasing Doppler indices and Doppler abnormality identifies those fetuses that are at greater risk for adverse perinatal outcome (Arduini & Rizzo, 1993). In addiction the middle cerebral artery evaluation and thus cerebroplacental ratio should be performed, as it improves the prediction of perinatal outcome compared with UA velocimetry alone. Changes in the cerebral vascular diastolic flow, are progressive after the presence of the brain-sparing effect, indicative of blood redistribution to vital organ, and usually reach a nadir just prior to the onset of an abnormal FHR pattern. Other vessels that should be investigated are that of the venous system such as the ductus venosus and umbelical vein (UV) which abnormalities, reversed flow and pulsations, respectively, reflect an advanced status of fetal compromise. Studies on the temporal sequence of changes in IUGR fetus showed that when Doppler changes occur, aggressive management of the fetus (delivery) is suggested despite the NST is normal. Ozcan et al. pointed out that in compromised IUGR fetuses Doppler changes occur as follow: abnormality in UA, MCA, UV pulsation, reversed flow in the ductus venosus and at last abnormalities in NST (Ozcan & al., 1998). Thus the IUGR fetus should be investigated by doppler velocimetry of the arterial system and venous system and by NST and BPP. Senat et al. shown that prior the evidence of fetal distress by means of NST, significant changes occur in the arterial (UA, MCA) and venous system (DV, UV) showing that other hemodynamic changes were not statistically significant (Senat & al., 2000). Other studies confirm the above findings, thus Doppler investigation is an important tool to use in the management of IUGR fetuses, as according to its findings conservative or aggressive management should be opted. Arterial and venous flow changes are the first to become evident prior to abnormal findings in FHR, and BPP, in the latter the first abnormality are represented by fetal breathing movements, AF, body movements and at least fetal tone. Moreover a recent study shown that there are early and late changes in Doppler velocimetry. The first are represented by abnormality in the UA (increased resistance, absent end diastolic flow) and MCA; the latter are changes in DV, reversed flow in UA, pulmonary vein abnormalities and DV reversed flow. The last changes in those fetuses were in FHR tracing while abnormality in the AF were not statistically significant. The early stage changes were correlated with a less rate of mortality if compared to the late one.

3. Outcome of IUGR infants

IUGR is the second leading cause of perinatal morbidity and mortality with a 10-fold greater risk of fetal death if compared to normal fetuses which are appropriate for gestational age (AGA) (Pallotto & Kilbride, 2006). Moreover the mortality and morbidity rates are correlated to the EFW of the fetus: the less is the percentile at a given gestational age, the higher is the morbidity and mortality rate. In fact the mortality and morbidity are increased among infants born at term whose birth weights are at or below the 5th percentile with an increase below the 3rd percentile for a given gestational age. In fact those fetuses share a greater risk for fetal demise, fetal distress, and could develop short term (hypoglycemia, hypocalcemia, hypothermia, polycythemia, necrotizing enterocolitis, pulmonary hypertension), and long-term (ischemic heart disease, stroke hypertension, Non-Insulin Dependent Diabetes) complications.

3.1 Short-term outcome

Infants with low birth weight as those born with IUGR have a risk significantly increased to provide a low Apgar score associated with respiratory, neurological and metabolic sequelae in the long term, thanks to the condition of acute and chronic deprivation of oxygen and nutrients. The risk of sudden death in utero in fetuses with EFW below the 10th percentile increased 2 to 6 times compared to fetuses with appropriate weight for gestational age, mainly due to the hepato-renal impairment (Baschat & al., 2007). Hence the importance of an early intrauterine diagnosis in order to programme for the best fetal monitoring and to identify the right time for the induction of labor. The negative outcome does not seem to depend on the underlying cause of the lack of growth, but appears rather "dose-related," as worse with the worsening of the disease, to generate a cascade mechanism of physiological effects chained together. Several authors have focused attention on the temporal sequence of hemodynamic changes that characterize the IUGR fetuses and affecting first the artery and then the venous compartment. Initially there is the increase >2SD of the pulsatility index (PI) of the umbelical artery (UA), then the reduction of middle cerebral artery PI (MCA), the absence of diastolic flow (AEDF) in UA, the reverse flow (RF) in UA and changes in ductus venosus (DV), with increased PI and absent or reverse flow of wave A (corresponding to atrial contraction) (Baschat & al., 2001). Observational studies carried out and especially the multicenter one performed at our Department of Gynecology and Obstetrics Sciences, has shown that the optimal timing for the delivery is the time when the fetus has no diastolic flow in the umbilical artery, gestational age> 28 weeks and fetal weight >600g. The morbidity due to IUGR occur both in the short and long term (Hecher & al., 2001). The first group includes the problems that the child must face in the post-partum (delivery outcomes), including the condition of prematurity, with its related complications. Among the complications of delivery outcomes appear: high risk of perinatal asphyxia (due to placental insufficiency and intrauterine chronic hypoxia), greater frequency of resuscitation's intervention in the delivery room, increased risk of developing hypothermia, greater incidence of hypoglycemia (blood glucose <40 mg/ dL) and other metabolic sequelae, especially the hypocalcemia ($[Ca2 +]$ <7 mg/dL) and hyperbilirubinemia, due to both impaired hepatic detoxifying function and hyperhemolysis. The morbidity related to them are respiratory, digestive, neurological or renal, and they complicate the neonatal period of these patients. All other changes are manifest in childhood or adulthood are considered rather long complications term.

3.2 Long-term outcome

The long term complications are numerous and involve several systems: first of all the cardiovascular one because these children frequently have hypertension, with a significant increase in systolic pressure and in intima-media thickness of the abdominal aortic wall. The "developmental origins of adult disease" hypothesis, often called "the Barker hypothesis"(Barker, 2006) proposes that these diseases originate through adaptations of the fetus when it is undernourished. These adaptations may be cardiovascular, metabolic or endocrine and they may permanently change the structure and function of the body, increasing coronary heart disease risk factors, such as hypertension, type 2 diabetes mellitus, insuline resistance and hyperlipidemia (Gillman, 2005). This hypothesis originally envolved from observation by Barker and colleagues that the regions in England with the highest rates of infant mortality in the early 20th century also had the highest rates of mortality from coronary heart disease decades later. As the most commonly registered cause of infant death at the start of 20th century was low birth weight, these observations led to the hypothesis that low birth weight babies who survived infancy and childhood might be at increased risk of coronary heart disease in later life (Barker, 2000). As Barker and his colleagues reported in several epidemiological and anthropological studies, in fetal life tissues and organs go through the so called "critical" periods of development. These may coincide with periods of rapid cell division. Although the fetal growth is influenced by its genes, several studies suggest that it is usually limited by intrauterine environment, in particular the nutrients and oxygen received from the mother. Influence linked to fetal and placental growth have an important effect on the risk of coronary heart disease and stroke. Thus this theory focusing on intrauterine life, offers a new point of departure for research in cardiovascular disease. According to the thrifty phenotype hypothesis, deficient fetal supply may be followed by a programming which includes circulatory adjustment and insulin resistance in liver and muscular tissue in order to spare the brain. In addiction post-natal over nutrition following intrauterine growth restriction may be pathogenetic for the development of obesity and type 2 diabetes, whereas the elevated cardiovascular mortality rate may be associated with rapid postnatal catch-up growth in early infancy (Barker & al., 2003). The many reports of relationship between birth size and disadvantageous glucose and insulin metabolism have widely been reviewed. In particular fetal growth retardation has been associated with increased insulin resistance, higher fasting insulin concentrations and increased incidence of type 2 diabetes. Neonatal abdominal circumference has been shown to predict plasma cholesterol and fibrinogen levels in adult in later life, which are both risk factors for cardiovascular disease. There is also an impaired renal function with increased risk of acute renal failure and metabolic disorders, especially a great incidence of insulin resistance, diabetes mellitus non-insulin-dependent, hyperlipidemia, hypercholesterolemia and a marked tendency to obesity. About the neuro-cognitive development, it is undermined by the delay of intrauterine growth, resulting in high incidence of brain dysfunction, cognitive and linguistic problems.

3.3 Incidence of arterial hypertension in infants born with IUGR

Recent epidemiological studies have shown the correlation between the insults occurred in the earliest stages of development of the individual, including the period in the uterus, and incidence of chronic diseases, especially cardiovascular diseases. Besides low birth weight, three other early factors that are considered to be important risk factors for developing high BP in adult life have been identified in individuals with IUGR. First, accelerated postnatal growth in weight and length is suggested to increase the risk for developing hypertension and type 2 diabetes in later life. Second, it was postulated that altered angiotensin activity was an important factor underlying the "fetal origins of adult diseases" hypothesis. Also, hypoxia increased sympathetic nerve activity and catecholamine production and proliferation of juxtaglomerular cells (and thus renin-producing cells) are suggested as factors in the pathogenesis (Huxley & al., 2000). A follow-up study recently published by Cosmi et al, demonstrates that systolic BP measuraments in 2 years-old children born intrauterine restricted are significantly higher than in appropriate for gestational age children at the same age (Zanardo & al., 2011). From a hystorical viewpoint, it is clear that the Barker hypothesis received significant support because of its public health implication. However it must be considered that may confounders are known to influence blood pressure in adult life apart from birth weight. In addiction a larger genetic heterogeneity of individuals enrolled may explain its results. However as stated by Gluckman and Hanson "it is no longer possible to ignore the developmental phase of life" and follow-up studies in early childhood will assist the medical community and public health to designing interventions in order to ensure the best possible fetal development (Gluckman & Hanson, 2008).

3.4 Fetal programming and renal consequences

According to the fetal programming also the kidneys appear to be extremely succeptible to intrauterine growth restriction and are often found small in proportion to body weight. Several studies in animals and humans have described a reduced number of nephron after IUGR (Manalich & al., 2000). This results in an inborn decreased glomerular filtration surface area, while renal blood flow per glomerulus is increased in attempt to maintain a normal overall glomerular filtration rate. According to the hyperfiltration hypothesis explained by Brenner and co-workers (Brenner & al., 1996), this leads to glomerular hypertension and hypertrophy, which causes systemic hypertension and higher sodium reabsorption and glomerular damage resulting in albuminuria (Figure 3) and glomeruloclerosis. Therefore IUGR can lead to impairment of renal function (Luyckx & Brenner, 2005). A kidney with a reduced nephron number has less renal reserve to adapt to dietary excesses or to compensate for renal injury. The pathway leading from small kidney to hypertension may include the renin - angiotensin system, which has been demonstrated to be altered in the early phase of primary hypertension. An increased activity of the renin - angiotensin system could be a compensatory mechanism in a decreased number of nephrons in order to maintain normal filtration.

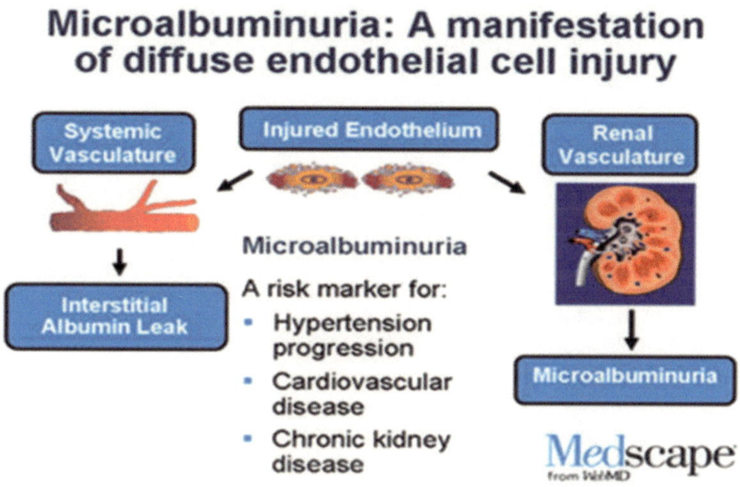

Fig. 3. Importance of microalbuminuria.

These mechanisms are well described in experimental study including IUGR male rats, whose presented higher blood pressure and fewer glomeruli at 22 weeks of age (Wlodek & al., 2008). In the last five years more clinical data are available regarding maturation of renal function in IUGR infants. Keijzer-Veen and colleagues in 2005 identified a positive association of birth weight and glomerular filtration rate (GFR) (Keijzer-Veen & al., 2005). The investigators also detected a negative association of birth weight and serum creatinine, suggesting that IUGR individuals are at greater risk to develop hypertension and progressive renal failure. This work made a significant contribution to understanding mechanism associated with the progression of cardiovascular disease and intrauterine retardation. In contrary Rakow at al found that glomerular filtration rate and urinary protein patterns were similar between IUGR 12 years-old children and controls, but kidney volume was smaller in the first group. A meta-analysis published by Teeninga et al in 2008, consisted in 201 patients (25 SGA, 176 AGA), showed that low birth weight has a strong influence in glomerular filtration rate and proteinuria, associated with a higher chance of developing several complications, including hypertension (Teeninga & al., 2008). A recent follow-up study demonstrated that 5 years- old children born IUGR showed higher BP, increased albuminuria, lower GRF and different urinary sodium excretion rate than controls. These observations support the contention that extrinsic renal injury is not a prerequisite for the initiation and perpetuation of renal injury and that certain circumstances, prenatally derived, intrinsic deficiencies in functioning renal mass may be sufficient to contribute to renal functional decline occurring with advancing age.

3.5 Endothelial dysfunction

The endothelium controls vascular tone, coagulation and inflammatory responses. Endothelial dysfunction is an early event of atherosclerosis (Figure 4), preceding structural changes in the vascular wall. Atherosclerosis is thought to begin in childhood and to develop silently before clinical events such as myocardial infarction or stroke occur (Jarvisalo & al., 2001). As with major cardiovascular risk factors, impaired growth in utero is associated with functional (endothelial dysfunction) and structural (increased wall thickness) changes to the arterial vasculare consistent with early atherosclerosis.

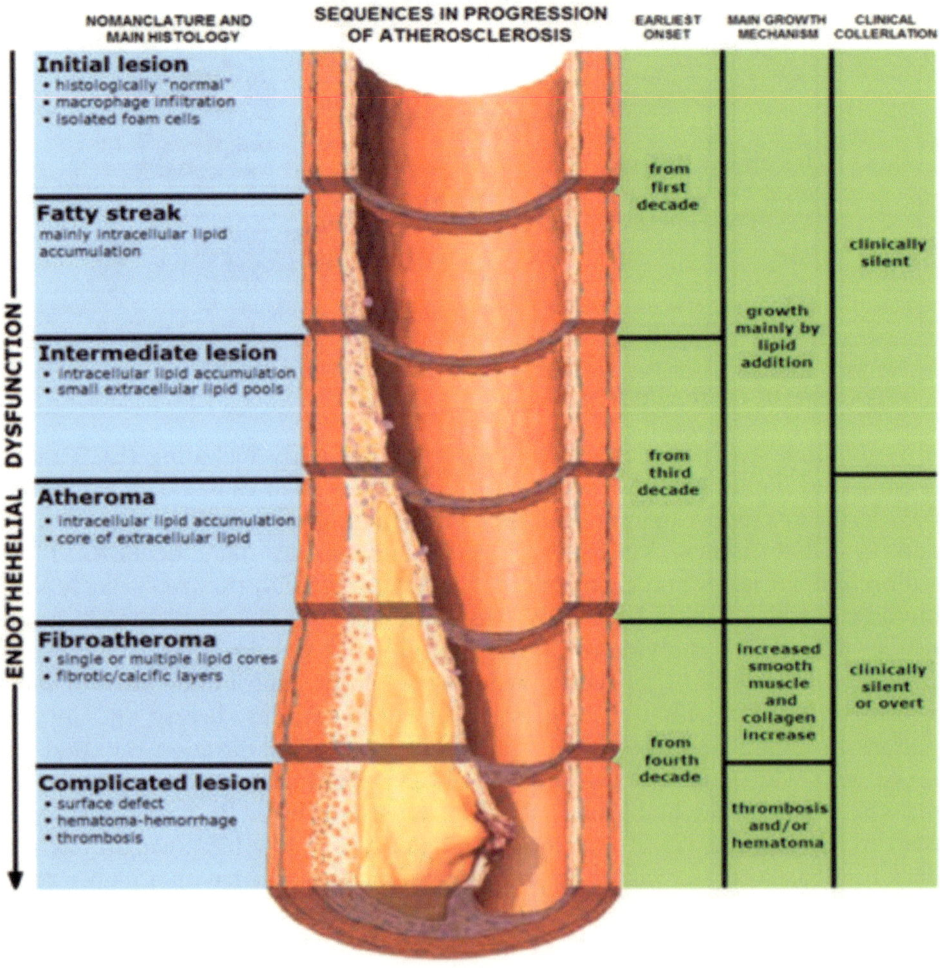

Fig. 4. Sequence in progression of atherosclerosis.

Impaired fetal growth in infants is associated with increased sympathetic tone and lipid concentration, and reduced concentration of insulin-like growth factor-1, all of which might contribute to arterial wall thickening. However, these findings are difficult to interpret because of potential confounding by, or interaction with, postnatal influences, so this hypothesis need further clarification. Tracy et al demonstrated atheromatous changes in the aorta of children (McGill & al., 2000). Atheromatous changes have been documented histopathologically by early childhood, and it has been assessed that the first atherosclerotic lesions actually begin to develop in the abdominal aorta. Nowadays many studies demonstrated atherosclerotic wall thickening in the arteries of children with cardiovascular risk factors using ultrasound imaging assessing noninvasively early vascular changes. In 2005 Skilton and co-workers add new interesting information to the Barker's hypothesis (Skilton & al., 2005). They compared intima-media thickness of the aortic wall in newborn infants with low birth weight with normal controls. In IUGR newborns aIMT was significantly greater than in the controls. On the basis of these finding they described the ultrasound-based measurement of abdominal aortic intima-media thickness in children as a feasible, accurate and sensitive marker of atherosclerosis risk and, as there was no confounding from childhood and adult exposures, they provide clear indications for a fetal contribution to later cardiovascular disease. Also Koklu et al in 2007 evaluated the potential use of aIMT in the study of high-risk neonates, concluding that aIMT measurement in IUGR newborns can help in the early identification of asymptomatic vascular dysfunction (Koklu & al., 2007). Recently Cosmi studied aIMT in fetuses for the first time and than in the same infants after a mean follow-up of 18 months. He found that aIMT measurements in IUGR fetuses are inversely related to estimated fetal weight, showing that low birth weight and Doppler abnormalities may be correlated to an altered vascular structure causing possible endothelial damage, consistent with the finding that atherosclerosis begins to develop first in the intima of the aorta. These differences remains also at the time of follow-up. Similarly, carotid intima-media thickness has been shown to be greater in children with low-birth weight. In a recent study Gratacos et al confirms the presence of increased carotid wall thickness in children with IUGR and that these changes persist into childhood (Crispi & al., 2010). The increased arterial wall thickness could be the result of vascular remodelling linked to metabolic programming in intrauterine life. They also highlighted that children with IUGR show changes in cardiac morphology, subclinical cardiac longitudinal dysfunction and hypertension, all of which increase linearly with the severity of growth restriction and are independent of gestational age at delivery, lipid profile or body mass index. The importance of early identification and intervention in pediatric risk factors for cardiovascular disease is now well recognized and this could open new opportunities for monitoring and intervention in newborns and children affected with intrauterine growth restriction.

3.6 IUGR Infant and their neurodevelopment

As said before intrauterine growth restriction plays a significant role in short and long term outcome ad reflected in high incidence of brain dysfunction and neurodevelopmental impairment, as well as in somatic growth failure. These clinical consequences could not be apparent until later in childhood development and could involve poor academic performance, memory, visuomotor and language difficulties and executive function problems. Several longitudinal studies have addressed the question of correlation between cognitive development and somatic growth in IUGR, using different questionnaire dealing with aspects of reading, writing, spelling and mathematics. An increased risk of cognitive impairment has been demonstrated in children with small head circumference. Shenkin et al found that birth weight is significantly related to IQ at age 11 (Shenkin & al., 2001). In other studies IUGR children have lower nonverbal and verbal IQ than controls. According to data from the National Collaborative Perinatal Project (1959-1976) the IQ scores of 2719 IUGR children tested at age 7 were 6 point lower than AGA children. Besides neurosensory handicaps, also behavioural sequelae are of serious concern. Behavioural problems, which might become manifested only at school age, can have a great impact on school performance and social competence and have a negative influence on quality of life (Van de Broek & al., 2010). Learning difficulties and behavioural problems are reported more often in IUGR preterm infants compared to AGA (Padilla & al., 2010). Management of these infants is controversial. They have an increased perinatal mortality and morbility including behavioural problems, minor developmental delay, poor neurosensory development and spastic cerebral palsy. Definition of these important long-term relationships invites research of pathological mechanism. Recent advanced magnetic resonance imaging studies have shown that IUGR is associated with structural differences that can be identified very early in life, such as reduction in cerebral cortical grey matter and hippocampal volume. These macrostructural alterations have been associated with microstructural and metabolic changes. As well explained from Baschat et al, the IUGR fetus "enables" sparing of the head while growing in a low-nutrient intrauterine environment and has neuroadaptative modification aimed at preserving brain oxygen supply in presence of chronic hypoxia (Baschat & al., 2009) . This process is identified clinically by a reduced Doppler pulsatility index (PI) in the middle cerebral artery (MCA). When multiple parameters are considered, such as gestational age and birth weight, umbilical artery reversed end diastolic velocity (UA-REDV) is identified as an important contributor to neurodevelopment. No similar effect could be demonstrated for abnormal venous Doppler findings. Brain sparing and cerebral arteries Doppler results are objects of study as predictors of adverse neurological outcome, but these relationships are not well assessed. These findings have important implications for the prognosis and the management of intrauterine growth restricted fetuses and children, who should be closely followed-up to identified individuals at risk.

4. Conclusion

The importance of IUGR in understanding adverse pregnancy outcome is relevant not only for clinicians, but also for public health service. During the last decade, knowledge of the short-term and long-term consequences of impaired fetal growth has increased at a very rapid rate and has involved lots of clinical aspects. At present, it is most important not only to develop efficient methods of preventing and diagnosing IUGR, recognizing at-risk fetuses, and screening fetal growth restriction among low-risk pregnancies, but to work out followup and adequate treatment programs for the control of the disorders which may follow this conditions. Programming the right time to deliver is the best method to avoid adverse perinatal outcome; indeed, proper postnatal feeding and infant growth may be essential for long-term outcome.

5. References

American College of Obstetricians and Gynecologists. ACOG practice bulletin. Intrauterine growth restriction. Obstet Gynecol 2001; 72: 85-96.

American College of Obstetricians and Gynecologists .ACOG. Utility of antepartum Umbelical artery Doppler velocimetry in intrauterine growth restriction. Committee Opinion. 1997; 188.

Arduini D, Rizzo G. Doppler studies of deteriorating growth retarded fetuses. Curr Opin Obstet Gynecol. 1993; 5: 195-203.

Barker DJ. In utero programming of cardiovascular disease. Therionol, 2000; 15;53(2):555-74.

Barker DJP, Eriksson JG, Forsen T, Osmond C. Fetal origins of adult disease:strength of effects and biological basis. Int J Epidemiology 2003; 31:1235-9.

Barker DJP: Adult consequences of fetal growth restriction. Clinical Obstetrics and Gynecology 2006; 49: 270–283.

Baschat AA, Viscardi RM, Hussey-Gardner B, Hashmi N, Harman C. Infant neurodevelopment following fetal growth restriction: relationship with antepartum surveillance parameters. Ultrasound Obstet Gynecol 2009;33:44-50.

Baschat AA, Cosmi E, Bilardo CM, Wolf H, Berg C, Rigano S, Germer U, Moyano D, Turan S, Hatung J, Bhide A, Muller T, Bower S, Nicolaides KH, Thilaganathan B, Gembruch U, Ferrazzi E, Hecher K, Galan HL, Harman CR: Predictors of Neonatal Outcome in Early-Onset Placental Dysfunction. Obstet Gynecol 2007; 109: 253-261.

Baschat AA: Pathophysiology of fetal growth restriction: implications for diagnosis and surveillance. Obstet Gynecol Survey 2004; 59: 617-627.

Baschat AA, Gembruch U, and Harman CR. The sequence of changes in Doppler and biophysical parameters as severe growth restriction worsens. Ultrasound Obstet Gynecol. 2001; 18 : 571-577.

Battaglia FC, Lubchenco LO: A practical classification of newborn infants by weight and gestational age. J Pediatr 1967; 71: 159-163.

Brenner BM, Lawler EV, Mackenzie HS. The hyperfiltration theory: a paradigm shift in nephrology. Kidney Int 1996;49:1774-1777.

Brodsky D, Christou H: Current concepts in intrauterine growth restriction. J Intensive Care Med 2004; 19: 307-319.

Cagnon R, Campbell K, Hunse C, Patrick J. patterns of human fetal heart rate acceleration from 26 week to term. Am J Obstet Gynecol. 1987; 157: 743-8.

Cosmi E, Ambrosini G, D'Antona D, Saccardi C, Mari G: Doppler, cardiotocography, and biophysical profile changes in growth-restricted fetuses. Obstet Gynecol 2005; 106: 1240-1245.

Crispi F, Bijnens B, Figueras F, Bartrons J, Eixarch E, Le Noble F, Ahmed A, Gratacos E. Fetal growth restriction results in remodelled and less efficient hearths in children. Circulation 2010;121:2427.36.

Dayal AK, Manning FA, Berk DJ, Mussalli JM, Avila C, Harman CR. Et al Fetal death after normal biophysical profile score: An eighteen year experience. Am J Obstet Gynecol. 1999; 181: 1231.

Dudley NJ: A systematic review of the ultrasound estimation of fetal weight. Ultrasound Obstet Gynecol 2005; 25: 80–89.

Froen JF, Gardosi JO, Thurmann A, Francis A, Stray-Pedersen B: Restricted fetal growth in sudden intrauterine unexplained death. Acta Obstet Gynecol Scand 2004; 83: 801–807.

Gillman MW: Developmental origins of health and disease. N Engl J Med 2005; 353: 1848-1850.

Gluckman PD, Hanson MA. Develompmental origins of health and disease: new insights. Basic Clin Pharmacol Toxicol. 2008 Feb;102(2):90-3.

Greiss FC Jr: Uterine blood flow in pregnancy: an overview. In: Uterine and placental blood flow. Moawad AH, Lindheimer MD eds Masson Publ 1982; pp 19-26.

Hadlock FP, Deter RL, Harrist RB, Park SK: Estimating fetal age: computerassisted analysis of multiple fetal growth parameters. Radiology 1984; 152: 497- 501.

Harkness U, Mari G: Diagnosis and management of intrauterine growth restriction. Clin in Perinatol 2004; 31: 743-764.

Hecher K, Bilardo CM, Stigter RH, Ville Y, Hackeoler BJ, Kok HJ, Senat MV and Visser GHA: Monitoring of fetuses with intrauterine growth restriction: a longitudinal study. Ultrasound Obstet Gynecol 2001; 18: 564-570.

Huxley RR, Shiell AW, Law CM. The role of size at birth and postnatal catch-up growth in determining systolic blood pressure: a systematic review in literature. J Hypertens 2000;18:815-31.

Jarvisalo MJ, Jartti L, Nanto-Salonen K. Increased aortic intima-media thickness: a marker of preclinical atherosclerosis in high-risk children. Circulation 2001;104:2943-7.

Keijzer-Veen MG, Schrevel M, Finken MJJ, Dekker FW, Nauta J, Hille ETM, Frolich M, van der Heijden BJ. Microalbuminuria and lower glomerular filtration rate at young adult age in subjects born very premature after intrauterine growth retardation. J Am Soc Nephrol 2005; 16:2762-2768.

Koklu E, Ozturk MA, Gunes T, Akcakus M, Kurtoglu S. Is increased intima-media thickness associated with preatherosclerotic changes in intrauterine growth restricted newborns? Acta Paediatr. 2007;96(12):1858.

Krebs C, Macara LM, Leiser R, Bowman AW, Greer IA, Kingdom JCP: Intrauterine growth restriction with absent end-diastolic flow velocity in the umbilical artery is associated with maldevelopment of the placental villous tree. Am J Obstet Gynecol 1996; 175: 1534-1542.

Lin CC, Santolaya-Forgas J: Current concepts of fetal growth restriction: part I. Causes, classification and pathophysiology. Obstet Gynecol 1998; 92: 1044-1055.

Luyckx VA, Brenner BM. Low birth weight, nephron number, and kidney disease. Kidney Int 2005;68:68-77.

Manalich R, Reyes L, Herrera M. Relationship between weight at birth and the number and the size of renal glomeruli in humans: a histomorphometric study. Kidney Int 2000;58: 770-773.

Mandruzzato G, Antsaklis A, Botet F, Chervenak FA, Figueras F, Grunebaum A, Puerto B, Skupski D, Stanojevic M: Intrauterine Growth Restriction (IUGR). J Perinat Med 2008; 36: 277–281.

Manning FA, Platt LD, Sipos L. Antepartum fetal evaluation : development of a biophysical profile score. Am J Obstet Gynecol. 1980; 136: 787-95.

McGill HCJ, McMahu CA, Herderick EE, Tracy RE, Malcom GT, Zieske AW, Strong JP. Effect of coronary heart disease risk factors on atherosclerosis of selected regions of the aorta and right coronary artery. PDAY Research Group. Pathobiological Detetrminants of Atherosclerosis in Youth. Ateriscler Thromb Vasc Biol. 2000; 20: 836,45.

McIntire DD, Bloom SL, Casey BM, Leveno KJ: Birth weight in relation with morbidity and mortality among newborn infants. N Engl J Med 1999; 340:1234-1238.

Ozcan T, Sbarcia M, d'Ancona L, Copel JA, and Mari G. Arterial and venous Doppler velocimetry in the severely growth-restricted fetus and associations with adverse perinatal outcome. Ultrasound Obstet Gynecol. 1998; 12: 39-44.

Padilla N, Perapoch J, Carrascosa A, Acosta-Rojas R, Botet F, Gratacos E. Twelve month neurodevelopmental out come in preterm infants with and without intrauterine growth restriction. Acta Pediatrica 2010;99:1498-1503.

Pallotto EK, Kilbride HW: Perinatal outcome and later implications of intrauterine growth restriction. Clin Obstet Gynecol 2006; 49: 257-269.

Senat MV, Schwarzler P, Alcais A, and Ville Y. Longitudinal changes in the ductus venosus, cerebral transverse sinus and cardiotocogram in fetal growth restriction. Ultrasound Obstet Gynecol. 2000; 16: 19-24.

Shenkin SD, Starr JM, Pattie A, Rush MA, Whalley LJ, Deary IJ. Birth weight and cognitive function at age 11: the Scottish Mental Survey 1932. Arch Dis Child 2001; 85(3):189-197.

Shepard MJ, Richards VA, Berkowitz RL, Warsof SL, Hobbins JC: An evaluation of two equations for predicting fetal weight by ultrasound. Am J Obste Gynecol 1982; 142: 47-54.

Skilton MR, Evans N, Griffiths KA, Harmer JA, Celermajer DS. Aortic wall thickness in newborns with intrauterine growth restriction. Lancet. 2005;365:1484-6.

Snijders RJ, Sherrod C, Golden CM, Nicolaides KH: Fetal growth retardation: associated malformations and chromosomal abnormalities. Am J Obstet Gynecol 1993; 168: 547-555.

Soothill PW, Bobrow CS, Holmes R: Small for gestational age is not a diagnosis (Editorial), Ultrasound Obstet Gynecol 1999; 33: 225–228.

Teeninga N, Schreuder M, Bokenkamp A, Delemarre-vam der Waal H, van Wijk J. influence of low birth weight on minimal change nephrotic syndrome in children, including a meta-analysis. Nephrol Dial Transplant 2008;23:1615-1620.

Van de Broek AJM, Kok JH, Houtzager A, Scherjon SA. Behavioural problems at the age of eleven years in preterm-born children with or without fetal brain sparing: A prospective cohort study. Early Human Development 2010;86:379-384.

Winick M: Cellular growth during early malnutrition. Pediatrics 1971; 47: 969-978.

Wlodek M, Westcott K, Siebel A, Owens J, Moritz K. Growth restriction before or after birth reduces nephron number and increases blood pressure in male rats. Kidney International 2008;74:187-195.

Zanardo V, Fanelli T, Weiner G, Fanos V, Zaninotto M, Visentin S, Cavallin F, Trevisanuto D, Cosmi E. Intrauterine growth restriction is associated with persistent aortic wall thickening and glomerular proteinuria during infancy. Kidney Int. 2011 Jul;80(1):119-23.

Zhang J, Bowes WA: Birth-weight-for-gestational-age patterns by race, sex and parity in the United States population. Obstet Gynecol 1995; 86: 200-208.

9

Pediatric Cardiac Surgery: A Challenge of Skill and Creativity in Constant Search Results

Miguel Angel Maluf
Cardiovascular Division,
São Paulo Federal University,
Brazil

1. Introduction

Pediatric cardiac surgery has been available for many years in several developing countries, thanks to the hard work and creative adaptation of individuals who were able to stretch the limits of their abilities in spite of the restricted resources. Limited resources were a constant problem forcing us to focus on short-term creativity about tomorrow's needs. A great deal of energy in the form of leadership and negotiations was used in order to encourage people to improve themselves and carry on working diligently despite the low pay.

Leadership, patience, perseverance, dedication, and the capacity to adapt to adversity have been the keys to success. Our sense of mission, commitment, enormous enthusiasm, dedication and clear objectives, supplemented the insufficient support of the institution that never fully met our needs. I have operated more than 4,500 children in Brazil since 1977 when I started my surgical training.

The Department of Pediatric Cardiology, Pediatric Cardiac Surgery and Pediatric Care Unit at São Paulo Federal University (SPFU) - Brazil, started in 1990, an Institutional Program for Diagnosis and Treatment of patients with Congenital Heart Disease.

This Institutional program development by SPFU was established to perform two elective and one emergency surgical procedure per week and complemented with electives operations in others two Private Institutions, performing: 20 operations per months or 250 operations a year.

This program was intended for the care of patients with congenital heart disease, development of protocols and conducts, during the pre-and postoperative period. On the other hand the surgeon's time, taking advantage of his own creativity conceived and developed new surgical techniques or preparation of biological tissue grafts for the construction of new models of heart valves for the remodeling of the right ventricle.

2. New technique in surgical procedure

2.1 Blalock-Taussig shunt in neonates using the brachiocephalic trunk (innominate artery) to ensure long patency

Placement of a Blalock-Taussig (BT) shunt is a "closed-heart" procedure performed as a first stage to correct Tetralogy of Fallot or others cyanotic congenital heart diseases. Placement of a shunt is usually a temporary measure designed to alleviate symptoms until such time that the patient is in better condition to undergo complete repair.The usual approach is performed by systemic-pulmonary shunts using right or left thoracotomy and today we used median sternotomy approach, for interposition of *polytetrafluoroethylene* (PTFE) vascular graft between the subclavian and pulmonary arteries.

In preterm or low birth weight children it is often found a subclavian artery of small diameter (2.5 to 3.0 mm), which could jeopardize the flow of the shunt due to difference in calibers between this vessel and the PTFE graft, compromising the patient's life. In order to overcome this anatomical difficulty, since 1986, we have been performing technical modifications of the B-T shunt, with PTFE prosthesis anastomosed to the brachiocephalic (innominate artery) trunk, always larger in diameter than the subclavian artery. To this end, the approach by thoracotomy was always done by other side of the descending aorta or the same side of the origin of the brachiocephalic trunk (BCT). This technique is an original contribution of our group.

This approach causes essentially a trauma to the lungs and some difficulty for dissection and definitive surgical ligation during later correction.

Since 1990 we have held the B-T shunt between the innominate artery and the right pulmonary artery, through a median thoracotomy, allowing a more comfortable procedure with hemodynamic and oximetric patient's control.

This technique is viable with advantages over lateral approach due to cutting easier access, vascular structure dissection, avoiding lung trauma; on the other hand, a rapid cardiopulmonary bypass is installed, if hypoxic crisis occurs during the surgical procedure. (Fig. 1)

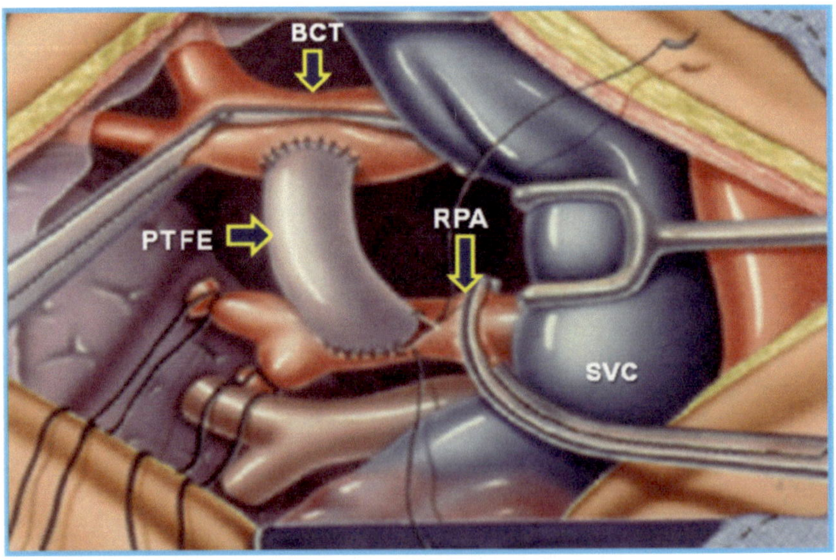

Fig. 1. Plot of the Blalock-Taussig shunt. Right thoracotomy approach and interposition of *polytetrafluoroethylene* (PTFE) graft between the brachiocephalic trunk (BCT) and the right pulmonary artery (RPA). SVC: superior vena cava.

2.2 Patient information

Sixty four patients; mean age of the patients was 29.3 ± 1.0 days (1 day to 17 years-old). Five neonates with mean weigh 2,600 gr (1,800 to 3,000 gr), were operated between 1987 and 1988, with interposition of PTFE graft between the BCT and right pulmonary artery (RPA), due to the reduced diameter of the subclavian artery. Four patients had hospital discharge with pervious BT shunt. The diagnosis of cardiac malformation was: T. of Fallot, pulmonary Atresia with intact ventricular septum, Tricuspid atresia and Univentricular heart.

These first 5 patients were operated by lateral thoracotomy, subsequently, 30 cases were operated using median thoracotomy approach. In all cases it was employed a PTFE graft (3.5 - 4.0 mm) , anastomosed to BCT. (Fig.2)

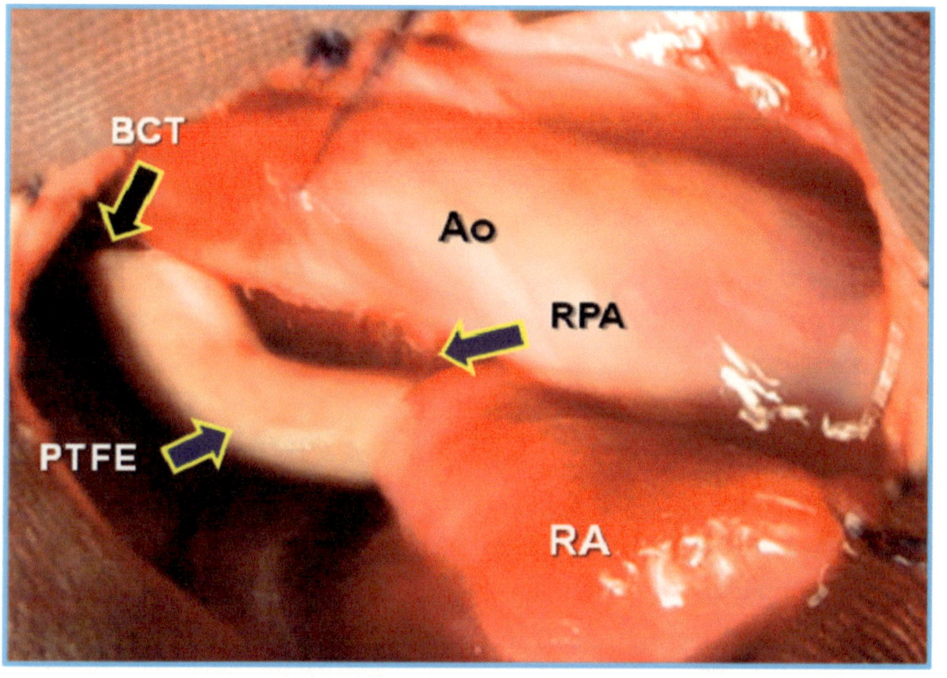

Fig. 2. Surgical picture of Blalock-Taussig shunt in a patient with pulmonary atresia with intact ventricular septum. Median thoracotomy approach: Interposition of polytetrafluoroethylene (PTFE) graft (arrow) between the brachiocephalic trunk (BCT) and the right pulmonary artery (RPA). RA: right atrium, Ao: aorta.

2.3 Results

There were 2 (5.7%) deaths in this group of 35 patients during the early postoperative period by sepsis and respiratory distress. Thirty three patients were submitted to Doppler-echocardiogram exam; all patients presented pervious B-T shunt.

3. Total cavopulmonary connection for treatment of the univentricular heart – *Staged strategy*

3.1 First stage: Bidirectional Glenn

The Fontan repair and its modifications can be performed in selected groups of patients which report relatively low rates of mortality. Among the later modifications of the Fontan-type procedure, a significant alteration was introduced by de Leval and associates when they described the Intracardiac cavopulmonary connection (ICPC). The modified Fontan procedure represents the final stage for the palliation of hearts with single-ventricle physiology.

The introduction of a bidirectional Glenn (BDG) procedure preceding an ICPC extends the indication for the Fontan procedure. High-risk Fontan candidates who have undergone BDG and staged ICPC (*staged strategy*) have exhibited excellent clinical results. However, the exact mechanism for the superiority of BDG is still poorly understood.

In addition, several management strategies have been incorporated in order to reduce the mortality: universal risk factors that have resulted in better patient selection; the use of tunnel fenestration; and the use of modified ultrafiltration after cardiopulmonary bypass (CPB).

Many reports discussed the importance of the pulmonary artery size and systemic ventricular function in Fontan candidates. A few studies undertaken to investigate in detail the hemodynamic conditions in Fontan circulation focusing on the ventricular efficiency.

When the ICPC was performed, the lower resting heart rate or the higher peak heart rate, are frequently part of the operation history which are each weakly associated with better physical function.

Cardiac arrhythmias are very common in patients submitted to intracardiac lateral tunnel using a long suture line on the right atrial wall.

3.2 Second stage: Inferior vena cava to pulmonary artery connection

3.2.1 Patient information

In our Institution, following the Great Ormond Street Hospital's protocol behavior the total cavopulmonary connection is performed in staged strategy: in March 1990, we performed the first BDG (1st stage) and in April, 1992 the same patient was completed to TCPC (2nd stage), with good results.

This successful technique was adopted, rapidly, by Institutions with Pediatric Cardiovascular Surgery, all over the country, and abandoning the atrio-pulmonary anastomosis.

Between March, 1990 and December, 2008; 105 patients were submitted to BDG in our Institution. In this study we included 52 patients of these series, consisting of 27 females and 25 males, mean age of the patients was 3.3 ± 1.0 years (1 to 8 years-old) and underwent ICPC. These patients were a consecutive series. Table1.

Diagnosis	Patients	(%)
Tricuspid Atresia	25	(48.2)
Single Ventricle	16	(30.7)
Pul. Atresia w / IVS	11	(21.1)

Pul. : pulmonary; w: with; IVS: intact ventricular septum

Table 1. Anatomic Diagnosis

3.3 Hemodynamic variables

The preoperative hemodynamic variables: heart rate, mean pulmonary artery pressure, ejection fraction and Nakata pulmonary arterial index were evaluated in all patients, according to the protocol established by our Institution.

The operative procedures before BDG were as follows: a modified Blalock-Taussig shunt was performed in 39 patients and pulmonary artery banding in 9 patients. In 52 (49.5%) patients the ICPC was indicated after the first stage of the BDG. Figure 3.

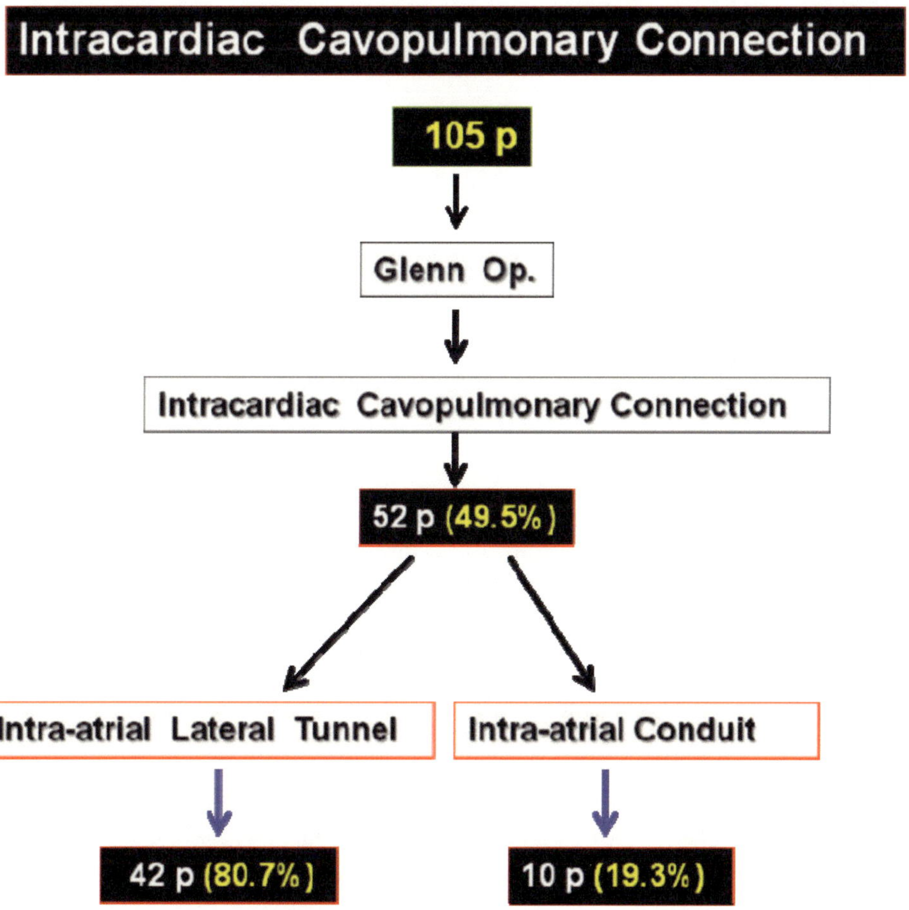

Fig. 3. Staged Intracardiac cavopulmonary connection.

3.4 Patient inclusion criteria

The indication for intra-atrial cavopulmonary anastomosis surgery included patients:

Diagnosed with univentricular heart.

- Previously submitted to BDG.
- Presenting cyanosis and decreased exercise tolerance
- Preserved ventricular function: EF >50 %, end-diastolic pressure of the systemic ventricle <11 mm Hg.
- Pulmonary pressure < 18 mmHg
- Pulmonary resistance < 2.0 wood units
- Nakata index > 250 mm^2 x m^2
- Staged period (BDG - ICPC) < 5 years
- New York Heart Association functional class I-II

3.5 Patient exclusion criteria

- Presence of pulmonary fistulae
- Low ventricle function: EF < 50 %, end-diastolic pressure of the systemic ventricle 11 mm Hg or higher
- Pulmonary pressure > 18 mmHg
- Pulmonary resistance > 2.0 wood units
- Nakata index < 250 mm^2 x m^2
- Staged period (BDG - ICPC) > 5 years
- New York Heart Association functional class III or higher

Fifty two patients had a previous bidirectional cavopulmonary shunt performed by direct end-to-side anastomosis between the SVC and the right pulmonary artery (RPA) (bidirectional Glenn). This group was referred to ICPC 1 to 5 years later: In 42 (80.7 %) cases it was indicated an intra-atrial lateral tunnel and in the last 10 (19.2%) consecutive patients, an intra-atrial conduit technique was performed.

3.6 Operative technique

Anesthesia was performed by the standard intravenous access with fentanyl, midazolam and pancuronium, for muscle relaxation. Although the ICPC was performed by Aortic SVC and inferior vena cava (IVC) cannulation to install a cardiopulmonary bypass (CPB) and perform the surgical approach with beating heart. When heart arrest was necessary, myocardial preservation was achieved with a cold blood cardioplegic solution. We reported our surgical technique in previous publications.

3.7 Intra-atrial lateral tunnel

Forty two (80.7%) patients had a previous BDG shunt performed by direct end-to-side anastomosis between the SVC and the RPA. Figure 4. These patients were operated by the intra-atrial lateral tunnel technique performed with a bovine pericardium patch. Figure 5.

The details of the surgical procedure employed are described as follows: After dissection of BDG, the operation was performed using CPB, moderated hypothermia and beating heart.

After the right atrium approach, the lateral tunnel was performed using a bovine pericardium patch sutured around the IVC *ostium* and on the lateral right atrium wall. The upper tip of the tunnel is connected to the SVC *ostium*. The RPA is open and stitched to the lateral tunnel by the proximal tip of the SVC. Finally, the anastomosis is enlarged using a bovine pericardium patch.

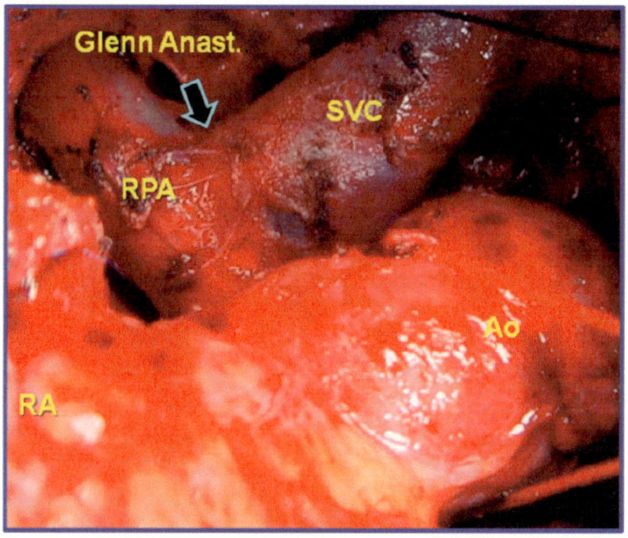

Fig. 4. Surgical photography- Bidirectional Glenn: Anastomosis between distal Superior Vena Cava (SVC) and Right Pulmonary Artery (RPA). RA: right atrium, Ao: aorta.

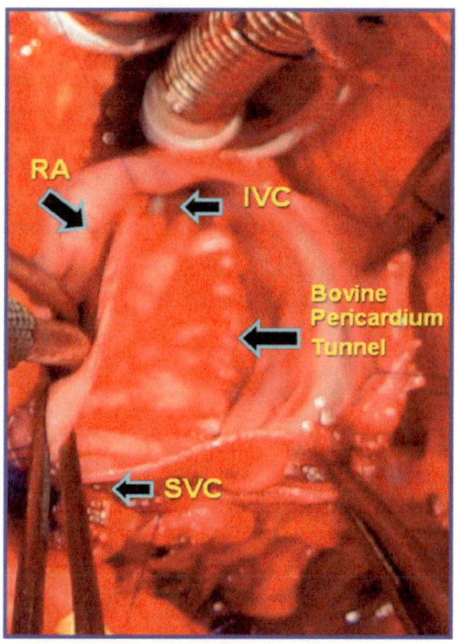

Fig. 5. Surgical photography- An intra-atrial lateral tunnel operation was performed suturing a bovine pericardium patch to the lateral right atrium wall. IVC: Inferior vena cava; SVC: Superior vena cava; RA: Right atrium.

3.8 Intra-atrial conduit

In the last 10 (19.2%) consecutive patients a technique modification was introduced to avoid the lateral suture in the free wall of the right atrium (RA) and cardiac arrhythmias. Figure 6.

After a longitudinal RA approach, a corrugated bovine pericardium tube, measuring 18 to 20 mm of diameter was sutured around the ostium of the IVC and SVC.

Finally, the connection with an RPA was performed using the same technique of the lateral tunnel. This technique is a original contribution of our group.

In both techniques a 4 mm trap-door type fenestration was performed promoting its spontaneous occlusion during the follow-up.

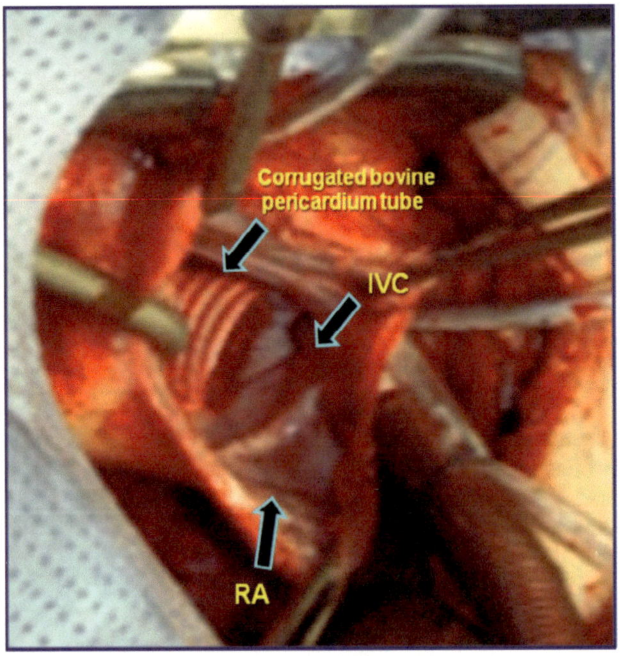

Fig. 6. Surgical photography- The intra-atrial conduit operation is performed, implanting a corrugated bovine pericardium tube around the ostium of the superior and inferior vena cava.

3.9 Statistical analysis

The relations of cardiac arrhythmias between two groups were evaluated with the exact Fisher test. A p value of less than 0.05 or 5% was considered to be significant.

3.10 Results

There were 2 hospital deaths (mortality 2.8%) in the intra-atrial lateral tunnel group: one patient presented acute renal insufficiency not reverted with peritoneal dialysis and compromised ventricular function, resulting in death 30 days after operation. The other patient presented multiple-organ failure resulting in death, 20 days after operation.

There were no records of mortality among the 10 (19.3%) patients submitted to intra-atrial conduit implant.

The mean cardiopulmonary bypass time was 114 ± 27 minutes (range 50 to 152). Thirty patients underwent aortic cross-clamping, and the mean aortic cross-clamp time was 42 ± 33 minutes (range 20 to 80). The mean duration of the mechanical ventilation was 12 hours (range 0 to 204). The average duration of intensive care unit stay was 5 days (range 3 to 29), the average duration of chest tube drainage was 6 days (range 2 to 38), the average duration of postoperative hospital stay was 16 days (range 7 to 60), and the average follow-up period was 87 ± 45 months (range 6 to 204). All of these patients received anti-platelet drug therapy during the follow-up. Table 2

	Variable Time	
	mean	range
CPB (min)	114 ± 27	50 - 152
Aortic Clamping (min)	42 ± 33	20 - 80
Mechanical ventilation (h)	12 ± 7	0 - 204
Intensive Care Unit (days)	5 ± 3	3 - 29
Chest tube drain (days)	6 ± 4	2 - 38
Hospital stay (days)	16 ± 8	7 - 60

CPB: cardiopulmonary bypass; min: minutes

Table 2. Operative date

Postoperative problems were minimal. Medication applied during the hospital stay for symptoms of fluid retention, congestive heart failure or both included digoxin, diuretics and captopril. Five patients had occasional early-morning facial edema; all of them remained on a regimen of diuretics, captopril and milrinone.

There was a significant improvement of O2 saturation after surgery in both groups: Intra-atrial lateral group, SO2: before M=78 %, after M= 92 %; Intra-atrial conduit, SO2: before M= 79 %, after M= 93 %.

The postoperative data were presented at Table 3.

Variables	Intra-atrial lateral tunnel	Intra-atrial conduit	p
Patients	42 pat	10 pat	----
BDG	42 pat	10 pat	----
Fenestration: tunnel/conduit	42 pat	10 pat.(trap-door)	----
Cardiac arrhythmias	13 pat. (30.9%)	0 pat. (0%)	0.048*
Take Down op.	0 pat	0 pat.	----
Death	2 pat	0 pat.	0.649
Mortality	4.76 %	0%	----

*Statistic significant. BDG: bidirectional Glenn; Sat: saturation; pat.: patients; Op: operation

Table 3. Post-operative data

In the intra-atrial lateral tunnel group: consisted of 40 (80%) surviving patients, it was observed the presence of cardiac arrhythmias in 13 (30.9%) cases and there were statistical differences (p=0.048) when comparing both groups. Ten (23.8%) patients received anti-arrhythmic drugs daily.

One patient developed late postoperative paroxysmal supraventricular tachycardia and was treated with a selective ß blocker.

However, no arrhythmias were detected in the intra-atrial conduit group.

All patients were submitted to periodic clinical and cardiac imaging exam: Doppler-echocardiogram each 6 month; MNR and CT after 2 years of operation. The details of the inta-atrial conduit are shown in the Magnetic nuclear resonance study; in this group there were no reports of open fenestration after 2 years of operation according to the MNR exam. Figure 7.

The Kaplan-Meier actuarial curve shows 96.1 % of surviving patients with Intra-atrial tunnel. In that period of time there had not been detected any thromboembolism events using Doppler-echocardiography criteria.

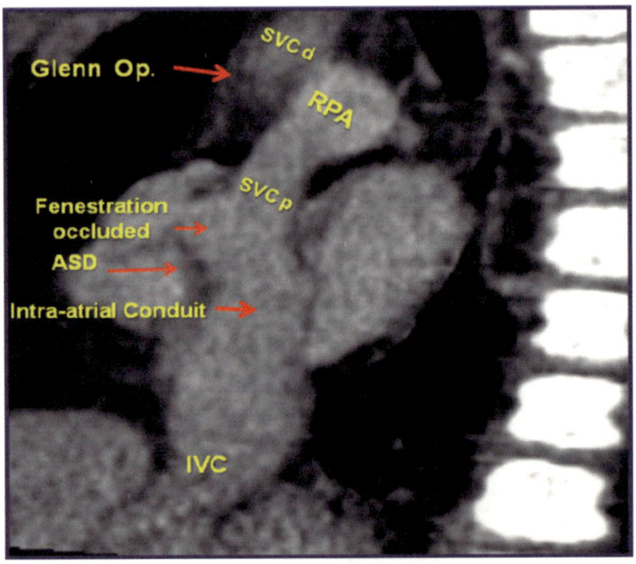

Fig. 7. Image of the Magnetic Nuclear Resonance performed in a patient 3 years after of Intra-atrial conduit implantation (a variant procedure technique). SVC: superior vena cava, p: proximal, d: distal; IVC: inferior vena cava; RPA: right pulmonary artery; ASD: atrial septal defect.

However, no reoperation had been performed at that moment. Figure 8,9.

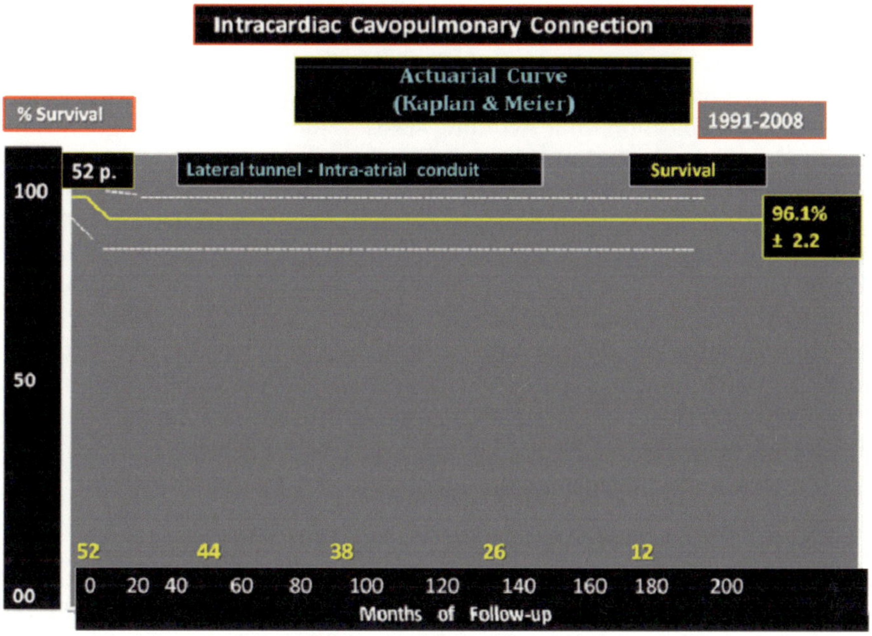

Fig. 8. Actuarial curve using the Kaplan-Meier method to analyze the surgical and follow-up results of Intracardiac cavopulmonary connection.

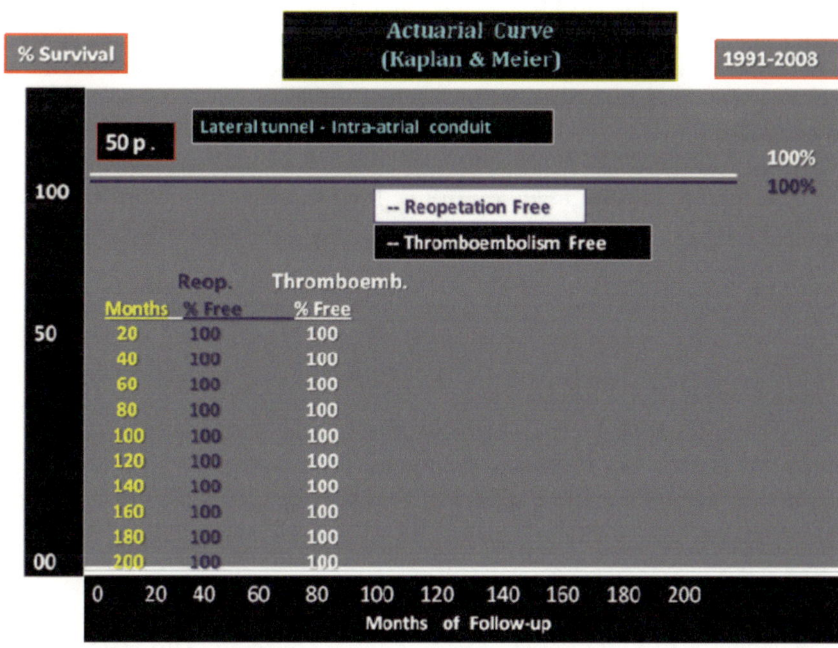

Fig. 9. Probability of overall reoperation and thromboembolism incidence in the last 9 years, after performing the lateral tunnel - Intracardiac conduit surgery.

3.11 Discussion

Throughout the years, the experience with Fontan operation has been increasing and has opened the way to a much wider application of this principle. The subsequent evolution of the cavopulmonary connection, thus avoiding stasis of the blood in the right atrium as seen in the atrial-pulmonary anastomosis or the turbulence seen in cases of atrial-ventricular-arterial connections. The hemodynamic concept of Jonas & Castaneda demonstrated the advantages of laminar flows, with less outflow and lower incidence of arrhythmias and thrombosis, introducing new surgical techniques. A number of major risk factors have been identified and managed by several modifications of the original Fontan procedure and late outcome of the Fontan circulation is encouraging. Ventricular morphology, surgical techniques and fenestration do not appear to influence early or late outcome. In the preoperative preparation of the patient is important to detect the impaired ventricular function and elevated pulmonary artery pressure because it has an adverse influence on both early and late outcome.

Reoperations are common with small preoperative pulmonary artery size being an additional risk factor.

This report focused its attention on the only two different variant options of intracardiac connection of the superior vena cava and inferior vena cava with the right pulmonary artery: intra-atrial lateral tunnel and intra-atrial conduit implantation, in order to reduce the cardiac arrhythmias and tunnel thrombosis.

In our Institution, the total cavopulmonary connection is performed in a staged strategy. An alternative approach is to make connections between both ends of the divided superior vena cava and the pulmonary artery and to place a patch within the right atrium at the entrance site of the superior vena cava. This procedure was performed at the São Paulo Federal University, being the first institution in the country to adopt this procedure, and then rapidly expand to other pediatric cardiac surgery centers in the country, looking for successful results. To complete the Fontan operation, the removal of this patch facilitates the connection between the IVC to RPA, with the construction of an intra-atrial tunnel or implantation of intra-atrial corrugated conduit of bovine pericardium, sutured to IVC and SVC ostium, facilitated by the proximal stump of the SVC with the RPA. This technique is an original contribution of our group.

In this series, 40 surviving patients with lateral tunnel Fontan presented 13 (30.9%) cases with cardiac arrhythmias. To prevent frequent cardiac arrhythmias we changed the lateral tunnel technique to the intra-atrial conduit implantation. A corrugated bovine pericardium tube is sutured around the ostium of the inferior vena cava and superior vena cava avoiding the right atrium wall stitched line. None of the last 10 patients, with intra-atrial conduit,submitted to Holter study during the follow-up, presented cardiac arrhythmias in 3 different moments: at rest, during exercise or sleeping. No patient was referred to pacemaker implant.

The postoperative period, early and late arrhythmias after a Fontan operation seem to be a consequence of adverse hemodynamic function. In the early follow-up is, therefore, poor even when the patient is restored to the sinus rhythm. Medical and surgical modifications in order to improve the hemodynamic disturbances associated with arrhythmias are therefore indicated.

Other authors described that Fontan conversion with concomitant arrhythmia surgery and permanent pacemaker placement are safe and improve the New York Heart Association functional class, and has a low incidence of recurrent arrhythmias. In most patients, concomitant permanent pacemakers are needed. The intra-atrial lateral tunnel (ILT) operation results in excellent midterm outcome even when used in patients with complex anatomy.

The incidence of postoperative atrial tachyarrhythmias is low and depends largely on the underlying cardiac morphology and incidence of preoperative arrhythmia. The good midterm outcome after an ILT operation should serve as a basis for comparison with other surgical alternatives to complete the Fontan circulation. Outcome after staged ILT operations is good, with comparable freedom from late re-operations and freedom from Fontan failure at 6-year follow-up. Right ventricular morphology was identified as a risk factor for arrhythmias.

The staged strategy is considered to be one of the most important factors for obtaining excellent clinical results in the treatment of high-risk Fontan candidates, with low mortality. The volume load reduction of bidirectional Glenn preceding intracardiac cavopulmonary connection allowed for any afterload mismatch to be corrected, thereby improving ventricular efficiency after staged intracardiac cavopulmonary connection in clinical patients.

The most significant findings in patients submitted to Fontan procedure who underwent a staged operation are: 1- The volume-load reduction of the systemic ventricle, resulted in an improvement of the contractility in both: after bidirectional Glenn and after staged intracardiac cavopulmonary connection; 2- Afterload increased both: after bidirectional Glenn and after staged intracardiac cavopulmonary connection and 3- These changes resulted in an improvement of ventricular efficiency during the interval period between bidirectional Glenn and intracardiac cavopulmonary connection.

Improved early morbidity and mortality after Fontan operation was presented in clinical experience of the Mayo Clinic, from 1987 to 1992.

In our Institution the study of the first 18 surviving patients submitted to bidirectional Glenn were available with cineangiographic exam showed a significant reduction in the total index of the left pulmonary artery after mean follow-up of 23.6 months.

An alternative approach to homogeneous distribution of SVC blood flow into RPA and LPA was performing of the hemi-Fontan operation that includes atriopulmonary anastomosis employing an atriopulmonary patch directs superior vena cava flow into both pulmonary arteries and inferior vena cava flow into the ventricle, thus maintaining cardiac output (modified Glenn physiology).

The extracardiac cavopulmonary connection is other alternative to cavopulmonary connection, utilizing a non-valved conduit is gradually becoming accepted as a new alternative for the surgical treatment of certain complex congenital heart diseases. Among the advantages of the use of an extracardiac conduit is the possibility of employing it under normothermic cardiopulmonary bypass with a beating heart, which is important for the preservation of the left ventricular function.

The extracardiac cavopulmonary connection, however, it is not always beneficial and among the complications that may arise are: thromboembolism, cellular hyperplasia, fibrosis and calcification and the absence of growth. All are severe complications, which can occur in the early follow-up or even months or years after the intervention and shadow the late evolution.

Another recent national experience shows: 18 consecutive patients with univentricular heart submitted to total cavopulmonary connection. These patients were operated using the extracardiac conduit procedure to make the connection between the inferior vena cava and the pulmonary circulation. Three patients died in the immediate post-operative period (hospital mortality rate: 16.6%). There were four cases of thrombosis with one case evolving to death. All the four cases were submitted to re-intervention. Apart from the case described above, a fifth case suffered from thrombosis and progressive calcification, which led to total occlusion of the conduit.

Due to this fact, the patients in this study were routinely prescribed warfarin sodium, using salicylic acetyl acid only when the use of the former was impossible or after the 12 post-operative month for the rest of their lives. This, however, did not prevent the occurrence of thrombosis in the conduit, initiating within 24 hours in one of the patients and with total occlusion of the tube, which forced replacement but this did not impede a lethal result of the complication.

The Fontan operation in its variant ways of performance was always associated with approximately 20% of thromboembolism in the post-operative period. The Kaplan & Meier actuarial curve in our series of 50 survival patients operated with the intra-atrial connection technique, followed-up by 12 to 204 months by Doppler-echocardiogram, MNR and CT reported survival of 96,1%, free of reoperations and we have not reported thromboembolism events in this period. Figure 6, 7, 8. All of our patients received anti-platelet drugs (salicylic acetyl acid), only.

3.12 Conclusion

The Bidirectional cavopulmonary anastomosis with intracardiac repair is a viable alternative for patients with RV hypoplasia. Early unloading of the functional univentricular heart by means of BDG allowed a good condition for completing the intra-atrial cavopulmonary connection.

Technical modifications of the intra-atrial operation (intra-atrial conduit implanted) have reported no cardiac arrhythmias and no prosthesis thrombosis during the follow-up. The modified surgical procedure can be a good alternative to the Fontan procedure in suitable patients.

4. Modified senning operation for surgical correction of simple transposition of the great arteries

Survival functional status and quality of life of patients with transposition of the great arteries (TGA), after an atrial switch operation (Senning or Mustard procedure) are reported to be reasonably good within the first two decades of life. However, in some cases the function of the systemic right ventricle deteriorates, severe tricuspid regurgitation develops or the patients suffer from arrhythmias.

Several strategies are proposed to handle those patients with failing right ventricle, such as: tricuspid valve repair, conversion to arterial switch or heart transplantation. In most of the cases, these procedures are performed after the right ventricular function has already deteriorated, as a consequence of high operative mortality In the present study we focused on the analysis of the long-term results of atrial switch procedure (Senning operation), to identify risk factors for long-term outcome and quality of life, in a group of patients with simple TGA.

4.1 Patient information

From July 1990 to December 2000, 40 consecutive patients with TGA were submitted to palliative atrial switch (Senning operation); 37 cases had atrial septal defect (ASD) and 3 cases had ASD associated to small muscular ventricular septal defect (VSD). These patients were operated the cardiovascular Division of São Paulo Federal University (UNIFESP).

Out of 39 (97.5%) surviving patients, thirty six (94.8%) cases were included in a retrospective follow-up study. Three patients, living overseas were excluded from this study.

The patients age at the moment of surgical correction was 1 to 11 months (mean 5.3 months); male 21 (52.4%). The clinic diagnostic was confirmed by Doppler-echocardiogram: d-TGA with ASD, in 37 (92.5%) cases, and ASD associated to small muscular VSD (size: 3 to 4 mm of diameter), in three (7,5%) cases, were present. All patients were submitted to Rashkind procedure prior to surgery. Table 3.

Characteristics	Patients(%)	Mean	(range)
Age (months)	---------------	5.3	(1-11)
Male	21 (52.4)	-----	-------
TGA + ASD	37 (92.5)	-----	-------
TGA + ASD + VSD *	03 (7.5)	-----	-------
Rashkind procedure	40 (100)	-----	-------

TGA: Transposition of the great arteries; ASD: Atrial septal defect; VSD: Ventricular septal defect. * Small muscular ventricular septal defect.

Table 3. Preoperative characteristics of patients

4.2 Operative technique

The surgical approach was performed by median sternotomy, employing hypothermic cardiopulmonary bypass (CPB), after vena cava and aortic cannulation; anterograte cold blood cardioplegia was used for myocardial protection, administrated every 20 minutes. During bypass assistance it was employed the conventional ultrafiltration (CUF) and after July 1996, it was associated with modified ultrafiltration (MUF), after the bypass was discontinued. In all patients it was used the Subramanian's technique modification using left atrial appendix flap, for reconstruction of the new atrial septum and dispense the use of any prosthetic tissue. Figure 10.In order to avoid tunnel stenosis, the Hegar dilator was used to measure the diameter of the vena cava ostium Figure 11. No patient required a more extensive enlargement of the right or left atrium Figure 12,13 and interrupted suture was applied, around the superior and inferior vena cava to avoid external restriction. Figure 4.

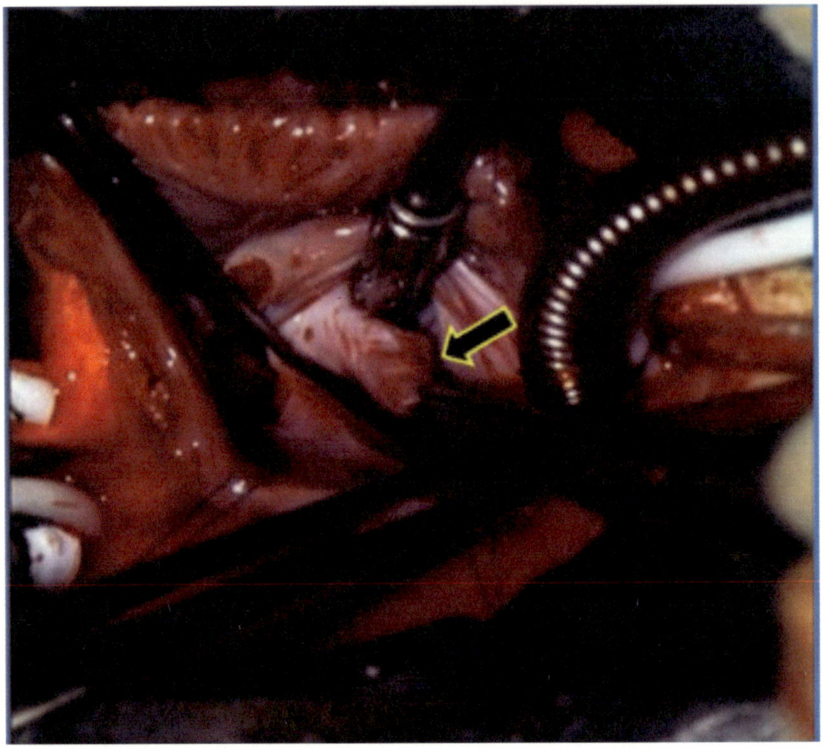

Fig. 10. Operative photography. Right atriotomy exposure of the left atrial appendix (arrow) used for the closure of the atrial septal defect and construction of the roof of the left atrial tunnel.

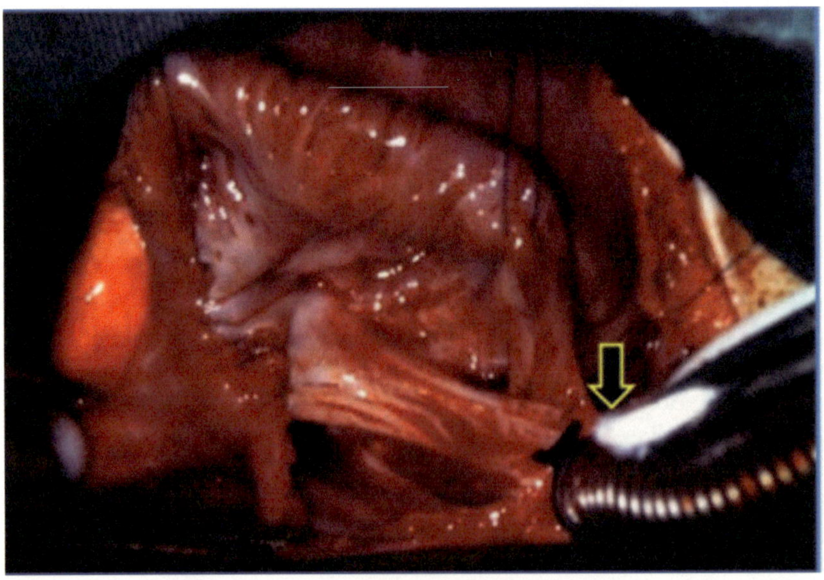

Fig. 11. Operative photography. Right atriotomy exposure of the vena cava tunnel. The Hegar dilator (arrow), was employed to measure the inferior vena cava ostium.

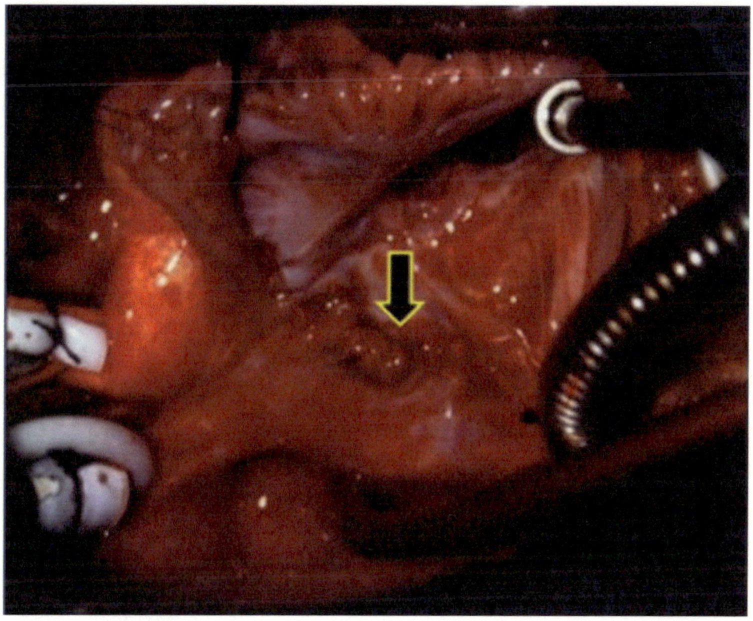

Fig. 12. Operative photography. Right atriotomy exposure of the vena cava tunnel finished. (arrow)

Small muscular VSD was kept open in three patients. The CPB was discontinued and whenever necessary administered inotropic drugs and temporary atrio-ventricular pacemaker stimulation in order to support the hemodynamic performance.

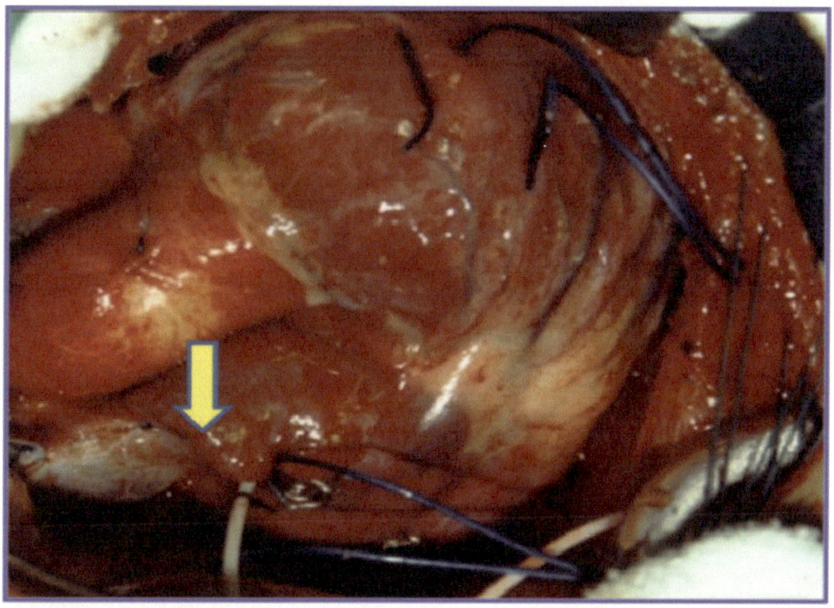

Fig. 13. Operative photography. Surgery conclusion; we can observe the Interrupted suture over the superior vena cava (arrow).

4.3 Statistical analysis

The surviving patients curve and relevant events, during the follow-up were performed according to the Kaplan-Meier's method, comparing 2or more functions by the long-rank test. For all tests, a *p* value of less than 0.05 was considered significant.

4.4 Results

There was only one death (1/39) (mortality=2.5%), during the follow-up time (mean: 14.7 +/- 3.1 years), a 16 year-old patient with bipolar disease that due to his disease committed suicide. The actuarial survival was 97.5% (simple or with little VSD, TGA). The probability of staying in sinus rhythm, in 38 surviving patients was 71.1% (11 cases lost sinus rhythm).Eight (21.0%) patients presented moderate dysfunction of RV; three cases have mild RV dysfunction in the pre-operative period.

Preserved RV function was observed in 30 (78.9%) cases, 10 to 20 years after operation. The incidence of lost sinus rhythm and right ventricular dysfunction, increased gradually over time. Right ventricular dysfunction and active arrhythmias were not risk factors for late death.

All patients are free of reoperations and definitive pacemaker implantation. Table 4.

Procedure	Patients	
	N°	(%)
Senning operation	40	(100)
Small muscular VSD (maintained open)	03	(7.5)
Moderated dysfunction of RV	03	(7.5)

VSD: Ventricular septal defect. RV: right ventricle

Table 4. Operative procedure: Senning operation

4.5 Late follow-up

Thirty eight (97.5%) surviving patients had mean follow-up of 177months. Three patients were lost during the follow-up (living overseas). Thirty five surviving patients (92.1%) were submitted to Doppler –echocardiogram study Figure 14, and Holter study, during 3 periods of follow-up: 0 to 60 months; 60 to 120 months and > 120 months and the results of exams were:

Tricuspid valve dysfunction in 7 (20.0%), 8 (22.8%) and 10 (28.5%) cases, respectively. Mean tricuspid insufficiency in 7 (70.0%) cases and moderate insufficiency in 3 (30.0%) cases.

Right ventricular dysfunction in 3 (8.5%), 6 (17.1%), 8 (22.8%) cases, in the respective period.

Cardiac arrhythmias in 5 (14.2%), 7 (20.0%) and 8 (22.8%)cases, of each respective period. Junction rhythm, in 5 (62.5%) cases, Atrial fibrillation in 2 (25.0%) cases and Atrial *flutter* in 1 (12.5%) case.

Functional status: 28 (80%) patients were in functional class I and 7 (20%) cases, in functional class II (NYHA).Table 5.

The Kaplan - Meier survival curve (Fig. 15) shows: late survival rate was 97.4 % in the mean period of 14.7 years of follow-up. All patients are free of definitive pacemaker implantation and free of reoperation by right or left atrial tunnel stenosis repair, tricuspid valve plastic repair or right ventricle dysfunction.

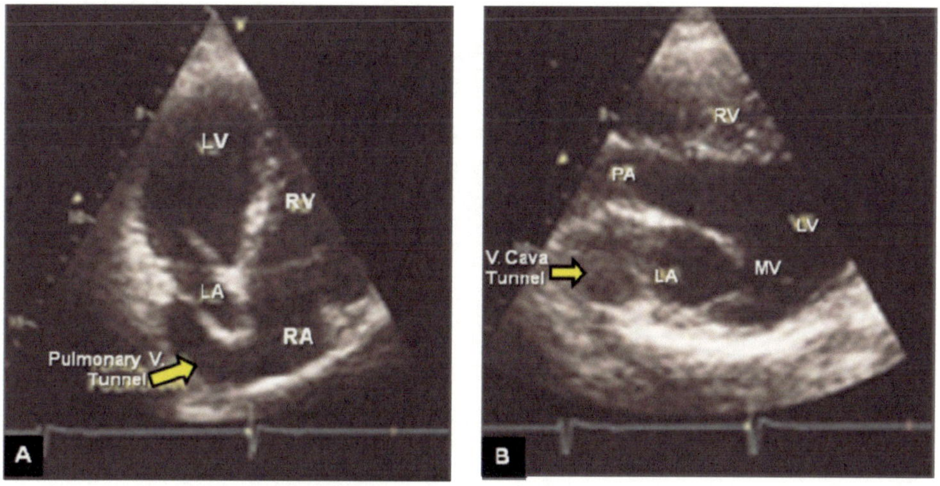

Fig. 14. Post-operative Doppler-echocardiogram study. Patient: male, 16 years-old, in late follow-up of Senning operation. A- Pulmonary vein tunnel draining into right atrium (arrow). B- Vena cava tunnel draining into the left atrium. RA: right atrium; LA: left atrium; RV: right ventricle; LV: left ventricle; V: vena .

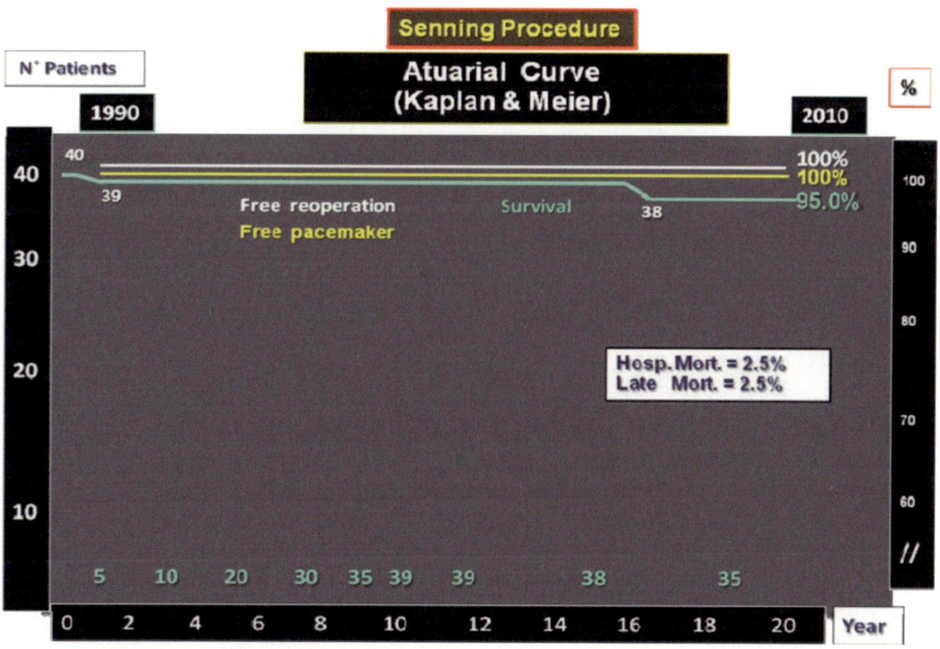

Fig. 15. Actuarial Kaplan & Meier curve. Late follow-up of patients submitted to Senning operation. Hosp. Mort.: hospital mortality

Time of	Tricuspid V. Function		RV function		Cardiac Arrhythmias	
Follow-up	Normal	Insufficiency	Normal	Dysfunction	Sinusal R	Arrhythmias
(months)	N° (%)	N° (%)	N° (%)	N° (%)	N° (%)	N° (%)
0- 60	28 (80.0)	7 (20.0)	32 (91.4)	3 (8.6)	30 (85.7)	5 (14.3)
60 – 120	27 (77.1)	8 (22.8)	29 (82.8)	6 (17.2)	28 (80.0)	7 (20.0)
120	25 (71.4)	10 (28.5)	27 (77.1)	8 (22.9)	27 (77.1)	8 (22.9)

* Total 38 patients; follow-up: 35 patients (three patients were excluded). V: valve; RV: right ventricle; R: rhythm

Table 5. Late follow-up patients with Senning operation (35 patients)*

4.6 Discussion

In the 1970s and 1980s, the atrial switch procedure was the treatment of choice for patients with TGA. After Quaegebeur et al reported favorable results with the Senning operation in 1977, many groups with arterial switch results not satisfactory, started a new surgical experience with Senning's operation, in infants.

In our Institution, from 1990 until the 2000's, the Senning's procedure was indicated for infant patients with TGA + ASD, using in all cases, the Subramanian's maneuver, with very satisfactory results.Baffle-related complications were the most frequent causes and accounted for 5.4% in the Senning a group. The curves for freedom of baffle re-intervention, were only slightly different within the first 15 years but began to diverge clearly after that time span. The study published by the Congenital Heart Surgeons Society in 2000 found the incidence of baffle-related complications in 173 Senning patients. All our patients were operated using the modified technique (Subramanian procedure) and no prosthetic material was used. Only two patients (2/40; 5.0%) presented stenosis of the IVC, during the early post-operative period; these patients were submitted to balloon angioplasty, with success. No patient of these series was re-operated during the late follow-up (mean 14.7 years).

In a recent publication, the inversion of the left atrial appendix, associated to autologous pericardium for venous pathway enlargement, presented retraction and calcification of the venous baffle with obstruction of the venous tunnel.

Surgery for RV dysfunction is the second most frequent indication for reoperation. Mortality associated with reoperations in general has been described to be as high as 36% in a previously published series, mainly because of conversion to the arterial switch operation.

Three (7.5%) patients in our series presented moderate RV dysfunction in the pre-operative period, but maintained the same RV dysfunction after Senning's operation, during the early and late follow- up; this patients are in functional class II (NYHA).

Loss of sinus rhythm at long term has been described in patients after atrial baffle procedures, with the incidence being the same after the Senning or the Mustard procedure. However, reports present series of patients with sinus rhythm in 80.8% of the cases, 17.4 years after the Senning's procedure.

In these published articles, patients free from pacemaker implantation, inthe Senning group, were 98.7%, at 10 years and, thus, it was comparable to the findings by others series: 91% to 92% at 10 years.

Patients freedom from pacemaker insertion, at 20 years, was still > 90%. This might be related to the fact that in these patients the coronary sinus was not incised as originally described by Senning, and the atrial suture line was placed posterior to the coronary sinus.

Our surgical technique to perform the Senning's operation included: 1- ASD closure using left atrial appendix and 2- The atrial suture line was placed posterior to the coronary sinus.

In 40 patients operated, the cardiac rhythm in the early post-operative period showed: sinus rhythm in 30 (85.7%) cases and cardiac arrhythmias in 5(14.3%) cases.

In 40 consecutive operations, we had one death (hospital mortality = 2.5%); these results are possible to compare to others reported series, with mortality ranging from 2% to 5.4%. Whereas, patients with simple TGA submitted to Senning's operation, resulted in a significant difference in the relative number of complex TGA. In addition, the surgical learning curve may have been a reason for the differences in mortality between the different published reports in international issues.

Thirty five (92.1%) surviving patients had mean follow-up of 177 months (other 3 surviving patients living overseas). During late follow-up, other 3 patients presented cardiac arrhythmias. Actually, 27 (77.1%) cases maintain sinus rhythm and 8 (22.9%) cases presented cardiac arrhythmias. No pacemaker was implanted in this group of patients.

Other series presented 90.9 ± 2.3 % of surviving patients in 25 years of follow-up, after the Senning procedure and 75.9 ± 4.8%, after the Mustard procedure and thus, it was significantly different in univariate analysis. The Mustard procedure remained a significant risk factor for late death in multivariate analysis fully adjusted for all variables that were statistically significant between the 2 groups. This difference in late survival between the 2 operative procedures is not confirmed in all investigations.

Whereas, authors have observed a significantly better survival rate of patients after the Senning's operation (94% versus 77% at 15 years).

The Senning's operation is a risk factor for late death. In contrast, authors reported a similar long-term outcome for the Toronto Mustard group and the Zurich Senning group, with ≈ 75% survival after 25 years. However, they found a difference in the mode of death between a the Mustard group and the Senning group. Similar to the results of the present study, relatively more Mustard patients died of sudden death compared with the Senning patients, who died preferentially of progressive congestive heart failure.

We had a previous published report, including only the first 17 patients, submitted to Senning's operation, for correction of the simple TGA, in our Institution. In this series we have one hospital death, (early mortality 2.5%).

In thirty nine surviving patients, no cardiac cause of death was observed (only one accidental death was observed). There was no sudden death in this group; the survival rate in our Institution was 95%, with mean follow-up of 14.7% years.

Regarding the type of atrial baffle procedure, patients with previous VSD carry a higher risk of late death than patients with intact ventricular septum. Reports show that: 90% of the patients with simple TGA but only 78% of the patients with complex TGA were alive 15 years after the Senning procedure. These data confirm the finding that the presence of a VSD is a significant risk factor for late death because VSD closure emerged as an dependent risk factor for late death in multivariate analysis.

From 1986, in our Institution, neonates with simple TGA, infants with TGA plus VSD or Taussig-Bing anomaly were referred to arterial switch operation (ASO) and VSD closure, but infants patients with diagnosis of simple TGA and simple TGA with small muscular VSD were referred to Senning's operation.

The question remains of whether the surgical procedure of VSDclosure or rather the hemodynamic consequences of a previous VSD account for the intrinsic risk of late mortality. Potential complications of VSD closure that may also lead to late RV dysfunction and consecutively to late death such as iatrogenic postoperative AV block or tricuspid insufficiency were no more frequent in patients after VSD closure.

However, freedom from pacemaker implantation was lower in patients who received VSD closure at the time of the atrial switch operation. The incidence of right bundle branch block (RBBB), which has been associated with late development of RV dysfunction, was increased. Hence, the surgical procedure of VSD closure may have an influence on mortality in the long term.

Deterioration of the function of the systemic ventricle (RV) is a major concern in patients after atrial switch procedures. The incidence of moderate or severe RV dysfunction shows a wide variation in the literature from 8% at 12 to 18 years and 20% at 20 to 28 years, respectively. Authors found a rapid increase of RV dysfunction, after 10 years, and described the probability of normal right ventricular function to be only 52% and 39%, 10 to 15 years after the Senning's procedure in patients with simple and complex TGA, respectively. In the Lange el al study, the incidence of RV dysfunction was 16.1% at 25 years. However, in our experience with 40 consecutive cases of Senning's operation, three patients presented mild RV dysfunction, before operation and maintaining after 15 years of follow-up, in functional class II. The RV variability in assessing right ventricular function and the lack of a uniform definition restrict comparison. The incidence of RV dysfunction in the long term has been shown to be associated with the complexity of the heart defect, which we confirmed that this dysfunction progressed to moderate dysfunction, but maintaining the functional class II.

In our series, actually, 8 (22.8%) patients presented mild or moderate RV dysfunction and tricuspid insufficiency; these patients are medicated with ß blocking drugs and patients with tachyarrhythmias are using anti-arrhythmic drugs.

4.7 Conclusions

Our results confirm that the patients with simple TGA submitted to the Senning's procedure in the late follow-up, presented a good quality of life functional class I-II), satisfactory results (low incidence of arrhythmias, free of pacemaker implantation or reoperation) and no risk of late sudden cardiac death.

5. Anomalous left coronary artery from the pulmonary artery. Autogenous arterial conduit technique

Anomalous left coronary artery from pulmonary artery (ALCAPA) is a rare cardiac malformation; whose clinical symptoms are expressed in the first months of life, by congestive heart failure (CHF) of difficult clinical improvement, followed by significant mortality. The symptoms of CHF associated with functional mitral insufficiency due to papillary muscle dysfunction and ischemic changes observed in the ECG are guidelines for the diagnosis of ALCAPA.

Doppler echocardiography diagnosis, depending on the operator may have difficulty in submitting images for reliable indication for surgery. Noninvasive diagnostic methods such as computerized tomography angiography (CT Angio) and magnetic resonance imaging (MRI) have enabled it to provide relevant information for a planned and safer surgical approach. These patients represent a model of our experience started in 1993 at the Department of Cardiovascular Surgery at São Paulo Federal University(UNIFESP), a group of 19 consecutive patients, all operated with the technique of direct re-implantation of left coronary artery from the ascending aorta and in the last three cases using the technique of autogenous arterial conduit.

5.1 Case report

Child, 9 years-old, male, with ALCAPA, who underwent corrective surgery in December 2001 with follow-up period of 9 years. The clinical examination, conducted in March 2010, showed an asymptomatic patient, without limitation during exercise, without medication in the last seven years in functional class I (NYHA). At 2 months of age, the patient was admitted to the Cardiology Department, of UNIFESP. On clinical examination the patient presented respiratory distress, tachycardia, thin wrists and pale complexion. He also presented enlarged liver and mitral systolic murmur. The ECG showed subendocardial injury current in precordial derivations, and the Doppler echocardiography showed lowered left ventricular function and moderate mitral insufficiency.

5.2 Surgical correction

After diagnosis of ALCAPA and moderate mitral insufficiency, the patient was submitted to surgical correction in December 2001 at two months of age, on cardiopulmonary bypass (CPB). During surgery it was confirmed cardiac malformation: the left coronary artery originated from the left posteriorsinus of the pulmonary valve. The heart chambers were found dilated and presented left ventricular dyskinesia, and it was observed in the epicardial surface, an exuberant intercoronary shunt between the right and left coronary system. Figure 16.

During CPB, clinical diagnostic was confirmed and was observed hypokinetic apical area of the left ventricle (LV). The patient was kept in moderate hypothermia at 28°C and the right and left pulmonary arteries were occluded. After aortic clamping was initiated the infusion of blood cardioplegic solution, injected into both vessels ascending aorta and pulmonary trunk. (Figure 17 a, b).

After dissecting the pulmonary trunk, the latter was cross-sectioned near the origin of the pulmonary arteries. We observed the ostium of the left coronary artery emerging from the left posterior sinus of the pulmonary valve, distant 25 to 30 mm from the ascending aorta.

The coronary ostium was removed from the posterior sinus of the left pulmonary sinus, along with a long flap, taken from the anterior wall of the proximal stump of the pulmonary trunk, while other similar flap was built on the side wall of the aorta below the aortic clamps, pedicle on the posterior wall of the aorta. (Figure 17 c)

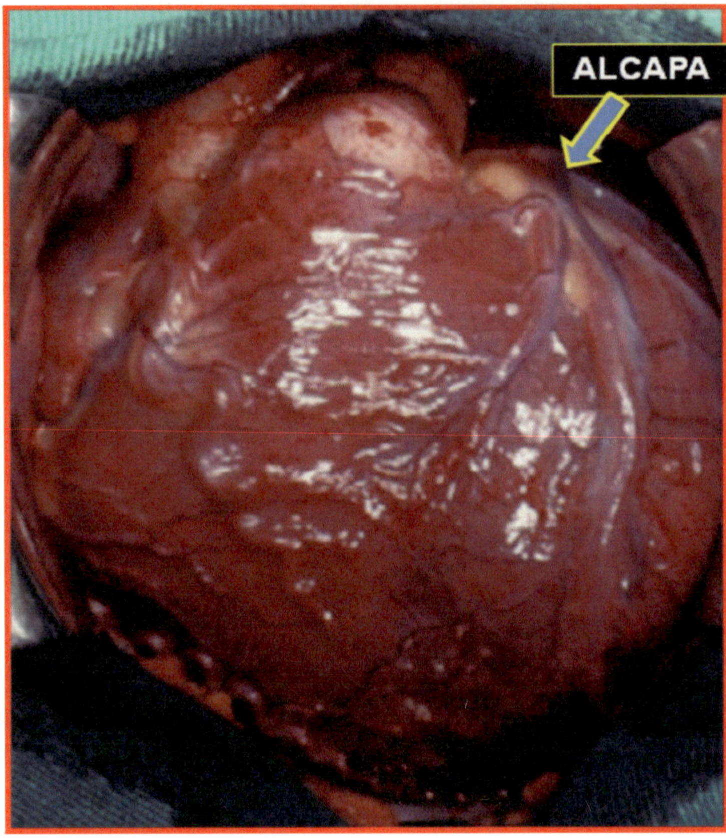

Fig. 16. Surgical image. External appearance of the heart, we observed the anomalous origin of left coronary artery from the pulmonary artery (ALCAPA) and significant intercoronary shunt.

The aortic and pulmonary flaps were sutured by their edges, using a 7-0 polypropylene thread, building an autogenous arterial conduit, anastomosed to the ascending aorta, about 2-3 cm above the left aortic sinus. (Figure 17 d).

No wire was needed for dissection or manipulation of the left coronary artery to approximate it to the aorta. The anterior wall of the pulmonary trunk was reconstructed with preserved bovine pericardium and there was no intervention on the mitral valve.

At the end of CPB, the patient underwent modified ultrafiltration (MUF) and administration of Dobutamine and Milrinone, with improvement of hemodynamic parameters.

The pediatric ICU stay was 96 hours and he had discharged on the 10th day after surgery, receiving medicated for CHF

This procedure was performed at the São Paulo Federal University, being the first Institution in the country to adopt this procedure, and then rapidly expand to other pediatric cardiac surgery centers in the country, looking for successful results and decide to abandon the intrapulmonary tunnel (Takeushi technique)

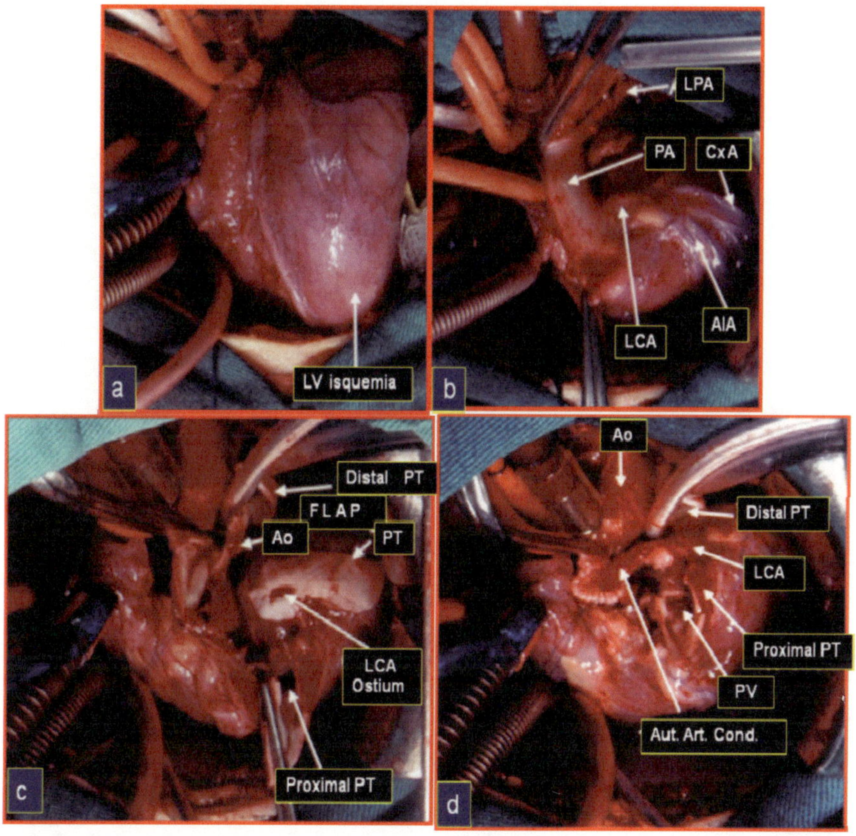

Fig. 17. Surgical image. Patient on cardiopulmonary bypass. a- Aspect of the ischemic anterior and apical region of the left ventricle b- Origin of the left coronary artery from the left posterior sinus of the pulmonary valve. Not was detected in previous pre- and postoperative tests. . c-: After section of the pulmonary trunk (PT) and resection of the *ostium* of the left coronary artery (LCA) along with flap from the wall of the PT; another pedicle was built on the lateral wall of the aorta (Ao). d- Implantation technique of the LCA in the ascending Ao. Manufacture of *autologous* arterial conduit (*Aut.* Art. Cond.) with flaps of pulmonary artery and aorta, sutured by their edges and side extremity anastomosed to the ascending aorta. . LV: left ventricle, PA: pulmonary artery, LPA: left pulmonary artery; Cx: circumflex artery; AIA: anterior interventricular artery PV: pulmonary valve.

5.3 Late postoperative follow-up

The patient had good postoperative evolution, returning for regular medical control. In October 2009, at eight years of age, the patient returned for clinical assessment: remained asymptomatic in Functional Class I (NYHA), without restriction to perform physical activities and without cardiac medication.

The clinical examination showed: regular heart rhythm without murmur; ECG: normal for the age; Doppler echocardiography: preserved left ventricular function, mitral valve competence and the presence of autogenous arterial conduit and patent left coronary artery.

Computerized Tomography Angiography showed images of implantation of autogenous arterial conduit in the ascending aorta above the aortic sinus (Figure 18 a), autogenous arterial conduit patency, with uniform diameter (Figure 18 b), reconstruction of the pulmonary artery (Figure 18 c) and the presence of a significant stenosis on the left pulmonary artery not detected inprevious pre-and postoperative tests. (Figure 18 d).

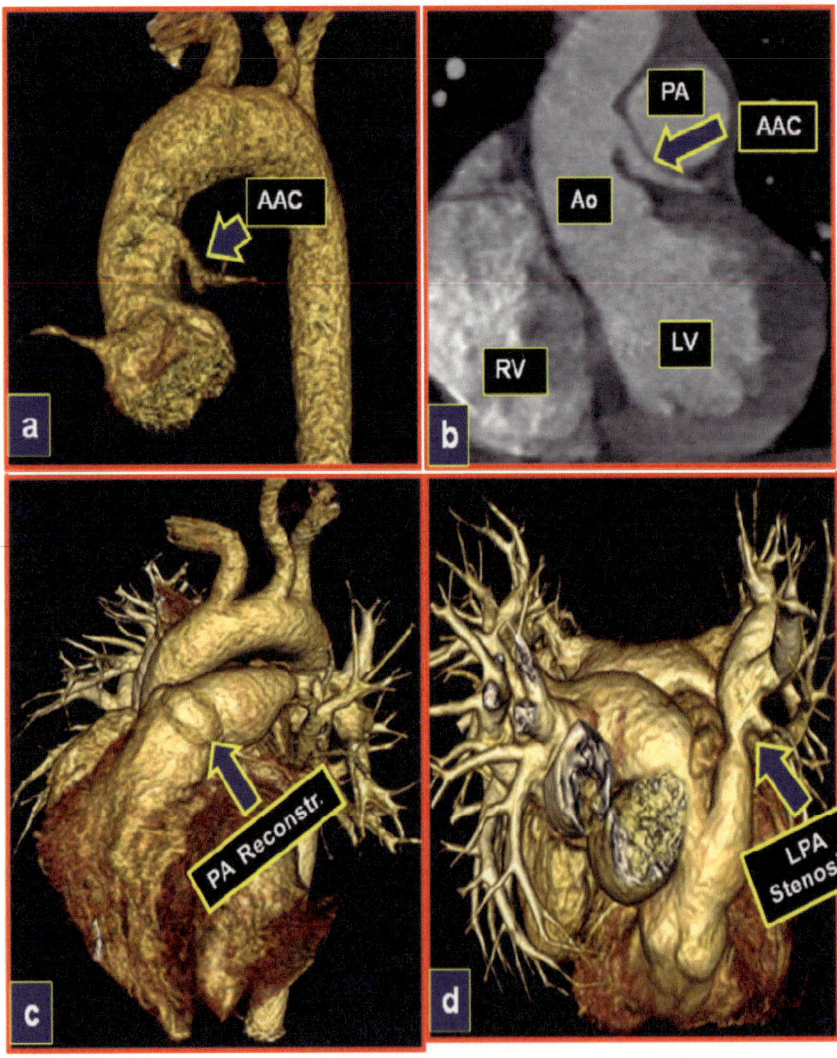

Fig. 18. Late follow-up of the 8th year. Postoperative image of CT angiography- a- Implantation of *Autologous* arterial conduit (ACC) in the ascending aorta above the aortic sinus. b- Autogenous arterial conduit patency, with uniform diameter. c- Reconstruction of the pulmonary artery . -d- Image of stenosis located in the distal left pulmonary artery. (LPA); RV: right ventricle; LV: left ventricle; PA: pulmonary artery; Ao; aorta

In February 2010 the patient was submitted to pulmonary angioplasty with balloon catheter (Figure 19 a), followed by stent implantation in the left pulmonary artery (Figure 19 b) with balloon expansion of the stent, successfully. (Figure 19 c).

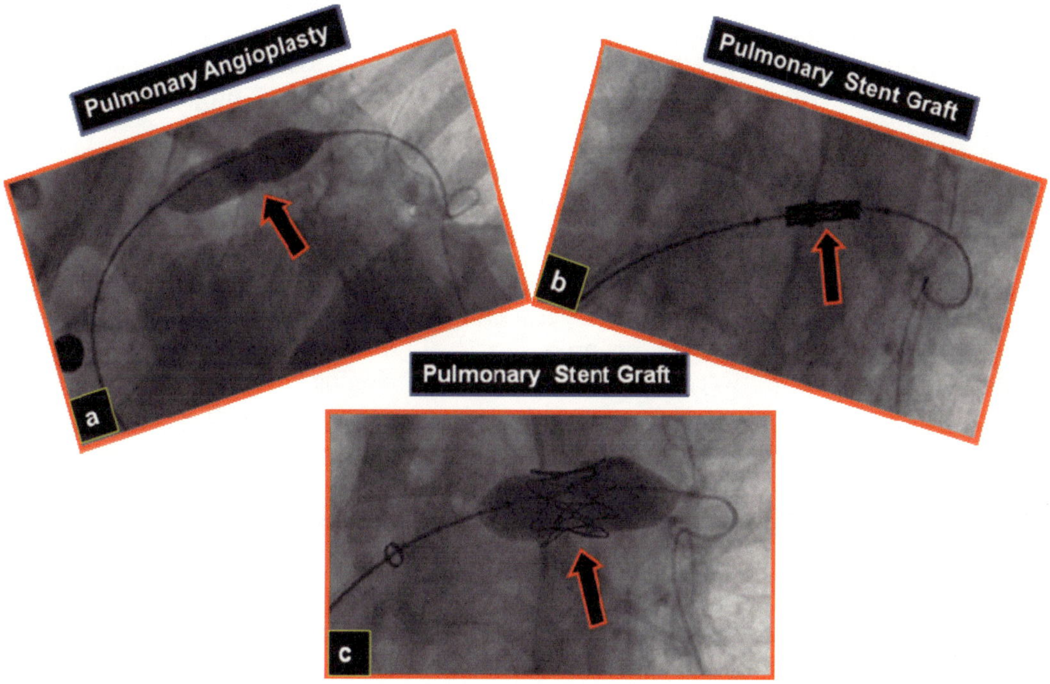

Fig. 19. Late follow-up of 8 years. Postoperative cardiac catheterization. Cineangiographic image a- Pulmonary angioplasty with balloon. b-Pulmonary stent implanted. c-Pulmonary stent dilatation, with balloon.

5.4 Comments

ALCAPA is a rare cardiac malformation described by Bland - White - Garland in 1933 and accompanied by high mortality in infants; Vouhe et al consider the mortality of about 90% in the first year of life.

This is a congenital defect where the myocardial function was deeply compromised due to myocardial ischemia, and as it occurred in our patient, it began at 2 months of life, immediately after the closure of the patent ductus arteriosus.

The most common local of origin of the left coronary artery ostium, as in our patient, occurred in the left posterior sinus of the pulmonary valve, standing away from the ascending aorta in any attempt for direct reimplantation into the aorta. During the external examination of the heart, we observed the presence of the main coronary arteries and their branches dilated and tortuous, the result of right to left coronary shunt.

The purpose of correction of ALCAPA is to create two separate coronary systems. However, the location of the left coronary ostium near or distant from the aorta, has raised interest and stimulated the creativity of the cardiac surgeon to develop new techniques and improve outcomes in the middle and long terms.

The direct re-implantation of the left coronary artery on the ascending aorta involves the dissection and movement of the coronary artery trunk and its main branches, but tension on the sutures compromise coronary flow and result in high mortality. In our series of patients we had two deaths due to ischemic dysfunction of the LV, probably due to tension in the anastomosis after aortic implantation of the left coronary artery, which originated within the left posterior sinus of the pulmonary valve.

Aiming to avoid such incidents and to improve the operative late outcome, this technique has been modified and now employs procedures to lengthen the proximal coronary artery and permit implantation in the aorta without tension.

Thus, Sese et al in 1992 described a new technique of stretching of the coronary artery, using a flap of the pulmonary artery wall and a pedicled flap of the aortic wall; this technique was called "trap-door." The criticism of this procedure is still the need for dissection of the main branches of the coronary artery, for its approach to the ascending aorta.

Similar procedures have been published by Tashiro et al in 1992 and Von Son et al in 1997. Katsumata et al in 1999 and Murthy et al in 2001, based on initial experience stretching the left coronary artery, now with aortic and pulmonary flaps, larger in width and length, built autogenous arterial conduits or tubs, to re-implant the left coronary artery originating from the left posterior sinus of the pulmonary valve, without tension and without dissection of the main coronary branches.

The experience of our group of congenital heart diseases at Unifesp started successfully in December 2001 and it was published six years later.

Nine years after the surgical correction, our patient presents good evolution and remains asymptomatic during physical activity and without medication (Functional Class I). The examinations of CT angiography, performed in December 2009, certifies the successful outcome of this technique, showing the autologous arterial graft patency and uniform diameter throughout its length.

Mitral regurgitation is a common finding in patients with ALCAPA, caused by ischemic papillary muscles and LV dilation. No case in our series had mitral valve surgery approach, being aware that after improvement of the ventricular function there would be regression of mitral valve dysfunction as documented in our patient. This conservative approach has been adopted by Vohue et al, with improvement of mitral dysfunction. This author reports that mitral valve repair is a procedure not very favorable in infants.

A recent report shows that a patient submitted to anomalous left coronary artery implanted in the aorta, followed by mitral valve repair by annuloplasty presented in the postoperative period, important mechanical hemolysis. This patient required a second intervention to remove a piece of bovine pericardium, .

Finally, the endothelized tube construction, performed in our patient, had the advantage of avoiding the use of bovine pericardial patch, employed by other authors or using the intrapulmonary tunnel technique, maintaining the patency during the late follow-up.

5.5 Conclusion

1. The coronary artery transference was technically safe and feasible. The endothelized inner conduit remains pervious during the late follow-up.
2. Long - term clinical outcome and left ventricular function are good despite severe left ventricular dysfunction at presentation.
3. Mitral valve repair was not necessary. Competent mitral valve was observed after the return of the normal left ventricle function.

6. Hypoplastic left heart syndrome. Hybrid procedure

Despite undeniable recent improvement in survival rates, the Norwood Stage I operation for hypoplastic left heart syndrome (HLHS) and related anomalies remains a high-risk endeavor. Neonates undergoing a stage I Norwood operation face a mortality of 10-20%,depending on the risk factors and the experience of the cardiac team. Current significant risk factors include birth weight < 2.5 kg, prematurity < 34 weeks gestational age, intact or restrictive atrial septum, additional cardiac anomalies and non-cardiac genetic malformations.

Lessons learned during the development of a novel hybrid approach have resulted in a reliable, reproducible alternative treatment for hypoplastic left heart syndrome (HLHS). Herein we report our results using this hybrid approach in a uniform risk cohort.

6.1 Methods

This is a review of prospectively collected data on patients treated for HLHS using a hybrid approach (n = 10) between July 1995 and June 2002. The hybrid approach includes pulmonary artery bands, a ductal stent, and atrial septostomy as a neonate, without cardiopulmonary bypass. (Figure 20,21)

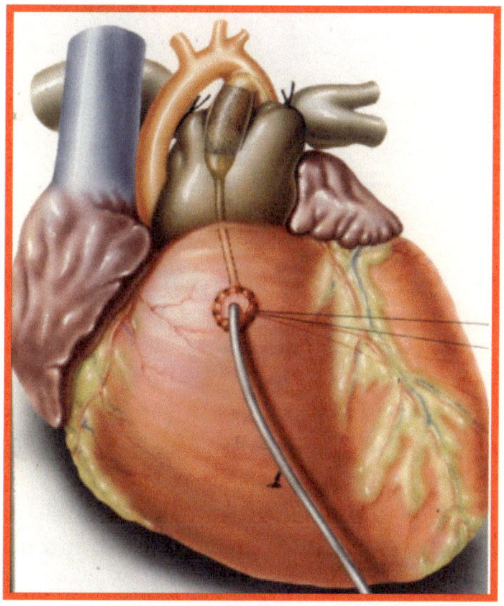

Fig. 20. Schematic drawing of surgical technique of hybrid procedure: stent implantation in the *ductus arteriosus* through the right ventricular infundibulum, associated with right and left pulmonary banding.

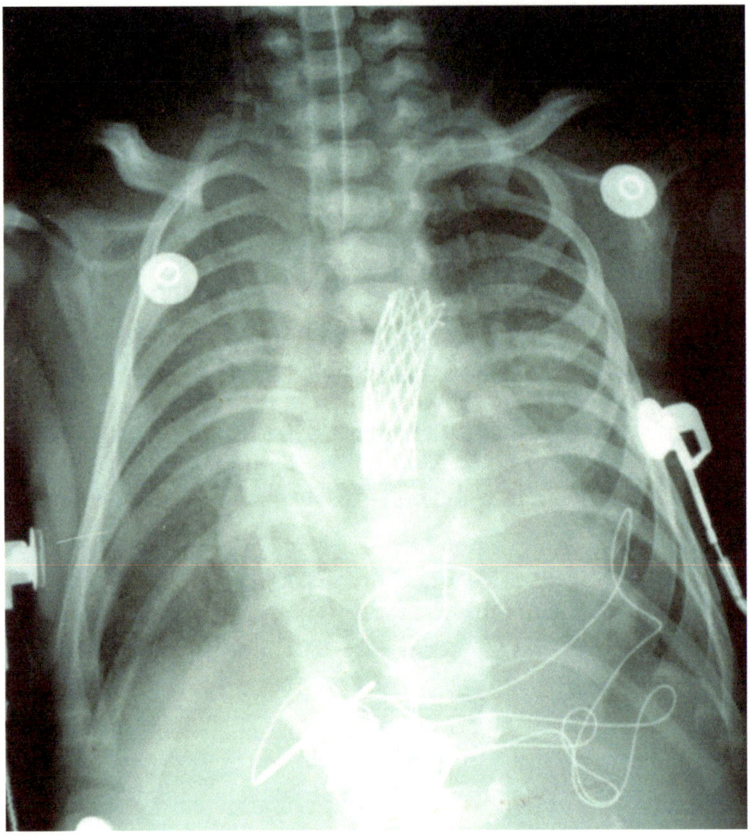

Fig. 21. Postoperative chest X-ray after hybrid procedure, showing stent implanted into the ductus arteriosus

This patient is getting prepared for stage 2 procedure resulting in Glenn shunt physiology at six months and stage 3, Fontan completion at two years.

6.2 Results

Ten patients had a hybrid stage 1 with survival rate between 1 day and 120 days. Unfortunately, no patient completed the stage 2 and 3.

This procedure was performed by the São Paulo Federal University, being the first institution in the country to adopt this procedure, and then rapidly expanding to other pediatric cardiac surgery centers in the country, seeking successful results.

Conclusion: The hybrid approach is still acceptable due to its intermediate results, but it is not comparable to a traditional Norwood strategy. Potential advantages of the hybrid approach include the avoidance of circulatory arrest and shifting the major surgical stage to a later time. These data provide the platform for a prospective trial comparing these two surgical options to assess whether there is less cumulative impact with the hybrid approach, thereby improving end organ function, quality, and quantity of life.

7. Hypoplastic left heart syndrome. Palliative surgical correction with beating heart

Hypoplastic left heart syndrome is a uniformly lethal cardiac abnormality if not surgically addressed. Since the description of surgical palliation by Norwood in the early 1980s and the description of allograft cardiac transplantation by Bailey in the mid 1980s, the interest in this lesion has remarkably increased. Currently, the Norwood surgical approach consists of a series of 3 operations: the Norwood procedure (stage I), the hemi-Fontan or bidirectional Glenn procedure (stage II), and the Fontan procedure (stage III). Orthotopic heart transplantation provides an alternative therapy, with results similar to those of the staged surgical palliation. Currently, the survival rate of infants treated with these surgical approaches is similar to that of infants with other complex forms of congenital heart disease in which a 2-ventricle repair is not possible.

7.1 Norwood operation

This surgery is complex and may vary slightly depending on the diagnosis and overall condition of the heart. The main pulmonary artery is separated from the left and right portions of the pulmonary artery and joined with the upper portion of the aorta. Widening of the pulmonary artery is often necessary, and may be accomplished by using the patient's existing biological tissue or appropriate animal tissue. This allows blood, a mixture of oxygenated and deoxygenated blood to be pumped to the body via the pulmonary valve.Since the remainder of the pulmonary artery is now disconnected from the heart, one of a few techniques must be used to supply blood to the lungs:With a modified Blalock-Taussig Shunt, a Gore-Tex conduit (a kind of plastic tubing) is used to connect the subclavian artery to the pulmonary artery. In this case, blood comes from the single ventricle, through the pulmonary valve, the reconstructed aorta, the subclavian artery, and the conduit, to the lungs. There are variations on this procedure where the origin of the shunt is elsewhere in the systemic circulation (e.g. from the aorta itself) rather than the subclavian artery.

7.2 Sano modification procedure

The Sano Modification of the Norwood involves the placement of a conduit (light blue tube below) between the pulmonary artery and the right ventricle instead of the Modified Blalock-Taussig Shunt.

7.3 Sano procedure

The first operation serves to make the right ventricle the main pumping chamber for blood flow to the body. The aorta is made larger to increase blood flow to the body. A connection is made to enable the blood traveling through the aorta towards the body to "shunt" through this connection and flow into the pulmonary artery to receive oxygen. This may be accomplished with a modified Blalock-Taussig shunt, which is a small tube placed between the aorta and the pulmonary arteries or by using the Sano modification procedure, in which a homograft (tissue) conduit is placed between the right ventricle and the pulmonary arteries. The choice of which procedure is best for your child can be discussed with your cardiologist and/or cardiovascular surgeon. However, even after the stage I procedure, the infant will still have some degree of cyanosis since oxygen-poor (blue) blood from the right atrium and oxygen-rich (red) blood from the left side of the heart mixes and flows through the aorta to the body.

7.4 The Sano shunt

Over the last few years, a number of centers around the world have begun to adopt a modification of the Norwood procedure that involves a different type of shunt. Introduced by Shunji Sano, MD, who was trained in congenital cardiac surgery in Melbourne, Australia, and is now working in his home country of Japan, this new modification indicates further improvement in the survival of newborn babies with hypoplastic left heart syndrome.

The Sano shunt modification avoids the problem of competitive flow between the lungs and coronary arteries. The shunt is constructed from a slightly larger gore-tex tube graft than that used for the modified Blalock shunt. Generally a 5 mm tube graft is selected in contrast to the 3.5 mm graft used for average size babies for a Blalock shunt. Distally, the graft is connected to the main pulmonary artery between the right and left pulmonary artery takeoffs. The proximal end of the shunt is connected to a limited infundibular incision in the right ventricle.

7.5 Norwood – Sano operation at São Paulo Federal University

The Norwood procedure has been replaced by the Norwood procedure-Sano in our institution since 2004. The surgical technique consists in the careful dissection of the ascending aorta (Hypoplasia}, vessels, pulmonary trunk, pulmonary branches and ductus arteriosus. (Figure 22)

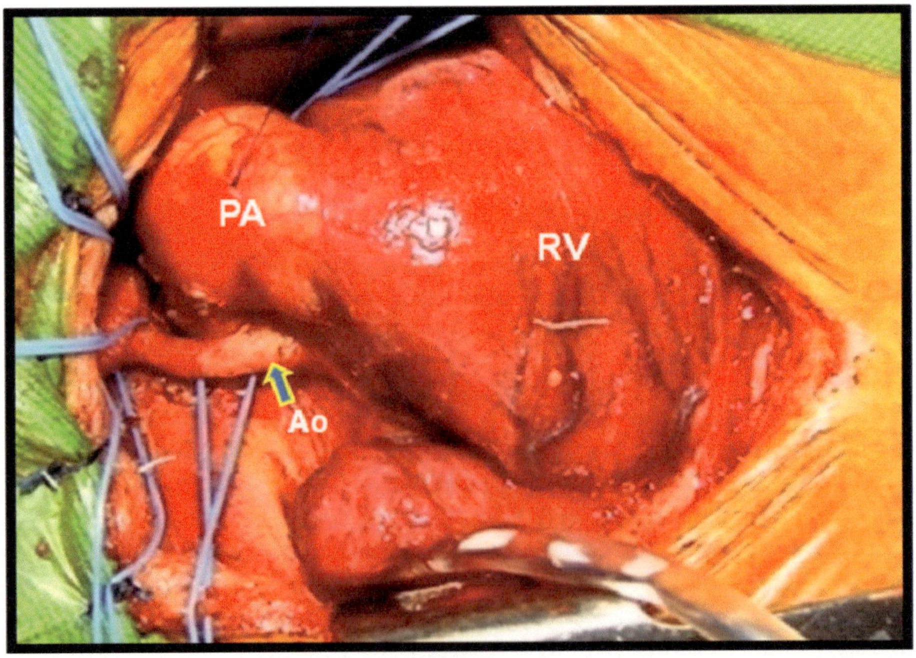

Fig. 22. Surgical image. Hipoplastic ascending aorta and dilated right ventricle (RV) and pulmonary artery (PA). Ao: aorta.

The establishment of cardiopulmonary bypass was performed by anastomosis of a gore-tex tube of 4.0mm in the brachiocephalic trunk where it will be held on cerebral and coronary arteries perfusion (fig. 23).The operation is performed with the aid of bypass and normothermic beating heart (without aortic clamping and without circulatory arrest).The perfusion of the descending aorta is performed by cannulation of the descending aorta using a Y-junction of the arterial line.

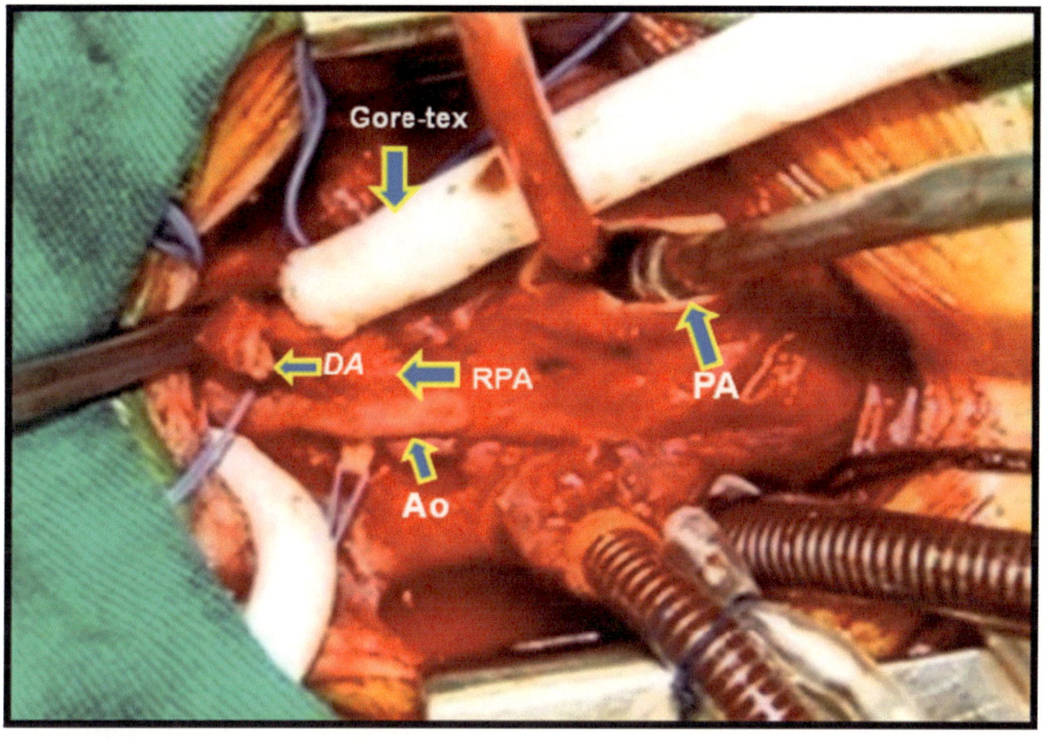

Fig. 23. Surgical image. Cardiopulmonary bypass installed: arterial perfusion by gore-tex prostheses anastomosed to braquiocephalic trunk. After ductus arteriosus and pulmonary artery (PA) sectioned, the pulmonary flow reconstructed with gore-tex tub (5.0mm), anastomosed to pulmonary arteries. Ao: aorta, RPA: right pulmonary artery, DA: ductus arteriosus.

With the clamping of the aortic arch near the innominate artery, and without interfering with the coronary and cerebral blood flow, and reconstruction of the neo-aorta by interposition of segment of porcine pulmonary trunk gauge similar to the pulmonary ring, interposed between the arch and isthmus and the pulmonary trunk in the region above the valve (modified Norwood Op.) figure 24.

Finally, the pulmonary blood flow is restored through the interposition of gore-tex prosthesis of 5.0 mm or 6.0 mm, between the infundibulum of the right ventricle and the pulmonary arteries (Sano modification) Figure 25.

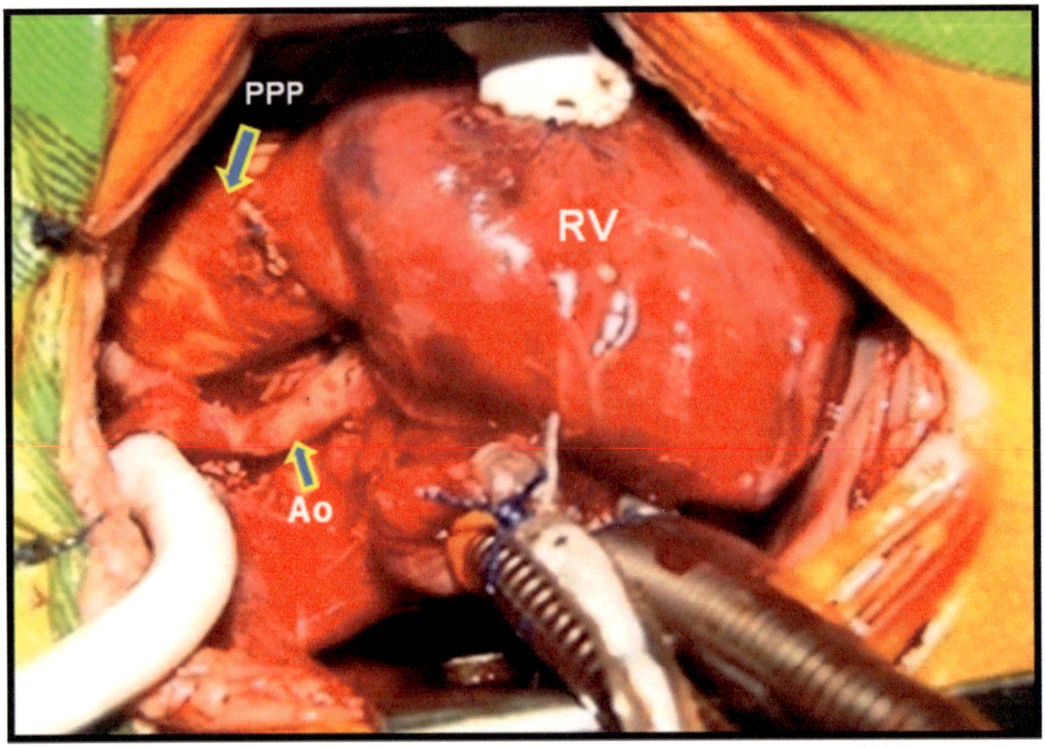

Fig. 24. Surgical image. Neoaorta reconstruction using a segment of porcine pulmonary prosthesis (PPP), implanted between pulmonary trunk and aortic arch. Ao: aorta, RV: right ventricle.

This kind of approach to HLHS is a unique technique developed at our institution, highlighting several advantages:

- Preservation of cerebral and myocardial function during the procedure, while maintaining continuous flow during CPB.- Minor metabolic disorders while maintaining normothermic CPB - Adequate flow without restriction and less chance of bleeding by using the neo-aortic porcine pulmonary prosthesis, anastomosed only their proximal and distal stumps.
- Preservation of cerebral and myocardial function during the procedure, while maintain continuous flow during CPB.
- Minor metabolic disorders while maintain CPB at normothermia.
- Adequate flow without restriction and less chance of bleeding by using the neo-aortic porcine pulmonary prosthesis, anastomosed only their proximal and distal stumps.

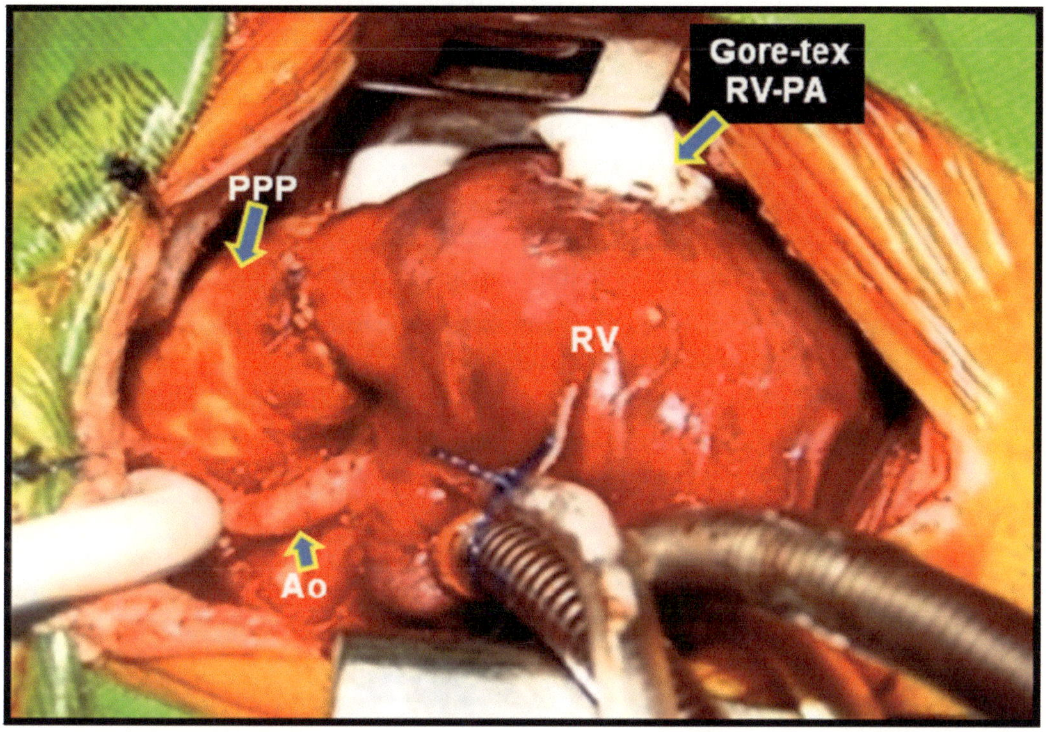

Fig. 25. Surgical image. Implant of a gore-tex prosthesis (5.0mm) between right ventricle (RV) and pulmonary artery (PA). Ao: aorta, PPP: porcine pulmonary prosthesis

8. New models of cardiac valves

8.1 Right ventricle remodeling surgery using porcine pulmonary prosthesis

The results of biventricular surgical repair of congenital heart disease with obstruction of the pulmonary ventricle are satisfactory. A surgical technique started over five decades ago is closely related to adequate pulmonary valve (PV) repair and right ventricular outflow tract (RVOT) reconstruction.

The use of prostheses with no valves induced the development of valvar pulmonary insufficiency (VPI), which for many years it was considered a benign residual lesion that patients tolerated reasonably well, but this selected technique and other causes that were responsible for ventricular dysfunction are now questioned.

With the increasing duration of follow-up, however, significant late morbidity and mortality have been observed in a portion of patients

More recently, the clinical relevance of VPI after enlargement of the hypoplastic pulmonary ring and trunk was confirmed once the medium and long-term results of the surgery were better known. Studies on the issue have established the need to repair the PV using valved prosthesis, minimizing or preventing VPI, which is considered to be the cause of late RV dysfunction.

Therefore, RV diastolic function should be carefully monitored in the long-term follow-up of patients undergoing correction of: tetralogy of Fallot (TOF) with trans-annular enlargement; *truncus arteriosus (TA);* pulmonary atresia (PA) with ventricular septal defect (VSD); PA with intact ventricular septum (IVS) and transposition of the great arteries (TGA) + VSD + left ventricle outflow tract obstruction (LVOTO).

The Doppler-echocardiography has shown the presence of diastolic flow in the pulmonary artery, synchronized with atrial systole and the respiratory cycle. The RV diastolic volume in the postoperative recovery, determines a diastolic compliance decrease and may be detected by a continuous laminar flow in the pulmonary artery

The VPI is known as one of the most important factors that cause RV dilation due to volume increase and ejection fraction decrease after surgical correction.

There is a spectrum of VPI quantified with more refined method of evaluation, utilizing magnetic resonance imaging (MRI) as well as exercise testing in the follow-up of patients submitted to operations to alleviate the pulmonary obstruction, associated with RV dilation and hypertrophy.

The development of akinetic regions and aneurysmatic dilation of the RVOT, related only in part to the trans-annular patching, is common and contributes to increase RV diastolic volumes (RVDV) and decrease RV ejection fraction (RVEF), related to the degree of VPI.

Left ventricular systolic dysfunction, aortic regurgitation and RV dilation and dysfunction exist in adults with TOF, *TA*, PA / VSD, TGA / VSD / LVOTO, PA / IVS etc. related to the length of palliation with arterial shunts.

Measures to maintain or restore pulmonary valve function and to avoid VPI, RVOT aneurysm or akinesia are mandatory for preserving RV and LV function late, after pulmonary ventricle repair.

This manuscript reviews our experience in 203 consecutive patients treated with RVOT remodeling utilizing a preserved porcine pulmonary prosthesis (bicuspid and trileaflet).

8.2 Patients and methods

8.2.1 Study group

This study reports the surgical technique and late follow-up of the pulmonary ventricle performance and preserved porcine pulmonary prosthesis, used to PV repair and RVOT reconstruction, in patients with pulmonary ventricle obstruction.

This clinical study was performed at the Cardiovascular Division of the São Paulo Federal University, between June 1991 and December 2008.

This prosthesis was initially tested in experimental model in March 1990 and after good performance, it was approved for clinical use by the Medical Ethical Committee of this Institution in June 1991.

In 2006, the Medical Ethical Committee at the São Paulo Federal University approved the Magnetic Resonance Images and Computerized Tomography study, in patients with follow-up over 10 years.

Two hundred and three consecutive patients, aged 4 months to 35 years (mean=3.0) were operated. The patients were classified in 5 groups according to the diagnosis of the cardiac malformation.

G1- TOF with pulmonary hypoplasia, 144 (70.9%) cases; G2- PA + VSD, 32 (15.7%) cases; G 3 - *TA*, 12 (5.9%) cases; G 4 - TGA + VSD + LVOTO, 8 (3.9%) cases and G 5 - PA + IVS, 7 (3.4%) cases. (Figure 26).

Preoperative pulmonary hypertension, defined as pulmonary artery pressure greater than 50% of the systemic pressure was noted in 12 (5.9%) patients with TA. Cardiac catheterization was performed in 80% of the patients; more recently, MRI and computerized tomography (CT) have been used for definition of the branch pulmonary anatomy, especially in patients with PA/VSD.

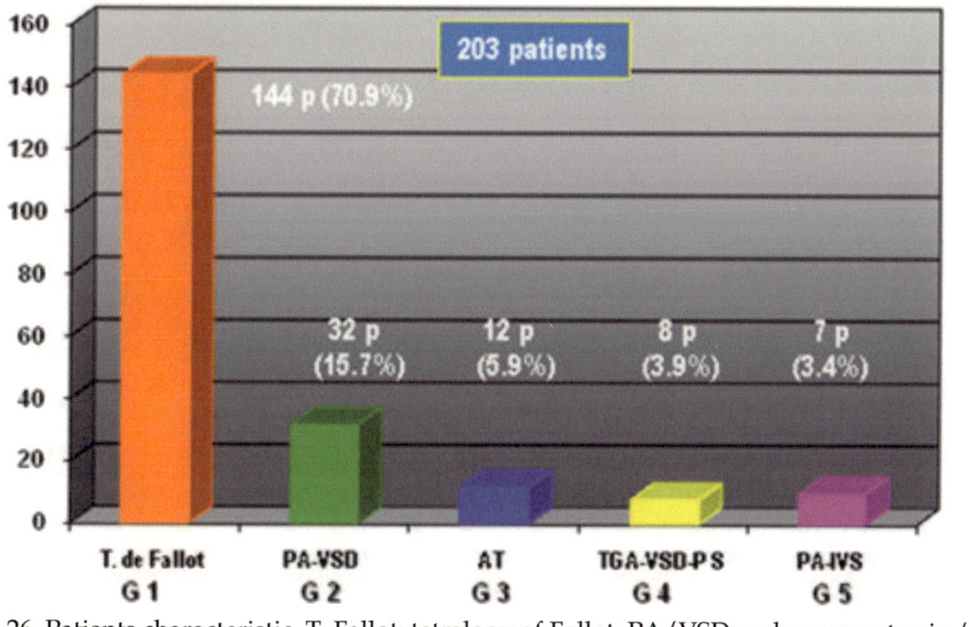

Fig. 26. Patients characteristic. T. Fallot: tetralogy of Fallot; PA/VSD: pulmonary atresia / ventricular septal defect; AT: arterial trunk; TGA / VSD / PS: transposition of the great arteries / ventricular septal defect / pulmonary stenosis; PA / IVS: pulmonary atresia / intact ventricular septum.

8.3 Prosthesis construction

The preparation of the biological material underwent several phases for the manufacture of the prosthesis: the valve and pulmonary trunk were isolated from the swine's heart, followed by cleaning, tanning and tissue conservation.

Four different models of prosthesis were manufactured, according to the anatomical type of RV reconstruction that was programmed. These prostheses were prepared in series according to Braile-Biomédica specifications with strict Medical Quality Control. These prostheses are available commercially at Braile Biomédica and were employed for RVOT reconstruction by Pediatric Cardiovascular Surgery groups, in Brazil. (Figure 27).

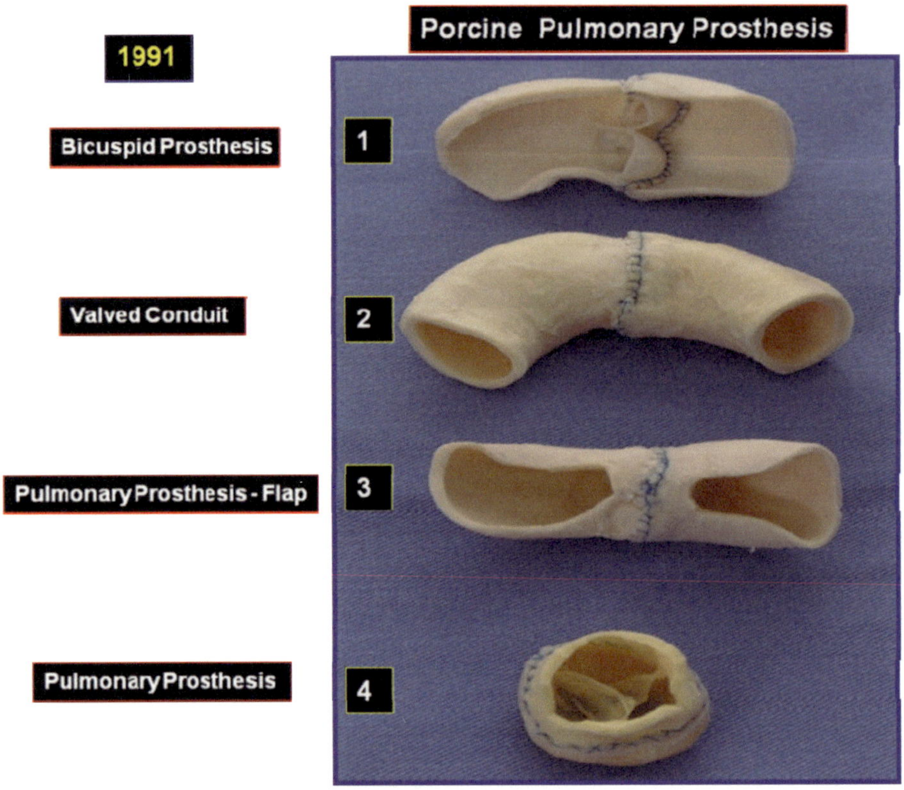

Fig. 27. Four different types of porcine pulmonary prosthesis

The pulmonary bicuspid prosthesis (PBP) was manufactured using two segments of the pulmonary artery, one including the trunk, ring and pulmonary valve and the other, only the pulmonary trunk (supravalvar area).The diameter of the pulmonary ring was measured using Hegar's dilator and the grafts were classified according to the size in millimeters. One longitudinal incision was made in the concave part, removing a slice of the wall with one of the pulmonary valve cusps. A proportional wall segment was removed from the non-valved portion.

Finally, the two structures were ligated by their proximal tips and were superposed in a 3 to 5 mm extension, with continuous anchored polypropylene 5-0 suture. The suture was started at the graft's concave face and followed the insertion of the fibromuscular ring cusp. A similar suture was performed in the convex side.

The pulmonary valved conduit (PVC) was manufactured using two entire segments of pulmonary trunk (one of these with trileaflet pulmonary valve); the tips of these segments were ligated with a running suture.

The pulmonary prosthesis with flap (PPF), was manufactured similarly to the CPP and two large flaps were performed at the pulmonary and ventricular tips.

The pulmonary prosthesis (PP) is performed by a short segment of the pulmonary artery, including the pulmonary valve

8.4 Surgical procedure

Our current strategy for RVOT remodeling utilized 4 types of preserved porcine pulmonary prosthesis: 1- Pulmonary bicuspid prosthesis (PBP) to repair the PV and RVOT reconstruction in patients under 1 year old (patients with narrow pulmonary ring and estimated pulmonary ring under 15 mm and **2-** Pulmonary valved conduit (PVC): trileaflet prosthesis used in patients over 1 year old with pulmonary atresia. 3- Pulmonary prosthesis with flap (PPF) used in patients over 1 year old and hypoplastic pulmonary ring and pulmonary trunk. 4- Pulmonary Prosthesis (PP) used in patients with regular pulmonary ring or absent pulmonary valve (estimated pulmonary ring over 15 mm).

Other associated procedures for remodeling of the RV included: ventricular septal defect repair or LV to Aorta tunnel, tricuspid repair, pulmonary artery branch plastic procedure.

8.5 Group 1: Tetralogy of fallot

This group had 144 (70.9%) patients aging 5 months to 35 years (mean= 3.2): 30 cases (20.8%) had systemic pulmonary shunt as a palliative procedure before the operation; 4 cases (2.7%) had absent PV and 15 cases (10.4%) had pulmonary atresia. (Table 6)

Characteristic	Data
N° Patients	144 p
Age (year)	5 m to 35 y (mean: 3.2)
Blalock -Taussig Shunt	30 p (20.8%)
Absent pulmonary valve	4 p (2.7%)
Pulmonary atresia	15 p (10.4%)

Table 6. Tetralogy of Fallot – Preoperative Patients data

The surgery was carried out using cardiopulmonary bypass, established with bicaval cannulation and mild hypothermia. Aortic cross-clamping with intermittent potassium cold blood cardioplegia employed for the intracardiac repair. Vacuum-assisted venous drainage routinely utilized.

The VSD was closed by right atriotomy or right ventriculotomy approach, using treated bovine pericardium patch and running suture. Relief of the RVOT obstruction was obtained by wide resection of all septum-parietal and parietal-parietal muscle bundles of the pulmonary infundibulum. In all cases where the pulmonary annulus itself seemed narrowed; the incision extended through the pulmonary annulus up to the main pulmonary artery and the whole area was primary or reoperation; were performed with the heart beating.

For the reconstruction of the pulmonary ventricle in patients under 1 year old, a PBP was implanted and adjusted to the rudimentary pulmonary valve of the patient. (Figure 28).

In patients over 1 year old, a PPF (trileaflet pulmonary valve) was implanted in the native pulmonary annulus with running suture. For the reconstruction of the pulmonary trunk and RV outlet tract, two flaps (pulmonary and ventricular flap) of this prosthesis were used.

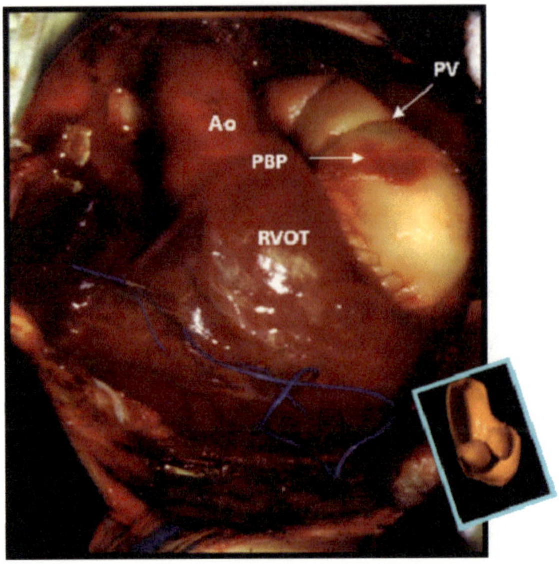

Fig. 28. Surgical photography. Patient with tetralogy of Fallot, submitted to remodeling of the right ventricle outlet tract (RVOT), using pulmonary bicuspid prosthesis (PBP) (in detail). Ao: aorta, PV: pulmonary valve.

Measurements were obtained by visualizing the heart images (including the prosthesis for the insertion of valves) and comparing them with the catheter's diameter in a superposed graded film with the identical magnification.

During the operation, the diameter of the pulmonary annulus was determined by classic normogram. The size graft was chosen according to the patient's weight: less than 10 kg, it was used 8 to 10 mm; and over 10 kg, it was used 12 to 20 mm.

In the cases with pulmonary atresia or absent pulmonary valve and under 1 year of age, a new cuspid was constructed using tissue from the pulmonary artery posterior wall, providing support for the PBP.

In patients over 2 years of age, the pulmonary valve and RVOT was reconstructed with porcine pulmonary prosthesis (Figure 29 a,b)

In cases with anomalous origin of coronary artery, crossing the infundibulum, the remodeling right ventricle surgery was performed with porcine pulmonary valved conduit. (Figure 30)

8.6 Group 2: Pulmonary atresia with ventricular septal defect

In this group, all thirty two (15.7%) patients were over 14 month of age. There were 3 cases with aortic-pulmonary collateral arteries submitted to previous unifocalization surgery plus Blalock-Taussig shunt. (Figure 31 a,b)

The surgical approach was performed by right ventriculotomy, after resection of the infundibulum muscle and closure of the VSD and finally was performed the right ventricle remodeling surgery, implanting a porcine pulmonary valved conduit, between right ventricle infundibulum and pulmonary artery

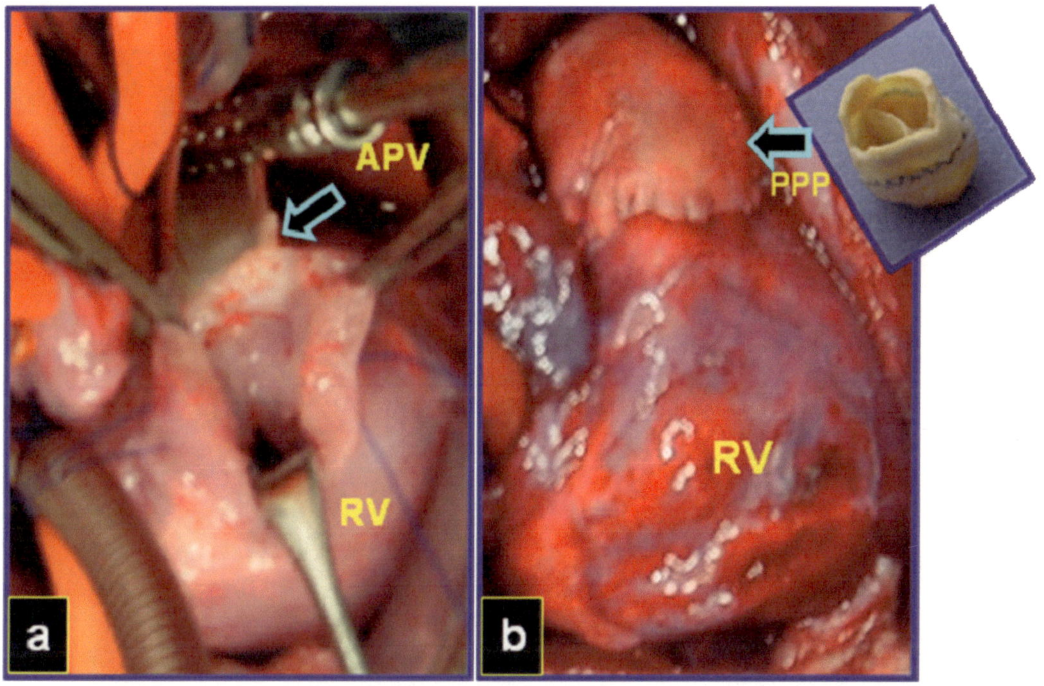

Fig. 29. Surgical photography. a- Patients with tetralogy of Fallot and absent pulmonary valve (arrow). b-Right ventricle (RV) remodeling with porcine pulmonary prosthesis (PPP) (arrow) (in detail)

8.7 Group 3: Truncus arteriosus

In this group, 12 (5.9%) patients under 6 months with TA type I, II were operated.

During the surgical approach, the pulmonary artery was disconnected from the ascending aorta and the left aortic sinus was reconstructed using a bovine pericardium patch; by the right ventricle approach, the VSD was closed, connecting the LV to the Aortic rout.

In ten patients, the posterior wall of RVOT was constructed with a pulmonary flap of the left pulmonary artery, but we did not use a monocuspid patch, according to the author`s technical specifications.

For the reconstruction of the pulmonary ventricle, we adjusted to the neo pulmonary annulus a PBP. In the remaining 2 patients, PVC was used for the reconstruction of the RVOT. PBP implantation was a surgical alternative for correcting TA type I and type II at early age (<6 months) using the technique without conduit.

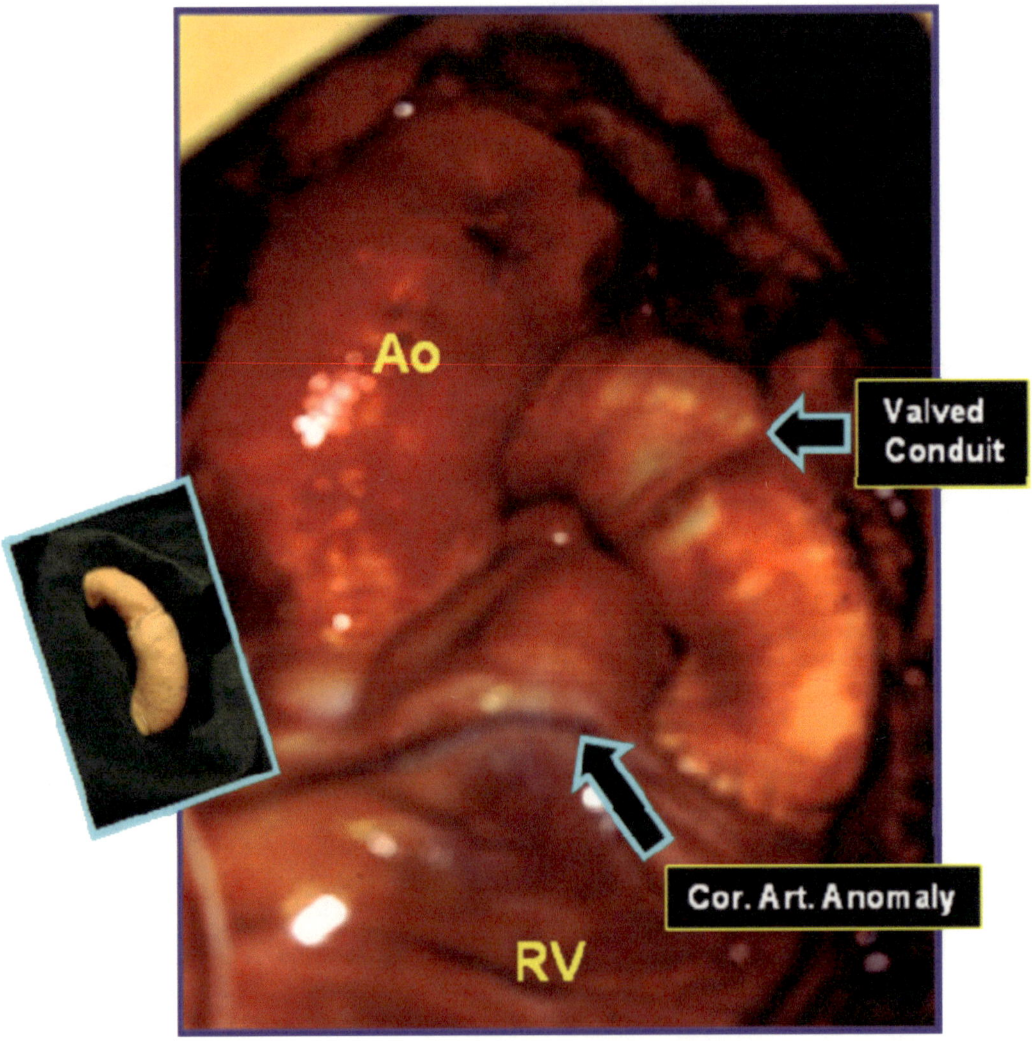

Fig. 30. Surgical photography. Patients with tetralogy of Fallot and anomalous origin of the coronary artery, crossing the Pulmonary infundibulum. The right ventricle remodeling surgery was performed with porcine pulmonary valved conduit (in detail). Ao: aorta, RV: right ventricle, Cor. Art.: coronary artery

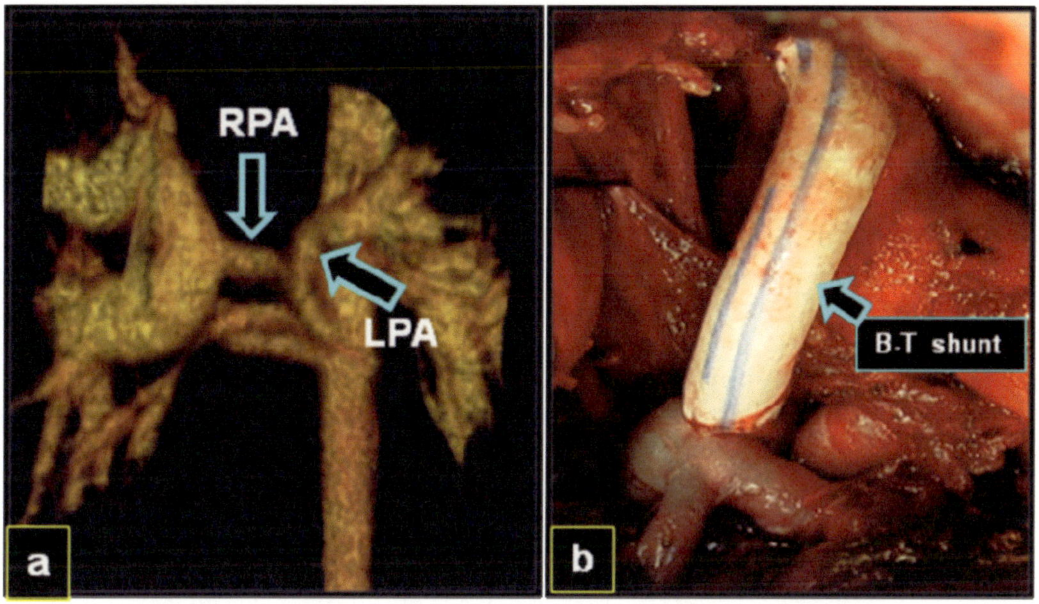

Fig. 31. a Computerized tomography showing pulmonary artery hypoplasia and aortic-pulmonary collaterals. b- Surgical photography : Unifocalization plus Blalok-Taussig (B-T) shunt.

8.8 Group 4: Transposition of the great arteries with pulmonary stenosis

Eight (3.9%) patients of this group, age ranging from 2 to 8 years old (mean= 3.0), had TGA, VSD and left ventricle outflow tract obstruction (LVOTO) (Fig 32 a).

The Lecompte technique, introduced for the treatment of TGA / VSD / LVOTO is called: REV (Réparation à l'Etage Ventriculaire) procedure.

The Lecompte technique was performed in all our cases, and consists in approaching the upper right ventriculotomy, extensive resection of the conal septum and enlargement of the VSD. Afterwards, with a pericardium or Polytetrafluoroethylene (PTFE) patch and running suture, a tunnel was performed connecting the left ventricle to the aortic route (LV-Ao). (Figure 32 b)

Later, the aorta and the pulmonary artery were sectioned, the pulmonary valve was closed, the Lecompte maneuver was performed and finally the aortic and pulmonary outflow tracts were reconstructed.

In 6 cases a porcine pulmonary prosthesis with flap was used for the RVOT reconstruction (Figure 32 c) and porcine pulmonary conduit , in 2 remaining cases. One patient who had been submitted to Rastelli procedure 3 years earlier, presented RV-PA prosthesis obstruction and severe RV failure. This case was operated in emergency state and converted to Lecompte operation: After aortic section, the Lecompte's maneuver was performed and the pulmonary artery was positioned in front of the aorta. A PBP was used for RVOT reconstruction.

8.9 Group 5: Pulmonary atresia with intact ventricular septum

Seven (3.4%) patients of this group, with ages between 1 and 12 years old (mean= 4.0), had pulmonary atresia with intact ventricular septum (PA/IVS). Three patients had the first stage of the operation (Blalock-Taussig shunt plus pulmonary valvotomy) performed in neonatal period and second stage (Glenn operation) at 1 year old .

In these patients a "normal" tricuspid valve (Z score more than - 4.0) and hypoplastic but potentially usable right ventricle was observed. The repair consisted in patch closure of the atrial septal defect, tricuspid valve plastic repair and reconstruction of the RVOT was performed with PBP (One and a half ventricle repair with pulsate bidirectional Glenn) (Figure 33)

The remaining 4 patients had pulmonary valvotomy in neonatal period. The tricuspid valve and RV had morphology, size and function near normality. In these patients it was implanted a PPF to reconstruct the RVOT.

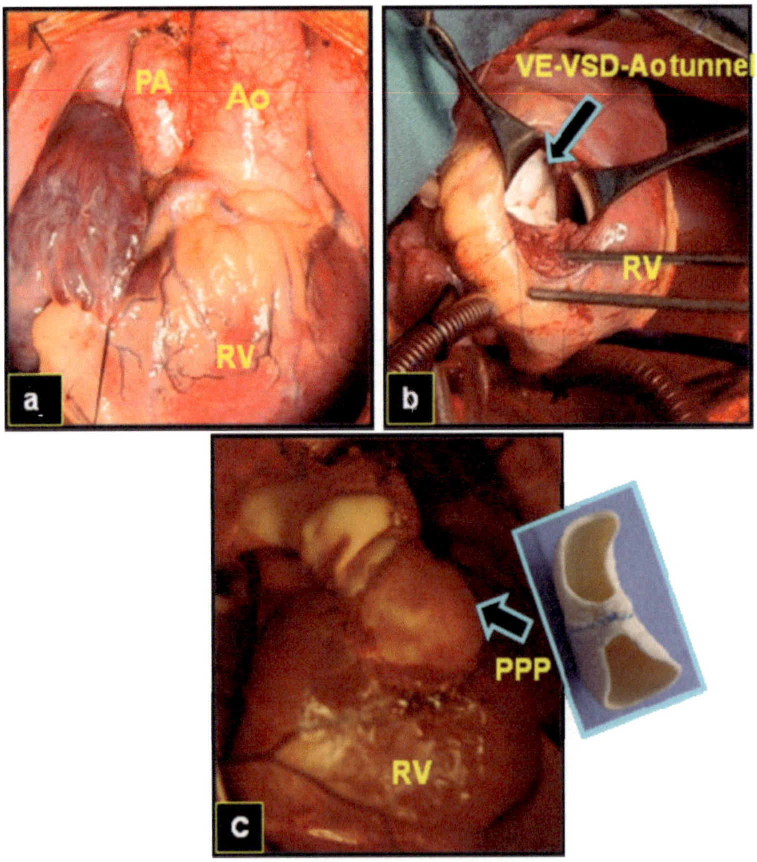

Fig. 32. Surgical photography. a- Transposition of the great arteries with ventricular septal defect (VSD) and left ventricle outlet tract obstruction. b- Lecompte operation : Left ventricle (LV) - ventricular septal defect (VSD) – aorta (Ao) tunnel is performed with polytetrafluoroethylene (PTFE) (in detail), and c- Right ventricle outlet tract reconstruction with porcine pulmonary prosthesis (PPP) with flap .

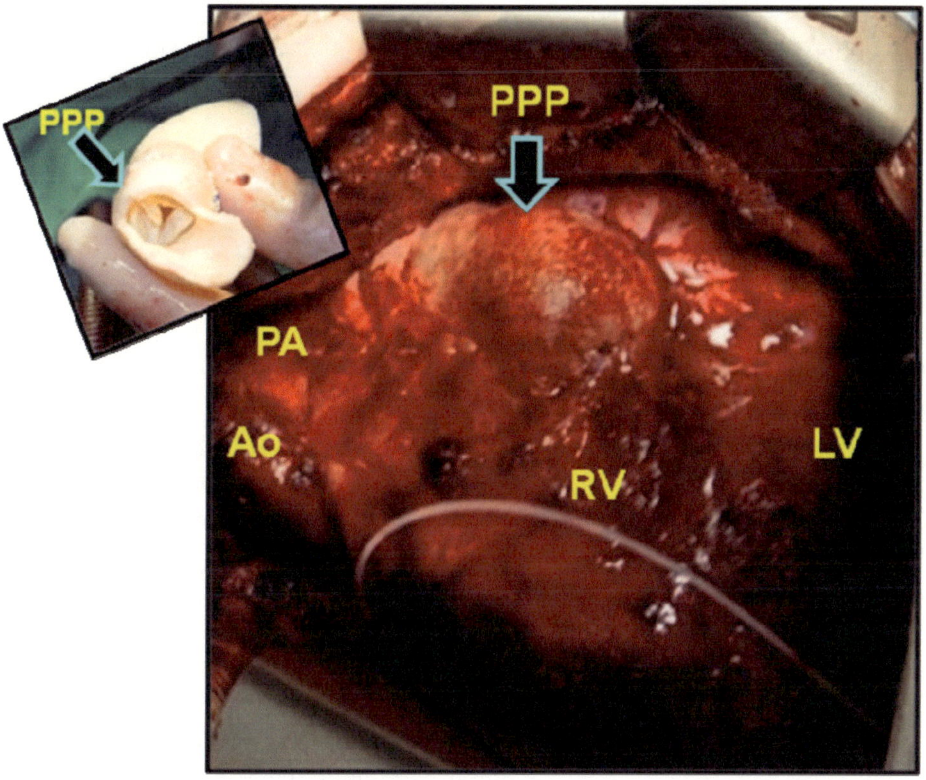

Fig. 33. Surgical photography. Pulmonary Atresia with Intact Ventricular Septum, submitted to surgical correction with: 1 ½ Ventricular Repair: Remodeling of the right ventricle (RV) outlet tract using valved porcine pulmonary prosthesis (PPP) (in detail); LV: left ventricle; Ao: aorta; PA: pulmonary artery.

8.10 Surgical recuperation

In all patients it was employed conventional ultrafiltration (CUF) during cardiopulmonary bypass (CPB) and in the last 12 years, modified ultrafiltration (MUF), after CPB was associated.

It was possible to discontinue CPB, in all cases and no patient had delayed sternum closure.

Sinus rhythm was maintained in all patients, before discharge from hospital. Temporary cardiac arrhythmias were detected, in 10 % of the cases, during hospital stay. No pacemaker was indicated or implanted in this group.

The most frequent cardiopulmonary support was performed with Dobutamine and Milrinone drugs.

8.11 Early and late mortality

There were 21 hospital deaths (10.3%); the mortality in different groups was: Group 1: TOF, 15 (10.4%) cases; Group 2: PA / VSD, 3 (9.3%) cases; Group 3: TA, 2 (16.6%) case; Group 4: TGA / VSD / LVOTO, 1 (12.5%) case. Group 5: PA / IVS, 0 (0.0%) cases.

There were 4 late deaths (2.1%): Two patients with TOF, caused by cardiac arrhythmia and bacterial endocarditis. Other two patients, with TA and PA/VSD, caused by ventricular dysfunction.

8.12 Morbidity

Forty (21.9%) nonfatal complications occurred in 182 early surviving patients.

In three patients it was detected residual pulmonary branch stenosis.

There were 159 (78.3%) patients free of reoperation.

8.13 Reintervention

Seventeen (9.6%) cases were submitted to reoperation due to residual defects or prosthesis dysfunction in an interval of 24 to 120 months after operation. Two patients developed aneurysmatic dilatation of the pulmonary prosthesis: after TOF correction and after "One and half ventricle" correction. Both patients died after reoperation due to ventricle dysfunction and surgical bleeding.

The pathologic study of the prosthesis removed shows: calcification islands compromising the external wall but preserving the integrity of its leaflet; nevertheless, two cases with aneurysmatic dilatation show sling wall and no presence of calcification. (Imperfection tissue fixation?).

Two patients presented residual pulmonary stenosis, located at the right and left branch origin. Both cases required placement of pulmonary stent implant.

8.14 Follow-up

Reconstruction of the PV and remodeling of the RV was an essential component in the treatment of many patients with congenital heart disease.

Fourteen patients (7.9%) were lost during the follow-up. One hundred and sixty two (79.8%) surviving patients were followed from 4 to 204 months (mean= 108). Actuarial survival curve at 204 month was estimated in 86.6%. (Figure 34)

The follow-up of these patients included: Clinical exam, exercise stress test, metabolic stress test, Doppler echocardiography study, Hemodynamic study, MRI and CT study.

We do not have all the complete data set on all of the above variables for the entire cohort of patients in this manuscript.

8.15 Doppler echocardiography study

This was the most frequent auxiliary study employed to analyze the results of cardiac surgery and prosthesis performance. This study was performed twice a year, during the follow-up. With the echocardiogram many parameters of the RV function were studied: RV performance, RV dimensions; and with the Doppler index: if tricuspid regurgitation (TR) is present an estimate of RV pressures, RV-PA gradients and pulmonary and tricuspid valves function.

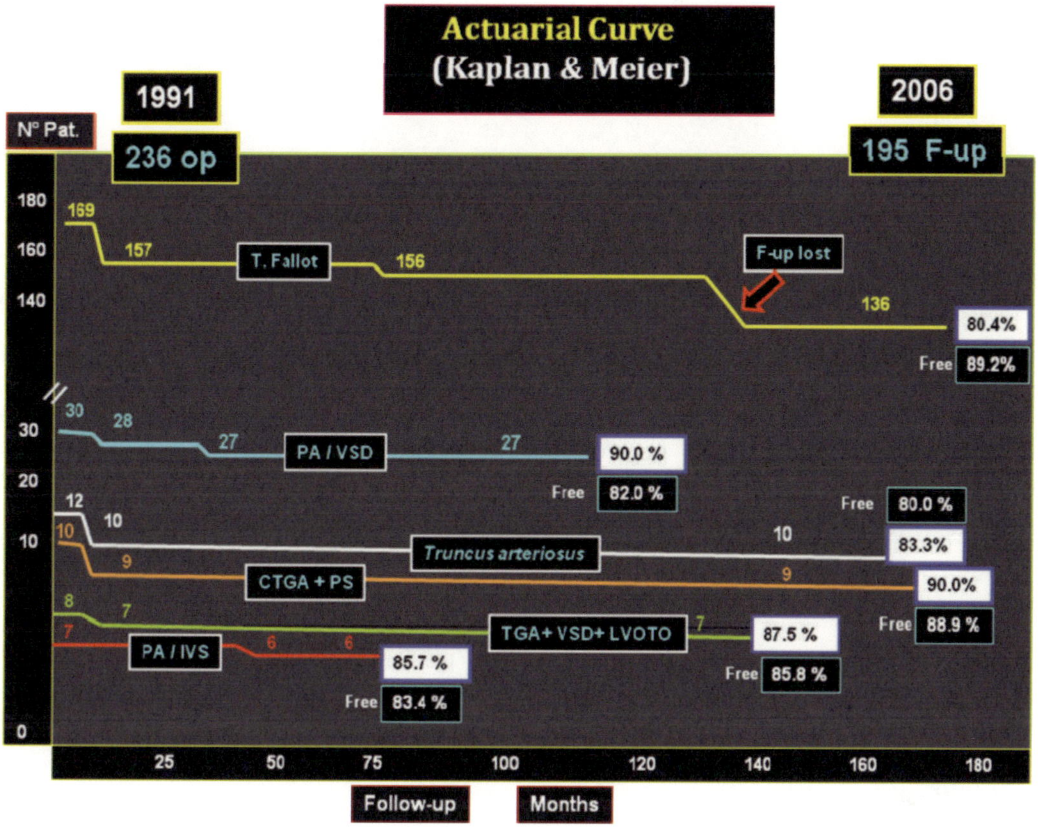

Fig. 34. Actuarial survival curve of patients undergoing right ventricle remodeling

One hundred and forty three surviving patients were discharged from hospital with RV-PA gradient less than 30.0 mmHg and trivial to moderated VPI. During the follow-up, in ten patients the Doppler-echocardiogram was decisive for reoperation and in other two patients, for the indication of hemodynamic procedure.

Among the 162 (79.8%) regular late follow-up patients, the degree of VPI that increased slightly was detected in 20 patients (12.3%), but only one patient had important pulmonary regurgitation

8.16 Hemodynamic evaluation

Hemodynamic studies were carried out in the first 15 (9.2%) cases of 162 survival patients with regular follow-up. All 15 patients had TOF and follow-up between 48 and 87 months (mean= 65.1). The patients age ranged from 5 to 16 years (mean= 8.2 years). Table 7.

Characteristic	Data
Age (years)	5 to 16 (mean=8.2)
Gender	F=6 (40.0%)
Weight (Kg)	16 to 49 (mean=23,6)
High (cm)	107 to 167 (mean=125.6)
Body surface (cm^2)	0.75 to 1.55 (mean=0.98.6)
PO Follow-up (month)	72 to 108 (mean=84)
Absent pulmonary valve	3 p (20.0%)
Pulmonary atresia	2 p (13.3%)

Table 7. Tetralogy of Fallot - Postoperative Hemodynamic study in 15 patients.

Right ventriculography in right anterior oblique (RAO) position and left anterior oblique (LAO) position and pulmonary arteriography in anterior posterior projection were carried out in all of the cases. The dimensions of the RV were established during cardiac cycle.

The measurements were obtained by visualization of the heart images (including the prosthesis for the insertion of valves) and superposed in a graded film with identical magnification which was compared to the catheter's diameter.

In some cases it was difficult to establish the position of the pulmonary ring due to the presence of RVOT prosthesis. The degree of VPI was evaluated by the quantitative method after injection of contrast solution in the pulmonary artery, and the VPI was classified as mild when regurgitation was lower than 50% (group A) and moderate when greater than 50% (group B).

8.17 Hemodynamic dates

Out of fifteen patients undergoing hemodynamic and angiocardiographyc evaluation, no residual blood flow from left to right ventricular camera or significant gradient between the RV and PA was observed.[14]

8.18 Magnetic Resonance Imaging and Computerized Tomography study of the heart

Cardiac MRI and CT study has become an available method of diagnostic and postoperative follow-up. (Fig 35, 36)

In order to assess the responses of PV reconstruction and remodeling of the RV with PBP or PPF, it was used CT imaging and PVI evaluation and biventricular function using a MRI in patients who underwent TOF, PA / VSD, AT, TGA / VSD / LVOTO and PA/IVS repair.

In 2006, 10 patients were submitted to MRI and CT study with follow-up over 10 years. The parameter of cardiac function was obtained at rest: RV ejection fraction was normal (>45%) in 8 (80%) patients, the MRI was well suited to assess cardiac response and findings revealed a discrete VPI in PBP and a trivial VPI in PPF.

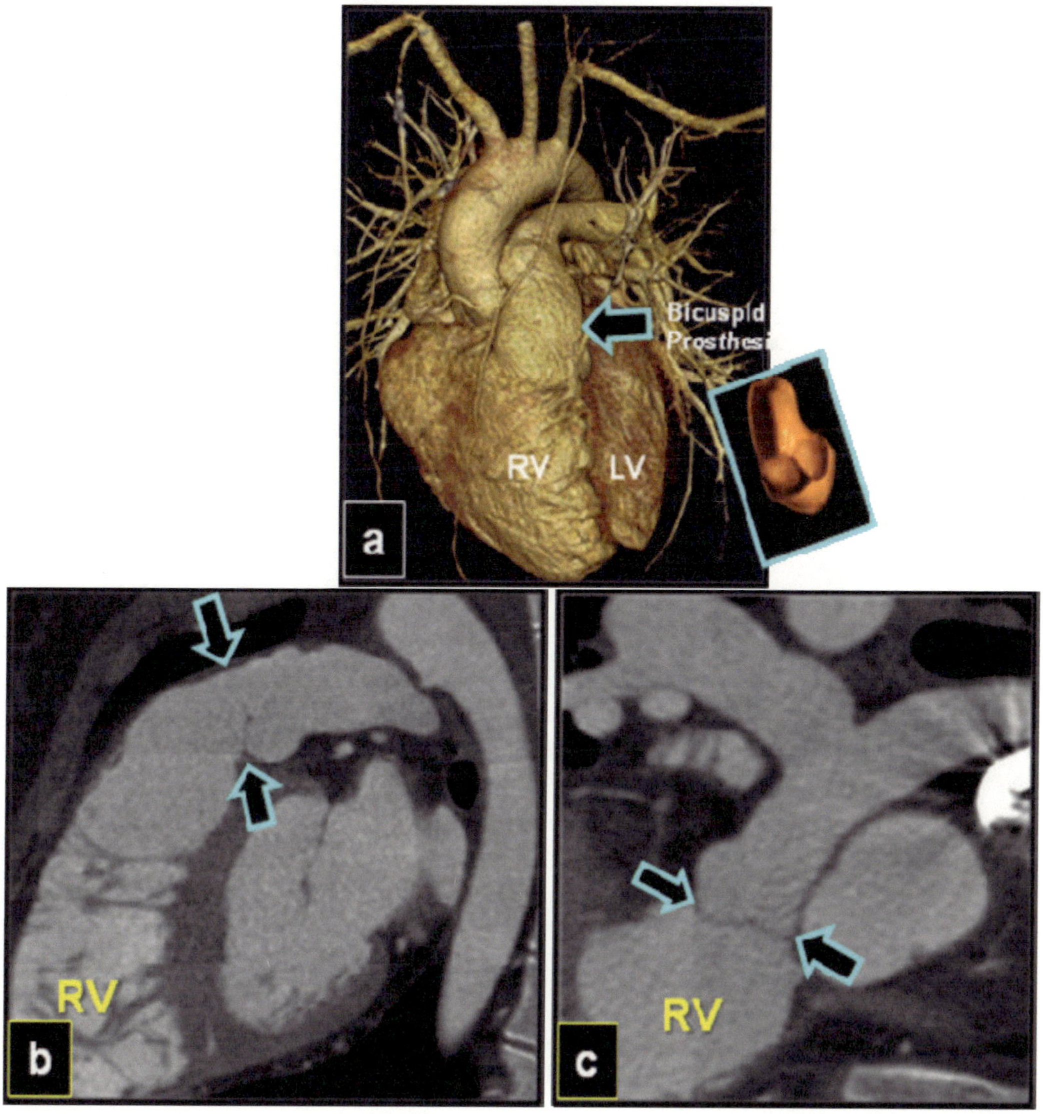

Fig. 35. Computerized tomography in a patient with tetralogy of Fallot submitted to surgical remodeling of the right ventricle (RV) outlet tract with an implant of a preserved porcine pulmonary bicuspid prosthesis (in detail), with 16 years of follow-up (arrows). LV: left ventricle

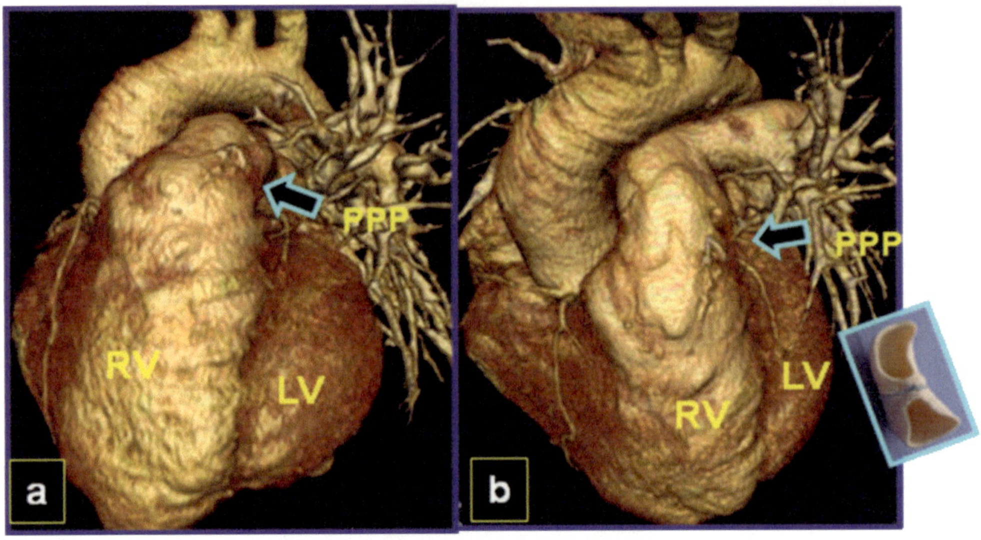

Fig. 36. Computerized tomography: a, b: Patient with tetralogy of Fallot and severe pulmonary insufficiency, after twenty years of follow-up., sububmitted to surgical remodeling of the right ventricle (RV) outlet tract with an implant of a preserved porcine pulmonary prosthesis (PPP) (in detail), with 7 years of follow-up (arrows). LV: left ventricle.

8.19 Statistical analysis

Statistical analyses of continuous variables were performed with both methods: by paired t test and the analysis of categorical variables performed by the Student's t test and $p<0.05$.was considered statistically significant. The surviving patients curve was prepared according to the Kaplan-Meier's method, comparing 2 or more functions by the long-rank test. For all tests, a p value of less than 0.05 was considered significant.

8.20 Comments

The patients undergoing TOF repair surgery have an excellent prognosis and good late survival in about 90% of the cases, ten years after the surgery. In 95% of the cases it is possible the patient's social reintegration and good physical ability during exercise and 79.3% practice sports.[20]

Reconstruction of the PV and remodeling of the RV using valved prostheses is an essential component in the treatment of patients with TOF and others congenital heart diseases with pulmonary ventricle obstruction.

It is difficult to establish the number of patients who had surgical correction of TOF and required reoperation. In general, it depends on the anatomical lesion of each patient and the kind of surgical approach used, as well as the kind of surgical reconstruction employed.

Multiple surgical options for PV reconstruction are available for these patients: mechanical valves, mechanical conduits, monocuspid homograft or patch, pulmonary and aortic homograft, stented and stentless heterograft, heterograft conduits, bovine jugular vein conduits and autologous pericardial valves.

The use of a mechanical valve in the pulmonary position has been reported in a few patients and had fallen out, due to frequent occurrence of thromboembolic phenomena and valve failure

In 1967, Marchand introduced a monocuspid homograft with excellent results. This type of RVOT repair was very well accepted and routinely adopted in several services, however, the presence of diastolic murmur and the early postoperative evaluation found out that different degrees of pulmonary insufficiency were interpreted as an inadequate alignment of the leaflet graft with the pulmonary valve native leaflets in the early postoperative follow-up.In 1968 Asano & Eguchi published their clinical experience with the use of a bicuspid pulmonary homograft and bicuspid pulmonary heterograft. An autologous pericardial segment sutured to pulmonary ring was used for the reconstruction of the RVOT. A posterior author's (publication28) performed, described aneurismal dilatation of autologous pericardial segment at late follow-up.

Therefore, when the enlargement of the pulmonary ring is strictly necessary, the use of open tile-shaped prosthesis, in patients under one year old, allowed the ring to grow at the expense of the posterior wall. On the other hand, once this is a valved prosthesis adjusted for the right closure at the time of the operation, the growth of the pulmonary ring might make the prosthesis less contingent. On the other hand, the growth of the native valve might also be expected, although it can hardly be clinically proven.

A larger experience with PTFE monocuspid for RVOT reconstruction in 115 patients with follow-up of 6 months to 8 years (mean=2.6), demonstrated significant development of VPI graded as moderate to severe after 35 months in this monocuspid study.

Homograft valves have become widely used for reconstruction of the right ventricular outflow tract in congenital heart disease. However, mid-term and long-term follow-up studies have clearly demonstrated conduit obstruction and early valve insufficiency, degeneration and progressive calcification, more frequent in aortic homograft.

Some authors suggest that possibly the durability of cryopreserved pulmonary homograft is similar to pulmonary homograft used for the Ross procedure. When the trileaflet prosthesis is implanted in the orthotopic position, as in the Ross aortic valve replacement patient, can be easily accommodated, maintaining valvar competence.

The limited durability of homograft conduits, especially in small sizes, supported the search for an alternative conduit as the PBP, bicuspid homograft and PTFE bicuspid valve, that allowed the growth of the posterior face of the pulmonary ring and posterior wall of the pulmonary trunk. The superiority of the bicuspid prostheses has been demonstrated in experimental studies for reconstruction of a hypoplastic pulmonary root, and this experience was confirmed in clinical experience.

Pulmonary valve insufficiency may have a negative impact on RV function leading to the need for reoperation for the insertion of a competent valve at the RVOT.

There are no ideal options for restoring the VPI. Studies including adult patients with TOF after pulmonary valve replacement with various prostheses, generally reported good long-term results with both porcine xenograft and homograft.

VSD or PS might impair the long-term results and significantly change the patient's prognosis. Beginning in 1991, we started to use a preserved PBP in infants and PPF in children for the reconstruction of PV and RVOT in patients with TOF aiming to decrease residual VPI.

This series of patients undergoing TOF repair surgery presented an excellent prognosis and good late survival rate in about 80% of the cases, seventeen years after the surgery. 78% of the surviving patients, with late follow-up, are free of reoperation and show good physical ability during exercise and practice of sports. The hemodynamic evaluation of these patients shows that average individual RV/LV length ratios did not increase over time.

Although the preliminary studies of a valved bovine jugular vein conduits had reported short to intermediate term durability, Boudjemline et al and Zavanella et al, reported similar findings of extensive fibrosis at the conduit pulmonary anastomosis by developing intimal proliferation.

In these patients, submitted to PPF implantation, a technical modification was introduced to reduce PS development by intimal proliferation at the conduit: It was performed an enlarged pulmonary anastomosis, after constructing a flap at the distal graft's tip.

This procedure was also used for the reconstruction of pulmonary ventricular outflow tract in another group of patients: PA / VSD, AT, PA / IVS, TGA / VSD / LVOTO.

In the PA/VSD group, all patients were over 14 months of age and only 18 cases had palliative procedure, type: Blalock-Taussig shunt and unifocalization procedure.

All patients were submitted to pulmonary arteriography; in order to study the diameter of the PA (trunk, right and left branches) it was determined the McGoon index. Although, other quantitative methods were employed to study the degree of pulmonary development, in order to measure the pulmonary area, it was determined the Nakata index or PA index (PAI). All patients of our series had PAI higher than 150 mm/m^2.

During the operation, it was possible to close the VSD in all patients and after cardiopulmonary bypass, the RV/LV ratio pressure was measured; in all cases this relationship was below 0.58%. Total deaths: one patient died after refractory low cardiac output and another by generalized infection.

In the AT group, two types of prostheses were used for the reconstruction of the PV and remodeling of the RVOT:

The implant of the PBP was a surgical alternative for the correction of the AT type I, II, at early age (under 6 months), using the technique without conduit. In 8 patients of our series, it was possible to use the RVOT reconstruction using a bicuspid prosthesis: Using a flap of the left pulmonary it was constructed the posterior wall of the RVOT and using one PBP and running suture this prosthesis was adjusted

There were two hospital deaths by pulmonary hypertension crises.

The PVI was trivial in all cases, at the immediate postoperative period, in 7 surviving patients. At this moment, no patient was submitted to re-intervention, but actually 3 patients are in functional class II (NYHA) and presented moderate VPI.

2 - In the second type of prosthesis, the PP was implanted in patients older than 6 months. Two patients underwent operation with this technique: One patient, who underwent operation with a valveless woven Dacron conduit 5 years earlier in another center for RV dysfunction with significant PVI, received a PP implant.

The pulmonary ventricle may be compromised by either morphologic or functional problems, or by both. The morphologic defect may be defined by tricuspid valve Z value. In general, this value also reflects the corresponding ventricle volume.

Right ventricle outflow tract is alleviated by a variety of techniques, including muscle resection, valvotomy with division of the pulmonary annulus along with the commissure and reconstruction of the RVOT with a trans-annular pericardial patch or biological valved prosthesis.

In our series, seven patients with PA /IVS were submitted to correction with "one and half ventricle" technique, with success. All cases had Glenn procedure previous and were performed with the same procedure: atrial septal defect (ASD) closure and reconstruction of the RVOT with PPF. One patient was submitted to trans-catheter closure of the residual Blalock-Taussig shunt. The right ventricle performance and RV - PA junction were evaluated with MRI and the RVOT reconstruction with CT study. (Fig 8 A,B) The gradient RV - PA in all three patients was lower than 30 mmHg.

The Lecompte[51] procedure introduced for the treatment of TGA / VSD / LVOTO, consisted in the construction of a LV to Ao tunnel, after conal septum resection, by ventricle approach. The RVOT reconstruction is performed after the pulmonary artery is transferred in front of aorta (Lecompte maneuver). A valved prosthesis is employed for the pulmonary valve reconstruction. This technique is called the REV procedure.

For the reconstruction of the pulmonary outflow tract there are two techniques:

When the aorta and the pulmonary artery are in anteroposterior position, the reconstruction of the RVOT is possible, after transversal aorta and pulmonary artery section and pulmonary valve reconstruction in front of the aorta.

When the aorta and the pulmonary artery are in side by side position, the Lecompte maneuver is dispensed and a valved conduit is necessary to reconstruct the pulmonary outflow tract.

In our series, when the great arteries had an anteroposterior relationship, it was not difficult to pull the pulmonary artery down to the right ventriculotomy site without tension in order to reconstruct the pulmonary outflow with a PBP. However, when the pulmonary artery and the aorta were in side by side position, the Lecompte maneuver was also employed and the pulmonary outflow tract was reconstructed with PPP.

8.21 Conclusion

The clinical follow-up of 176 (86.6%) patients from 4 to 204 months (mean=108) allowed the following conclusions:

Right ventricle remodeling constitutes a safe and standardized technique.

The early reconstruction of the pulmonary valve and right ventricle outlet tract could be able to preserve ventricular performance for a long period.

The prosthesis function could be analyzed during the follow-up.

The porcine pulmonary prosthesis has shown satisfactory results for a long time.

9. New technique in Cardiopulmonary bypass

9.1 Conventional and Modified Ultrafiltration during cardiac surgery in high-risk congenital heart disease.

The use of cardiopulmonary bypass (CPB), with hypothermia and hemodilution, in the pediatric age group is associated with the accumulation of an excessive amount of water. The ratio of prime volume to patient blood volume may be twice as high in smaller patients. However the inflammatory capillary leak is probably responsible for tissue edema and malfunction of several organs. Dilution of plasma proteins increases water transfer to the extravascular compartment and postoperative blood loss as a result of clotting disturbances.

Several methods are in use in order to reduce this water accumulation such as reduction of circuit diameter and prime volume, anti-inflammatory therapy, continuous diuretic and peritoneal dialysis. In 1991, Elliott's group from The Hospital for Sick Children at Great Ormond Street (London), reports an alternative technique of modified ultrafiltration (MUF) after CPB, through a filter with semi-permeable membrane, to remove water, electrolytes and other low molecular weight substances.

Conventional ultrafiltration (CUF), performed during CPB is associated with a statistically significant prime ultrafiltration but with clinically poor results.

Early studies with CPB in children demonstrated clinical improvement due to inflammatory agent removal, including endothelin–1 (a potent pulmonary vasoconstrictor) and other cytokines released during the warming period of CPB.

Efforts to reduce the detrimental effects of the capillary leak syndrome after CPB include ultrafiltration during CPB.

This prospective study was therefore undertaken to compare the effects of CUF + MUF with those of CUF during surgery for congenital heart disease.

9.2 Patients and methods

Forty-one children with complex congenital heart disease who underwent operations using CPB at Cardiovascular Division of the São Paulo Federal University .

Our service is the first service in the country in implementing this technique. To day, the MUF is used routinely in all patients submitted to surgery with CPB

Patients operated between January 1996 and March 1998 were included in this study. The Ethics Committee of the Institution approved the study protocol and informed consent was obtained from the parents of each child.

9.3 Patient group

This was a prospective, consecutive and nonrandomized study. We assigned 41 patients to one of two groups as follows: control group (n = 21) in which CUF during CPB was used.

Pediatric cardiac surgeries were performed between January 1996 and April 1997 (CUF group); and the experimental group (n = 20) in which CUF was associated with MUF after CPB, with surgeries performed between May 1997 and March 1998 (CUF + MUF group)

The patient characteristics are shown in Table 8. Both groups included patients with ages between 9 and 36 months. These groups were homogeneous and no significant differences were observed between them.

1996 - 1997 CUF 21 patients		1997 - 1998 CUF+MUF 20 patients	p
10/11	Sex (M/F)	10/10	----
15.0 ± 11.8	Mean age (mo)	9.2 ± 8.5	0.08
1 (4.7%)	Neonates	3 (15.0%)	----
7.2 + 3.0	Mean weight (kg)	5.7 ± 2.5	0.09

CUF: conventional ultrafiltration; CUF+MUF: modified ultrafiltration; mo.: months

Table 8. Patients characteristics

The preoperative diagnoses for each group were classified into 4 different degrees according to the operative complexity (Jenkins et al), as shown in Figure 37.

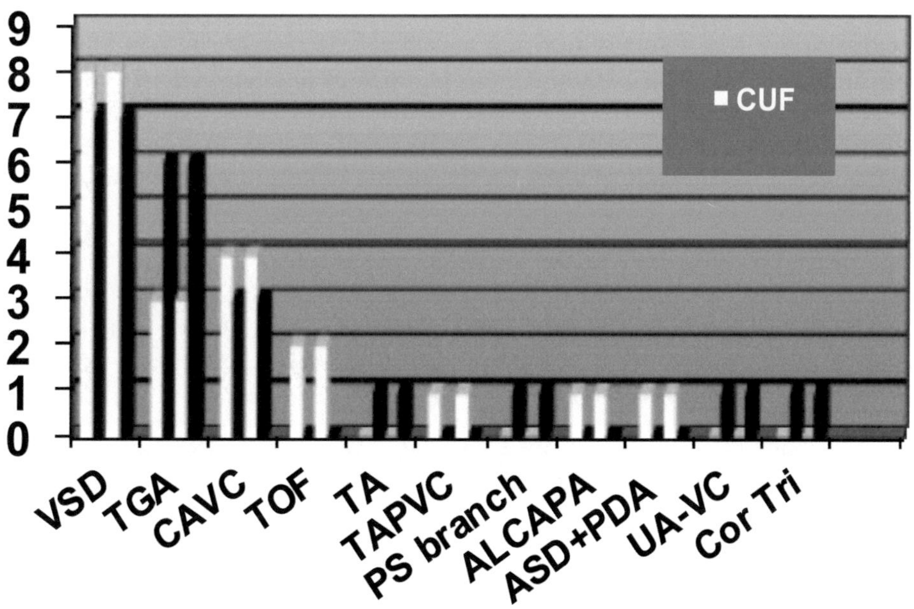

*Jenkins et al. (1995)

Fig. 37. 4 Operative Complexity

Figure 1: VSD: ventricular septal defect; TGA: transposition of great arteries; CAVC: complete atrioventricular canal; TOF: tetralogy of Fallot; TAPVC: total anomalous pulmonary vein connection; ASD: atrial septal defect; PDA: patent ductus arteriosus; TA: truncus arteriosus; ALCAPA: anomalous left coronary artery from pulmonary artery; PS: pulmonary stenosis; UA-VC: univentricular atrioventricular connection; Cor Tri: Cor-triatriatum.

9.4 Preoperative evaluation

Preoperative evaluation was performed by cardiac catheterization in all patients with moderate and severe pulmonary hypertension (PH), using a 40-biplane angioscope (Siemens). Preoperative PH was defined as a systolic pulmonary pressure/systolic systemic pressure > 60. PH was present in 15 patients (71.4%) of the CUF group and in 14 patients (70.0%) of the CUF + MUF group.

Transthoracic Doppler echocardiography was performed in the patients using ATL Ultramark 9 with a 3-5 MHz transducer.

9.5 Surgical technique

Surgical management was standardized by cannulation of the ascending aorta for inflow, separate caval cannulae being inserted through the right atrium. CPB was instituted after 400 U/kg heparin infusion. A flow rate of 2.4 l/min/m2 at normothermia was reduced to 1.8 l/min/m2 during moderate hypothermia (25°C to 28°C).

Deep hypothermia (< 24°C) and circulatory arrest were not required. The left side of the heart was vented with a catheter inserted in the apex through the right upper pulmonary vein.

The pump prime was composed of 500 to 900 ml electrolyte solution with 5% glucose (Darrow Imagem S/A, Brazil), sodium bicarbonate 10 to 30 mEq/l, 25% albumin (12.4 g/250 ml of prime), 2% mannitol 2.0 ml/kg and washed packed red blood cells to maintain a hematocrit value of 25%. Partial arterial pressure of carbon dioxide was recorded. The infusion of blood cardioplegic solution was repeated at 20-minute intervals.

9.6 Technique of conventional ultrafiltration

In the CUF group, patients were treated with ultrafiltration during CPB, at the warming stage, which removed excess fluid and hemoconcentrated the patient's blood. A hemoconcentrator (model HPH 400, Minntech, Minneapolis, MN) was also inserted in parallel in the cardioplegic line (connected to the recirculation line).

The total amount of fluid filtered by CUF was 19.7 ml/kg. After CPB, blood from the extracorporeal circuit was centrifuged for red cell salvage.

9.7 Modified ultrafiltration technique

The MUF group was submitted to the CUF procedure during CPB and then an arteriovenous ultrafiltration via the cardioplegia circuit was used according to Groom's technique, with some adjustments introduced in the system (Fig. 38).

Following the last dose of cardioplegia, the hemofilter is placed in the cardioplegia circuit after the cardioplegia (sucker) roller pump but before the heat exchanger. The cardioplegia line is clamped and CPB is discontinued but the heparin is not reverted.

The venous cannulae are removed from the right atrium and the blood within the venous line is siphoned into the venous reservoir. The clamp on the arterial filter bypass line is removed and placed just prior to the filter. A 10 F to 12 F cannula is attached to the cardioplegia line and placed in the atrium. The cardioplegia pump is turned on and the flow is slowly increased.

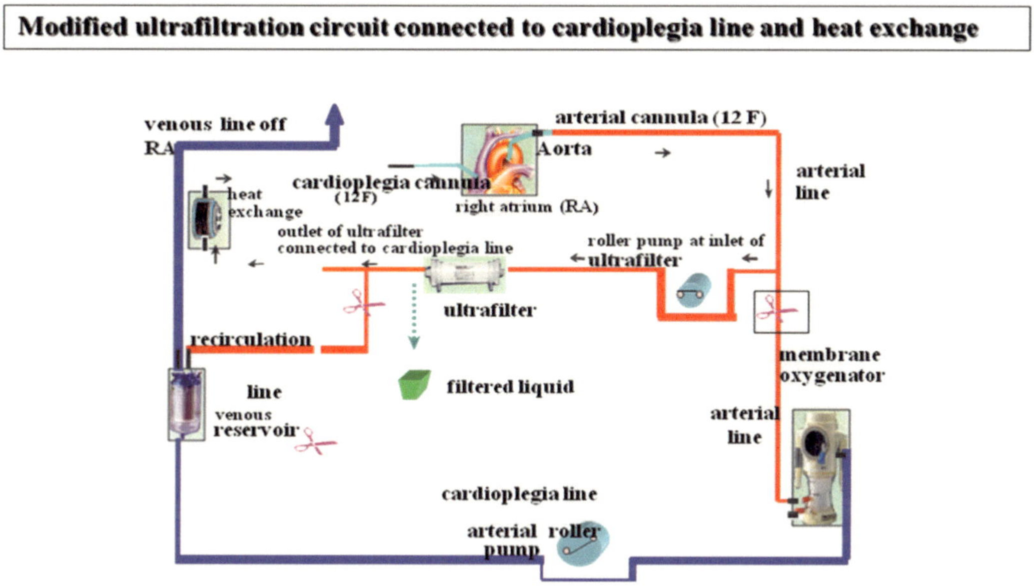

Fig. 38. Modified Ultrafiltration Circuit

This maneuver pumps blood from the aorta through the hemofilter and cardioplegia system and then Returns, the warm blood, to the RA after passing through the heat exange of the cardioplegia line.

When the target flow of 100 to 200 ml/min is reached, the clamp of the filtrate line is removed, allowing the ultrafiltration process to begin. No suction was applied to the filtrate line. As plasma water is removed, it is necessary to maintain the patient's volemic status by transfusing the content of the pump circuit at a rate equal to the filtration rate.

After this process continues for approximately ten minutes, the cannulae are removed and protamine is administered. The total amount of fluid filtered by conventional and modified ultrafiltration in this group was 39.3 ml/kg.

Intraoperative monitoring

Left atrial catheter was used in all patients and pulmonary arterial catheter was used in-patients with preoperative PH. When the systolic pulmonary artery pressure was higher than 40 mmHg, nitroprusside at a dose of 0.5 to 1.5 µg/kg/min, or nitroglycerin at a dose of 1 to 10 µg/kg/min was used.

If dobutamine or dopamine was required, a dose of 5 to 10 µg/kg/min was used; or in the case of epinephrine, a dose of 1 µg/kg/min.

9.8 Postoperative pulmonary hypertension control

Patients with preoperative PH were curarized and moderate hyperventilation was used. These patients also received nitroprusside, nitroglycerin and nitric oxide.

9.9 Postoperative management

All patients were followed-up in the Pediatric Intensive Care Unit (PICU).

9.9.1 Strategy for extubation

The respiratory management consisted of mechanical ventilation support to maintain the arterial oxygen tension at > 100 mmHg, the arterial carbon dioxide tension at 30 to 35 mmHg and the pH at 7.45 to 7.50. Once the children exhibited hemodynamic stability, they were weaned from mechanical ventilatory support and sedation.

Once the children demonstrated the ability to sustain adequate spontaneous respiration effort and required minimal supplemental oxygen as reflected by normal arterial blood gases, they were extubated. Neonatal patients at high-risk for post-operative PH required longer ventilatory support. Strategy for blood or hemoderivate replacement

No patient in this study received aprotinin. Washed packed cells were transfused to maintain hematocrit at 40% for patients with cyanotic congenital heart disease and 35% for those without cyanotic heart disease. Platelets, fresh frozen plasma, cryoprecipitate and albumin were transfused as required postoperatively.

9.10 Statistical analysis

Comparison between the two groups regarding duration of ventilator support, PICU stay and hospital stay data was performed by means of Student's t test.

Repeated measures analysis of variance was employed to evaluate the two groups during pre- and perioperative periods regarding hematocrit and platelet counts.

The hospital discharge probability was estimated using the Kaplan-Meier method. The log-rank test was employed to compare the two groups.

9.11 Results

9.11.1 Operative outcome

There were no MUF related complications. In all the patients it was possible to close the chest. No patient required reexploration for bleeding.

There were four postoperative deaths in the CUF + MUF group. All patients had PH and the main causes were cardiac arrhythmia, low cardiac output, ventilation problems, vasoactive agent handling and pulmonary infection.

There were six postoperative deaths in the CUF group. Five patients had PH and the main cause were coagulopathy, low cardiac output, ventilation problems, vasoactive agent handling and pulmonary infection.

9.11.2 Duration of ventilator support

Mean and standard deviation of duration of ventilator support in surviving patients of the CUF group were 94.8± 66.20 h for the CUF group and 95.67 ± 90.29 h, and for the CUF+MUF group. No significant difference was observed between the two groups (p= 0.976) Table 9.

9.11.3 PICU stay

Mean and standard deviation of the time of PICU stay in surviving patients of the CUF group were 169.60 ± 90.61 h and 157.81 ± 150.80 h for the CUF+MUF group. No significant difference was observed between PH groups (p= 0.795) Table II.

9.11.4 Hospital stay

The time of hospital stay in surviving patients of the CUF group were 14.87 ± 5.57 days and in surviving patients of the CUF+MUF group it was 14.69 ± 9.67 days. No significant difference was observed between PH groups (p= 0.950) (Table II). The estimated probability discharge from hospital after the 15th postoperative (PO) day was approximately 85% for both groups (Fig. 39)

Variables (Group)	N°	Minimum	Maximum	Mean	Standard deviation	P*
Ventilation support (hours)						
- CUF	15	24.00	192.00	94.80	66.20	0.976
- CUF+MUF	16	12.00	288.00	95.67	90.90	
PICU stay** (hours):						
- CUF	15	66.00	312.00	169.60	90.61	0.795
- CUF+MUF	16	24.00	576.00	157.81	150.80	
Hospital stay** (days)						
- CUF	15	5.00	28.00	14.87	5.57	0.950
- CUF+MUF	16	4.00	43.00	14.69	9.67	

*Student's "t" test.

** Only alive patients were included In this Analysis

Table 9. Comparative results regarding studies variables of the CUF and CUF+MUF groups.

9.11.5 Blood transfusion

The CUF group presented significantly higher values of hematocrit than the CUF+MUF groups at the different times during the perioperative periods (p= 0.032). A significant decrease was observed after the surgery (p= 0.037), mainly in the CUF+MUF group.

The analysis of platelet counts at the different times during the perioperative period. There were no significant differences between groups (p= 0.673). A significant decrease was observed in platelet counts after the surgery (p< 0.001).

Requirements for red blood cell and coagulation factors (platelet, fresh frozen plasma and cryoprecipitate) were similar in both groups.

Only 15.8% of the CUF group (3 of 21) did not require red blood cell transfusion, whereas 16.7% patients (3 of 20) in the CUF+MUF group were free of red blood cell transfusion.

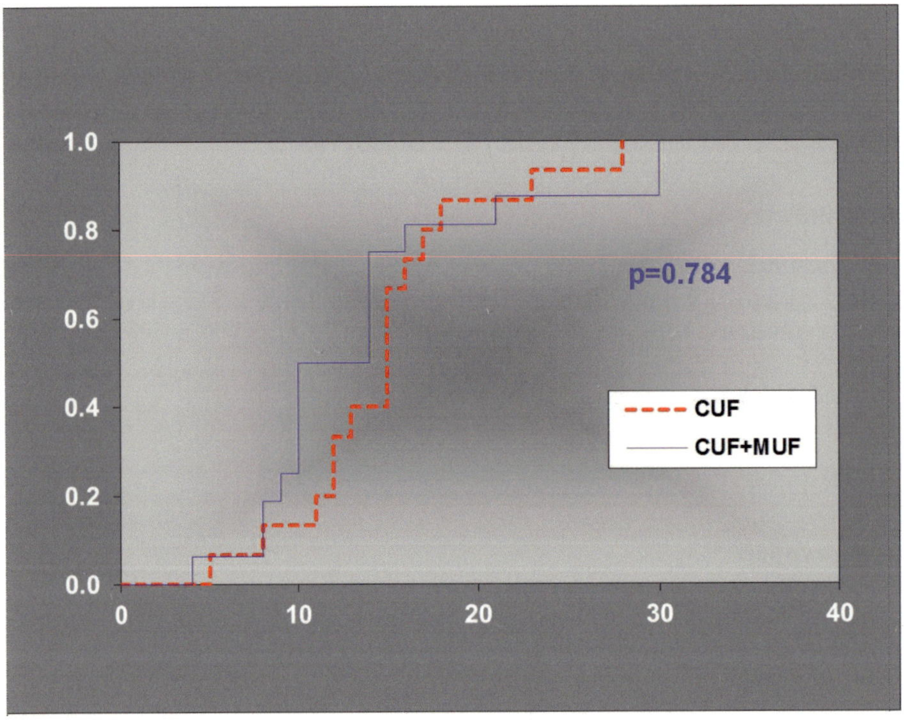

Fig. 39. Effective Hospital Stay or calculated probability

9.12 Discussion

Surgical correction of complex congenital heart disease in children requires long times of CPB and moderate or deep hypothermia inducing water retention, hypervolemia and distribution of liquid in the extravascular compartment. On the other hand, the generalized inflammatory reaction due to protein mediator release contributes to increase in capillary permeability and tissular edema, impairing organs such as the heart, lung and brain.

Accumulation of body water occurs due to intravenous administration of solutions and the contact of the prime with the patient's blood. On the other hand, CPB induces a generalized inflammatory reaction with unbalance of the patient's internal environment, increasing body water retention. These effects have a greater impact in low weight children who require correction of complex heart defects.

Based on studies of ultrafiltration in adult's, in 1990 we started to use CUF in children during the warming stage of CPB with satisfactory results. The purpose of CUF was: removal of excess water from the priming of the CPB and hemoconcentration of erythrocytes and coagulation factors increasing hematocrit, decreasing bleeding in the postoperative period, thus reducing the need for transfusions of the patient.

Introduction of MUF, after CPB, has avoided excessive accumulation of body water and improving the patient's clinical conditions, allowed decrease in bleeding and reduction of blood replacement and ultrafiltration of protein mediators responsible for the inflammatory response, aiming at PH control, reduction in time of use of vasoactive drugs, of pulmonary ventilation and of hospitalization.

In this study, 20 patients below the age of 36 months, who on surgical correction were submitted to the association of ultrafiltration methods (CUF + MUF) with follow-up until discharge from hospital, were compared to a similarly operated group previously and submitted to CUF. Therefore this is a comparative, prospective and consecutive, nonrandomized study like others in the literature.

Randomization of patients undoubtedly represents an ideal situation because it allows an accurate evaluation of the results, as shown by other studies on this subject. However, other comparative studies present restrictions to the evaluation of the benefits of MUF use.

Studies, equal to the present, one comparing CUF + MUF with CUF in two similar groups of pediatric patients, have been carried out by other authors.

The design of our research offered equal ultrafiltration opportunity to both groups, whose age, weight surgical complexity profile characterized them as being at high risk. All patients received CUF, thus allowing ultrafiltration of inflammatory reaction mediators primarily released during the warming stage of CPB.

Initially the MUF technique we used was similar to that presented by Elliott. However, due to the need to keep the ultrafiltered blood returning to the right atrium warm, as in Groom's study, we introduced changes in the outlet of the hemoconcentrator, substituting it for the cardioplegia line and thus allowing passage of ultrafiltered blood through the heat exchange.

Use of MUF after CPB, allows improvement in the systolic function of the left ventricle (LV) in children submitted to correction of congenital defects. There is an increase in the final diastolic diameter and fall in final diastolic pressure of the LV after MUF due to improvement in ventricular compliance, as a result of the reduction of myocardial edema. The hemodynamic improvement could be related to this reduction and the neutralization of the inflammatory response because of ultrafiltration of protein mediators.

Interest in the use of the MUF technique, benefits to the patients and possible intercurrences are increasing and justifying further studies by multiple centers. Despite the acquired experience, technical complications, which should not be discarded, have been detected.

The need for the evaluation of results in children at high surgical risk has led us to define our research in children aged 0 to 36 months, as has been done by other studies.

Patients submitted to prolonged CPB, hemodilution and hypothermia might develop a substantial myocardial edema, making chest closing difficult if they are not adequately ultrafiltered . In our study all patients were led to the PICU with a closed chest.

Association of CUF + MUF was efficient, significantly increasing the total volume of ultrafiltration (227 + 71.4 ml) when compared with CUF alone (143.3 + 54.3 ml) ($p < 0.001$).

In spite of the significant hemodynamic improvement through the use of CUF + MUF in our study, as well as in others, no significant differences were found regarding number and time of use of inotropic drugs when compared with the control group.

Reduction in pulmonary ventilation time and time of stay in the PICU is evident with use of MUF, although in our study no significant difference has been found.

There was a proportional fall in the Ht of both groups during the postoperative period and, according to the established criteria to maintain the Ht at 35% in acyanotic children and at 40% in cyanotic children, 84.2% of the patients of the CUF group and 83.3% of the patients of the CUF + MUF group, received blood, but there was no statistically significant difference between the groups.

Classification of the patients according to the degree of surgical complexity allowed the analysis of impact of hospital mortality in relation to the different variables. Despite the fact that there was no statistically significant difference regarding degree of complexity of the CUF and CUF + MUF groups, there were 50% of the CUF + MUF patients in category 3 and 4 (more severe) while in the CUF group, 76.2% of the cases belonged to category 2 (less severe).

Regarding duration of hospital stay, there was no significant difference between the groups, analyzed at 5 different times, 90% of the patients of both groups being discharged from hospital on the 20th day of postoperative period. Duration of hospital stay of patients submitted to surgical correction of complex congenital heart disease is usually prolonged, significantly increasing hospital costs. A detailed analysis of treatment time in this group of patients submitted to ultrafiltration will allow the assessment of reduction in hospital costs.

Association of congenital cardiopathies with severe PH (ratio pulmonary pressure/systemic pressure > 60%) represents a group at higher surgical risk requiring effective treatment for PH control. The PH associated with high pulmonary vascular resistance is responsible for the long periods of mechanical ventilation, stay in PICU and high morbidity and mortality, after correction of cardiac defects using CPB.

Endothelin-1 produced by the cells of the vascular endothelium is a vasoactive agent, which participates, in the pathophysiological mechanism of PH. Studies have shown that the use of total hemodilution during CPB, associated with MUF, in children submitted to correction of cardiac malformations and PH, allow the elimination of excess body water and ultrafiltration of endothelin-1.

In our study, in the CUF + MUF group, consisting of 20 patients, 14 (70%) presented PH and in the CUF group, consisting of 21 patients, 15 (71.4%) had PH.

Despite the tendency to improvement of the results in the CUF + MUF group, there were 4/20 deaths (20%) as compared to the CUF group with 6/21 (28.5%) deaths.

9.13 Conclusion

We obtained those of Groom's group, a circuit design using cardioplegia line, have shown to be safe and equally efficient, with a significant filtered volume in the CUF + MUF group. Probably the efficacy of the CUF used in all patients and the lack of adjustment of the preoperative care protocol did not allow establishing more consistent results in the studied groups. These results should be examined with caution because they refer to a nonrandomized group with a small number of patients with high-risk congenital heart disease.

Currently we routinely use CUF + MUF in all pediatric patients undergoing heart surgery in our Institution. With ultrafiltration methods, in the future, pediatric patients should equally benefit from controlling their water balance, neutralizing the inflammatory response and reducing transfusion volumes.

10. Philantropic activities

10.1 Pediatric cardiac surgery as a philanthropic activity in the country and foreign humanitarian mission

In Brazil each year are born 30,000 new patients with congenital heart disease, 50% of which need surgical correction in the first year of life. The statistics show data that are published yearly by Associação Nacional de Saúde (ANS) of Brazil, that only 6,000 - 7,000 patients undergo cardiac corrective or palliative surgery each year. These figures do not include the patients holding health insurance operated in hospitals associated to the medical insurance network; although it is a small contingent.

This reality shows that due to the fast technological development process in Medicine, the particularity of each patient was completely disregarded and his illness became an object of scientific study. The medical procedures, therefore, became inhuman.

In the same process, some changes have occurred in medicine graduation and in the work conditions, increasingly specialized, restricting the availability of physicians either for contact with the patient or for the search of a more specialized formation.

The actual conditions of medicine practice have not contributed to the betterment in the relationship between physicians and patients, and for a humanized assistance with good quality (this applies for both professionals in the area and health care institutions).

Nowadays, several actions have been proposed aiming the implementation of humanizing programs in health institutions, especially in pediatric assistance in hospitals; several projects and actions develop activities associated with plastic arts, music, theater, leisure and entertainment.

There are some Institutions that claim to be already humanized, but in some cases, this humanization applies only to architectural improvements and medical assistance aiming fiscal benefits. Undoubtedly, these are relevant measures in an Institution; however, they can be merely superficial factors unless they are inserted in a vast process of Humanizing Institutional Relationships.

When pondering about the Assistance Duties it can also lead us to Ethics. The ethic matters appear when one worries about the consequences of his actions upon others.

The work of a professional, whatever his activity might be, depends on both technical quality and interaction quality. In medicine, quality is a must that makes each specialty aim to develop its technical capacity that is part of what it is called relative abilities and knowledge of the technical area. In order to internationally capacitate the physician, of any specialty, it becomes necessary the instrumentalization to recognize and deal with the emotional aspects of assistance, that is, developing attitude.

Humanization is a vast, slow and complex process to which many definitely offer some resistance, because it involves changes of behavior that often promote insecurity. The already established standards seem rather safer, in addition, the new ones are not currently legal and do not have general characteristics, because each professional, each institution has its own particular humanization process. In this process many instances must be involved: Professionals of all areas, Institution Directory Board, politicians and public attorneys, a Professional Counsel and Philanthropic Entities.

There are a few public and private hospitals, in the country, that offer conditions for a complete assistance to children, in order to perform high complexity procedures.

Therefore, the pediatric assistance fails to meet the special needs of patients due to the long lines in ERs, shortage of vacancies in nurseries, ICU, etc; on the other hand, children that need to be transferred to more complex hospitals end up missing the opportunity due to the unavailability of rooms, which in its turn leads to a natural selection of patients.

These examples allow us to see the complexity in health management in the pediatric department.

In 1994, our pediatric cardiac surgery group, working at the Hospital Israelita Albert Einstein (HIAE), was invited by the Assistance Pediatric Directory to perform, in a philanthropic way, surgical corrections in children presenting cardiac defects, being followed up at the institution.

A similar experience with fewer patients was performed through the project Multi Assistance Association (AMA) at the Hospital Samaritano (HS).

Due to the success of this experience and sympathetic to the technical difficulties of colleagues in the same specialty belonging to the "Instituto para la Salud del Niño (ISN)" of Lima, Peru and also the social and economical difficulties of the country (Peru), we decided to accept this new challenge by initiating Humanitarian Missions to the ISN where professionals from the institution would perform operations for the surgical correction of complex cardiac defects. In this mission some theoretical and practical courses have been scheduled aiming a multidisciplinary training.

The recent meeting of pediatric cardiac surgeons in the World Summit on Pediatric and Congenital Heart Surgery held in Montreal (Canada) in June 2008, made possible some Cardiac Surgery Groups and Multidisciplinary Groups of wealthy countries to plan and perform humanitarian missions in third world countries.

More and more often a Health Institution is becoming an integrated system, consisting of a number of organizations, in search of a more harmonious joint action: Community / Physician / Hospital; more adequate to the current reality and without frontiers.

In the period between July 1994 and December 2008, 204 patients presenting congenital heart diseases were submitted to corrective or palliative surgery of cardiac defects.

Among these, 153 (75.0%) patients were operated in the philanthropic category, at the HIAE 20 p. (9,9%) at the HS, and the remaining 51 (25.0%) under humanitarian mission at the ISN (Table 10)

Data	Participating Institutions	Country	N °patients	(%)
1994 - 1999	HIAE	Brasil	133	(65.1)
2000 - 2003	H S	Brasil	20	(09.9)
2004 - 2008	ISN	Peru	51	(25.0)
Total			204	(100)

Table 10. Participating Institutions and patients enrolled in the Philanthropic and Humanitarian Project.

The characteristics of the patients were the following: Age: 1 day-old - 18 years-old (M=2.5); Gender: Female 52.6% of the cases; Operation: first operation in 163 (80%) cases and reoperation in 41(20%) cases.

All the patients were evaluated by the pediatric cardiologist that requested the complementary examinations and performed all the pre-operative procedures, post-operative follow-up and intensive care of the patients.

In the 3 institutions that participated in the study, the intensive care structure was held in Pediatric ICU and the intensive physicians were pediatricians. All the patients with surgical recommendation were presented in the specialty meeting.

The patients were rated according severity of their cardiac defects and surgical risk, according to international rules: Risk Adjustment Congenital Heart Surgery (RACHS) (Table 11)

Risk I (Mortality accepted: 0 - 3%)
ASD: Atrial Septal Defect; PDA: Patent Ductus Arteriosus (> 30d); CO-Ao: Coarctation of Aorta (> 30d); PAPVC: Partial Anomalous Pulmonary Venous Connection.
Risk II (Mortality accepted: 3 - 9%)
VSD: Ventricular Septal Defect; Sub Ao S: Sub aortic Stenosis; Tetralogy of Fallot; BDG: Bidirectional Glenn; AVC: Atrio-Ventricular Channel; Aortic Valvar Stenosis.
Risk III (Mortality accepted: 9 - 20%)
Ross Op.; Mitral Valve Op.; Co-Ao + VSD; Anomalous Coronary Artery Origin; Fontan Op.; PCA (<30d).
Risk IV (Mortality accepted: 20 - 25%)
Kono Op; Rastelli Op; Jatene Op; Unifocalization Pulmonary Artery Op.; TAPVD: Total Anomalous Pulmonary Veins Drain.
Risk V (Mortality accepted: 25 - 35%)
Ebstein Anomaly (<30d); Truncus Arteriosus;Aortic Arch Interruption.

Table 11. Risk Adjustment Congenital Heart Surgery (RACHS)

10.2 Statistical analysis

The relationships between hospital mortality and these risk factors were examined with Q2 (Siegel-2006). A p value of less than 0.05 or 5% was considered to be significant.

In the total analysis of result, there were 28 (13.7%) deaths in the immediate post-operative period. (Fig. 40) When we analyzed the results of each institution separately, it was observed: HIAE: 20 (15.0%) deaths; HS: 1 (5.0%) deaths and ISN: 7 (13.7%) deaths.(Table 12). (Fig. 41,42,43,44)

Classification of the Patients
"Risk Ajustment Congenital Heart Surgery"
(RACHS)

Risk 1
ASD, PDA (>30d), Ao-C (>30d), PAPVC

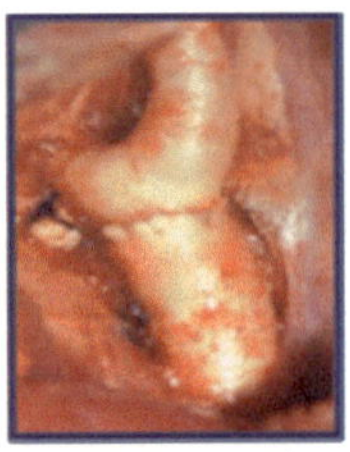

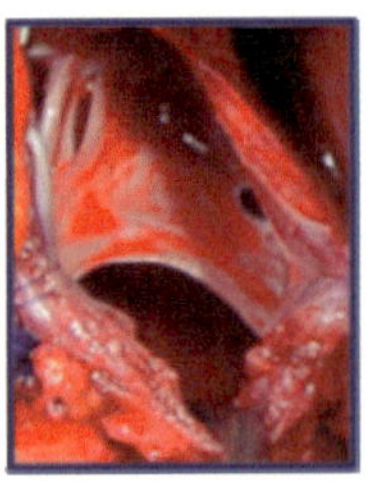

INSTITUTION	N° Pat.	N° Death	Mort. (%)
HIAE:	37	1	2,7
H. S. :	5	0	0
ISN :	1	0	0
	43	1	2,3

Fig. 40. Surgical results in patients operated in Risk Group 1, at 3 referred Institutions . PAPVC: Partial Anomalous Pulmonary Vein Connection; PDA: *Patent Ductus Arteriosus*; Ao C: Aortic Coarctation; ASD: Atrial Septal Defect.

There aren't statistic significance in this group.(p=0.147)

Institution	Patients	(%)	Deaths	Mortality (%)	p
HIAE	133	(65.2)	20	(15.0)	ns
HS	20	(09.8)	01	(5.0)	ns
ISN	51	(25.0)	07	(13.7)	ns
Total	204	(100)	28	(13.7)	0.147

Table 12. Immediate post-operative results.

When we analyzed the results according to the severity of cardiac malformation and the complexity of the surgical correction, we observed that the Risk Group I, consisting of 43 patients, there was only 1 death (Mortality 2.3%) at the Institution HIAE. (Table 13). There aren't statistic significance in this group.(p=0.748).

Institution	Patients	Deaths	Mortality	p
	N° (%)	N°	(%)	
HIAE	37 (27.8)	1	(2.7)	ns
HS	05 (25.0)	0	(0.0)	ns
ISN	01 (01.9)	0	(0.0)	ns
Total	43 (21.0)	1	(2.3)	0.748

Table 13. Immediate Post-operative Results - Risk I

The Risk Group II consisted of 68 patients and there were 5 deaths (Mortality 7.3%). All this 5 deaths occurred in the HIAE Institution (Table 14) (Fig 41). There was no statistical significance in this group. (p=0.202)

Institution	Patients	Deaths	Mortality	p
	N° (%)	N°	(%)	
HIAE	44 (33.0)	5	(11.3)	ns
HS	10 (50.0)	0	(0.0)	ns
ISN	14 (27.5)	0	(0.0)	ns
Total	68 (33.3)	5	(7.3)	0.202

Table 14. Immediate Post-operative Results - Risk II

The Risk Group III was the most numerous, consisting of 74 patients, there were15 deaths (Mortality20.2%). The deaths occurred at the HIAE: 12 cases; HS: 1 case and at the ISN: 2 cases (Table 16) Figure 42. There was no statistical significance in this group. (p= 0.06)

nstitution	Patients	Deaths	Mortality	p
	N° (%)	N°	(%)	
HIAE	43 (32.3)	12	(27.9)	ns
HS	05 (25.0)	01	(20.0)	ns
ISN	26 (19.5)	02	(7.6)	ns
Total	74 (36.2)	15	(20.2)	0.060

Table 15. Immediate Post-operative Results - Risk III

Risk 2

Ao V. Surg, Sub Ao VSD clos., T. Fallot, Glenn op., A-V C D

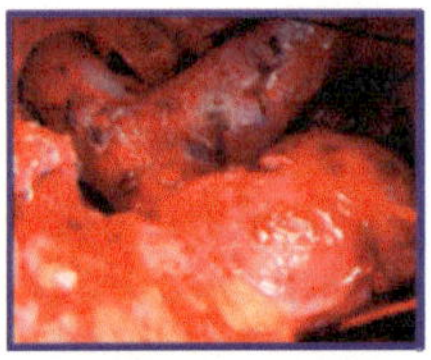

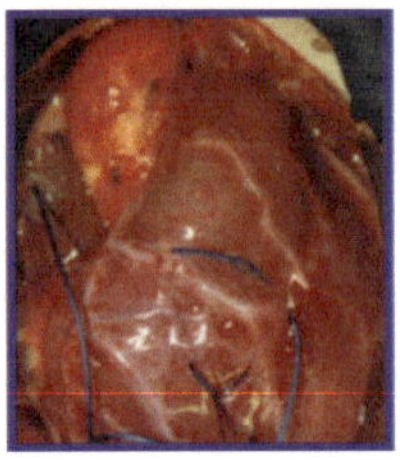

INSTITUTION	N° Pat.	N° Death	Mort. (%)
HIAE :	44	5	11,3
H. S.:	10	0	0
ISN:	14	0	0
	68	5	7,3

Fig. 41. Surgical result in patients operated in Risk Group 2, at 3 referred Institution. Ao V Surg.: Aortic Valve Surgery; Sub Ao VSD Clos.: Sub-aortic Ventricular Septal Defect Closure; T: Tetralogy; Op: Operation; Atrio Ventricular Canal Defect

Risk 3

Ao v. Subst., Ross Op., Mitral v. subst., Ao-C + VSD op., Cor. Art. An.; Fontan Op.

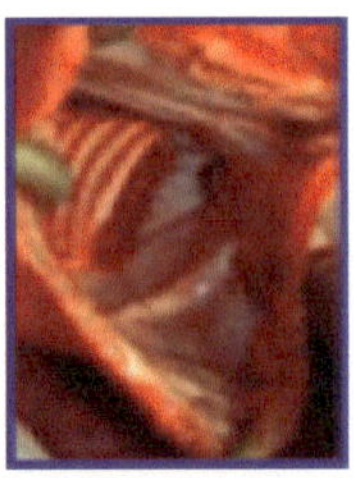

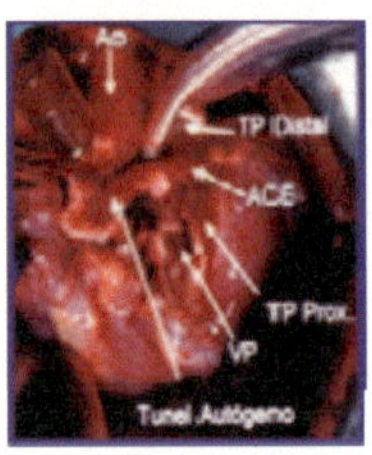

INSTITUTION	N° Pat.	N° Death	Mort. (%)
HIAE :	43	12	27,9
H. S.:	5	1	20,0
ISN :	26	2	7,6
	74	15	20,2

Fig. 42. Surgical Result in patients operated in Risk Group 3, at 3 referred Institutions. Aortic Valve Substitution; Op.: operation; v. : valve; Ao-C +VSD Op.: Aortic Coarctation + Ventricular Septal Defect operation; Cor. Art. An.: Coronary artery Anomaly.

The Risk Group IV consisted of 13 patients; there were 3 deaths (Mortality 23.0%). The deaths occurred at the HIAE: 1case and at the ISN: 2 cases (Table 16) Figure 43. There was no statistical significance in this group. (p= 0.600).

Institution	Patients	Deaths	Mortality	p
	N° (%)	N°	(%)	
HIAE	7 (3.4)	1	(14.2)	ns
HS	0 (0.0)	0	(0.0)	ns
ISN	6 (2.9)	2	(33.3)	ns
Total	13 (6.3)	3	(23.0)	0.600

Table 16. Immediate Post-operative Results - Risk IV

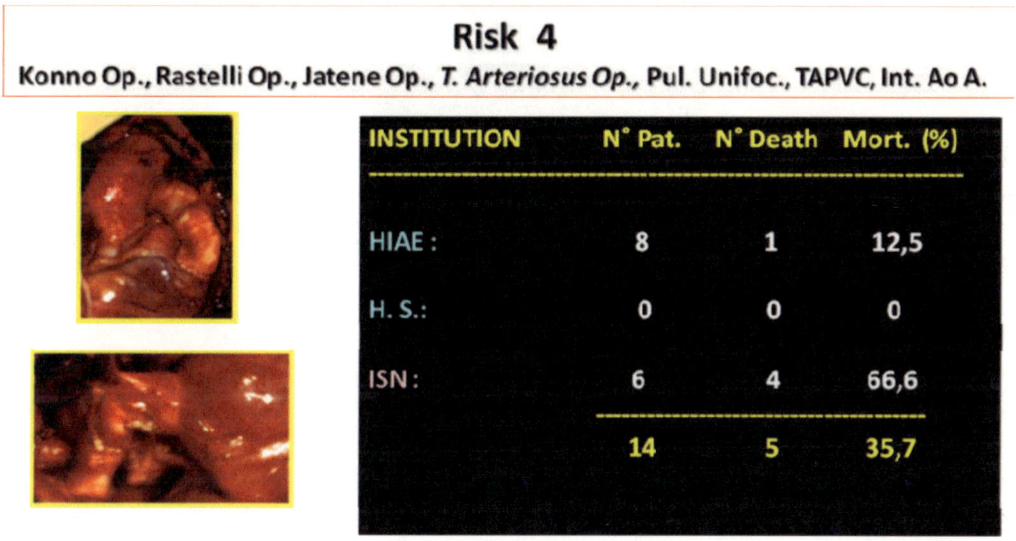

Fig. 43. Surgical outcome of patients operated in Risk Group 4, the three participating institutions. Op: operation; T: truncus; Pul. Unifocal.: pulmonary unifocalization; TAPVC: total anomalous pulmonary venous connection ; Int. A. Ao: Interrupted aortic arch

The Risk Group V consisted of 6 patients, there were 3 deaths (Mortality 50.0%).These deaths occurred: HIAE: 1 case and at the ISN: 2 cases (Table 17) (Fig.44). There was no statistical significance in this group. (p= 0,187).

Institution	Patients	Deaths	Mortality	p
	N° (%)	N°	(%)	
HIAE	2 (0.9)	1	(50.0)	ns
HS	0 (0.0)	0	(0.0)	---
ISN	4 (1.9)	2	(50.0)	ns
Total	6 (2.9)	3	(50.0)	0.187

Table 17. Immediate Post-operative Results - Risk V

Risk 5

Ebstein A. (< 30 d), *T. Arteriosus* + A. Ao Interr.

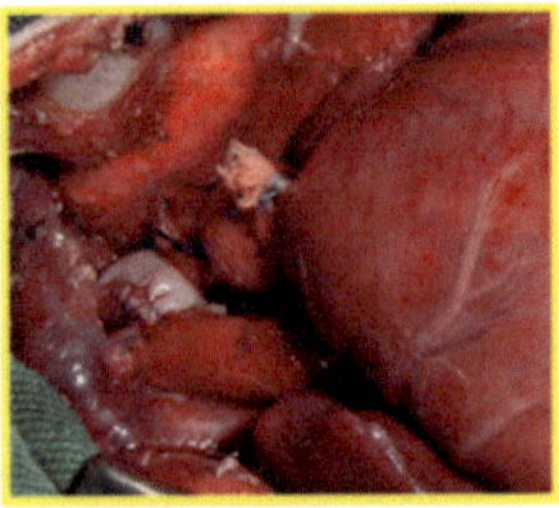

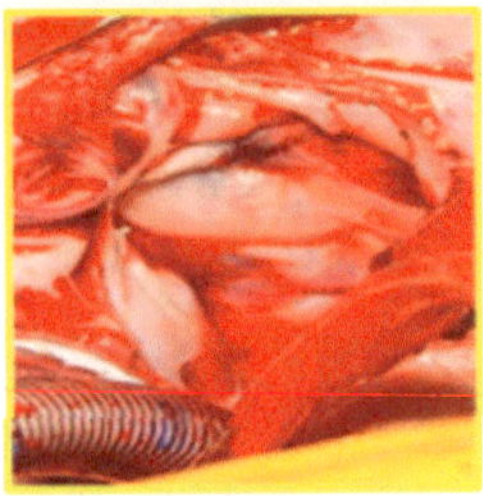

INSTITUTION	N° Pat.	N° Death	Mort. (%)
HIAE :	1	1	100
H. S.:	0	0	0
ISN :	4	0	0
	5	1	20

Fig. 44. Surgical outcome of patients operated in Risk Group 5, the three participating institutions: A: Anomaly, T.: truncus; Ao A Inter: : aortic arch interruption

10.3 Discussion

Even though the incidence of congenital heart disease not being significantly high, the restrict number of specialized centers, as well as the number of professionals and the high costs of procedures, make the surgical referrals increase proportionally with the population growth, though the amount of surgeries does not increase in the same proportion and many patients miss the opportunity to have surgical correction or simply end up dying.

Although the number of pediatric cardiac surgeries performed in public Institutions is noticeably increasing, unfortunately it is still not sufficient in order to put an end to the prolonged lines awaiting an opportunity for treatment.

In our field, many private hospitals well structured, sympathizing with this situation and motivated by the exemption of income tax, perform an important Welfare Work in the pediatric area. Undoubtedly, multiplying these services throughout the country is necessary, and by doing so, it would definitely have an immediate impact on the quality of assistance, the training of professionals and the surgical results.

Our group initiated its Philanthropic Activities in 1994 at the HIAE, supported by the Directory in effect, aiming the implementation of a Pediatric Cardiac Surgery Program, followed by the philanthropic assistance of children with cardiac malformation referred by the Pediatric Assistance Service originating from the poorest areas of the city and state of São Paulo. The immediate results of this philanthropic program for the treatment of more complex cardiac malformations allowed the access of patients from other states in the country.

Alongside with the theoretical and practical training of professionals in the area enabled the establishment of work regulations and protocols of conduct in the specialty.

Pediatric Cardiac Surgery Services are frequently in deficit or poorly developed in many countries around the world and currently there are several active foundations with services of cardiovascular support, specialized in the pediatric area, in business for 15 years, aiming to give humanitarian assistance, in the 4 continents, to a very restricted number of excluded patients.

The experience acquired with philanthropic assistance activities enabled the attainment of some experience which constituted an essential tool in order to embrace programs of humanitarian assistance. Between June, 2004 and December, 2007; 7 missions to Lima-Peru were realized, supported by the Ministério de La Salud of that country and we operated an average of 8 patients per mission.

Despite the well structured institutions assisting patients of the specialty, the technical resources for diagnosis and therapy, as well as the human resources ones were somewhat different for the philanthropic patients operated in the country, taking advantage of a more advanced technology, when compared to the one present in the humanitarian missions. As expected, the majority of the operated patients belong to the philanthropic group (75%) (HIAE= 65.1% and HS= 9.9 %), when compared to the humanitarian mission group (25%) (ISN= 25.0%).

When the operated patients were classified considering the surgical risk, according RACHS, we observed that the majority is in the Risk Group II and III (69.6%) and that none of the patients in Risk Group VII was operated.

10.4 Conclusions

Patients operated belonged to the 5 categories of Rachs risk, being that the Risk Group III was the most numerous (36.2%) - The results obtained at the HIAE and at the ISN, are justified by the number of patients, complexity of cardiac defects operated and structural difficulties in the implementation stage of the Pediatric Cardiac Surgery Service. The mortality in the Risk Group V, was higher than estimated by the Rachs study. On the other hand, in this study, neither did we consider the social-economical conditions of the patient nor the clinical ones, such as: malnutrition, pulmonary infection, type of clinical treatment that largely interfere in the final results in our experience.

11. References

Ad N, Snir E, Katk J, Birk E, Vidne BA. Use of the modified technique of ultrafiltration in pediatric open-heart Surgery: a prospective study Isr J Med Sci 1996;32;1326-31.

Agnetti A, Carano N, Cavalli C, Tchana B, Bini M, Squarcia U, Frigiola A. Long-term outcome after Senning operation for transposition of the great arteries. *Clin Cardiol. 2004; 27: 611–614.*

Albert JD, Bishop DA, Fullerton DA, Campbell DN, Clarck DR. Conduit reconstruction of the right ventricle outflow tract. Lessons learned in a twenty-year experience. J Thorac Cardiovasc Surg 1993;106:228-35.

Andreason S, Gothberg S, Berggren H, Bengstsoon A, Erikson E, Risburg B. Hemofiltration modifies complement activation after extracorporeal circulation in infants. Ann Thorac Surg 1993;56:1515-7.

Ballard G, Tibby S, Miller O, Krasemann T, Rosenthal E, Anderson D, Austin C, Qureshi S, Simpson J. Growth of left heart structures following the hybrid procedure for borderline hypoplastic left heart. Eur J Echocardiogr, 2010; 11(10): 870 - 874.

Bando K, Danielson GK, Schaff HV, Mair DD, Julsreed PR, Puga FJ. Outcome pulmonary and aortic homograft for right ventricular outflow tract reconstruction. J Thorac Cardiovasc Surg 1995;109:509-17.

Bando K, Turrentine MW, Vijay P, Sharp TG, Sekine Y, Lalone BJ, et al. Effect of modified ultrafiltration in high risk patients undergoing operation for congenital heart disease. Ann Thorac Surg 1998;66(3): 821-8.

Barbero-Marcial ML, Riso A, Verginelli G et al. Técnica para correção do truncus arteriosus I, II sem conduto extracardíaco.

Bender HW Jr, Stewart JR, Merrill WH, Hammon JW Jr, Graham TP Jr. Ten years' experience with the Senning operation for transposition of the great arteries: physiological results and late follow-up. *Ann Thorac Surg. 1989; 47: 218–223.*

Birnie D, Tometzki A, Curzio J, Houston A, Hood S, Swan L, Doig W, Wilson N, Jamieson M, Pollock J, Hillis WS. Outcomes of transposition of the great arteries in the era of atrial inflow correction. *Heart. 1998; 80: 170–173.*

Blalock A, Taussig H- Surgical treatment of malformations of the heart in which there is stenosis or pulmonary atresia. *JAMA, 1945; 128: 189-202*

Bockeria L, Alekyan B, Berishvili D, Pursanov M, Krupianko SM, Zarginava G, Grigoryanz A. A modified hybrid stage I procedure for treatment of hypoplastic left heart syndrome: an original surgical approach. Interactive CardioVascular and Thoracic Surgery, 2010; 11(2): 142 - 145.

Boudjemline Y, Bonnet D, Agnoletti G, Vouhe P. Aneurysm of the right ventricular outflow following bovine valved venous conduit insertion. Eur J Cardiovasc Surg 2003;23:122-124.

Bove T, Demanet H, Wauthy P, et al. Early results of valved bovine jugular vein conduit versus bicuspid homograft for right ventricular outflow tract reconstruction. Ann Thorac Surg 2002; 74:536-541.

Bricker JT. Sudden death and tetralogy of Fallot: risks, markers and causes. Circulation 1995;92:158-159 .

Brown JW, Ruzmetov M, Rodefeld MD, Vijay P, Darragh RK. Valved bovine jugular vein conduit for right ventricular outflow tract reconstruction in children: An attractive alternative to pulmonary homograft. Ann Thorac Surg 2006;82:909-916.

Bull C, Mccartney FJ, and Horvath P et al. Evolution of long-term results of homograft and heterograft valves in extracardiac conduits . J Thorac Cardiocasc Surg 1987;94:12-9

Caliani J; Machado A; Marinho J; Simões L; Barbosa O. Correção da origem anômala de artéria coronária esquerda com insuficiência mitral e hemólise mecânica. Rev Bras Cir Cardiovasc 2004; 19 (4): 405-408.

Canêo L, Lourenço D, Silva R, Franchi S, Afiune J, Afiune C, Mocelin A, Barbero-Marcial M, Jatene F. Senning operation with autologous tissue for atrial septum augmentation or pulmonary venous pathway enlargement. Bras J Cardiovasc Surg 1999; 14 (4):298-302.

Carvalho JS, Shinebourne EA, Busst C, Rigby ML, Redington AN. Exercise capacity after complete repair of tetralogy of Fallot: deleterious effects of residual pulmonary regurgitation. Br Heart J 1992;67:470-473

Carvalho MV, Maluf MA, Catani R, La Rotta CA, Gomes WJ, Salomon R, Silva C, Carvalho AC, Branco JN, Buffolo E. Cytokines and pediatric open heart surgery with cardiopulmonary bypass. Cardiol Young 2001; 11: 36-43

Chen Q, Parry. The current role of hybrid procedures in the stage 1 palliation of patients with hypoplastic left heart syndrome. Eur. J. Cardiothorac. Surg., 2009; 36(1): 77 - 83.

Cochrane AD, Karl TR, Mee RB. Staged conversion to arterial switch for late failure of the systemic right ventricle. *Ann Thorac Surg. 1993; 56: 854–861.*

Croti U; Braile D; Resende C; Beani L. Origem anômala de artéria coronária da artéria pulmonar: operação de Takeuchi. Rev Bras Cir Cardiovasc 2006; 21 (4): 305-306.

Davies MJ, Nguyen K, Gaynor JW, Elliott MJ. Modified ultrafiltration improves left ventricular systolic function in infants after cardiopulmonary bypass. J Thorac Cardiovasc Surg 1988; 115: 361-70

Davlouros PA, Kilner PJ, Hornung TS, Li W, Francis JM, Moon JCC, Smith GC, Tat T, Pennell DJ, Gatzoulis MA. Right ventricular function in adults with repaired tetralogy of Fallot assessed with cardiovascular magnetic resonance imaging: detrimental role of right ventricular outflow aneurisms or akinesia and adverse right-to-left ventricular interaction. J Am Coll Cardiol 2002;40(11):2044-52.

De Leval MR, Mc Kay R, Jones M, Stark J, Macartney FJ - Modified Blalock-Taussig shunt J thorac Cardiovasc Surg, 1981;81:112-9

De Leval MR.. Evolution of the Fontan-Kreutzer procedure. Semin Thorac Cardiovasc Surg Pediatr 2010;13(1):91-

De Leval, MR, Kilner P, Gewillig M, Bull C, Total cavopulmonary connection: a logical alternative to atriopulmonary connection for complex Fontan operation: Experimental studies and early clinical. J Thorac Cardiovasc Surg. 1988; 96(5):682-95.

Eguchi S & Asano K. Homograft of pulmonary artery or ascending aorta with valve as a right ventricular outflow. J Thorac Cardiovasc Surg 1968;56:413-20

Eguchi S, Irisawa T, Asano K. Use of valve-retaining homograft and heterograft patch for reconstruction of right ventricular outflow tract. Ann Thorac Surg 1972;14:615-25

Elliott MJ. Ultrafiltration and modified ultrafitration in pediatric open heart operations, Ann Thorac Surgery 1993; 56: 1518-22.

Finn A, Naik S, Klein N, Levinsky RJ, Strobel S, Elliott MJ. Interleukin release and neutrophil degranulation after pediatric cardiopulmonary bypass Thorac Cardiovasc Surg 1993; 105:234-41.

Fontan F, Baudet E. Surgical repair of tricuspid atresia. Thorax 1971;26:240-8.

Friesen RH, Campbell DN, Clarke DR, Tornabene MA. Modified ultrafiltration attempted dilutional coagulopathy in pediatric open heart operations. Ann Thoracic Surg 1997;64:1787-9.

Gelatt M, Hamilton RM, McCrindle BW, Connelly M, Davis A, Harris L, Gow RM, Williams WG, Trusler GA, Freedom RM. Arrhythmia and mortality after the Mustard procedure: a 30-year single-center experience. *J Am Coll Cardiol. 1997; 29: 194–201.*

Gewilling M, Wyse RK, de Leval MR, Deanfield JE. Early and late arrhythmias after the Fontan operation: predisposing factors and clinical consequences. Br Heart J 1992; 67(1):72-9

Graham TP, Cordell D, Atward GF, Boucek RJ, Boerth RC, Bender HW, Nelson JA, Vaughn WR. Right ventricle volume characteristics before and after palliative and reparative operation in tetralogy of Fallot. Circulation 1976,54:417-423

Groom RC, Akl B, Albus RA, Hill A, Munoz R, Lefrak EA. Alternative method of ultrafiltration after cardiopulmonary bypass. Ann Thorac Surg; 58:573-576.

Gurbuz AT, Novick WM, Pierce CA, Watson DC. Impact of ultrafiltration or blood use for atrial septal defect closure in infants and children . Ann Thorac Surg 1998, 65: 1105-9.

Harrison DA, Harris L, Isu SC, Mc Laughin CJ, Connelly MS, Wehog D, Downar E, Mc Laughin PR, Williams WG. Sustained ventricular tachycardia in adult patients late after repair of tetralogy of Fallot. Am J Coll Cardiol 1997;30:1368-1373

Hazekamp MG, Kurvers MM, Schoof PH, et al. Pulmonary Valve insertion late after repair of Fallot's tetralogy. Eur J Cardiothorac Surg 2001;19:667-70

Helbing WA, Hansen B, Ottenkamp J, Rohmer J, Chin JG, Brom AG, Quaegebeur JM. Long-term results of atrial correction for transposition of the great arteries: comparison of Mustard and Senning operations. *J Thorac Cardiovasc Surg. 1994; 108: 363–372.*

Howkins JA, Bailey WW, Dillon T, Schwartz DC. Midterm results with cryopreserved allograft valved conduits from the right ventricle to the pulmonary arteries. J Thorac Cardiovasc Surg 1992;104:910-6.

Ilbawi MW, Idriss FS, Deleon SY, Muster AJ, Gidding SS, Berry TE, Paul MH: Factors that exaggerate the deleterious effects of pulmonary insufficiency on the deleterious effects of pulmonary insufficiency on the right ventricle after tetralogy repair. Surgical implications. J Thorac Cardiovasc Surg 1987;93:36-44.

Jenkins KJ - Risk adjustment for congenital heart surgery: 1 metrhod Semin Thorac Cardiovasc Surg Pediatr Card Surg Annu 2004;7:180-4

Jenkins KJ. Newburger JW, Lock JE, Davis RB, Coffman A, Lezzoni LI. The hospital mortality of variation by care load. Pediatrics,1995,95:323-30.

Jonas RA, Castaneda AR. Modified Fontan procedure: atrial baffle and systemic venous to pulmonary artery anastomotic techniques. J Card Surg 1988;3: 91-6.

Journois D, Pouard P, Greeley WJ, Mauriat P, Vouhe P, Safran D. Hemofiltration during cardiopulmonary bypass in pediatric cardiac surgery . Effects on homeostasis, cytokines, and complement components Anesthesiology 1944; 81:1181-9.

Katsumata T, Westaby S. Anomalous left coronary artery from the pulmonary artery: A simple method for aortic implantation with autogenous arterial tissue. Ann Thorac Surg1999; 68:1090-1.

Keenan HT, Thiagarajan R, Stephens KE, Williams G, Romamoorthg C, Lupinetti FM. Pulmonary function after modified venousvenous ultrafiltration in infants: a prospective randomized trial J Thorac Cardiovasc Surg 2000; 119: 501-7.

Kirjavainen M, Happonen JM, Louhimo I. Late results of Senning operation. *J Thorac Cardiovasc Surg. 1999; 117: 488–495.*

Kirklin JW, Barrat-Boyes BG. Anatomy, dimensions and terminology: Cardiac Surgery, 2nd ed. New York: Churchill Livingstone, 1993.

Kitahori K, Murakami A, Takaoka T, Takamoto S, Ono MPrecise evaluation of bilateral pulmonary artery banding for initial palliation in high-risk hypoplastic left heart syndrome. J. Thorac. Cardiovasc. Surg., 2010; 140(5): 1084 - 1091.

Kiyota Y, Shiroyama T, Akamatsu T, Yokota Y, Ban T. In Vitro closing behavior of the St Jude Medical Herat valve in the pulmonary position. Valve incompetence originating in the prosthesis itself. J Thorac Cardiovasc Surg 1992; 104:779-85.

Kocica MJ, Corno AF, Carreras-Costa F, Ballester-Rodes M, Moghbel MC, Cueva CNC, Lackovic V, Kanjuh V I, Torrent-Guasp F. The helical ventricular myocardial band: global, three-dimensional, functional architecture of the ventricular myocardium. Eur J Cardiothorac Surg 2006; 295:S21-40.

Koutlas TC, Gaynor JW, Nicolson SC, Steven JM, Wernovsky G, Spray TL. Modified ultrafiltration reduces postoperative morbidity after cavopulmonary connection. Ann Thorac Surg 1997; 64 ;37-43.

Kreutzer GO, Schlichter AJ, Kreutzer C. The Fontan/Kreutzer procedure at 40: an operation for the correction of tricuspid atresia. Semin Thorac Cardiovasc Surg Pediatr Card Surg Annu. 2010;13(1):84-90.

Lange R, Hörer J, Kostolny M, Cleuziou J, Vogt M, Busch R, Holper K, Meisner H, Hess J, Schreiber C. Presence of a Ventricular Septal Defect and the Mustard Operation Are Risk Factors for Late Mortality After the *Atrial Switch Operation.* Circulation. *2006;114:1905-1913.*

Lecompte Y. Réparation á l'etage ventriculaire - The REV procedure: technique and clinical results. Cardiol Young 1991 ;1:63-70.

Levinsky L, Srinivasan V, Alvarez-Diaz F, Subramanian S - Reconstruction of the new atrial septum in the Senning operation. New technique. J Thorac Cardiovasc Surg, 1981;81(1):131-4.

Lillehei, CW; Cohen, M; Warden, HE; Warco, RL: Complete anatomical correction of the tetralogy of Fallot defects. Report of successful surgical case. Arch Surg 1956;73:526-31.

Lillehei, CW; Levy, M; Adams, P; Anderson, RL: Corrective surgery for tetralogy of Fallot. Long term follow-up by postoperative recatheterization in 69 cases and certain surgical considerations. J Thorac Cardiovasc Surg 1964; 48:556-76..

Lima LC. Resultados tardios da correção da transposição das grandes artérias com comunicação interatrial com a técnica de Senning. Tese Mestrado, *UNIFESP, 2001.*

Maluf MA, Mangia CM, Diogenes MS. Carvalho AC, Buffolo E. Anomalous coronary artery from pulmonary artery: Autogenous arterial tube for aortic implantation. J Cardiovasc Surg 2004;45:577-9.

Maluf M, Andrade JC, Catani R, Carvalho A C, Andrade JL, Silva C, Carvalho WB, Negrini N, Buffolo E. Avaliação dos Resultados Tardios da Operação de Derivação Cavo-Pulmonar Bidirecional no Tratamento Paliativo de Cardiopatias Congênitas com Câmara Ventricular Única Funcionante. Rev Bras Cir Cardiovasc 1994;9:95-103.

Maluf M, Mangia C, Bertuccez J, Silva C, Catani R, Carvalho W, Carvalho A, Buffolo E. Estudo comparativo de associação de ultrafiltração convencional e modificada na correção de cardiopatias congênitas de alto risco. Rev Bras Cir Cardiovasc 1999;14(3):221-36.

Maluf M; Franzoni M; Melgar E; Hernandez A; Perez R -. The Pediatric Cardiac Surgery as a Phylantropic Activities in the Country and Foreign Humanitarian Mission. Rev Bras Cir Cardiovasc, 2009; 24(3): VII - IX.

Maluf M; AndradeJ C; Catani R; Carvalho AC; Lima W; Andrade JL; Leão LEV; Buffolo E. Derivação Sistêmico-Pulmonar em Cardiopatias Congênitas com Hipofluxo Pulmonar: Análise Crítica da Técnica Cirúrgica e resultados Imediatos. Arq. Bras. Cardiol. 1991,56(4): 281-286.

Maluf MA, Braile DM, Silva C, Catani R, Carvalho AC, Buffolo E: Reconstruction of the pulmonary valve and right ventricular outflow tract with bicuspid prosthesis in tetralogy of Fallot. Ann Thorac Surg 2000;70:1911-1917

Maluf MA, Carvalho AC, Carvalho WB -Use of right ventricular remodeling surgery with a porcine pulmonary prosthesis for congenital heart disease. Heart Surg Forum, 2011;14:E40.

Maluf MA, Mangia C, Silva C, Carvalho WB, Carvalho AC, Buffolo E. Conventional and conventional plus modified ultrafiltration during cardiac surgery in high-risk congenital heart disease. J Cardiovasc Surg 2001; 42:465-73.

Maluf MA. Comparative study between conventional and association of the conventional and modified ultrafiltration, during cardiac surgery in high-risk congenital heart disease. Tese Livre Docencia. São Paulo: UNIFESP, 1998;10:120.

Maluf MA: Reconstruction of the pulmonary valve and right ventricular outflow tract with porcine pulmonary bicuspid and tricuspid prosthesis. Experimental study in sheeps. PhD tesis - São Paulo - UNIFESP 1991.

Maluf MA; Cal RG- *Tratamento Paliativo das Cardiopatias Congênitas* - Condutas em Cirurgia do Departamento de Cirurgia da *UNIFESP-EPM - 2001: cap.27, pg. 479-490. Ed. Atheneu*

Maluf MA; Carvalho AC; Carvalho WB.- Intracardiac Cavopulmonary Connection in patients with Univentricular Heart using Intra-atrial lateral Tunnel and Intra-atrial conduit technique. The Heart Surgery Forum 2010; 13(6): 362-369.

Maluf MA; Carvalho AC; Carvalho WB.- One and a half ventricular repair as na alternative for hypoplastic right ventricle. Rev Bras Cir Cardiovasc 2010; 25(4): 466-473

Maluf, MA *Tratamento Cirúrgico das Cardiopatias Congênitas* - Guia de Medicina Ambulatorial e Hospitalar da UNIFESP - EPM - 2ª Ed.2009, pg. 491-503. *Ed. Manole*

Maluf, MA; Andrade, JC; Catani, R; Carvalho, AC; Lima, W; Andrade, JL; Leão, LV; Buffolo, E - *Derivação sistêmico – pulmonar em cardiopatias congênitas com hipofluxo pulmonar: Análise crítica da técnica cirúrgica e resultados imediatos. Arq Bras Cardiol 56(4):281-286,1991.*

Marcelletti C, Corno A, Giannico S, Marino B. Inferior vena cava-pulmonary artery extracardiac conduit: a new form of right heart bypass. J Thorac Cardiovasc Surg 1990; 100:228-32.

Marchand P: The use of a cusp-bearing homograph patch the outflow tract and pulmonary artery in Fallot's Tetralogy and pulmonary valvular stenosis. Thorax 1967;22:497-509.

Marie PY, Marcon F, Brunorte F, Briancon S, Dauchin N, Worms AM, Robert J, Pernot C. Right ventricular overload and induced sustained ventricular tachycardia in operatively "repaired" tetralogy of Fallot. Am J Coll Cardiol 1994;69:785-789.

Mc Elhinney DB, Reddy VM, Moore P, Hanley FL. Revision of previous Fontan connections to extracardiac or intraatrial conduit cavopulmonary anastomosis. Ann Thorac Surg. 1996, 62(5):1276-82.

McGoon DC, Baird DK, Davis GD. Surgical management of large bronchial collateral arteries with pulmonary stenosis or atresia Circulation 1975;52:109-18.

McKay R, De Leval MR, Rees P – Post –operative angiographic assessment of modified Blalock-Taussig shunts using expanded polytetrafluioroethylene (Gore - tex). Ann thorac Surg, 1980;30:137-45

Messmer K; Sunder-Plassman L; Klovekorn WP; Holper K. Circulatory significance of hemodilution: rheological changes and limitations. Adv. Microcirc 1972; 4: 1-77.

Miyamura H, Kanazawa H, Hayashi J, Eguchi S. Thrombosed St Jude Medical valve prosthesis in the right side of the heart in patents with tetralogy of Fallot. J Thorac Cardiovasc Surg 1987;94:148-50.

Moons P, Gewillig M, Sluysmans T, Verhaaren H, Viart P, Massin M, Suys B, Budts W, Pasquet A, De Wolf D, Vliers A. Long term outcome up to 30 years after the Mustard or Senning operation: a nationwide multicentre study in Belgium. *Heart. 2004; 90: 307–313.*

Murphy JG, Gersh BJ, Mair DD, Fuster V, Mc Goon MD, Ilstrup DM, Mc Goon DC, Kirklin JW, Danielson GK. Long-term outcome in patients under-going surgical repair of tetralogy of Fallot. N Engl J Med 1993;329:593-599.

Murthy KS, Krishnanaik S, Mohanty SR, Varghese R, Cherian KM. A new repair for anomalous left coronary artery. Ann Thorac Surg 2001; 71:1384-6.

Naik SK, Knight A, Elliott MJ. A prospective randomized study of a modified technique of ultrafiltration during pediatric open-heart surgery. Circulation 1991;84 (Suppl 3): 422-31.

Nakata S, Imai Y, Takanashi Y, Kurosawa H, Tezuka K, Nakazawa M, Ando M, Takao A- A new method for the quantitative standardization of cross-sectional areas of the pulmonary arteries in congenital heart diseases with decreased pulmonary blood flow. J Thorac Cardiovasc Surg 1984; 88:610-9.

Nakata S, Imai Y, Takanashi Y, Kurosawa H, Tezuka K, Nakazawa N, Ando M, Takao A. A new method for the quantitative standardization of cross-sectional areas of the pulmonary arteries in congenital heart disease with decreased pulmonary blood flow. J Thorac Cardiovasc Surg 1984;88:610-19.

Niwaya K, Knott-Graig CJ, Lane MM, Chandrasekaren K, Overholt ED, Elkins RC. Cryopreserved homograft valves in the pulmonary position: risk analysis for intermediate-term failure. J Thorac Cardiovasc Surg 1999; 117:141-6.

Nollest G, Fischlein T, Bouterwek S, Bohmer C, Klinner W, Reichart B. Long-term survival in patients with repair of tetralogy of Fallot: 36-year after surgical repair. J Am Coll Cardiol 1997;30:1374-1383.

Norvick WM, Stidham GL, Guillory KL, Ivancan V, Malicic I, Sandoval N, Reid RW, Lazorishisnets VV, Davis MG, Baum VC, Di Sessa TG. Are we improving after 10 years of humanitarian paediatric cardiac assistance?- Cardiology in the Young 2005,15:379-384.

Norwood WI, Lang P, Castaneda AR, Campbell DN. Experience with operations for hypoplastic left heart syndrome. J Thorac Cardiovasc Surg, 1981;82(4):511-9.

Norwood WI, Lang P, Hansen DD. Physiologic repair of aortic atresia-hypoplastic left heart syndrome. N Engl J Med, 1983;308(1):23-6.

Oechslin E, Jenni R. 40 years after the first atrial switch procedure in patients with transposition of the great arteries: long-term results in Toronto and Zurich. *Thorac Cardiovasc Surg. 2000; 48: 233–237.*

Oku, H; Shirotani, H; Sunakawa, A; Yokoyama, T: Postoperative long-term results in total correction of tetralogy of Fallot: hemodynamics and cardiac function. Ann Thorac Surg 1986;41:413-18.

Oury JH, Hiro SP, Maxwell JM, Lamberti JS, Duran CM. The Ross procedure: current registry results. Ann Thorac Surg 1998; 66: S162-5.

Owen AR, Gatzoulis AM. Tetralogy of Fallot: late outcome after repair and surgical implications. Semin Thorac Cardiovasc Surg 2000;3:216-26.

Pacifico, AD; Kirklin, JW; Blackstone, EH: Surgical management of pulmonary stenosis in tetralogy of Fallot. J Thorac Cardiovasc Surg 1977,74:382-95.

Pearl JM, Mannig PB, ME Namara JL, Sancier MM, Thomas DW. Effect of modified ultrafiltration on plasma thromboxane B2, Leukotriene B4, and eudothelin-1 in infants undergoing cardiopulmonary bypass. Ann Thorac Surg 1999, 68: 1369-75.

Quintessenza JA, Jacobs JP, Morell VO, Giroud JM, Boucek RJ. Initial experience with a bicuspid polytetrafluoroethylene pulmonary valve in children and adults: A new option for right ventricular outflow tract reconstruction. Ann Thorac Surg 2005;79:924-931.

Rastelli GC, McGoon DC, Wallace RB. Anatomic correction of transposition of great arteries with ventricular septal defect and subpulmonary stenosis. J Thorac Cardiovasc Surg 1969; 58:545-52.

Rastelli or Lecompte procedure? J Thorac Cardiovasc Surg 1992; 103:428-36.

Reich O, Voriskova M, Ruth C, Krejcir M, Marek J, Skovranek J, Hucin B, Samanek M. Long-term ventricular performance after intra-atrial correction of transposition: left ventricular filling is the major limitation. *Heart. 1997; 78: 376–381.*

Rost L, Murz B, Colle AM, Festa P, Rodaelli S, Frigiola A. Pulmonary valve replacement: a role for mechanical prostheses? Ann Thorac Surg 1998; 65:889-90.

Sakurai T, Kado H, Nakano T, Hinokiyama H, Shiose, M. Kajimoto, K. Joo, and Y. Ueda. Early results of bilateral pulmonary artery banding for hypoplastic left heart syndrome. Eur. J. Cardiothorac. Surg., December 1, 2009; 36(6): 973 - 979.

Sano S, Kawada M, Yoshida H, Kino K, Irie H, Aoki A, et al. Norwood procedure to hypoplastic left heart syndrome. Jpn J Thorac Cardiovasc Surg. 1998;46(12):1311-6.

Sarkar D, Bull C, Yates R, Wright D, Cullen S, Gewillig M, Clayton R, Tunstill A, Deanfield J. Comparison of long-term outcomes of atrial repair of simple transposition with implications for a late arterial switch strategy. *Circulation. 1999; 100: II-176–II-181.*

Senning A- Surgical correction of transposition of the great vessels. Surgery, 1959;45: 966-999.

Sese A, Omoto Y. New technique in the transfer of an anomalously originated left coronary artery to the aorta. Ann Thorac Surg 1992; 53:527-9.

Sievens HH, Storde U, Rohwedder EB, et al. Superior function of a bicuspid over a monocuspid patch for reconstruction of a bicuspid over a monocuspid patch for reconstruction of a hypoplastic pulmonary root in pigs. J Thorac Cardiovasc Surg 1993;105:580-90.

Stark J, Bull C, Stajevic M, Jothi M, Elliott M, de Leval M. Fate of subpulmonary homograft conduits: determinants of late homograft failure. J Thorac Cardiovasc Surg 1998;115:506-14.

Stoica SC, Philips AB, Egan M, Rodeman R, Chisolm J, Hill S, Cheatham JP, E. Galantowicz ME. The retrograde aortic arch in the hybrid approach to hypoplastic left heart syndrome. Ann. Thorac. Surg., 2009; 88(6): 1939 - 1947.

Tashiro T, Todo K, Hamta Y, Yasunaga H, Nagata M, Nakamura M. Anomalous origin of the left coronary artery from the pulmonary artery: new operative technique. J Thorac Cardiovasc Surg 1993; 106:718-22.

Therrien J, Marx GR, Gatzoulis AM. Late problems in tetralogy of Fallot-recognition, management and prevention. Cardiol Clin 2002, 20:395-404.

Thompson LD, Mc Elhinney DB, Findlay P, Miller- Hance W, Chen MJ; Minami M; Petrossian E , Parry AJ; Reddy VM, Hanley FL. A prospective randomized study comparing volume-standardized modified and conventional ultrafiltration in pediatric cardiac surgery. Thorac Cardiovasc Surg 2001; 122 (2): 220-28.

Turina M, Siebenmann R, Nussbaumer P, Senning A. Long-term outlook after atrial correction of transposition of great arteries. *J Thorac Cardiovasc Surg. 1988; 95: 828–835.*

Turrentine MW, McCarthy RP, Vijay P, McConnell KW, Brown JW. Polytetrafluoroethylene monocusp valve reconstruction of the right ventricular outflow tract. Ann Thorac Surg 2002;73:871-9.

Vliegen HW, van Straten A, de Roos A, et al. Magnetic resonance imaging to assess the hemodynamic effects of pulmonary valve replacement in adults late after repair of tetralogy of Fallot. Circulation 2002; 106:1703-7.

Vohue PR, Tamisier D, Sidi D, Vernant F, Mauriat P, Pouard P. Leca F. Anomalous left coronary artery from the pulmonary artery: Results of isolated aortic reimplantation. Ann Thorac Surg 1992; 54: 621-7.

Von Son JA, Mohr FW. Repair of anomalous connection of the left coronary artery to the pulmonary artery using native aorta and pumnonary tissue flaps. Eur J Cardiothorac surg 1997; 12:322-9.

Vougpatanasin W, Hillis LD, Lange RA. Prosthetic heart valves. N Engl J Med 1996;335:407-16.

Wells WJ, Arroyo Jr H, Bremner RM, Woog J, Starnes VA. Homograft conduit failure in infants is not due to somatic out growth. J Thorac Cardiovasc Surg 2002;124:88-96.

Wells WJ, Blackstone E. Intermediate outcome after Mustard and Senning procedures: a study by the Congenital Heart Surgeons Society. *Semin Thorac Cardiovasc Surg Pediatr Card Surg Annu. 2000; 3: 186–197.*

Westphal FL, Maluf MA, Silva CM, Carvalho ACC, Buffolo E. Estudo angiográfico comparativo da artéria pulmonar no pré e pós-operatório de pacientes submetidos a operação de derivação cavopulmonar bidirecional. Rev Bras Cir Cardiovasc 2001; 16 (4): 305-20.

Williams WG, Mc Crindle BW, Ashburn DA, Jonas RA, Mavroudis C, Blackstone EH. Outcomes of 829 neonates with complete transposition of the great arteries 12–17 years after repair. *Eur J Cardiothorac Surg. 2003; 24: 1–9.*

World Summit on Pediatric and Congenital Heart Surgery . Services, Education and Cardiac Care in Children and Adults with Congenital Heart Disease. Global Coalition to Improve Cardiac Care for Children and Adults with Pediatric and Congenital Heart Disease across the World. Montreal - Canada; June, 2008.

Yamagishi M, Kurosawa H. Outflow reconstruction of tetralogy of Fallot using a Gore-Tex valve. Ann Thorac Surg 1993;56:1414-6.
Zavanella C, Portela F. Early failure of bovine jugular vein conduit. J Thorac Cardiovasc Surg 2004; 127:610.

Part 4

Pediatric Hemato–Oncology

10

Alpha Thalassemia Disorders

Vefik Arica and Secil Gunher Arica
Mustafa Kemal University Medical Faculty
Turkey

1. Introduction

1.1 Alpha thalassaemia and new developments

The thalassaemias, the commonest monogenic diseases, are a family of inherited disorders of haemoglobin synthesis characterised by a reduced output of one or other of the globin chains of adult haemoglobin. They are likely to pose an increasing health problem for many developing countries during the early part of the new millennium (1). This review focuses mainly on their control and management, a subject of increasing importance not only for parts of the world in which the disease is particularly common but for any country which has an immigrant population from these regions.

1.2 Genetic control of haemoglobin

All the human haemoglobins consist of two different pairs of globin chains combined with haemoglobin, the iron containing moiety that binds oxygen. Fetal haemoglobin, the synthesis of which continues throughout fetal life and declines after birth, has alpha 2-gama 2, and in adults there is a major component called haemoglobin A (alpha 2-beta 2) and a minor fraction, haemoglobin A2.

The sequence of DNA that comprises the globin genes and the chromosomal regions around them has been determined. Each gene consists of three coding regions (exons) and two non-coding regions (introns). When a globin gene is transcribed, a mirror image molecule called messenger RNA is copied from one of the strands of DNA of the particular gene. While it is still in the nucleus of the red cell precursor, the intron sequences are removed and the exon sequences spliced together in the correct order to form the template for the production of a globin chain. This processed molecule moves into the cytoplasm, where it acts as the blueprint whereby appropriate amino acids are strung together to form a definitive globin chain. In adult red cells alpha and beta chains synthesised in this way combine with haem to form definitive haemoglobin molecules. There are also critical regulatory regions of DNA that are involved in ensuring that globin chains are produced in appropriate amounts in the correct tissues at the right time of development. The thalassaemias result from mutations or gene deletions that involve one or other of these complex steps.

1.3 Definitions and classification

The alpha and beta thalassaemias are by far the most important. In many populations in which thalassaemia is common, the genes for structural haemoglobin variants such as haemoglobins S, C, and E are also common, so it is not unusual for individuals to inherit a gene for thalassaemia from one parent and that for a haemoglobin variant from the other. The most important diseases of this type are sickle cell thalassaemia and haemoglobin E thalassaemia. Most of the important forms of thalassaemia are inherited in a Mendelian recessive fashion; carrier parents who are symptomless have a one in four chance of having a severely affected child.

1.4 Population distribution

The thalassaemias are distributed across the Mediterranean region, the Middle East, the Indian subcontinent, and throughout southeast Asia. In many of these countries gene frequencies for the different thalassaemias and structural haemoglobin variants are excess of alpha globin chains that are produced, and a genetically determined ability to produce high levels of fetal haemoglobin, are important factors (2). Heterozygotes for beta thalassaemia have mild hypochromic anaemia with small red cells and a raised concentration of haemoglobin A2.

2. Epidemiology

Like all common globin gene disorders (sickle cell trait and β thalassaemia) alpha thalassaemia occurs at high frequencies throughout all tropical and subtropical regions of the world. In some areas, the carrier frequency of alpha thalassaemia may be as high as 80-90% of the population, almost at fixation (3-7). It is thought that all of these globin gene disorders (including alpha thalassaemia) have been selected because in some way they protect carriers from the ravages of falciparum malaria. The micro epidemiological evidence supporting this is very strong (8, 9). The mechanisms underlying this protection have been extensively studied but remain unknown. Of all globin disorders, alpha thalassaemia is the most widely distributed and therefore many individuals in these areas have interacting combinations of these variants (e.g. both alpha and β thalassaemia). Due to differences in the interactions between the various molecular defects underlying alpha thalassaemia HbH disease is predominantly seen in South East Asia, the Middle East and the Mediterranean. In passing it should be mentioned that ATR16, ATR-X and ATMDS syndromes show no geographical bias in their distributions.

Although the previously established distribution of alpha thalassaemia, over the past few decades there have been massive population movements so that now the globin gene disorders, thought to be rarities in North European and North American clinical practice, have become major diagnostic and therapeutic challenges for our current health care systems (10).

2.1 Screening and prevention

The carrier states for all the important thalassaemias can be identified (11, 12) and methods for their prenatal diagnosis are well established. Where this approach is acceptable to families on religious and other grounds it is being adopted as a way of controlling thalassaemia. Control programmes require screening, either at the population level if the disease is particularly common or, more usually, at the first visit to the antenatal clinic. Every woman of appropriate racial background should be screened for thalassaemia by a standard blood count with particular reference to the red cell indices. All the important carrier states for the different forms of thalassaemia are associated with a reduced mean cell haemoglobin concentration and cell volume. When a blood picture of this kind is encountered it should be followed by the estimation of the haemoglobin A2 concentration, which is raised in all the common forms of beta thalassaemia. It is important therefore to obtain the help of an expert laboratory to distinguish between these possibilities. If a mother is a carrier for alpha thalassaemia her pregnancy is at risk for the Bart's hydrops fetalis syndrome, whereas the worst possible outcome of a pregnancy involving a woman homozygous for alpha thalassaemia is the much milder condition, haemoglobin H disease. The forms of beta thalassaemia with normal haemoglobin A2 concentrations may interact with the other thalassaemia genes to produce a severe phenotype.

Once a woman has been diagnosed as a carrier for one or other forms of thalassaemia her partner should be tested and the couple referred for expert genetic counselling. If they opt for prenatal diagnosis they should be referred as early as possible.

Early prenatal diagnosis, first by fetal blood sampling and later by chorion villus biopsy and direct analysis of the globin genes, is now extremely effective (13). The error rate in experienced centres is now well under 1%, most of the mistakes resulting from either contamination of the fetal DNA by maternal tissue, nonpaternity, or technical problems of DNA analysis (14).

Alpha thalassaemias (15, 16) show several important differences from beta thalassaemia. Because alpha chains are shared by fetal and adult haemoglobin the disease is manifest in both fetal and adult life. Furthermore, excess gama and beta chains do not precipitate immediately in the bone marrow like alpha chains but produce the physiologically useless and unstable tetramers: haemoglobin Bart's and haemoglobin H. Since the alpha genes are duplicated the genetics of alpha thalassaemia is more complicated than that of beta thalassaemia. Usually these alpha genes are lost by deletion, though sometimes they are inactivated by a point mutation, as is the case in the beta thalassaemias.

The homozygous state for alpha thalassaemia produces intrauterine death with a profoundly anaemic and hydropic fetus: the haemoglobin Bart's hydrops fetalis syndrome. Mothers carrying babies of this type commonly have toxaemia of pregnancy and post partum bleeding.

Alpha thalassaemia is certainly not a rare genetic trait. On the contrary, it is one of the most common human genetic abnormalities known. Carriers of alpha thalassaemia are found at polymorphic frequency (>1%) in all tropical and subtropical populations that have been studied and, in some areas, the carrier state has almost gone to fixation. This is because carriers of alpha thalassaemia are thought to be at a selective advantage in areas where falciparum malaria is or has been endemic. In areas where the carrier state is common, two clinically important diseases (HbH disease and Hb Bart's hydrops foetalis) occur in compound heterozygotes and homozygotes. The reason for discussing this here is therefore not because these diseases are rare, rather that they may be rarely considered by physicians outside of the regions where thalassaemia commonly occurs. For example, a retrospective study of obstetric records in the U.K. by Petrou et al. revealed an underdiagnosis of both alpha-thalassaemia trait and alpha-thalassaemia hydrops foetalis (17).

With the massive migrations that have occurred over the past few decades it is important to bring these rarely considered diseases to the general attention of clinicians in Northern Europe and North America.

2.2 Disease names and synonyms

The generic term alpha thalassaemia encompasses all of those conditions in which there is a deficit in the production of the alpha globin chains of haemoglobin (Hb) which is a tetrameric molecule including two alpha-like and two β-like globin chains (alpha2β2). Underproduction of alpha globin chains gives rise to excess β-like globin chains which form γ4 tetramers, called Hb Bart's (in foetal life) and β4 tetramers, called HbH (in adult life). Individuals who carry mutations affecting the alpha globin genes on one chromosome, associated with minimal anaemia, are said to have alpha thalassaemia trait. Compound heterozygotes and some homozygotes for alpha thalassaemia have a moderately severe anaemia characterised by the presence of HbH in the peripheral blood. This condition is referred to as HbH disease. Finally some individuals who make very little or no alpha globin chains have a very severe form of anaemia which, if untreated, causes death in the neonatal period. This condition is called the Hb Bart's hydrops foetalis syndrome (18-21).

Rarely patients have been seen with very large deletions which remove the alpha globin genes but also remove many other genes that surround them. This condition is associated with developmental abnormalities (including intellectual disability) and is referred to as the alpha thalassaemia/mental retardation syndrome on chromosome 16 (ATR16 syndrome: OMIM:141750, reviewed in Higgs et al., 2009 (22) and Wilkie et al., 1990 (23)). Also patients with a rare form of syndromal X-linked mental retardation associated with alpha thalassaemia have been described, in which the intellectual disability is more severe and the dysmorphic features show striking similarities among patients. This rare condition is called ATR-X syndrome and has been found to involve mutations in a chromatin associated protein called ATRX on the X-chromosome (ATR-X syndrome: OMIM:301040, reviewed elsewhere)(22, 24-27).

Finally, an acquired form of alpha-thalassaemia referred to as the ATMDS syndrome has been described. This predominantly occurs in elderly males with a pre-malignant, clonal haematopoietic disease called myelodysplasia (MDS). This rare syndrome involves acquired mutations in the ATRX gene causing alpha thalassaemia (OMIM:300448, reviewed in Gibbons et al., 2003;Higgs et al., 2009) (22, 28). Since these rare conditions have all been reviewed elsewhere they will not be discussed further in this synopsis.

2.3 Definition/diagnostic criteria

Alpha thalassaemia is most frequently suspected initially on the basis of a routine full blood count. All affected individuals have a variable degree of anaemia (Hb), reduced mean corpuscular haemoglobin (MCH/pg), reduced mean corpuscular volume (MCV/fl) and a normal or slightly reduced level of the minor HbA2. These parameters are discussed in greater detail below. When the level of alpha globin synthesis falls below ~70% of normal, in the foetal period, excess γ globin chains form Hb Bart's which can be detected on routine Hb analysis (29-35). In adult life, excess β globin chains form β4 tetramers of HbH in the cell and these can be identified by staining the peripheral blood with 1% brilliant cresyl blue (BCB) (36-38), or when present in sufficient quantity by routine Hb analysis (36, 39). Previously alpha thalassaemia was confirmed by globin chain biosynthesis, when the alpha/β globin chain biosynthesis ratio was reduced to less than ~0.8 (40-44).

All of these parameters are reduced in alpha thalassaemia but none of them alone or in combination can accurately or consistently predict the genotype for which directed molecular analysis of the alpha globin cluster is required and this is discussed below.

2.4 Clinical description

The clinical phenotypes of most individuals with alpha thalassaemia are very mild and may not be noticed during life other than when a routine full blood count is examined. Patients with HbH disease have a variable phenotype and those with Hb Bart's hydrops foetalis have a lethal form of anaemia.

2.5 Alpha thalassaemia trait

Apart from mild to moderate microcytic hypochromic anaemia (detected on a routine blood count), carriers (heterozygotes) of alpha thalassaemia, whatever the molecular basis (see below), are clinically asymptomatic and the diagnosis (when made) is often established during a regular health check or during antenatal screening. Complaints related to more severe anaemias, such as fatigue, listlessness and shortness of breath are uncommon and almost certainly related to other concomitant disorders.

Carriers of alpha$^+$- or alpha^0-thalassaemia alleles generally do not need treatment, because their anaemia is either very mild or absent due to a compensating high red blood cell count. On the other hand, once a diagnosis of alpha thalassaemia trait is made, there is a tendency to discard iron-deficiency as a subsequent cause of anaemia. Carriers of alpha thalassaemia can be anaemic as a consequence of coexisting nutritional deficiencies, such as iron deficiency, folate or vitamin B12 deficiencies and should be managed correctly from this point of view. Of course prophylactic iron should never be given to carriers of alpha thalassaemia who are at risk of developing iron overload if treated inappropriately.

2.6 Genotype/phenotype correlations

Although there are now 128 different molecular defects known to cause alpha thalassaemia and an ever increasing number of potential interactions, the clinical phenotypes (broadly classified as alpha thalassaemia trait, HbH disease and Hb Bart's hydrops foetalis) resulting from the interactions between these various molecular defects. The severity of the clinical phenotype correlates very well with the degree of alpha globin chain deficiency. An important additional point is that, in general, interactions involving non-deletional forms of alpha$^+$-thalassaemia result in a more severe phenotype than in those with deletional forms of alpha$^+$-thalassaemia (45-59).

2.7 Diagnosis and diagnostic methods

Initial laboratory testing should include a complete blood count with red cell indices, HPLC or Hb electrophoresis and eventually alpha/β-globin chain synthesis ratio measurement.

The latter procedure, however, is sometimes by passed by DNA analysis as a less complicated method to diagnose alpha-thalassaemia.

2.8 Molecular analysis

Over the past 30 years it has become increasingly possible to diagnose alpha thalassaemia accurately and define the precise defects underlying these disorders using a variety of molecular genetic approaches. Ultimately, most alpha globin rearrangements have been characterised by Southern blotting and DNA sequence analysis. However, for today's diagnostic demands these techniques are far too laborious to apply in each case, and from the original work defining these mutations, rapid screening assays have been developed.

2.9 Differential diagnosis

Sometimes carriers of alpha^{+}-thalassaemia present with normal haematology, especially carriers of –alpha 3.7 and non deletional mutations affecting the alpha1-gene. Such individuals may be normocytic or borderline hypochromic without anaemia. These can only be found by chance during routine molecular analysis for haemoglobinopathies.

2.10 Prognosis

There is no reason to think that carriers for alpha thalassaemia have any altered prognosis for life compared to the normal population. The prognosis for patients with HbH disease who are newly emerging in previously nonendemic countries, like Northern Europe and Northern America, is less clear. Anecdotally many patients with HbH disease appear to lead a normal life in all respects. Some even remain undiagnosed throughout their lives. However, detailed actuarial studies are not available. When complications arise, of course the outcome depends on the awareness and availability of health care systems. Certainly some complications suffered by patients with HbH disease are life threatening in the absence of adequate medical care (21, 60, 61). A long term problem for all patients with HbH disease is the unwanted accumulation of iron which may be more of a problem for those with severe HbH disease with nondeletional alpha- thalassaemia (62, 63).

Clearly, previously undiagnosed and untreated infants with the Hb Bart's hydrops foetalis syndrome die in the perinatal period. The recent attempts to rescue infants with this syndrome either by intra-uterine transfusion or by transfusion in the perinatal period have met with variable success. As discussed above many infants develop other irreversible abnormalities during foetal life and even with rescue the infant will be required, either to receive lifelong blood transfusion and iron chelation therapy, or bone marrow transplantation with its attendant risks.

3. Therapy and management of Alpha-thalassemia

Alpha-thalassemia silent carrier and alpha-thalassemia trait:

Alpha globin is made by four genes, two on each strand of chromosome 16. Individuals who have one or two abnormal alpha globin genes have alpha thalassemia trait. An individual with one abnormal alpha globin gene is said to be a silent carrier of alpha thalassemia. This condition, in which one of the four alpha globin genes is missing or defective, generally causes no health problems because the lack of alpha globin protein is so small that there is no anemia. It is called "silent carrier" because of how difficult it is to detect. Silent carrier state is "diagnosed" by deduction when an apparently normal individual has a child with hemoglobin H disease or alpha thalassemia minor. It can also be diagnosed by special DNA testing.

Hb H disease:

Hemoglobin H disease is an inherited hemoglobin disorder in which three of the four alpha globin genes normally present are deleted or have a mutation which impairs alpha globin chain production. This leads to an excess of beta globin chains, which are unstable, precipitate within the cell and lead to destruction of the red blood cells. Hemoglobin H is a thalassemia-like syndrome characterized by hemolysis as well as ineffective red cell production. Co-inheritance of HbH with other globin gene defects can affect the severity of the condition. Hemoglobin H disease has a wide spectrum of clinical severity in patients, therefore, early diagnosis is important so patients can be followed. Hemoglobin levels and the patient's growth and development should be regularly monitored. Complications related to chronic hemolysis also need to be assessed. Infections should to be monitored closely so any severe drop in hemoglobin can be recognized and treated. Health care monitoring and maintenance with appropriate immunizations are important as well.

Hb Bart hydrops fetalis:

Hydrops fetalis is a serious disorder, usually indicative of an ominous prognosis for the affected fetus. There are many causes, including both hereditary and acquired diseases. With population migrations during the past decades, this syndrome is now seen in increasing numbers in other parts of the world. Hydrops fetalis can be diagnosed and monitored by ultrasound scans. Prenatal ultrasound scanning enables early recognition of hydrops fetalis and has been enhanced with the introduction of MCA Doppler. Recent advances in molecular genetics have provided insights into the mutations and pathophysiology causing α-thalassemias, as well as definitive clinical diagnostic tests for adult carrier detection and prenatal diagnosis. Severely anemic fetuses can be treated with blood transfusions while still in the womb.

4. Future expectations in Alpha thalassaemia

Alpha thalassemia severity ranges from asymptomatic to fatal in utero. Hemoglobin H disease, a mutation of three alpha globin genes, is more severe than previously recognized. New developments in the epidemiology, treatment and prognosis of thalassemia have dramatically altered the approach to the care of affected patients, and these developments are likely to have an even greater impact in the next few years. Alpha thalassemia is being recognized with increasing frequency in Turkey, and newborn screening for Hemoglobin Barts in some states is leading to early detection of Hb H disease. New data clarify the importance of distinguishing these two disorders because of the increased severity associated with Hb H. The use of intrauterine transfusions to sustain the viability of fetuses with homozygous alpha thalassemia has created a new population of patients with severe thalassemia and has raised new and complex issues in genetic counseling for parents with alpha thalassemia trait. Demographic changes have required an awareness and understanding of the unique features of alpha thalassemia disorders that were previously uncommon in Turkey but are now seen more frequently in children and recognized more consistently in adults. Anemia, hypersplenism, hemosiderosis, growth failure, and osteoporosis are commonly noted as the patient ages. Alpha thalassemia major, a usually fatal in utero disease, is now recognized to have a complex molecular and phenotypic expression with increasing births being reported. Surviving newborns without intrauterine transfusion often have congenital anomalies and neurocognitive injury. Serious maternal complications often accompany pregnancy. Doppler ultrasonography with intrauterine transfusion ameliorates these complications. The high incidence in many populations mandates population screening and prenatal diagnosis of at-risk couples. Universal newborn screening has been adopted in several regions with DNA confirmatory testing. These advances have resulted in ethical dilemmas for the family and the provider.

5. References

[1] Weatherall DJ, Clegg JB. Thalassemia—a global public health problem. Nature Med 1996;3:479.

[2] Weatherall DJ. The molecular basis for phenotypic variability of the common thalassaemias. Mol Med Today 1996;1:1520.

[3] Bernini L: Geographic distribution of alpha-thalassemia. In Disorders of Hemoglobin first edition. Edited by: Steinberg MH, Forget BG, Higgs DR, Nagel RL. Cambridge University Press; 2001:878-894.

[4] Flint J, Harding RM, Clegg JB, Boyce AJ: Why are some genetic diseases common? Distinguishing selection from other processes by molecular analysis of globin gene variants. Hum Genet 1993, 91:91-117.

[5] Flint J, Harding RM, Boyce AJ, Clegg JB: The population genetics of the haemoglobinopathies. Baillieres Clin Haematol 1993, 6:215-262.

[6] Fodde R, Losekoot M, Broek MH van den, Oldenburg M, Rashida N, Schreuder A, Wijnen JT, Giordano PC, Nayudu NV, Khan PM, et al.: Prevalence and molecular heterogeneity of alfa+ thalassemia in two tribal populations from Andhra Pradesh, India. Hum Genet 1988, 80:157-160.

[7] Modiano G, Morpurgo G, Terrenato L, Novelletto A, Di RA, Colombo B, Purpura M, Mariani M, Santachiara-Benerecetti S, Brega A, et al.: Protection against malaria morbidity: near-fixation of the alpha-thalassemia gene in a Nepalese population. Am J Hum Genet 1991, 48:390-397.

[8] Higgs DR, Weatherall DJ: The alpha thalassaemias. Cell Mol Life Sci 2009, 66:1154-1162.

[9] Weatherall DJ: Genetic variation and susceptibility to infection: the red cell and malaria. Br J Haematol 2008, 141:276-286.

[10] Harteveld CL, Beijer C, Van DP, Zanardini R, Bernini LF, Giordano PC: alpha thalassaemia as a result of a novel splice donor site mutation of the alpha1-globin gene. Br J Haematol 2000, 110:694-698.

[11] Weatherall DJ, Letsky EA. Screening and prenatal diagnosis of haematological disorders. In: Wald N, ed. Antenatal and neonatal screening. 2nd ed. Oxford: Oxford University Press.

[12] World Health Organisation. Working Group on the Community Control of Hereditary Anaemias. Bull WHO 1983;61:6380.

[13] Cao A, Rosatelli MC. Screening and prenatal diagnosis of the haemoglobinopathies. Clin Haematol 1993;6:26386.
[14] Modell BMP, Layton M, Petrou M, Layton M, Varnavides L, Ward RHT, Rodeck C, et al. Audit of prenatal diagnosis for haemoglobin disorders in the United Kingdom: the first 20 years. BMJ.
[15] Huisman THJ. Molecular genetics of áthalassemia. In: McArthur RJ, Lee SH, Wong JEL, Ong YW, eds. Haematology 1996. Education Programme of the 26th congress of the International Society of Haematology. Singapore: ICH, 1996:2336.
[16] Higgs DR. AlphaThalassaemia. Clin Haematol 1993;6:11750.
[17] Petrou M, Brugiatelli M, Old J, Hurley P, Ward RH, Wong KP, Rodeck C, Modell B: Alpha thalassaemia hydrops fetalis in the UK: the importance of screening pregnant women of Chinese, other South East Asian and Mediterranean extraction for alpha thalassaemia trait. Br J Obstet Gynaecol 1992, 99:985-989.
[18] Chui DH, Waye JS: Hydrops fetalis caused by alpha-thalassemia: an emerging health care problem. Blood 1998, 91:2213-2222.
[19] Liang ST, Wong VC, So WW, Ma HK, Chan V, Todd D: Homozygous alpha thalassaemia: clinical presentation, diagnosis and management. A review of 46 cases. Br J Obstet Gynaecol 1985, 92:680-684.
[20] Nakayama R, Yamada D, Steinmiller V, Hsia E, Hale RW: Hydrops fetalis secondary to Bart hemoglobinopathy. Obstet Gynecol 1986, 67:176-180.
[21] Weatherall DJ, Clegg JB: The Thalassaemia Syndromes 2001.
[22] Higgs DR, Buckle V, Gibbons R, Steensma D: Unusual Types of Alpha Thalassaemia. In Disorders of Hemoglobin second edition. Cambridge University Press; 2009.
[23] Wilkie AO, Buckle VJ, Harris PC, Lamb J, Barton NJ, Reeders ST, Lindenbaum RH, Nicholls RD, Barrow M, Bethlenfalvay NC, et al.: Clinical features and molecular analysis of the alpha thalassemia/mental retardation syndromes. I. Cases due to deletions involving chromosome band 16p13.3. Am J Hum Genet 1990, 46:1112-1126.
[24] Gibbons R: Alpha thalassaemia-mental retardation, X linked. Orphanet J Rare Dis 2006, 1:15.
[25] Gibbons RJ, Picketts DJ, Villard L, Higgs DR: Mutations in a putative global transcriptional regulator cause X-linked mental retardation with alpha-thalassemia (ATR-X syndrome). Cell 1995, 80:837-845.
[26] Wilkie AO, Zeitlin HC, Lindenbaum RH, Buckle VJ, Fischel-Ghodsian N, Chui DH, Gardner-Medwin D, MacGillivray MH, Weatherall DJ, Higgs DR: Clinical features and molecular analysis of the alpha thalassemia/ mental retardation syndromes. II. Cases without detectable abnormality of the alpha globin complex. Am J Hum Genet 1990, 46:1127-1140.
[27] Wilkie AO, Gibbons RJ, Higgs DR, Pembrey ME: X linked alpha thalassaemia/mental retardation: spectrum of clinical features in three related males. J Med Genet 1991, 28:738-741.
[28] Gibbons RJ, Pellagatti A, Garrick D, Wood WG, Malik N, Ayyub H, Langford C, Boultwood J, Wainscoat JS, Higgs DR: Identification of acquired somatic mutations in the gene encoding chromatin-remodeling factor ATRX in the alpha-thalassemia myelodysplasia syndrome (ATMDS). Nat Genet 2003, 34:446-449.

[29] Kutlar F, Reese AL, Hsia YE, Kleman KM, Huisman TH: The types of hemoglobins and globin chains in hydrops fetalis. Hemoglobin 1989, 13:671-683.
[30] Lie-Injo LE, Jo BH: A fast-moving haemoglobin in hydrops foetalis. Nature 1960, 185:698.
[31] Lin TM, Eng HL, Kuo PL, Wu HL: Neonatal screening for alpha thalassemia in southern Taiwan. J Formos Med Assoc 1992, 91:1213-1215.
[32] Todd D, Lai MC, Beaven GH, Huehns ER: The abnormal haemoglobins in homozygous alpha-thalassaemia. Br J Haematol 1970, 19:27-31.
[33] Velati C, Sampietro M, Sciariada L, Allievi E, Mosconi L, Cappellini MD, Fiorelli G: Neonatal screening for Hb Bart's in Italian subjects of heterogeneous regional origin born in Lombardy. Haematologica 1983, 68:20-29.
[34] Weatherall DJ, Clegg JB, Boon WH: The haemoglobin constitution of infants with the haemoglobin Bart's hydrops foetalis syndrome. Br J Haematol 1970, 18:357-367.
[35] Zorai A, Harteveld CL, Bakir A, Van DP, Falfoul A, Dellagi K, Abbes S, Giordano PC: Molecular spectrum of alpha-thalassemia in Tunisia: epidemiology and detection at birth. Hemoglobin 2002, 26:353-362.
[36] Chui DH: Alpha-thalassemia: Hb H disease and Hb Barts hydrops fetalis. Ann N Y Acad Sci 2005, 1054:25-32.
[37] Galanello R, Paglietti E, Melis MA, Giagu L, Cao A: Hemoglobin inclusions in heterozygous alpha-thalassemia according to their alpha-globin genotype. Acta Haematol 1984, 72:34-36.
[38] Pan LL, Eng HL, Kuo CY, Chen WJ, Huang HY: Usefulness of brilliant cresyl blue staining as an auxiliary method of screening for alpha thalassemia. J Lab Clin Med 2005, 145:94-97.
[39] Ingram VM, Stretton AO: Genetic basis of the thalassaemia diseases. Nature 1959, 184:1903-1909.
[40] Clegg JB, Weatherall DJ: Haemoglobin synthesis in alpha-thalassaemia (haemoglobin H disease). Nature 1967, 215:1241-1243.
[41] Giordano PC, van Delft P, Batelaan D, Harteveld CL, Bernini LF: Haemoglobinopathy analyses in the Netherlands: a report of an in vitro globin chain biosynthesis survey using a rapid, modified method. Clin Lab Haematol 1999, 21:247-256.
[42] Hunt DM, Higgs DR, Old JM, Clegg JB, Weatherall DJ, Marsh GW: Determination of alpha-thalassaemia phenotypes by messenger RNA analysis. Br J Haematol 1980, 45:53.
[43] Weatherall DJ, Clegg JB, Naughton MA: Globin synthesis in thalassaemia: an in vitro study. Nature 1965, 208:1061-1065.
[44] Weatherall DJ, Clegg JB: Haemoglobin synthesis in thalassaemia. Biochem J 1970, 119:68P.
[45] Higgs DR: The molecular basis of alpha -thalassemia. In Disorders of Hemoglobin second edition. Edited by: Steinberg MH, Forget BG, Higgs DR, Nagel RL. Cambridge University Press; 2009.
[46] Cao A, Rosatelli C, Pirastu M, Galanello R: Thalassemias in Sardinia: molecular pathology, phenotype-genotype correlation, and prevention. Am J Pediatr Hematol Oncol 1991, 13:179-188.

[47] Eng B, Patterson M, Walker L, Hoppe C, Azimi M, Lee H, Giordano PC, Waye JS: Three new alpha-thalassemia point mutations ascertained through newborn screening. Hemoglobin 2006, 30:149-153.
[48] Galanello R, Aru B, Dessi C, Addis M, Paglietti E, Melis MA, Cocco S, Massa P, Giagu N, Barella S, et al.: HbH disease in Sardinia: molecular, hematological and clinical aspects. Acta Haematol 1992, 88:1-6.
[49] Harteveld CL, Beijer C, Van DP, Zanardini R, Bernini LF, Giordano PC: alpha thalassaemia as a result of a novel splice donor site mutation of the alpha1-globin gene. Br J Haematol 2000, 110:694-698.
[50] Henderson S, Chapple M, Rugless M, Fisher C, Kinsey S, Old J: Haemoglobin H hydrops fetalis syndrome associated with homozygosity for the alpha2-globin gene polyadenylation signal mutation AATAAA-->. Br J Haematol 2006, 135:743-745.
[51] Moi P, Cash FE, Liebhaber SA, Cao A, Pirastu M: An initiation codon mutation (AUG----GUG) of the human alpha 1-globin gene. Structural characterization and evidence for a mild thalassemic phenotype. J Clin Invest 1987, 80:1416-1421.
[52] Noguera NI, Gonzalez FA, Davoli RA, Milani AC, Villegas A: A novel splice acceptor site mutation of the alpha2-globin gene causing alpha thalassemia. Hemoglobin 2001, 25:311-315.
[53] Olivieri NF, Chang LS, Poon AO, Michelson AM, Orkin SH: An alpha-globin gene initiation codon mutation in a black family with HbH disease. Blood 1987, 70:729-732.
[54] Pressley L, Higgs DR, Clegg JB, Perrine RP, Pembrey ME, Weatherall DJ: A new genetic basis for hemoglobin-H disease. N Engl J Med 1980, 303:1383-1388.
[55] Tabone P, Henni T, Belhani M, Colonna P, Verdier G, Godet J: Hemoglobin H disease from Algeria: genetic and molecular characterization. Acta Haematol 1981, 65:26-31.
[56] Thein SL, Wallace RB, Pressley L, Clegg JB, Weatherall DJ, Higgs DR: The polyadenylation site mutation in the alpha-globin gene cluster. Blood 1988, 71:313-319.
[57] Traeger-Synodinos J, Papassotiriou I, Karagiorga M, Premetis E, Kanavakis E, Stamoulakatou A: Unusual phenotypic observations associated with a rare HbH disease genotype (- -Med/alphaTSaudialpha): implications for clinical management. Br J Haematol 2002, 119:265-267.
[58] Viprakasit V, Green S, Height S, Ayyub H, Higgs DR: Hb H hydrops fetalis syndrome associated with the interaction of two common determinants of alpha thalassaemia. Br J Haematol 2002, 117:759-762.
[59] Whitelaw E, Proudfoot N: Alpha-thalassaemia caused by a poly(A) site mutation reveals that transcriptional termination is linked to 3' end processing in the human alpha 2 globin gene. EMBO J 1986, 5:2915-2922.
[60] Slomp J, Bosschaart A, Dousma M, van ZR, Giordano PC, Bergh FA van den: [Acute anaemia in a Vietnamese patient with alpha-thalassaemia and a parvovirus infection]. Ned Tijdschr Geneeskd 2006, 150:1577-1582.
[61] Chen FE, Ooi C, Ha SY, Cheung BM, Todd D, Liang R, Chan TK, Chan V: Genetic and clinical features of hemoglobin H disease in Chinese patients. N Engl J Med 2000, 343:544-550.

[62] Chan V, Wong MS, Ooi C, Chen FE, Chim CS, Liang RH, Todd D, Chan TK: Can defects in transferrin receptor 2 and hereditary hemochromatosis genes account for iron overload in HbH disease? Blood Cells Mol Dis 2003, 30:107-111.
[63] Ooi GC, Chen FE, Chan KN, Tsang KW, Wong YH, Liang R, Chan V, Ngan H: Qualitative and quantitative magnetic resonance imaging in haemoglobin H disease: screening for iron overload. Clin Radiol 1999, 54:98-102.

11

Neuroblastoma and Whole Genome Searches

Mario Capasso
University of Naples Federico II,
Department of Biochemistry and Medical Biotechnology,
CEINGE Biotecnologie Avanzate,
Italy

1. Introduction

Neuroblastoma is the most frequent solid cancer of early childhood, its incidence is 10.2 cases per million children under 15 years of age. Neuroblastoma is thought to be an embryonal tumor that is derived from precursor cells of the peripheral (sympathetic) nervous system (Hoehner et al., 1996; Maris, 2010). The tumor can arise anywhere along the sympathetic chain but is most frequently in the adrenal medulla and paraspinal ganglia (Maris, 2010).

The most fascinating feature of neuroblastoma is its remarkable biological heterogeneity, which becomes apparent in the broad of the clinical courses of the disease. While some patients experience spontaneous regression or differentiation of the tumor into benign ganglioneuroma, others are affected by rapid and fatal tumor progression despite increasingly intensive strategies. This highly heterogeneous clinical behavior of disease makes the prediction of each patient's individual risk at the time of diagnosis the major goal to choose the most adequate therapeutic approach.

So far, the well-known tumor-specific genetic markers (amplification of the MYCN oncogene, DNA ploidy, chromosome 1p and 11q losses, and gains of chromosome 17q), patient age at diagnosis with two cut-offs of 12 and 18 months, the histopathological assessment (Shimada system), disease stage defined by the international neuroblastoma staging system (INSS) have been crucial determinants for the assignment of the risk class and the treatment plan. Currently, clinical trials stratify patients into four prognostic subgroups with expected very low risk, low risk, intermediate risk, and high risk of death from disease, and sixteen pretreatment designations (Cohn et al., 2009).

However, according to the Surveillance, Epidemiology, and End Results databases (www.seer.cancer.gov), the survival rates, during the period from 1999 through 2005, have improved only for patients with the more benign form of the disease, the rates among children with high-risk neuroblastoma have shown only modest improvement, despite dramatic escalations in the intensity of therapy provided. The incorporation in clinical decision of additional genetic prognostic markers, including gene copy number aberrations, common genetic polymorphisms as well as gene expression and epigenetic markers is believed to be crucial in the development of a more accurate classification of patients in distinct prognostic risk categories and so in making treatment decisions.

The completion of the human genome sequence and the development of high throughput technology present exciting opportunities for the study of cancer. Recent technological advances based on whole genome approaches have made possible to discover a lot of new genetic markers in neuroblastoma which could be of substantial clinical importance in the relatively near future (Capasso and Diskin, 2010; Maris, 2010). Genome-wide analysis of amplification, deletion of genomic regions, somatically acquired genetic variations, common predisposing genetic variants, and mRNA expression profiles is a critical step to resolving the mechanisms of neuroblastoma tumorigenesis, might have implications towards better risk assessment and offer possibilities for target therapy. In this chapter, we will summarize the new discoveries related to the underlying molecular pathogenesis of this tumour with a special focus on advances that are translatable to the clinic. We will also present some recent, exciting findings from studies that have used a whole genome analysis technique such as comparative genomic hybridization (CGH), genome-wide association studies (GWAS), gene expression profiling (GEP) and next generation sequencing (NGS). We will finally discuss the clinical application of these whole genome searches and, the challenges and future directions for the genome-wide approaches to study the genetics of neuroblastoma.

2. Comparative Genomic Hybridization (CGH) of neuroblastoma

Genetic alternations such as amplifications and deletions frequently contribute to tumorigenesis. These alternations change the level of gene expression, which modify normal growth control and survival pathways. Characterization of these DNA copy-number changes is important for both the basic understanding of cancer and its diagnosis (Pinkel and Albertson, 2005). CGH was developed to survey DNA copy-number variations across a whole genome. With CGH, differentially labeled test (i.e. tumor) and reference (i.e. normal individual) genomic DNAs are cohybridized to normal metaphase chromosomes, and fluorescence ratios along the length of chromosomes provide a cytogenetic representation of the relative DNA copy-number variation. Chromosomal CGH resolution is limited to 10-20 Mb – therefore, anything smaller than that will not be detected. In the few years, diverse studies have used in-house bacterial artificial chromosome array or cDNA microarray to identify novel cancer related genes or crucial genome copy number alterations that determine distinct genetic subgroups for risk stratification of neuroblastoma (Mosse et al., 2005; Wang et al., 2006).

In a most recent paper, investigating 165 primary neuroblastomas, Caren and colleagues have compared the survival of patient subgroups defined by genomic alterations (Caren et al., 2010). They have demonstrated that patients with only numerical chromosomal aberrations and no other alteration had a favorable long-term outcome. On the other hand, the survival of patients characterized by MYCN amplification, loss of 11q or gain of 17q was considerably worse, whereas no death or disease was observed in patients with tumors harboring segmental chromosome alterations other than those previously mentioned. The main significance of these results is that a small number of predictive genomic alterations is sufficient for risk assessment of neuroblastoma patients.

Another study conducted by Janoueix-Lerosey et al. examined almost 500 primary neuroblastomas by bacterial artificial chromosome array-CGH and indicated that global genomic profiles may add significant prognostic information to current neuroblastoma risk estimation (Janoueix-Lerosey et al., 2009). The analysis showed that two distinct genetic classes of neuroblastoma might be related to two different mechanisms of instability. One, characterized by whole chromosome changes without any segmental alteration, is associated with an excellent outcome even in patients older than 18 months or with advanced stages of disease. The other class presents segmental chromosome imbalances that mainly arise through unbalanced chromosome translocations leading to concomitant loss and gain of chromosome fragments. Patients included in this last class, regardless the MYCN amplification, have an increased risk of relapse and in general they show a worse prognosis.

Another interesting CGH analysis has been performed on 236 primary neuroblastomas in Japan (Tomioka et al., 2008). The authors demonstrated that three major groups of genomic alterations in sporadic neuroblastomas could well define the prognoses of neuroblastomas:

- GG-S (n=23): a genetic group of silent with no obvious losses and gains except MYCN amplification (5-year cumulative survival rate: 68%; DNA ploidy: 87% diploidy);
- GG-P (n=53): a genetic group of partial chromosomal gains and / or losses (43% survival; 77% diploidy);
- GG-W (n=36): a genetic group of whole chromosomal gains and / or losses (80% survival; 22% diploidy).

In general, even if the results of these three excellent studies highlight the importance of prognostic classification of neuroblastoma using CGH, the clinical significance of global genomic alterations needs to be further evaluated in independent studies and compared with current risk estimation strategies.

Currently, the clinical significance of this advanced technology is monitoring cancer progression and distinguishing between mild and metastatic censorious lesions using FISH (Florescence in situ hybridization) probes on regions of recurrent copy number aberrations in several tumor types. It can be also used to reveal more regional copy number markers that can be used for cancer prediction. Finally, identifying and understanding the genes that are involved in cancer will help to design therapeutic drugs that target the dysfunction genes and/or avoid therapies that cause tumor resistance. However, one of the limitations of CGH analysis is due to the contamination of stromal cells that can affect the copy number detection. The routine application of CGH in clinical practice might be considerably limited by the issue of contaminating stromal cells, because defined thresholds of tumor content will *a priori* exclude a substantial fraction of samples from the analysis.

3. Gene Expression Profiling (GEP) of neuroblastoma

Microarray-based gene expression profiling enables the rapid, simultaneous measurement of gene expression on a genome-wide scale and consequently this technology represents an exciting development in genomic marker research that has been enthusiastically embraced by researchers worldwide.

Comparison between neuroblastoma subsets with good and poor prognosis, or based on neuronal functions has indicated diverse gene expression markers such as the genes whose mRNA expression is high in the favorable type of neuroblastoma include TRKA, CD44, pleiotrophin, N-cadherin, H-RAS, ECEL1, NLRR3, BMCC1, NEDL1 and ZNF423, and those in the unfavorable ones include TRKB, TERT, CDC10, NLRR1, HEN2 and LMO3 (Ohira and Nakagawara, 2010). There are evidences in literature that indicate the tyrosine kinase receptors as tractable theraupetic targets due to their cell surface localization and limited normal tissue distribution (Maris, 2005). A phase I trial of lestaurtinib, a multi-kinase inhibitor that strongly inhibits TrkB, has recently been completed in children with refractory neuroblastoma (Minturn et al., 2011). This study has identified a well-tolerated oral dose that results in effective TrkB inhibition, and its efficacy will be studied in future pediatric clinical trials. However, none of the above mentioned candidate genes alone could sufficiently explain the different biological behavior of neuroblastoma tumors, or could be considered as a prognostic marker in a clinical setting.

Global gene expression analysis can reveal significant information about the nature and state of cells, including disease progression, pharmacological response, and biological phenomena such as growth and development. These discoveries often point to sets of genes and gene pathways that are specifically associated with the state or change in state induced by disease. It also leads to the identification of gene sets associated with disease outcome and prognosis, as well as drug-induced responses. In many cases, only a small number of genes in the total genome (e.g., 25–500 genes) respond in a statistically significant way. The set can be further reduced by removing redundant genes. The resulting smaller subset becomes a true signature for diagnosis of the biological state and a predictor of therapeutic response. The identification of gene expression signatures is proving to be a powerful tool for disease diagnosis and drug discovery. For example, in oncology, microarray analysis is now being broadly applied toward the diagnosis and classification of a host of different cancers, including breast (van 't Veer et al., 2002), kidney (Vasselli et al., 2003), prostate (Best et al., 2003), and childhood cancers (Khan et al., 2001). Microarray analysis has also been used to categorize chemotherapy response and potentially direct the course of chemotherapy, for example, in acute myeloid leukemia (Okutsu et al., 2002).

In the past few years, several reports have provided irrefutable, evidence that specific gene-expression patterns can predict the natural courses of neuroblastoma patients with high accuracy. In the 2004, the first study showed a gene-expression-based classifier able to predict the prognosis of patients efficiently by profiling 56 tumors using cDNA microarrays containing 42 578 cDNA clones (classification accuracy was 95% for 21 test samples) (Wei et al., 2004). However, this study shows important limitations that prevented a diagnostic application of the proposed classifier: the low number of cases analyzed and the lack of validation analyses in independent sets of neuroblstomas. Since this first report on gene-expression-based risk classification, there have been multiple attempts to define and validate an optimal mRNA prognostic expression signature in neuroblastoma.

Ohira and colleagues, in the 2005, published a prognostic gene-expression signature for neuroblastoma patients that was derived from a large cohort of 136 primary neuroblastomas diagnosed in Japan (Ohira et al., 2005). They utilized an algorithm calculating survival probabilities of each patient at 2 years or 5 years after diagnosis, which is indicated by a "posterior" value range from 0 to 1. The gene expression signature was able to predict patient prognosis with high efficiency (90% accuracy, 96% sensitivity and 90% specificity). Of note, an intermediate-risk group (stage 3 or 4 without MYCN amplification) was classified with an accuracy of 86% better than the current clinical markers (age, stage and MYCN) that exhibited 64% accuracy. The authors also made a "mini-chip" carrying the top-ranked 200 genes for clinical use. It was tested on 50 independent tumor samples of all stages indicating high reproducibility as well as high efficiency. This 'mini-chip' is now under clinical validation in a larger cohort in Japan.

In the 2006, Asgharzadeh et al. have built a classifier comprising 55 genes using 102 patients with metastatic, MYCN non-amplified neuroblastoma, that was able to separate patients into two groups with statistically different event-free survival rates (Asgharzadeh et al., 2006). Regardless of MYCN status, all patients 18 months or older with metastatic neuroblastoma are currently considered high risk, and receive intensive therapies. The use of a molecular risk classification based on each tumor's gene expression signature may be able to identify a subgroup with less aggressive disease that may not require intensive, high-risk therapy. However, the 55-gene signature determined by Asgharzadeh et al. has not been validated in independent data sets, no trial for the this sub-group of patients is prospectively assessing the use of the 55-gene signature, so its clinical application is still far.

Oberthuer *et* al., in the 2006, published a gene signature including 144-genes able to improve the risk estimation of current neuroblastoma trials (Oberthuer et al., 2006). They utilized a customized oligonucleotide microarray comprising 10,163 probes. The 144-gene signature obtained by analyzing 77 samples could classify 174 patients more accurately than risk stratification of current trials from Germany, Japan and the United States. To further evaluate the impact of this 144-gene expression-based classifier on the neuroblasotma risk classification, Oberthuer et al., in the 2010, determined its prognostic value in a validation cohort of 440 internationally collected neuroblastoma specimens, 125 of which were examined prospectively (Oberthuer et al., 2010). The results demonstrated that the 144-gene classifier improved the accuracy of discrimination of true low-risk patients who may need no chemotherapy at all from patient's aggressive tumors who require intense cytotoxic treatment. The main limitation of these two studies is that a large number of genes has been included in the classifier and this might negatively influence its translation to the clinical routine as the costs to perform a gene expression analysis of 144 genes will be likely high. Even if the high number of genes analyzed can balance the outlying values of individual transcripts, and thus yield more stable classification results, the future directions for this kind of study will be construct small gene signatures with high accuracy and specificity of outcome prediction. This study strategy can more quickly facilitate the introduction of gene-based classifiers into the clinical routine use.

Another interesting gene signature was recently built (De Preter et al., 2010; Vermeulen et al., 2009). Based on an innovative data-mining strategy, the authors identified a 59-signature that was built using 30 training samples, tested on 313 test samples, and subsequently validated in a blind study on an independent set of 236 tumors. This gene signature can act as an independent risk predictor enabling the identification of patients with increased risk in the current European treatment group. This 59-gene classifier shows three important advantages compared to the previously published gene expression classifiers: the small amounts of starting material, the low number of genes, high cost-efficiency and speed of the quantification method (real-time quantitative polymerase chain reaction) and the possibility of cross lab data comparison. This gene expression based classifier mostly responds to criteria for facing future studies to identify gene signatures that may be rapidly translated into the clinical management of neuroblastoma.

In one study published in the 2010, (Fardin et al., 2010) and co-workers investigated the prognostic potential of hypoxia induced genes in neuroblastoma tumors. Hypoxia, a condition of low oxygen tension occurring in poorly vascularized areas, has profound effects on tumor cell growth, susceptibility to apoptosis, and resistance to radio- and chemotherapy. A biology-driven approach was chosen to define the hypoxia signature. The authors obtained a 62 probsets neuroblastoma hypoxia signature (NB-hypo) by performing a systematic analysis of the transcriptome of neuroblastoma cell lines cultured under hypoxic or normoxic conditions. NB-hypo signature efficiency were tested on 88 neuroblastomas, it resulted be an independent prognostic factor for neuroblastoma. This study also supports the view that hypoxia is negatively correlated with tumors' outcome. However the performance of this signature has been assessed only in a modest set of patients and of course it needs to be tested in diverse and larger cohorts of neuroblastoma patients.

3.1 Gene expression profiles of non-coding RNA

MicroRNA (miRNA), a class of small non-coding RNA that regulates gene expression at a post-trascriptional level, has been studied in the context of cancer, and promising miRNA biomarkers have been identified for numerous major cancer types. miRNA are molecules comprising 22-25 nucleotide and function as negative regulators of gene expression. Literature data show that miRNAs can have a role in neuroblastoma and their expression correlates to prognosis, diagnosis and response to treatment. A recent whole genome search for MYCN target miRNA promoters differentially repressed under high MYCN conditions has indicated two miRs, miR-591 and miR-558, as potent tumor suppressors (Shohet et al., 2011). An other interesting study, conducted by Lin and co-workers, has analyzed 66 neuroblastoma tumors using a plausible neural networks to select a combination of 15 biomarkers that consist of 12 miRNAs' signature, expression levels of Dicer and Drosha (miRNA processing enzymes that are required for the maturation of miRNAs), and age at diagnosis, were able to segregate all patients into four distinct patterns that were highly predictive of clinical outcome (Lin et al., 2010).

4. Genome Wide Association Studies (GWAS) of neuroblastoma

GWAS is indicated as an unbiased approach to revealing the risk alleles for genetically complex non-Mendelian disorders. One important characteristic of this advance technology is rapidly scanning markers across the complete sets of DNA, or genomes, of many people to find genetic variations associated with a particular disease. Indeed, during the past few years, this methodological approach has identified several affordable associations between specific chromosomal loci and common complex human disease. So far, GAWS have identified more than 200 new common low-penetrance susceptibility loci for cancers (NHGRI GWAS Catalog; http://www.genome.gov/gwastudies/). The discovery of new genetic associations is particularly useful in determining the genetic risk profile for a specific disease and so to develop better strategies to detect, treat and prevent the disease.

Moreover, GWAS analysis is very useful in identifying new disease genes and so to understand the functional consequences of these genes.

Recently, by using a GWAS approach, we have identified multiple genetic risk factors associated with the neuroblastoma development and its clinical phenotypes (Table 1). Our data unequivocally demonstrate that multiple common DNA variations cooperate to increase the risk for neuroblastic malignant transformation. In the 2008, we identified the first predisposition locus by genotyping over 550,000 germline DNA SNPs from 1,752 neuroblastoma pantients and 4.171 controls of European descent (Maris et al., 2008). Three common SNPs located in intronic region of the predicted genes LINC00340 (chromosome 6p22) were strongly associated with the development of sporadic neuroblastoma. Of particular interest was the finding that not only were the three 6p22 SNPs associated with the likelihood of developing neuroblastoma, but patients who carried the 6p22 risk alleles were more likely to develop the clinically aggressive form of the disease and suffer tumor recurrence (Maris et al., 2008). We therefore performed a second genetic analysis, this time limiting the cases to those patients with high-risk neuroblastoma; we were able to identify a

Table 1. Neuroblastoma susceptibility genes and variants identified by GWAS

Gene	Most Associated genetic variant	Type	Location	Risk allele	§Estimated odds ratio	§P-value	Protein function	References
LINC00340 *FLJ22536*	rs6939340	SNP	6p22	A	1.37	9.33×10^{-15}	°Long intergenic non-protein coding RNA 340	Maris et al., 2008
BARD1	rs6435862	SNP	2q35	G	1.68	$8.65X10^{-18}$	Binding partner of BRCA1; BRCA1–BARD1 heterodimer has tumour-suppressor functions; splice variant BARD1β has oncogenic functions	Capasso et al., 2009
LMO1	rs110419	SNP	11p15	A	1.34	$5.2x10^{-16}$	Cysteine-rich transcriptional regulator with two LIM zinc-binding domains	Wang et al., 2011
DUSP12	rs1027702	SNP	1q23	T	2.01	$3.38x10^{-06}$	Member of the dual specificity protein phosphatase subfamily	Nguyen le et al., 2011
DDX4	rs2619046	SNP	5q11	T	1.48	$5.70x10^{-05}$	DEAD box proteins, characterized by the conserved motif Asp-Glu-Ala-Asp (DEAD), are putative RNA helicases	Nguyen le et al., 2011
IL31RA	rs10055201	SNP	5q11	A	1.49	$3.85x10^{-05}$	Type I cytokine receptor family	Nguyen le et al., 2011
HSD17B12	rs11037575	SNP	11p11	C	1.67	$1.07x10^{-06}$	Multifunctional isoenzyme functional in the conversion of estrone to estradiol (E2), and elongation of long-chain fatty acids	Nguyen le et al., 2011
NBPF23	*rs11579261-rs3853524	CNV	1q21	-	2.49	$2.97x10^{-17}$	Novel member of the NBPF (neuroblastoma breakpoint family)	Diskin et al., 2009

°Official full name provided by HUGO Gene Nomenclature Committee (HGNC)
*Start point SNP and end point SNP of the CN
§Odds Ratios and P-values as reported in the corresponding published research article
Abbrevations: SNP, single nucleotide polymorphism; copy number variation

Table 1. Neuroblastoma susceptibility genes and variants identified by GWAS

new association with common intronic and nonsynonymous SNPs at the BARD1 tumor-suppressor gene (Capasso et al., 2009). In this GAWS, we compared the allelic frequencies between more than 500 high-risk patients and 2043 controls, six SNPs at chromosome 2q35 located within introns 1, 3 and 4 of BARD1 reached the genome-wide significant level. Furthermore, by TaqMan based genotyping in 540 high-risk neuroblastoma cases and 1,142 controls, we demonstrated that also four nonsynonymous SNPs were genetic risk factors for the susceptibility to the development of high-risk neuroblastoma. BARD1 has been previously implicated in several cancers due to its association with BRCA1, a well-known breast cancer susceptibility gene. BARD1 heterodimerizes with BRCA1 and is thought to be necessary for the tumor suppressive function of BRCA1. Studies are ongoing to understand how sequence variations within BARD1 influence neuroblastoma tumorigenesis.

Most recently, increasing of the number of cases and controls of the original GWAS cohort allowed us to identify a further predisposition locus at 11p15, within LIM domain only 1 (LMO1) gene, a transcriptional regulator (using 1,627 neuroblastoma patients and 3,254 controls) (Wang et al., 2011). Two SNPs were found to be associated with neuroblastoma in general and with high-risk neuroblastoma. Additional genomic analyses of DNA from 701 primary neuroblastoma tumors demonstrated that a duplication of the LMO1, presents in 12% of tumors, resulted in increased expression of LMO1 in cell lines and tumors and was associated with more advanced disease. Further functional experiments indicated LMO1 as an oncogene involved in the pathogenesis of neuroblastoma.

To confirm the validity of these findings beyond the Caucasian population, an association test was performed by using the genotype data from 326 self-reported African-American neuroblastoma patients and 2500 African-American unaffected children. Devoto and co-workers showed the first preliminary results at 60th annual meeting of The American Society of Human Genetics in November 2010. Among the known loci, the one that was most consistently replicated was BARD1, with six SNPs showing p-value less than 0.05 (smallest p-value equal to 0.0004 for rs7587476). Two SNPs in the LINC00340 region had nominally significant p-value, and only one in LMO1. Overall these results support the hypothesis that the same genetic factors affect risk of neuroblastoma in both populations.

An other published article that utilized a GWAS approach to detect allelic risk variants suggested again that neuroblastoma is both phenotypically and genetically heterogeneous. Indeed, an analysis restricted to low-risk neuroblastoma cases identified predisposing loci for less aggressive disease within four additional genes: *DUSP12* at 1q23.3, *DDX4* and IL21RA both at 5q11.2 and *HSD17B12* at 11p11.2 (Nguyen le et al., 2011). Interestingly, the same risk alleles resulted to be not associated with high-risk neuroblastoma. Furthermore, a single SNP replication analysis in an Italian cohort of 115 low-risk cases and 680 controls showed that the three most significant SNPs (rs1027702, rs2619046, rs11037575) in the three loci that contain DUSP12, DDX4/IL31RA, and HSD17B12, respectively were confirmed to be genetic risk factors for the susceptibility to the development of low-risk neuroblastoma. Together, these results suggest that genetic initiating events may predispose not only to neuroblastoma, but to clinically relevant sub-phenotypes as well.

We are currently adding new cases and controls to our data sets for both United States population and Italian population. Moreover, we are utilizing alternative strategies for finding those genetic risk loci hidden among signals discarded by multiple testing corrections needed in the analysis of GWAS data. Toghether these two approaches will allow us to identify new genetic variants associated with neuroblastoma.

The next few years will see the completion and publication of additional genome-wide scans that involve higher resolution tools and substantially larger DNA collections than have been used before. Even when performed with exquisite resolution, however, association and epidemiology studies are limited in their power to prove causation. Thus, effective functional studies will be required that connect genetic variation with disease pathophysiology. Furthermore, while GWAS are a valuable tool for assessment of the effects of common polymorphisms, the aggregate role of low-frequency rare functional gene variants in neuroblastoma has not been properly evaluated. Uncommon variants with relatively large effects might account for part of the unexplained heritability in neuroblastoma. Moreover, some of these rare variants might reside in genes previously identified in GWAS. Rare genetic variation is not well represented in current databases or commercially available fixed arrays, and can be only ascertained by targeted deep sequencing of samples from affected individuals (Nejentsev et al., 2009).

4.1 Copy Number Variations (CNVs) based GWAS

In addition to SNP genotypes, CNVs (deletion or duplication of segments of germline DNA) represent a significant source of genetic diversity that may influence disease susceptibility. An analysis of copy number at 550,000 SNPs in germiline DNA from 1,441 neuroblastoma cases and 4,160 controls identified a common deletion polymorphism spanning less than 145-Kb at 1q21.1 associated with neuroblastoma, no duplications reached genome-wide significance (Diskin et al., 2009). A novel member of the NBPF ("neuroblastoma breakpoint family") gene family mapping within the CNV was cloned and sequenced. Expression of this transcript, termed NBPF23, was found to be significantly correlated with the underlying CNV genotype in neuroblastoma tumors and cell lines, further supporting the biological relevance of the CNV association (Diskin et al., 2009). The highest levels of NBPF23 expression were seen in fetal brain and sympathetic ganglia and expression was directly correlated with CNV status in neuroblastoma cells, implicating NBPF23 in the molecular pathogenesis of neuroblastoma. Further CNVs-based GWAS analyses are ongoing and it is likely that other CNVs affect the neuroblstoma development.

The results from GWAS are clearly telling us that common, heritable genetic variants contribute to the predisposition for sporadic neuroblastoma (Figure 1). We now can state that the neuroblastoma belongs to the group of complex genetic diseases, which are common disorders characterized by modest disease-risk heritability and multifaceted interactions between genetic and environmental factors. The full list of disease genes (susceptibility and modifiers) and environmental triggers in neuroblastoma remains incomplete (Figure 1). Moreover these studies are giving an important contribution in understanding the complex genetic architecture of neuroblastoma and in providing valuable insight into the underlying tumor biology. Identifying the genes and pathways involved in predisposing individuals to neuroblastoma may also lead us to the development of novel treatments. On the other hand, we can not state that there is an immediate clinical utility of knowing an individual genotype at these disease variants. However it is plausible to prefigure that the discovery of many others single disease risk variants, disease risk gene-gene and gene-environment interactions toghether with the development of new statistical methods (able to construct reliable disease predictor) will make feasible the clinical application of these GWAS findings in the relatively near future. Indeed, predictive modeling might be substantially created if more-penetrant variants are identified, and transcriptional signatures and accurate environmental exposures are taken into account. The translational potential of such modeling might extend to redefining disease classification, prognosticating progression, and predicting treatment responses and/or adverse effects.

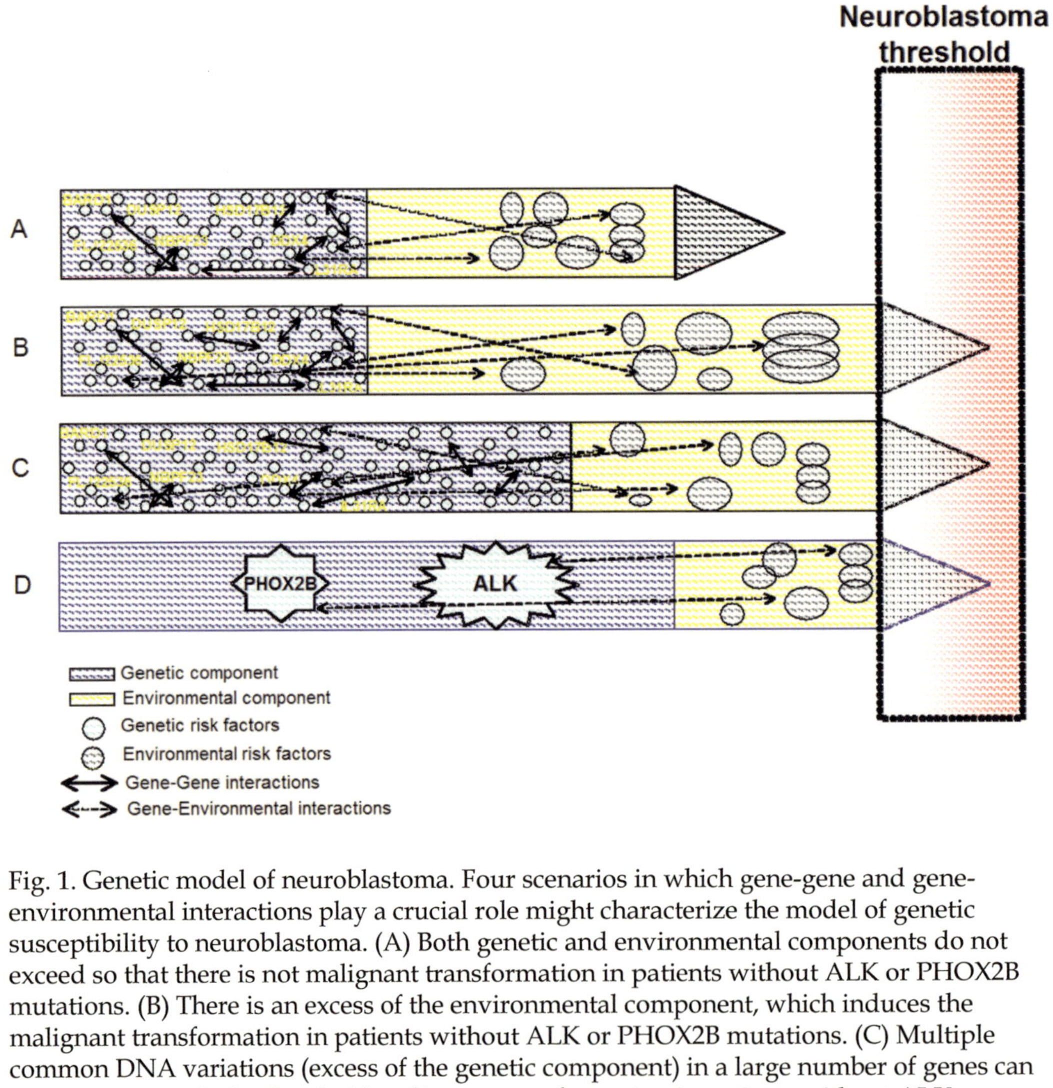

Fig. 1. Genetic model of neuroblastoma. Four scenarios in which gene-gene and gene-environmental interactions play a crucial role might characterize the model of genetic susceptibility to neuroblastoma. (A) Both genetic and environmental components do not exceed so that there is not malignant transformation in patients without ALK or PHOX2B mutations. (B) There is an excess of the environmental component, which induces the malignant transformation in patients without ALK or PHOX2B mutations. (C) Multiple common DNA variations (excess of the genetic component) in a large number of genes can cooperate to reach the threshold malignant transformation in patients without ALK or PHOX2B mutations. (D) A mutation in the ALK or PHOX2B gene results in a single, highly penetrant risk allele that interacting with environmental factors allows a malignant transformation.

5. Genome-wide linkage analysis of familial neuroblastoma

An other important genome-wide approach, utilizing high density SNP-based microarray technology, made possible the identification of three separate missense mutations within coding exons of the anaplastic lymphoma kinase (ALK) gene which were responsible for familial neuroblastoma (Mosse et al., 2008). While almost 99% of neuroblastoma occurs sporadically the remaining 1-2% of neuroblastoma has a familial history (Maris, 2010). This genome-wide approach was utilized in an attempt to identify linkage signals that might identify predisposition loci for the majority of hereditary neuroblastoma pedigrees, which do not harbor germline PHOX2B mutations (explaining only a small subset of cases). Six thousands SNPs were genotyped in 176 individuals from 20 families with hereditary neuroblastoma. ALK gene which maps to 2p23 is a receptor protein-tyrosine kinase which functions as an oncogene in many human cancers, most notably through translocations resulting in constitutive activation of the ALK kinase domain as seen in anaplastic large cell lymphomas (Morris et al., 1994), inflammatory myofibroblastic tumors (Griffin et al., 1999), squamous cell carcinomas (Jazii et al., 2006), and non-small cell lung cancers (Soda et al., 2007). The ALK and PHOX2B mutations are responsible for approximately 90% of hereditary neuroblastoma. Based on these data a genetic testing could be created for facilitating the identification of unaffected siblings who carry highly penetrant germline mutations and would justify screening in an attempt to ensure early detection of neuroblastoma. By using an exome high-throughput sequencing, researchers are now attempting to find the heritable genetic etiology in the remaining rare families with evidence of hereditary neuroblastoma that do not harbor ALK or PHOX2B germline mutations.

Of note, somatic ALK mutations or amplifications were also identified in 6-9% of sporadic cases (Chen et al., 2008; George et al., 2008; Janoueix-Lerosey et al., 2008). According to the recent success of small molecule tyrosine kinase inhibitors in a certain subset of cancers, such as gefitinib in non-small-cell lung carcinoma with epidermal growth factor receptor (EGFR) mutations, a similar therapeutic approach based on inhibition of ALK-mediated signaling will be expected to target oncogenic ALK mutations in neuroblastoma (Li and Morris, 2008).

In a recent study a novel activating mutation in ALK (F1174) in a neuroblastoma patient in the course of analysis of genomic DNA from patient biopsy samples has been identified (Martinsson et al., 2011). The appearance of this novel F1174S ALK mutant correlated with the development of aggressive disease at the patient level with emergence of therapy resistance and fatal outcome. This study points out an important issue regarding the possibility of the occurrence of genomic mutation events during the disease outcome. So, the initial screening in the first tumor biopsy of a patient is not sufficient and further molecular analyses of the ALK locus, in particular in tumor progression and/or tumor relapse, is warranted for better understanding of the treatment of neuroblastoma patients.

6. Next Generation Sequencing (NGS) of neuroblastoma

Over the past four years, there has been a fundamental shift away from the application of automated Sanger sequencing for genome analysis. The automated Sanger method is now considered as a 'first-generation' technology, and newer methods are referred to as next generation sequencing. This sequencing method that has emerged since 2005 parallelizes the sequencing process and produces millions of typically short sequence reads (50–400 bases) from amplified DNA clones. In general, the field of cancer genomics has been impacted most profoundly by the application of next generation sequencing technology, which has tremendously accelerated the pace of discovery while dramatically reducing the cost of data production. Hence, there has been a rapid progression from targeted gene re-sequencing using PCR and Sanger sequencing to either targeted, whole genome, or whole transcriptome sequencing using these massively parallel sequencing platforms, coupled with the requisite bioinformatics-based approaches to analyze the data. There are particular challenges for the detection and diagnosis of cancer genome alterations. For example, some genomic alterations in cancer are prevalent at a low frequency in clinical samples, often owing to substantial admixture with non-malignant cells. Second-generation sequencing can solve such problems (Thomas et al., 2006). Furthermore, these new sequencing methods make it feasible to discover novel chromosomal rearrangements (Campbell et al., 2008) and microbial infections (MacConaill and Meyerson, 2008) and to resolve copy number alterations at very high resolution (Campbell et al., 2008; Chiang et al., 2009).

So far, only a few studies have utilized this advanced methodology to search genetic alterations responsible of the neuroblastoma initiation. To identify potential drug targets against recurrent neuroblastoma, Morozova and colleagues used next generation RNA sequencing and/or human exon arrays to profile the transcriptomes of 11 tumor-initiating cells from six neuroblastoma patients, revealing genes that are highly expressed in the tumor-initiating cells compared with normal neural crest-like cells and unrelated cancer tissues (Morozova et al., 2010). This analysis revealed 30 targets with an available inhibitor, six of which have never been implicated in neuroblastoma. Further validation analyses were performed on one of the six novel drug targets, AURKB. Interestingly, a selective AURKB inhibitor, AZD1152, was cytotoxic to neuroblastoma tumor-initiating cells used in the study but not to normal pediatric neural crest-like precursor cells. This is the first report of AURKB inhibitors as potential therapeutics for neuroblastoma. However, AURKB inhibitors are currently in clinical trials so it is reasonable to forecast a rapid translation of this observation to neuroblastoma therapy.

Another recently published study shows that miRNA-based classifiers can be used to stratify neuroblastoma patients according to clinical course (Schulte et al., 2010). The small RNA transcriptomes of five favorable and five unfavorable neuroblastomas were analyzed using SOLiD next-generation sequencing, generating a total of more than 188,000,000 reads. Favorable and unfavorable neuroblastomas were distinguishable by hierarchical clustering of miRNA patterns. Expression of single miRNAs also differed significantly between the two groups. The authors then identified 13 candidates for novel miRNAs of which three were further validated in 70 primary neuroblastomas using RT-qPCR.

However, in literature, there is no published research article showing the use of next generation sequencing to search for somatically acquired DNA mutations in sporadic neuroblastoma. The most significant impact of next generation sequencing on cancer genomics has been the ability to re-sequence, analyze and compare the matched tumor and normal genomes of a single patient. Many studies have identified several mutations responsible of the development of diverse cancers (Bass et al., 2011; Puente et al.; Wei et al., 2011). About neuroblastoma, a large collaborative effort, the Therapeutically Applicable Research to Generate Effective Treatments (TARGET) project (http://target.cancer.gov), is leveraging genomic profiling techniques to help identify the molecular mechanisms that drive oncogenesis and to discover new therapeutic targets. The first results have been shown at 102nd Annual Meeting of American Association for Cancer Research in April 2011. So far, the exome sequencing of 81 tumor/normal pairs from high-risk neuroblasotma patients has been completed. Pugh and colleagues reported that several genes resulted significantly mutated including ALK (6 tumors) and PTPN11 (3 tumors). Interestingly, there were 27 other genes with candidate mutation frequencies in the 4-10% range, but no single gene was identified with a mutation frequency greater than 10%. Morozova and co-authors instead presented a study about a whole genome shotgun sequencing of six stage 4 MYCN-non-amplified and four stage 4 MYCN-amplified neuroblastomas cases and matched peripheral blood, as well as whole transcriptome sequencing of the corresponding tumor RNA. The analysis of tumor and normal genomes revealed an average of 1664 candidate somatic mutations per case, the majority of which were single nucleotide variants and small indels falling within introns or intergenic sequence. Moreover, an average of 10% of candidate somatic mutations in coding sequence was expressed in the transcriptome representing candidate oncogenic events. Of note, two novel somatic gene fusions, between TRIM37 on chromosome 17 and RNF121 on chromosome 11, and between LSAMP and STAG1 on chromosome 3, previously uncharacterized in neuroblastoma, were identified.

It is likely that the biggest impact of second-generation sequencing of cancer genomes will be in cancer diagnostics. The major challenge will be to make biological sense of the mountains of genomic data. This will require computational, biological and clinical analyses of the genome data. These developments might potentiate accurate genome-based diagnosis for patients with neuroblastoma. Moreover, this advanced technology will rapidly identify therapeutic targets that will have implications in developing new and effective treatments for this devastating disease.

7. Whole genome searches to open the door to the personalized medicine

Recent advances in genomics are likely to change the molecular characterization of cancer and provide a path for the personalized treatment of patients with cancer. The generation of comprehensive catalogs of genetic alterations could inform strategies for effective prevention and early detection, as well as guiding the development of therapeutics in the appropriate patient subpopulation. Genome searches also hold great potential to inform the prognosis and guide evidence-based management of early stage diseases, which comprise an increasing proportion of cancer diagnoses. It is likely that whole genome searches will drive the transition from a morphology-based to a genetics-based taxonomy of cancer, point of care decisions will become increasingly customized to the unique genomic and proteomic features of a patient's tumor. These molecular changes might be evaluated in circulating tumor cells or in tumor biopsies or in body fluids (plasma, lymph and ascites) using specific diagnostic tests that can predict the probability of clinical benefit for all treatment options.

Genome searches have provided an important contribution in the risk stratification of neuroblastoma. To date, the International Neuroblastoma Risk Group (INRG) Task Force has assessed several potential prognostic factors in 8800 patients. These factors included stage, age, lactate dehydrogenase, as well as certain genetic markers such as MYCN amplification, chromosome 1p, 17q, and 11q aberration, and ploidy. After appropriate statistical analyses, four risk groups were established and the current consensus scheme includes stage, age, histologic category, grade of tumor differentiation, MYCN status, 11q aberration, and tumor cell ploidy as final criteria (Cohn et al., 2009). According to the INRG Task Force, these four risk groups were designed to stratify children into more homogenous pretreatment groups. Despite these efforts, more needs to be done to decrease the death rates of children with neurobalstoma and the upcoming whole genome searches might play a main role in both improving risk stratification and developing more appropriate treatments. Indeed, genome-wide analyses have already identified diverse therapeutic targets and biological agents are currently tested. They include small molecule inhibitors of genetic pathways implicated in tumor growth, such as inhibitor of the phosphoinositide 3-kinase/mammalian target of rapamycin pathway; insulin-like growth factor 1 receptor; ALK; Aurora kinase A and B; tyrosine receptor kinase, and histone deacetylase inhibitors. It is plausible that by the inclusion of biological end points in large cooperative studies, further insight will be gained about the underlying pathways in the tumorigenesis of neuroblastoma, which will lead to new therapies to improve outcome.

8. Future directions

Since the publication of the Human Genome Project data, medical practice and research have entered the genome era. From a predominant focus on single genes and disease-related mutations has emerged the technology to assay the genome in its entirety and the first means to interpret findings in a comprehensive manner. Several genome-wide approaches have been used to study neuroblastoma and several information about molecular mechanisms underlying the neuroblastic malignant transformation, and genomic or genetic abnormalities associated with neuroblastoma and its clinical phenotypes have been obtained. This allows us to understand how to ameliorate therapeutic treatments of neuroblstoma and how to optimize risk group classification. However, despite extensive research, relatively few genomic markers have been implemented into routine clinical use and the survival rate for neuroblastoma high-risk patients is still low (~ 40%). Integrative genomic approaches incorporating data from high-throughput genomic technologies are needed, on the one hand, to facilitate our understanding of neuroblastoma pathogenesis and consequently to accelerate the development of more effective therapies, on the other hand, to improve risk estimation of children with neuroblastoma (Figure 2). To give strong push for the achievement of these two objectives, inter and intra-disciplinary collaborations of biologists, chemists, clinicians, computer scientists, and mathematicians are strongly warranted. Furthermore, sharing and availability on public depositories of scientific results from neuroblastoma whole genome studies and in general from cancer studies are very important start points to get the main aim of research work: increasing the percentage of children who beat this devastating disease.

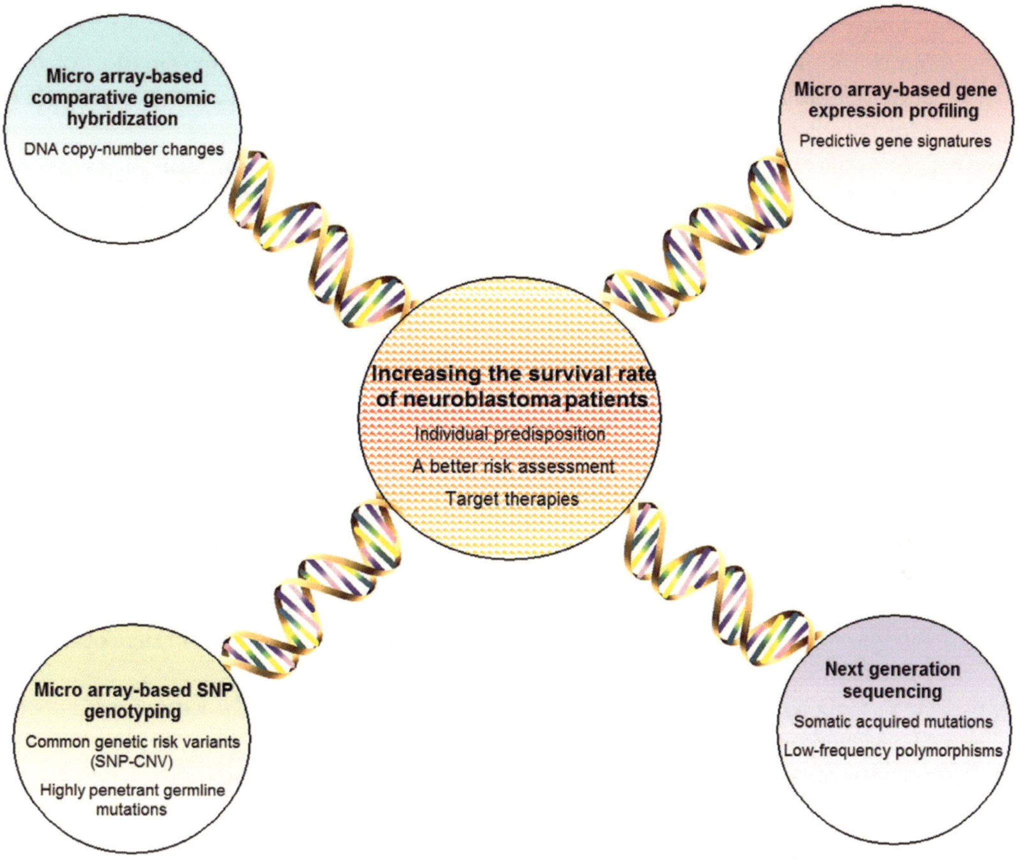

Fig. 2. Integrated genome-wide approaches in neuroblastoma. The integration of diverse genome-wide-based analyses will provide a large amount of biological and genetic information that presumably will determinate the identification of individual predisposition to the clinical sub-groups of neuroblastoma, the refinement of risk stratification and development of new and effective cures. Overall the integrated application of these approaches will lead us to improve the survival of children with high-risk neuroblastoma.

9. References

Asgharzadeh, S., Pique-Regi, R., Sposto, R., Wang, H., Yang, Y., Shimada, H., Matthay, K., Buckley, J., Ortega, A., and Seeger, R. C. (2006). Prognostic significance of gene expression profiles of metastatic neuroblastomas lacking MYCN gene amplification. J Natl Cancer Inst *98*, 1193-1203.

Bass, A. J., Lawrence, M. S., Brace, L. E., Ramos, A. H., Drier, Y., Cibulskis, K., Sougnez, C., Voet, D., Saksena, G., Sivachenko, A., *et al.* (2011). Genomic sequencing of colorectal adenocarcinomas identifies a recurrent VTI1A-TCF7L2 fusion. Nat Genet *43*, 964-968.

Best, C. J., Leiva, I. M., Chuaqui, R. F., Gillespie, J. W., Duray, P. H., Murgai, M., Zhao, Y., Simon, R., Kang, J. J., Green, J. E., *et al.* (2003). Molecular differentiation of high- and moderate-grade human prostate cancer by cDNA microarray analysis. Diagn Mol Pathol *12*, 63-70.

Campbell, P. J., Stephens, P. J., Pleasance, E. D., O'Meara, S., Li, H., Santarius, T., Stebbings, L. A., Leroy, C., Edkins, S., Hardy, C., *et al.* (2008). Identification of somatically acquired rearrangements in cancer using genome-wide massively parallel paired-end sequencing. Nat Genet *40*, 722-729.

Capasso, M., Devoto, M., Hou, C., Asgharzadeh, S., Glessner, J. T., Attiyeh, E. F., Mosse, Y. P., Kim, C., Diskin, S. J., Cole, K. A., *et al.* (2009). Common variations in BARD1 influence susceptibility to high-risk neuroblastoma. Nat Genet *41*, 718-723.

Capasso, M., and Diskin, S. J. (2010). Genetics and genomics of neuroblastoma. Cancer Treat Res *155*, 65-84.

Caren, H., Kryh, H., Nethander, M., Sjoberg, R. M., Trager, C., Nilsson, S., Abrahamsson, J., Kogner, P., and Martinsson, T. (2010). High-risk neuroblastoma tumors with 11q-deletion display a poor prognostic, chromosome instability phenotype with later onset. Proc Natl Acad Sci U S A *107*, 4323-4328.

Chen, Y., Takita, J., Choi, Y. L., Kato, M., Ohira, M., Sanada, M., Wang, L., Soda, M., Kikuchi, A., Igarashi, T., *et al.* (2008). Oncogenic mutations of ALK kinase in neuroblastoma. Nature *455*, 971-974.

Chiang, D. Y., Getz, G., Jaffe, D. B., O'Kelly, M. J., Zhao, X., Carter, S. L., Russ, C., Nusbaum, C., Meyerson, M., and Lander, E. S. (2009). High-resolution mapping of copy-number alterations with massively parallel sequencing. Nat Methods *6*, 99-103.

Cohn, S. L., Pearson, A. D., London, W. B., Monclair, T., Ambros, P. F., Brodeur, G. M., Faldum, A., Hero, B., Iehara, T., Machin, D., *et al.* (2009). The International Neuroblastoma Risk Group (INRG) classification system: an INRG Task Force report. J Clin Oncol *27*, 289-297.

De Preter, K., Vermeulen, J., Brors, B., Delattre, O., Eggert, A., Fischer, M., Janoueix-Lerosey, I., Lavarino, C., Maris, J. M., Mora, J., *et al.* (2010). Accurate outcome prediction in neuroblastoma across independent data sets using a multigene signature. Clin Cancer Res *16*, 1532-1541.

Diskin, S. J., Hou, C., Glessner, J. T., Attiyeh, E. F., Laudenslager, M., Bosse, K., Cole, K., Mosse, Y. P., Wood, A., Lynch, J. E., *et al.* (2009). Copy number variation at 1q21.1 associated with neuroblastoma. Nature *459*, 987-991.

Fardin, P., Barla, A., Mosci, S., Rosasco, L., Verri, A., Versteeg, R., Caron, H. N., Molenaar, J. J., Ora, I., Eva, A., *et al.* (2010). A biology-driven approach identifies the hypoxia gene signature as a predictor of the outcome of neuroblastoma patients. Mol Cancer *9*, 185.

George, R. E., Sanda, T., Hanna, M., Frohling, S., Luther, W., 2nd, Zhang, J., Ahn, Y., Zhou, W., London, W. B., McGrady, P., *et al.* (2008). Activating mutations in ALK provide a therapeutic target in neuroblastoma. Nature *455*, 975-978.

Griffin, C. A., Hawkins, A. L., Dvorak, C., Henkle, C., Ellingham, T., and Perlman, E. J. (1999). Recurrent involvement of 2p23 in inflammatory myofibroblastic tumors. Cancer Res *59*, 2776-2780.

Hoehner, J. C., Gestblom, C., Hedborg, F., Sandstedt, B., Olsen, L., and Pahlman, S. (1996). A developmental model of neuroblastoma: differentiating stroma-poor tumors' progress along an extra-adrenal chromaffin lineage. Lab Invest *75*, 659-675.

Janoueix-Lerosey, I., Lequin, D., Brugieres, L., Ribeiro, A., de Pontual, L., Combaret, V., Raynal, V., Puisieux, A., Schleiermacher, G., Pierron, G., *et al.* (2008). Somatic and germline activating mutations of the ALK kinase receptor in neuroblastoma. Nature *455*, 967-970.

Janoueix-Lerosey, I., Schleiermacher, G., Michels, E., Mosseri, V., Ribeiro, A., Lequin, D., Vermeulen, J., Couturier, J., Peuchmaur, M., Valent, A., *et al.* (2009). Overall genomic pattern is a predictor of outcome in neuroblastoma. J Clin Oncol *27*, 1026-1033.

Jazii, F. R., Najafi, Z., Malekzadeh, R., Conrads, T. P., Ziaee, A. A., Abnet, C., Yazdznbod, M., Karkhane, A. A., and Salekdeh, G. H. (2006). Identification of squamous cell carcinoma associated proteins by proteomics and loss of beta tropomyosin expression in esophageal cancer. World J Gastroenterol *12*, 7104-7112.

Khan, J., Wei, J. S., Ringner, M., Saal, L. H., Ladanyi, M., Westermann, F., Berthold, F., Schwab, M., Antonescu, C. R., Peterson, C., and Meltzer, P. S. (2001). Classification and diagnostic prediction of cancers using gene expression profiling and artificial neural networks. Nat Med *7*, 673-679.

Li, R., and Morris, S. W. (2008). Development of anaplastic lymphoma kinase (ALK) small-molecule inhibitors for cancer therapy. Med Res Rev *28*, 372-412.

Lin, R. J., Lin, Y. C., Chen, J., Kuo, H. H., Chen, Y. Y., Diccianni, M. B., London, W. B., Chang, C. H., and Yu, A. L. (2010). microRNA signature and expression of Dicer and Drosha can predict prognosis and delineate risk groups in neuroblastoma. Cancer Res *70*, 7841-7850.

MacConaill, L., and Meyerson, M. (2008). Adding pathogens by genomic subtraction. Nat Genet *40*, 380-382.

Maris, J. M. (2005). The biologic basis for neuroblastoma heterogeneity and risk stratification. Curr Opin Pediatr *17*, 7-13.

Maris, J. M. (2010). Recent advances in neuroblastoma. N Engl J Med *362*, 2202-2211.

Maris, J. M., Mosse, Y. P., Bradfield, J. P., Hou, C., Monni, S., Scott, R. H., Asgharzadeh, S., Attiyeh, E. F., Diskin, S. J., Laudenslager, M., *et al.* (2008). Chromosome 6p22 locus associated with clinically aggressive neuroblastoma. N Engl J Med *358*, 2585-2593.

Martinsson, T., Eriksson, T., Abrahamsson, J., Caren, H., Hansson, M., Kogner, P., Kamaraj, S., Schonherr, C., Weinmar, J., Ruuth, K., *et al.* (2011). Appearance of the novel activating F1174S ALK mutation in neuroblastoma correlates with aggressive tumor progression and unresponsiveness to therapy. Cancer Res *71*, 98-105.

Minturn, J. E., Evans, A. E., Villablanca, J. G., Yanik, G. A., Park, J. R., Shusterman, S., Groshen, S., Hellriegel, E. T., Bensen-Kennedy, D., Matthay, K. K., *et al.* (2011). Phase I trial of lestaurtinib for children with refractory neuroblastoma: a new approaches to neuroblastoma therapy consortium study. Cancer Chemother Pharmacol *68*, 1057-1065.

Morozova, O., Vojvodic, M., Grinshtein, N., Hansford, L. M., Blakely, K. M., Maslova, A., Hirst, M., Cezard, T., Morin, R. D., Moore, R., *et al.* (2010). System-level analysis of neuroblastoma tumor-initiating cells implicates AURKB as a novel drug target for neuroblastoma. Clin Cancer Res *16*, 4572-4582.

Morris, S. W., Kirstein, M. N., Valentine, M. B., Dittmer, K. G., Shapiro, D. N., Saltman, D. L., and Look, A. T. (1994). Fusion of a kinase gene, ALK, to a nucleolar protein gene, NPM, in non-Hodgkin's lymphoma. Science *263*, 1281-1284.

Mosse, Y. P., Greshock, J., Margolin, A., Naylor, T., Cole, K., Khazi, D., Hii, G., Winter, C., Shahzad, S., Asziz, M. U., *et al.* (2005). High-resolution detection and mapping of genomic DNA alterations in neuroblastoma. Genes Chromosomes Cancer *43*, 390-403.

Mosse, Y. P., Laudenslager, M., Longo, L., Cole, K. A., Wood, A., Attiyeh, E. F., Laquaglia, M. J., Sennett, R., Lynch, J. E., Perri, P., *et al.* (2008). Identification of ALK as a major familial neuroblastoma predisposition gene. Nature *455*, 930-935.

Nejentsev, S., Walker, N., Riches, D., Egholm, M., and Todd, J. A. (2009). Rare variants of IFIH1, a gene implicated in antiviral responses, protect against type 1 diabetes. Science *324*, 387-389.

Nguyen le, B., Diskin, S. J., Capasso, M., Wang, K., Diamond, M. A., Glessner, J., Kim, C., Attiyeh, E. F., Mosse, Y. P., Cole, K., *et al.* (2011). Phenotype restricted genome-wide association study using a gene-centric approach identifies three low-risk neuroblastoma susceptibility Loci. PLoS Genet *7*, e1002026.

Oberthuer, A., Berthold, F., Warnat, P., Hero, B., Kahlert, Y., Spitz, R., Ernestus, K., Konig, R., Haas, S., Eils, R., *et al.* (2006). Customized oligonucleotide microarray gene expression-based classification of neuroblastoma patients outperforms current clinical risk stratification. J Clin Oncol *24*, 5070-5078.

Oberthuer, A., Hero, B., Berthold, F., Juraeva, D., Faldum, A., Kahlert, Y., Asgharzadeh, S., Seeger, R., Scaruffi, P., Tonini, G. P., *et al.* (2010). Prognostic impact of gene expression-based classification for neuroblastoma. J Clin Oncol *28*, 3506-3515.

Ohira, M., and Nakagawara, A. (2010). Global genomic and RNA profiles for novel risk stratification of neuroblastoma. Cancer Sci *101*, 2295-2301.

Ohira, M., Oba, S., Nakamura, Y., Isogai, E., Kaneko, S., Nakagawa, A., Hirata, T., Kubo, H., Goto, T., Yamada, S., *et al.* (2005). Expression profiling using a tumor-specific cDNA microarray predicts the prognosis of intermediate risk neuroblastomas. Cancer Cell *7*, 337-350.

Okutsu, J., Tsunoda, T., Kaneta, Y., Katagiri, T., Kitahara, O., Zembutsu, H., Yanagawa, R., Miyawaki, S., Kuriyama, K., Kubota, N., *et al.* (2002). Prediction of chemosensitivity for patients with acute myeloid leukemia, according to expression levels of 28 genes selected by genome-wide complementary DNA microarray analysis. Mol Cancer Ther *1*, 1035-1042.

Pinkel, D., and Albertson, D. G. (2005). Array comparative genomic hybridization and its applications in cancer. Nat Genet *37 Suppl*, S11-17.

Puente, X. S., Pinyol, M., Quesada, V., Conde, L., Ordonez, G. R., Villamor, N., Escaramis, G., Jares, P., Bea, S., Gonzalez-Diaz, M., *et al.* Whole-genome sequencing identifies recurrent mutations in chronic lymphocytic leukaemia. Nature *475*, 101-105.

Schulte, J. H., Marschall, T., Martin, M., Rosenstiel, P., Mestdagh, P., Schlierf, S., Thor, T., Vandesompele, J., Eggert, A., Schreiber, S., *et al.* (2010). Deep sequencing reveals differential expression of microRNAs in favorable versus unfavorable neuroblastoma. Nucleic Acids Res *38*, 5919-5928.

Shohet, J. M., Ghosh, R., Coarfa, C., Ludwig, A., Benham, A. L., Chen, Z., Patterson, D. M., Barbieri, E., Mestdagh, P., Sikorski, D. N., *et al.* (2011). A genome-wide search for promoters that respond to increased MYCN reveals both new oncogenic and tumor suppressor microRNAs associated with aggressive neuroblastoma. Cancer Res *71*, 3841-3851.

Soda, M., Choi, Y. L., Enomoto, M., Takada, S., Yamashita, Y., Ishikawa, S., Fujiwara, S., Watanabe, H., Kurashina, K., Hatanaka, H., *et al.* (2007). Identification of the transforming EML4-ALK fusion gene in non-small-cell lung cancer. Nature *448*, 561-566.

Thomas, R. K., Nickerson, E., Simons, J. F., Janne, P. A., Tengs, T., Yuza, Y., Garraway, L. A., LaFramboise, T., Lee, J. C., Shah, K., *et al.* (2006). Sensitive mutation detection in heterogeneous cancer specimens by massively parallel picoliter reactor sequencing. Nat Med *12*, 852-855.

Tomioka, N., Oba, S., Ohira, M., Misra, A., Fridlyand, J., Ishii, S., Nakamura, Y., Isogai, E., Hirata, T., Yoshida, Y., *et al.* (2008). Novel risk stratification of patients with neuroblastoma by genomic signature, which is independent of molecular signature. Oncogene *27*, 441-449.

van 't Veer, L. J., Dai, H., van de Vijver, M. J., He, Y. D., Hart, A. A., Mao, M., Peterse, H. L., van der Kooy, K., Marton, M. J., Witteveen, A. T., *et al.* (2002). Gene expression profiling predicts clinical outcome of breast cancer. Nature *415*, 530-536.

Vasselli, J. R., Shih, J. H., Iyengar, S. R., Maranchie, J., Riss, J., Worrell, R., Torres-Cabala, C., Tabios, R., Mariotti, A., Stearman, R., *et al.* (2003). Predicting survival in patients with metastatic kidney cancer by gene-expression profiling in the primary tumor. Proc Natl Acad Sci U S A *100*, 6958-6963.

Vermeulen, J., De Preter, K., Naranjo, A., Vercruysse, L., Van Roy, N., Hellemans, J., Swerts, K., Bravo, S., Scaruffi, P., Tonini, G. P., *et al.* (2009). Predicting outcomes for children with neuroblastoma using a multigene-expression signature: a retrospective SIOPEN/COG/GPOH study. Lancet Oncol *10*, 663-671.

Wang, K., Diskin, S. J., Zhang, H., Attiyeh, E. F., Winter, C., Hou, C., Schnepp, R. W., Diamond, M., Bosse, K., Mayes, P. A., *et al.* (2011). Integrative genomics identifies LMO1 as a neuroblastoma oncogene. Nature *469*, 216-220.

Wang, Q., Diskin, S., Rappaport, E., Attiyeh, E., Mosse, Y., Shue, D., Seiser, E., Jagannathan, J., Shusterman, S., Bansal, M., *et al.* (2006). Integrative genomics identifies distinct molecular classes of neuroblastoma and shows that multiple genes are targeted by regional alterations in DNA copy number. Cancer Res *66*, 6050-6062.

Wei, J. S., Greer, B. T., Westermann, F., Steinberg, S. M., Son, C. G., Chen, Q. R., Whiteford, C. C., Bilke, S., Krasnoselsky, A. L., Cenacchi, N., *et al.* (2004). Prediction of clinical outcome using gene expression profiling and artificial neural networks for patients with neuroblastoma. Cancer Res *64*, 6883-6891.

Wei, X., Walia, V., Lin, J. C., Teer, J. K., Prickett, T. D., Gartner, J., Davis, S., Stemke-Hale, K., Davies, M. A., Gershenwald, J. E., *et al.* (2011). Exome sequencing identifies GRIN2A as frequently mutated in melanoma. Nat Genet *43*, 442-446.

12

Neuroblastoma – Molecular Basis for Diagnosis and Staging System

Priscila Torres Babié, Ramón de J. Ropero Toirac,
Jesús de los Santos Renó and Samira Proveyer Derich
National Cancer Registry Department,
National Oncology and Radiobiology Institute, Havana,
National Cancer Control Unit of the Cuban Ministry of Public Health,
Cuba

1. Introduction

The origin of neuroblastoma was first described in Berlin, by Virchow in 1864, when he gave it the name "Glioma". In 1891, Marchand observed similarities between this tumor and the ganglia of the Sympathetic Nervous System in its developmental phase, and Wright demonstrated that the cellular type of this tumor was similar to the one observed in the embryonic stage of the medulla of the adrenal glands. The name Neuroblastoma was proposed by James Homer Wright in 1910, while Morgan observed microscopically an adrenal tumor with fibrillar characteristics. In 1914, Herxheimer, using Bielschowsky's method of silver staining, showed that the fibrillar structures were nerves fibers originating in the nerve cell proper, and not in the cells of the sheaths nerve as it has been noted in the case of a benign ganglioneuroma. Robertson indicated that any important series of these tumors of the neural crest were characterized by a variety of histological grades ranging from benign, with well differentiated cellular elements, to highly anaplastic forms. Rinscheid observed little fibrillar elements inside the tumor cells that were similar to those observed in normal neuroblasts. These findings were later confirmed by Murray and Stout in investigations done in vitro cultures of Neuroblastoma cells. Pepper described a supposed propensity for hepatic metastases (Pepper Metastases) in young children with Neuroblastoma, and Hutchison described a predilection for skeletal metastases(especially in the skull) from a primary Adrenal lesion in older children (Hutchinson metastases) In 1916, William Barlett, in Missouri, achieved the first successful tumor resection in a boy that survived for more than 15 years. Cushing and Worbach reported in 1922, in a 10 review, the progression of neuroblastoma to ganglioneuroblastoma. In 1928, Fill and Dresser used radiotherapy as treatment for neuroblastoma without success. Cytotoxic agents were introduced in 1940 without therapeutic results. In 1957, Mason published a report of a boy with neuroblastoma whose urine contained amine vasoconstrictors. This discovery contributed to the best understanding of neuroblastoma and its possible origin in the sympathetic nervous system [1].

He noted that it was common to have spontaneous regression of microscopic group of cells within the Neuroblastoma, called Neuroblastoma in Situ. According to Beckwith and Perrin, in 1963, this spontaneous regression occurred almost 40 times more frequently than the number of well defined true clinical cases.

In 1965, James and colleagues (St Jude's Children Hospital), using combination chemotherapy appeared to have a small effect on the survival of these patients.

2. Epidemiology

The incidence of cancer children is analyzed according to the International Classification of Cancer in Childhood [2], which since its first edition has taken into account the classification of Birch and Marsden [3] which divides all the morphologies in twelve groups and forty seven diagnostic subgroups. The third edition of the International Classification of Cancer of Childhood is based on the third edition of the International Classification for Oncology (CIE-OR 3) [4], where all the morphological changes published in this classification have been upgraded. Neuroblastoma and Ganglioneuroblastoma are within group IVa of this classification.

Neuroblastoma (NB) is the most common neural crest derived extra cranial solid tumour of childhood and arises from sympathetic nervous tissue origins. It's the most common solid tumour in children younger than 5 years of age. It is the fourth most common paediatric malignancy, accounting for 7-10% of all childhood cancers and the most common cancer diagnosed during infancy with a median age at diagnosis of 18 months. Neuroblastoma is the fourth pediatric most frequent tumor and it burdens 6-10% of all cancers of the childhood. The highest incidence is during the first year of life, when about 1-2% of the cases are congenital tumors. It is often described as enigmatic and unpredictable disease and the incidence of spontaneous regressions is much greater than in any other human cancer [5, 6]. The age range is wide, including children older than 5 years of age, in which only 10% of the cases are reported [5].

There are geographical differences in the incidence of Neuroblastoma. In the United States the frequency is reported to be 8-9: 1000000 children, while a screening of the population in Japan in the years 1984-2002 estimated the incidence to be approximately 180:1 000 0000 [6]. In the United Kingdom only around 75 new cases have been diagnosed every year, in general, about 6 of each 100 cases of cancer in children younger than 15 years in that country [5,6,7]. In Germany, one of each 5000 children is affected, that is to say that in that country, every year, about 150 children are diagnosed with this disease. In Cuba, between the years 2000-2003, it represented 3,3% of tumors in infants [8].

Neuroblastoma is more common in Caucasian children with a slight prevalence in boys. The ratio of male to female is 1.3: 1 [12].

It is difficult to find population data about the mortality for this tumor because the data on mortality, published by the statistical registrations at world level, are based on the anatomical localization of the tumor and not related to its morphology, This makes it difficult to obtain accurate data to evaluate the mortality rate of Neuroblastoma, due to its propensity to present itself in multiple anatomical locations. Therefore we suggest that the information about infant mortality be reported by diagnostic groups as well as the incidence.

3. Cytogenetic and molecular characteristics

According to Knudson and Strong (1972), 20% of All neuroblastomas are inherited through an autosomal dominant pattern, whether solitary, bilateral or multifocal tumors. It can have several abnormalities in the karyotype, but the deletion of the short arm of chromosome number 1 is found in 70-80% of all patients with neuroblastoma14. The malignant transformation and persistence of the state of differentiated cells of the neural crest can be the result of the failure of these cells to respond to the normal signals that are responsible for the normal morphological differentiation. The factors involved in the cascade of events are not well known, but probably involve one or more lines of the binding receptor. One of the more popular and well studied lines is the Nerve Growth Factor (NGF) and its receptor (NGFR).

Tumours with N-myc amplification or loss of heterozygosis for chromosome 1p generally have a poor prognosis. NB cells vary in relation to their differentiation stage, with aggressive NB tumors deriving from more immature NB cells. These NB tumors may be present as phenotypically distinct groups of NB cell types (i.e.neuroblastic, neuroendocrine) organized in lobular structures with a central necrotic/hypoxic zone. Recent evidence has demonstrated that NB cells growing in these necrotic/hypoxic zones undergo a gene expression switch involving decreased expression of neuronal/neuroendocrine marker genes, but induced gene expression of neural crest sympathetic progenitor markers. These data, indicating that hypoxia causes dedifferentiation of NB cells to proliferative immature neuroblast-like cells, suggest potential activation of epithelial mesenchyme transition mechanisms (EMT). Although EMTs occur during critical phases of embryonic development in many animal species, it is now well recognized that EMT is a potential mechanism for cancer progression. However, the activation of these events in hypoxic NB cells remains largely undetermined [16].

Recently, continuous lines of human NB cells in culture have established that enzyme activities associated with neurotransmitter biosynthesis have been detected in approximately 10 independently derived cell lines [10]. The unresolved questions are whether and to what extent an individual tumour consists of a mixture of functionally differing neuronal phenotypes and whether and to what extent a single NB cell may have the potential for synthesis of more than one transmitter. Results of several combined clinical and biochemical studies suggest that the cells established in culture reflect the characteristics of the tumour from which they were derived. Although karyotype analysis of the human cell lines has revealed the presence of consistent marker chromosomes suggestive of clonal origin of individual neuroblastomas, the possibility of functional diversity and multipotentiality of the tumor cells in vivo cannot be explored by studying the tumour cell population as a whole. To obtain evidence regarding functional properties as well as phenotypic stability of human NB cells, it was isolated clones from the NB lines SK-N-SH and SK-N-MC and began their characterization. These 2 parental lines were compared to a hitherto uncharacterized set of NB lines, SK-N-BE(1) and SK-N-BE(2), isolated at different times from the same patient and possessing several biological and biochemical features in common [17].

Genetic studies have an important role in formulating the prognosis in children with neuroblastoma, because certain acquired genetic abnormalities in the tumour cells correlate closely with the clinical outcome. Established indicators of the aggressiveness of the tumour and poor outcome include the deletion of the short arm of chromosome 1 (1p), the amplification of the N -myc gene, and near diploidy or near tetraploidy. Conversely, the presence of 1p, single copies of N -myc, near triploidy, and expression of the TRK gene are significantly associated with a favorable prognosis. Recent methods revealed that the gain of material from chromosome 17 is the most frequent genetic abnormality of NB cells, with an incidence ranging from 63 to 83 percent. This gain may consist of an entire chromosome 17 (e.g., tetrasomy17 in a triploid tumour) or of only the distal segment of the long arm, 17q21–qter. Such a partial gain is strongly associated with risk factors: age of more than one year, presence of advanced disease, deletion of 1p, amplification of the N -myc gene, and unfavourable ploidy. The principal mechanism underlying partial gain of 17q is an unbalanced translocation, with a variety of partner chromosomes. The segment on the partner chromosome distal to the breakpoint is lost, and a segment of 17q translocates to that site [18].

It is also found on virtually all unipotent and multipotent colony-forming cells, on blast colony-forming cells, and on precursors of colony-forming cells detectable in long-term marrow culture. This antigen has been identified by antibodies MY-10, BI-3C5, ICH3, and 12-8. Previous work has demonstrated that isolated autologous CD34+ marrow cells can engraft lethally irradiated baboon, It has been observed that the CD34 antigen is not detected on tumour cells from patients with most solid tumors including breast cancer and neuroblastoma. In viitro studies have demonstrated that immunoadsorption with antibody 12-8 can be used to separate normal marrow progenitors from tumor cells. There is considerable evidence suggesting that ATP functions as an extracellular signaling molecule in neural and nonneural mammalian tissues. In central and peripheral synapses, ATP mediates fast excitatory neurotransmission. In the autonomic nervous system, ATP is a major purinergic cotransmitter that is often colocalized in secretory vesicles with norepinephrine or acetylcholine. In the vascular system, aggregating platelets secrete ATP and ADP, which stimulate the release of nitric oxide and other vasodilators from the endothelium. In the immune system, ATP modulates macrophage phagocytosis and mast cell degranulation. In the human airway epithelium, ATP stimulates trans-epithelial ion transport, an effect that may underlie the therapeutic effect of ATP and UTP in the treatment of cystic fibrosis-related lung disease. It has been postulated that these responses to extracellular ATP are mediated by specific plasma membrane receptors, called P2 purinergic receptors. Based on agonist selectivity and signalling properties, five subclasses of P2 receptor have been tentatively defined: three subclasses of receptors (P2T, P2U, and P2y) that are believed to signal through G proteins, one subclass (P2X) that is believed to be a ligand-gated cation channel, and one subclass (P2z) that is present on mast cells, macrophages, and fibroblasts, but whose signalling mechanism is less well understood. G protein-coupled P2 receptors are found in numerous cultured cell lines, where they have been shown to activate signal transduction systems that involve the breakdown of membrane phospholipids and the elevation of cytoplasmic free Ca2+. Ionotropic P2X receptors carry Na+, K+, and Ca2+ currents and appear to be predominantly expressed in neural and neuromuscular tissues. A more complete characterization of this putative family of P2 purinergic receptors has been hampered by the complete lack of specific P2 receptor antagonists, radioligands, and cloned receptor cDNAs. To circumvent this difficulty, we have used a Xenopus laevis oocyte expression cloning strategy to isolate a cDNA encoding a functional P2U receptor from NG108-15 neuroblastoma x glioma hybrid cells [19].

Of considerable interest in connection of herpes simplex virus 1 (HSV-1) with this disease are the genes that confer the capacity to replicate in the central nervous system (CNS) tissues. The y134.5 gene is located in the inverted repeats flanking the long component of viral DNA and therefore the gene is present in two copies per genome Its location is consistent with previous reports showing that a locus that affected the capacity of the virus to multiply in the CNS tissues mapped at the right end of the long component of HSV DNA in the prototype arrangement [20].

4. Forms of clinical presentation

Neuroblastoma has been called the great imitator due to its varied clinical presentations, related to the anatomical distribution of the Sympathetic Nervous System, location of the primary tumor, metastasis and metabolic byproduct of the tumor.

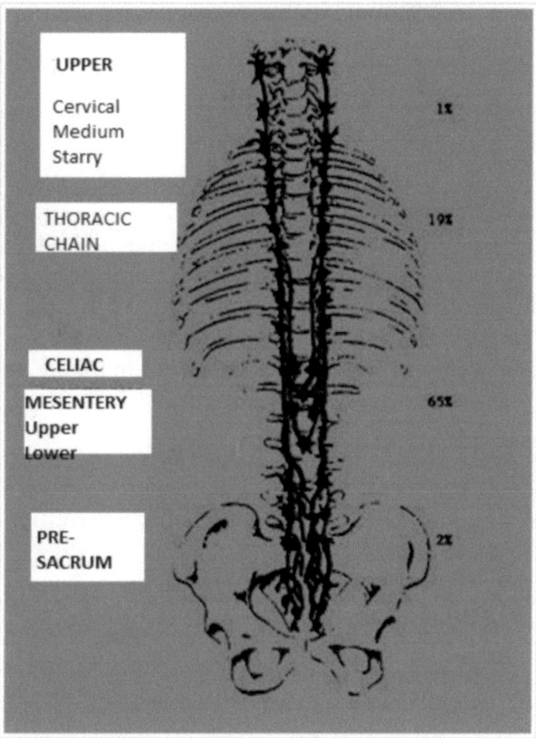

From: Bowman LC et to 1994 J. Clin Oncol 9: 1599 - 1608

Fig. 1. Anatomical distribution of the sympathetic nervous system and frequency of localization of Neuroblastoma according to regions.

Seventy five percent of primary Neuroblastoma occur in the abdomen, and most of these happen in the Adrenal (50%) Glands. As a result, most of the children affected complain of abdominal discomfort, such as fullness and, or abdominal distension. The most common symptoms are related to pain in the abdominal mass and the bones, secondary to metastatic neuroblastoma. The complaints of fatigue, pain in bones, and changes in intestinal habits can contribute to the exact diagnosis. The physical findings could include hepatomegaly, hypopigmented subcutaneous nodules, big, firm irregular abdominal mass.

Typically children with localized disease are asymptomatic, while {the} children with disseminated neuroblastoma are generally sick and they can have systemic manifestations, including fever of unknown origin, marked weight loss, anorexia, diarrhea, growth problems, general malaise, irritability and bone pain, difficulty walking, subcutaneous nodules, hepatomegaly, adenopathy, asthenia, paleness, proptosis, periorbital hematoma, hypertension, paraparesis, paraplegia, cerebellar ataxia [9,10].

At the time of diagnosis, the site of the neuroblastoma is predictable depending on the patient's age. Infants often present with compression of the Sympathetic Ganglia in the thoracic region which could manifest, for example, as a Horner's Syndrome (myosis, anhydrosis, and palpebral ptosis palpebral) or as a Superior Vena Cava Syndrome. Older children typically present with abdominal pain because as it was mentioned previously, more than {of} 40% of neuroblastomas originate in the adrenals. More than 50% of the patients who present with neuroblastomas have metastatic disease. The most frequent sites of involvement are, the bone marrow, bones, liver, lymph nodes and skin [10].

The appearance of other syndromes also related to neuroblastoma is not surprising; Pepper's Syndrome, for example, occurs in infants with liver metastasis which causes respiratory insufficiency. Described by William Pepper in 1901, it was identified as a primary localized tumor with metastatic disease limited to the skin, liver, and bone marrow; in children it has been associated with neuroblastoma stage IVs. This syndrome is the only entity that only occurs in children younger than 1 year of age. It generally confers a better prognosis when spontaneous regression is associated with this entity; however some children with stage IVs can die from massive hepatomegaly, respiratoty failure, and generalized sepsis. Hepatoblastoma should be considered in the differential diagnosis [9,10].

Babies called "Blueberry muffin" are infants whose neuroblastoma has randomly metastasized to subcutaneous areas. These nodules become intensely red when first touched followed by blanching, lasting several minutes. This response is probably secondary to the discharge of vasoconstrictors derived from metabolic byproduct of the tumor. These nodules can be the diagnosis of neuroblastoma [11].

Extensive metastases of neuroblastoma to bone can produce bone pain and as consequence, limping and pathological fractures. Neuroblastoma involving the paravertebral ganglia can extend through nerve foramina, and cause spinal cord compression with subsequent paralysis. Infrequently, neuroblastoma can metastasize to the retrobulbar region, progressing quickly to a unilateral proptosis without pain, to periorbital edema, and to ecchymosis of the superior part of the eye, characterized as the syndrome of Hutchinson. Those signs can be mistaken for trauma in a child [23]. This syndrome can also be characterized by preauricular, ipsilateral sub maxillary and upper cervical adenopathy, as well as metastasis to lymph nodes of the retroperitoneum, mediastinum and supraclavicular region.

Most neuroblastomas produce catecholamine like substances as metabolic byproducts that are responsible for some of the most interesting manifestations observed in children with this disease. For example, Kerner-Morrison's syndrome causes secretory refractory diarrhea, producing hypovolemia, hypokalemia, and prostration. This is secondary to the vasoactive intestinal peptide (VIP) secreted by the tumor. This syndrome is usually associated with ganglioneuroblastoma or ganglioneuroma [11].

The diagnosis of neuroblastoma requires the participation of pathologists who are well familiarized with children's tumors. Some of the cells cannot be differentiated from small, round, blue cells found in other childhood tumors (such as lymphomas, primitive neuroectodermal tumors and rhabdomyosarcoma) by simple light microscopy. The evidence necessary to make the differentiation of neurosympathetic origin should be demonstrated by immunohistochemistry, electron microscopy, elevated levels of serum catecholamines (dopamine, noradrenaline) or catecholamine metabolites in the urine, vanillylmandelic acid (VMA) or homovanillyc acid (HVA) [10].

The minimum criteria required to determine a diagnosis definition of Neuroblastoma has been recently established by an international group of experts and the corresponding participants. These are unequivocal pathological diagnosis or the unequivocal presence of scyncytium cells in the bone marrow, as mentioned before [10, 32].

The staging and monitoring of disease in patients with NB are major areas of application for diagnostic imaging methods. Thus, diagnostic studies that enable accurate tumour staging should help in treatment planning and reduce unnecessary surgery. The current staging evaluation of patients with NB consists of computed tomography (CT) or magnetic resonance (MR) imaging of the primary tumour, a skeletal survey and either bone scintigraphy or metaiodobenzylguanidine scintigraphy for skeletal metastases, and bone marrow aspiration and biopsy for marrow disease. CT has a reported accuracy of about 80% in tumor staging; when CT is complemented with scintigraphy or bone marrow aspiration, the accuracy has been reported to increase to 97% (15). MR imaging has also yielded high sensitivities (85%–100%) in the detection of abdominal disease and distant metastases [33].

There are organized systems to classify Neuroblastomas. Historically, each organized system has represented a temporary improvement in the understanding of this tumor. However, the existence of so many systems has not only confused the literature, but it has also complicated the comparison of studies among the different institutions27. A standard of clinical criteria exists for diagnosis, staging and response to therapy known as The International Neuroblastoma Staging System (INSS), determining the necessity to obtain biological (histopathological and genetic) data to create therapeutic new groups internationally. In 1984, Shimada classified the neuroblastomas correlating their histopathological features with their clinical behavior. With this purpose, Shimada divided neuroblastomas into favorable and unfavorable categories, depending on the grade of differentiation of the neuroblasts, quantity of Schwannian spindle cell stroma, the index of mitosis- karyorrhexis, and the age at diagnosis [12].

It has been observed that there are two types of Neuroblastoma with very different prognosis, which do not differ either biochemically or histologically, but from the genetic molecular aspect which allows the determination of unfavorable risk factors Amplified N-myc, deletion of 1p, DNA euploidy, CD44 and N-level. These risk factors are rarely found in children younger than 1 year of age, but they are present in one third of Stages III and IV Neuroblastoma in children older than 1 year of age [13].

At this moment N-myc is considered to be the best genetic molecular parameter to define risk groups. For many years the patient's age and the stage of the disease at the moment of diagnosis were the two variables most significant in predicting prognosis in neuroblastoma. Evans found that the nursing infants younger than 1 year old with stages I, II and IV-s had significantly better prognosis. Patients older than 1 year of age and those with more advanced stages, that is to say, III and IV, had worse prognosis. The worst survival prognosis is observed in children older than 1 year of age, in stage IV and with cortical bone metastasis. The site of the primary tumor was also considered a predictor of survival according to some investigators. The patients with tumors in neck, pelvis and mediastinum have better prognosis when compared with those that present with tumors in the retroperitoneal space (paraspinal or Adrenal Glands) [9,13].

CCG or Evans System	POG* System	INNS** System
Stage I Tumor confined to the organ or structure of origin	Stage A Complete microscopic resection of primary tumor with or without residual microscopy. Intracavitary lymph nodes not adhered to the primary tumor and histologically free of tumor. Positive lymph nodes adhered to the surface or inside the tumor.	Stage 1 Localized tumor, microscopic complete resection, with or without microscopic residual disease. Ipsilateral lymph nodes negatives for microscopic tumor. Positive lymph nodes adhered to the resected tumor
Stage II Tumor that extends {for} by continuity beyond the original organ, but it doesn't cross the midline. Positive regional ipsilateral lymph nodes.	Stage B Microscopic incomplete resection of the primary tumor. Lymph nodes and liver similar to stage A.	Stage 2 A Localized tumor, with microscopic incomplete resection. Representative ipsilateral lymph nodes not adhered, negatives for microscopic tumor. Stage 2B Localized tumor, microscopic complete or incomplete resection, ipsilateral lymph nodes or adhered positive nodes Contralateral lymph nodes negative for microscopic tumor.
Stage III Tumor that extends {for} by continuity beyond the midline, positive bilateral lymph nodes.	Stage C Complete or incomplete resection of the primary tumor. Lymph nodes not adhered to the primary tumor, histologically positive for tumor, liver similar to the stage A	Stage 3 Unilateral unresectable tumor that crosses the midline, with or without positive regional lymph nodes; or unilateral tumor that is localized, with positive regional contralateral lymph nodes; or tumor in the midline that has extended bilaterally by continuity or by involving lymph nodes.
Stage IV Metastasis to Bone, bone marrow, soft tissue and distant lymph nodes.	Stage D Disease spreading beyond Intracavitary lymph nodes	Stage 4 Any primary tumor with distant metastasis to lymph nodes, bone, liver, skin, bone marrow or other organ (except the defined by Stage IVs).
Stage IV-S Defined as Stages I or II, except for the presence of distant disease confined to skin, liver or bone marrow (without bone metastases) or both.	Stage D-S Nursing children younger than 1 year-old, with Stage IVs disease (CCG Staging	Stage 4 S Localized primary tumor (as define in the Stage 2A or 2B, with limited spread to liver, skin, bone marrow). Nursing infants younger than one year old.

Classification by Shimada and Jhosi (1992 and 1999) establishes a prognostic classification based on histological features, the patient's age, presence or absence of stroma, the grade of differentiation and the index of Mitosis-Karyorrhesis (MKI).

Table 1. Neuroblastoma Staging System. Comparison of the three systems

Poor stroma	Favourable histology Well differentiated Intermediate	Unfavourable histology Nodular
Poor stroma	MKI < 200/5000	MKI <100/5000
Age < 18m	MKI >100/5000	MKI < 100/5000
Age 18- 60m	Differentiated	Undifferentiated
Age <5 years old	None	All

FROM: Grosfeld JL et to 2002 Cir. Pediatr 12: 1345-46

Table 2.

5. Diagnosis

To carry out the diagnosis of this disease, it is necessary to keep it in mind, to take into account the epidemiological aspects described before, the signs and symptoms described in the forms of clinical presentation, added together to the study of the catecholamines, the blood chemistry result: complete hemogram with differential, glycaemia, urea, creatinine, study of {the} hepatic (TGP, TGO, alkaline phosphatase) function, radiological study of the thorax including CAT Scan and MRI. If needed, abdominal ultrasound, bone scan included the bone gammagraphy, bone marrow examination, histological study (included immunohistochemistry) of a biopsy of the lesion.

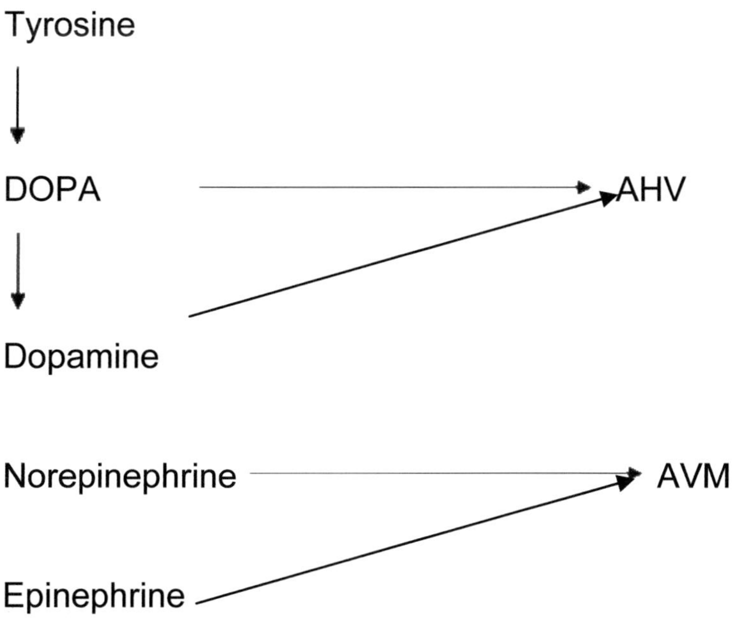

The following studies are being referred to due to their significant importance. [10]:

- The examination of the bone marrow aspirate is characterized by the presence of malignant cells, that can present a diffuse pattern or, in its characteristic way of rosettes (Homer-Wright rossetes). They appear in nests or islands of atypical cells separated by septa , disseminated among the normal cells of the bone marrow.
- Study of levels of Catecholamines in blood and in urine. With sensitive technique, in more than 95% of these tumors elevated urinary metabolites can be detected: homovanilic acid (AHV) and {the} vanillylmandelic acid (AVM).

Catecholamine is the generic name of the amines derived from catechol or 1,2-bencenodiol; being the most important epinephrine, norepinephrine and their precursor, DOPA (dihydrophenylalanine), of sympaticomimetic action. In the following figure it is show in a simplified manner [10]:

- By means of a biopsy it is possible to obtain the two histological varieties of this tumor: Ganglioneuroblastoma (morphological code 9490/3) and Neuroblastoma (morphological code 9500/3)

In half of the cases, metastasis is already present at the time of diagnosis, especially in regional organs and distant lymph nodes, in the bone marrow, bone, liver, skin, and rarely in the Central Nervous System.

6. Differential diagnosis

Fundamentally with: non Hodgkin lymphomas, Ewing sarcoma and rhabdomyosarcoma [10, 14].

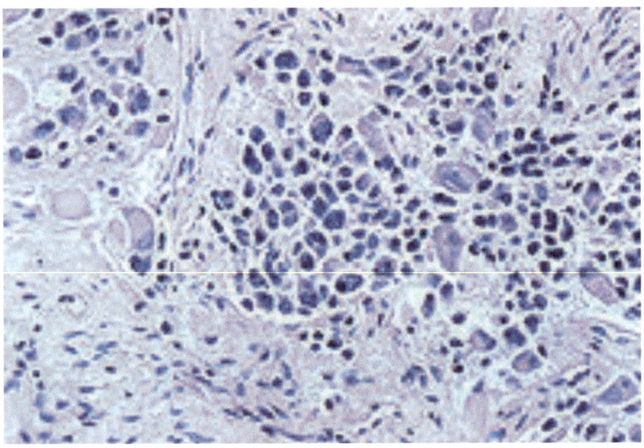

Fig. 2. Cells of a nerve ganglion with neuroblastoma.

7. Prognostic factors

Certain biological variables have been identified that affect the prognosis of children with neuroblastoma. The specific examples include the aneuploidia of the DNA in the tumor and the amplification of the oncogene N-myc. The amplification of N-myc happens in 20% of the primary neuroblastoma and it is associated with a neuroblastoma subset that has a high metastatic potential and a POOR prognosis. It is thought that N-myc contributes to the aggressive behavior of neuroblastoma. However, the precise role of non-amplified N-myc in tumors is unknown [9,15,16].

The hyperdiploidity of the DNA in tumors is associated with a favorable prognosis. The amplification of N-myc is associated with a POOR prognosis in children older than 1 year of age, but not in children younger than 1 year of age. The amplification of N-myc is associated with the deletion of the short arm of chromosome 1p and a gain on the long arm of the chromosome 1755. In neuroblastoma, areas consistently showing heterogenecity of the chromosome (LOH) include bands of the chromosomes 1p36, 11q23, and 14Q23qter. In 2000, Maris et al. informed the Children's Cancer Group (CCG) that the deletion of the 1p predicted a lower survival independently, but not the overall survival. The clinical relevance of 14q LOH is uncertain at this time. There are other prognostic variables such as the level of ferritin in serum, of neuron-specific enolase (NSE), and the nutritional status of the patient [17, 18].

Different prognostic factors have been described in Neuroblastoma, but most of the reviewed authors classify them as favorable factors and unfavorable factors [10, 19, 20].

Favorable factors:

1. Early clinical stages (I, II, IVS)
2. Location: thorax, pelvis, and neck
3. Age: younger than one year of age
4. Favorable histological pattern of Shimada:
   - STROMA rich in cells of Schwann, diffuse
   - Neuroblasts with nuclear and cytoplasmic differentiation toward node cells.
   - MKI Index (mitosis / karioresis) related to age: younger than 18 months: MKI < 200/5000; from 18 to 24 months < 100/50.000 and from 2 to 5 years not
5. Normal homovanillic acid (HVA) in urine.
6. Normal serum levels of ferritin and neuron-specific enolase.
7. Negative intestinal vasoactive peptide.
8. Good Nutritional State
9. DNA aneuploidy.
10. Oncogene N-myc < 10 amplifications
11. Absence of metastasis.

Other factors associated separately, to a favorable evolution and inversely related to the amplification of the gene N-myc they are:

- The expression of the gene that codes the receptor of the factor of High Neural Affinity named proto oncogene TRK-TO
- The expression of the receptor Low Neural Affinity (LNGFR)
- .H-ras p21 oncogene expression

Unfavorable factors:

1. Stage: III and IV
2. Location: retroperitoneum
3. Age: older than 1 year old
4. Histologic pattern: undifferentiated neuroblastoma

5. Increase in the index homovanillic acid/ vanillylmandelic acid.
6. Increase in serum level of ferritin, neuron-specific enolase and LDH.
7. Increase of intestinal vasoactive peptide.
8. Malnutrition.
9. DNA diploidy
10. Oncogene N-myc with> 10 amplifications
11. The loss of expression of the glycoprotein CD44 on the surface of the tumor.
12. Metastasis to regional lymph nodes.
13. Increased levels of p-glycoprotein after chemotherapy
14. The activation of gelatinase A is related with high expression of MT-MMP-1 (membrane-type matrix metalloproteinase-1) in neuroblastoma cells, and in turn it is related with advanced stages and with worse outcome.

NOTE: p-glycoprotein is the protein produced by the gene that code for drug multiresistance.

Contrary to what has happened {to} with other embryonic tumors in children, in which the combined treatment of the different therapeutic modalities of the cancer has achieved a considerable increase in survival, the prognosis of neuroblastoma continues to be uncertain.

8. Treatment

The treatment of NB is determined by the stage of the tumor at time of diagnosis. Disease that is regionally limited is potentially resectable, while disease that is locally extensive or disseminated is usually not resectable.

In 1988, the Pediatric Oncology Group (POG) carried out a study that revealed that 89% of patient with localized neuroblastoma that were treated by surgical resection had a survival of only 2 years. Additionally, chemotherapy seemed to have offered no advantage residual disease was present in these patients 34. Therefore, for patients with favorable stage, surgery is the main form of therapy. The most important goals of surgery are: to determine an exact diagnosis, to excise completely the entire primary tumor, to provide the exact surgical findings, the adjuvant therapy in delayed primary surgery, and to remove residual disease in second look surgery[21].

Since surgery is only done in early stages of neuroblastoma (stages I and II) multi agent chemotherapy is the conventional therapy for patients in the most advanced stages of neuroblastoma. In children younger than one year of age with disseminated neuroblastoma, favorable results have been obtained with the combination of chemotherapy and surgery. In contrast, children older than 1 year of age with neuroblastoma in advanced stage have a very low survival rate, despite intensive multimodality therapy [36]. Due to these observations, in Japan, during the 1980's it was proclaimed that an aggressive exploration in children younger than 6 months with catecholamines in the urine could uncover earlier neuroblastoma which could result in better outcome. In Europe and North Americ controlled clinical tests were carried out in the affected population and when comparing results with those of the Japanese study , no benefits were found with this investigation [22].

In spite of these confusing studies, symptomatic treatments are available for patients with neuroblastoma. The Adrenocortical Hormone (ACTH) is thought to be quite effective, although some patients are resistant. Plasmapheresis and gamma globulin have been used in the treatment of selected patients with neuroblastoma; however, it is thought that treatment with chemotherapeutic agents produce better neurological results [23].

The common chemotherapeutic agents used to treat Neuroblastoma include cisplatin, doxorubicin, cyclophosphamide, and the epipodophyllotoxins (teniposide and etoposide). The protocols with combination of narcotics have used strategies that take advantage of drug synergism, mechanism of toxicity, and variety of adverse effects. Despite the different drug combinations, the rate of cure has not been significantly affected. The long term survival of patient with metastatic neuroblastoma is low. It is believed that this is due to the presence of a large number of non-proliferating cells in the tumor. However, in neuroblastoma treated with chemotherapeutic agents a reduction in the size of the primary tumor, occasional sterilization of the bone marrow, and, rarely, transformation of the neuroblastoma into a benign ganglioneuroma have been observed [24].

The current tendencies for the use of chemotherapy in the treatment of neuroblastoma include: dose-intensive chemotherapy followed by surgical excision of residual disease myeloablative therapy by combination of chemotherapeutic agents , followed by Autologous Bone Marrow Transplantationand biological responder modifiers, to bring about differentiation of the tumor and to reduce the degree of bone marrow infiltration [40]. The multimodal therapeutic protocols outlined by POG are the norm of care for children diagnosed with neuroblastoma.

Topotecan, an inhibitor of the topoisomerasa I, alone or in combination with Cyclophosphamide, has shown to have activity against recurrent neuroblastoma. This information has recently prompted the Children's Oncology Group to design a study to prove the clinical effectiveness of incorporating Topotecan in an intensive induction régimen for patients with high-risk neuroblastoma.

Retinoic acid (RA), a biologically active form of vitamin A, plays a central role as a signaling molecule in the early stages of embryonic development and the generation of multiple organs and systems, including the Nervous System [59]. In vitro culture it has been demonstrated a decrease in the regulation of the expression of the N-myc messenger RNA which obstructs the proliferation of tumor cells. These observations taken to clinical trials demonstrated the efficacy of 13-cis RA in children with neuroblastoma in relapse. The results of phase I and II trials didn't show benefits in patients with high tumor load; however in patient with minimal disease, phase III randomized trials involving , 13-cis RA produced an improved rate of survival from 20% - 40% in patient with high risk neuroblastoma [24].

Indirect immunotherapy has been evaluated as part of multimodal treatment of microscopic resistant neuroblastoma. Diasilganglioside (GD2) is an excellent target for immunotherapy because this antigen is overexpressed in the majority of human neuroblastoma. The response rate is reinforced for those that have used cytosine combinations along with anti-GD2 antibodies, increasing the antibody dependent cellular cytotoxicity (ADCC). Other immunotherapies like cytotoxic T lymphocytes, modified dendritic cells, fusion protein Hu 14.18-IL2 (immnunocytokine), GM-CSF, and interleukine-2 (IL-2) have shown promising results against neuroblastoma.

The clinical trials in Europe and North America are delineating the effectiveness of the radio-tagged methyliodobenzylguanidine (MIBG) with I-131 with or without combination myelobastic chemotherapy, followed by rescue with autologous stem cells. The optimal doses, schedules, and best timing for MIBG therapy are the goals of these clinical trials [25].

On the other hand, the therapy with antiangiogenesis has more than a theoretical role in the treatment of neuroblastoma. In fact, the preclinical studies have demonstrated that these agents inhibit the growth of neuroblastoma in vivo, mainly in minimal residual disease. Phase I protocols that test inhibitors of angiogenesis allow the determination if a very vascular neuroblastoma responds to these agents.

In vitro cultures have demonstrated that neuroblastoma is radiosensitive, but the clinical trials carried out have been unclear and inconclusive. As a primary modality of treatment, radiation therapy still has a limited role. In metastatic regional lymph nodes sequential chemotherapy with cyclophosphamide can be used.

Intensive multimodal treatment of patient with neuroblastoma has shown an increase in survival rate. However, the risk of therapy related delayed manifestations must be taken into consideration because of adverse, devastating effects. Survivors should be closely followed and supervised by multidisciplinary Centers to detect and document any long term sequelae. The Oncological Pediatric (GOP) Group recently developed a classification system named Neuroblastoma Risk Stratification System (NRSS). This new classification includes biological and clinical characteristics to predict behavior, similar to the Shimada Index and it is also used with the purpose of stratifying the treatment. The patients are classified in the categories of low, intermediate or high-risk according with the age at the diagnosis, the staging according to INSS, the histopathological features, the state of amplified N-myc and the DNA index.

9. Protocols of treatments

Low Risk Disease (Protocol I)

Cyclophosphamide	400 mg / m^2 /BS/ IV	Day 1
Vincristine	1.5 mg/ m^2 /BS /IV	Day 1
Adriamycin	30 mg/m^2 /BS/ IV	Day 8

4 weeks rest.

Total number of cycles: 6

Intermediate risk (Protocol II)

Block A*	Dose	Day
Cyclophosphamide	1500 mg / m^2 /BS/ IV	Day 1
Vincristine	1 mg / m^2 /BS/ IV	Day 1 and 2
Rest 3 weeks		
Block B		
Cisplatin	120 mg / m^2 /BS/ IV	Day 1
Etoposide	100 mg / m^2 /BS /IV	Day 1,2 and 3
Rest 3 weeks Total of cycle: 6		

*In stage III, the use of radiotherapy is recommended to help in the reduction of the primary tumor volume during the weeks of the first cycle of Block A plus 2 more weeks.

Considerations for surgery are taken as soon as the cytoreduction of the tumor is achieved. It is recommended to start evaluation for surgery from the third cycle.

High risk disease (Protocol III)

Block A*	Dose	Day
Cyclophosphamide	1500 mg /m^2 /BS/ IV	Day 1
Vincristine	1 mg /m^2 /BS/ IV	Day 1 and 2
Rest 3 weeks		
Bloque B		
Cisplatin	120 mg /m^2 /BS/ IV	Day 1
Etoposide	100 mg /m^2 /BS /IV	Day 1,2 and 3
Block C	Dose	Day
Adriamycin	60 mg /m^2 /BS/ IV	Day 1 and 2

Rest 4 weeks

Total cycles: 6

Protocol according to clinical stages (Protocol IV, V, VI, VII)

STAGE	Surgery	Chemotherapy	DAY	Radiotherapy (Total Dose)
I	Complete resection of tumor			
II	Complete resection of tumor	VCR: 1.5 mg/ m^2 /BS /IV* CFM:400 mg/ m^2 /BS /IV*	1,8,29 1,3,7	20 Gy*
III	1 Partial resection or biopsy ** 2 Rescue surgery***	VCR:1.5 mg/m^2 /BS/ IV** CFM:300mg/ m^2 /BS IV** ACTD:600mcg/m^2/BS/ IV*** ADM: 100mg/m^2 /BS IV**	1,8,29 1,3,7 1,2,3,4 28	
		VCR:1.5mg/ m^2 /BS /EV** CFM:300mg/ m^2 / BS EV** DTIC:300mg/m^2 / BS EV** ADM: 40mg/ m^2 / BS /EV** CDDP:100mg/m^2/ BS EV**	1,8,29 2,3,4 1,2,3,4 8,29 28	20 Gy*
IV		VCR:1.5 mg/m^2 / BS /EV** CFM:300mg/ m^2/ BS /EV** ACTD:600mcg/m^2/ BS EV** ADM:100mg/ m^2 / BS EV**	1,8,29 1,3,7 1,2,3,4 28	20 Gy*
	Alternative	VCR: 1.5 mg/m/BS/IV** CFM:300mg/m^2/BS /IV** DTIC:300/mg/m^2/BS / IV** ADM: 40 mg/ m^2/BS/ IV** CDDP:100mg/m^2/BS/IV**		20 Gy

STAGE	Surgery	Chemotherapy	DAY	Radiotherapy (Total Dose)
IVS	Total resection or CAFF	CFM*** ADM***	1,2,3,4,5,6,7 8	

Abbreviations:
VCR: Vincristine
CFM: Cyclophosphamide
ACTD; Actinomycin D
ADM: Doxorubicin
DTIC: Dacarbazine
CDDP: Cisplatin
Surgery:
*In the event of existing doubts that it is a true stage I, treatment should be done with chemotherapy using the proposed outline for stage II cases.
**It is preferably recommended to carry out fine needle aspiration biopsy (FNAB) of the primary tumor
*** Surgery for biopsy specimen if there is cytoreduction of the initial tumor
Chemotherapy:
*Weekly treatment for 8 cycles, then biweekly for 8 cycles and then repeats the protocol until completing one year of treatment.
**Rest for 3 weeks and then repeat a cycle every 3 weeks, to complete 4 cycles.
*** give a cycle every 3 weeks for 1 year.
*VCR: 1.5 mg m2 BS IV
*CFM: 300 mg m2 BS IV
NOTE: When concluding the radiotherapy treatment , rest for 3 weeks and then continue with the initial chemotherapy protocol, 1 cycle every 4 weeks until giving 4 cycles, and later on 1 cycle every 6 weeks until giving 4 cycles, followed by 1 cycle every 8 weeks until completing 2 cycles.

10. Radiotherapy

For patient with low risk or neuroblastoma intermission in the plan of current treatment of COG (COG-ANBL0531), radiation therapy is reserved for patients with a symptomatic life-threatening tumor which does not respond to chemotherapy. The treatment of children with low-risk stage 4S disease depends on clinical presentation - those who are clinically stable may not require therapy. However, the disease complications, such as respiratory distress from massive hepatomegaly may need a low intensity chemotherapy regimen (low dose cyclophosphamide). Resection of the primary tumor is not associated with improved outcome.

In patients classified as intermediate risk with unfavorable biologic features, radiation therapy is given if residual viable tumor remains after 24 weeks of chemotherapy and secondlook surgery.

For patients classified as high risk, the use of radiation therapy for local control after surgical resection is recommended whether or not complete tumor removal was obtained

Schema of Hayes (Protocol VIII)

Cyclophosphamide	150 mg / m^2 / BS / IV	Day 1 to 7
Adriamycin	35 mg / m^2 / BS / IV	Day 8

Rest for {of} 3 weeks

Total of cycles: 6

Protocol OPEJ / OJEC (Protocol IX)

OPEC		
Vincristine	1.5 mg m^2 /BS /IV	Day 1
Cisplatin	80 mg m^2 / BS/IV	Day 1
Etoposide	200 mg m^2 / BS /IV	Day 3
Cyclophosphamide	500 mg m^2 / BS /IV	Day 1
OJEC		
Vincristine	1.5 mg m^2 /BS /IV	Day 1
Carboplatin	500 mg m^2 /BS /IV	Day 1
Etoposide	200 mg m^2 /BS /IV	Day 1
Cyclophosphamide	500 mg m^2 /BS /IV	Day 1

Rest for 3 weeks

Total of cycles: 7

11. References

[1] Carmen Gloria Rostión, Lorena Jáuregui, Valentina Broussain, Karol Gac y Angélica Paulos, Internas Mariana Hepp y Daniela Cortez. Neuroblastoma: Forma de presentación y probabilidad de resección quirúrgica. Rev. Ped. Elec. [en linea] 2005, Vol2, No2 ISSN 0718-0918

[2] Birch JM, Marsden HB. A classification scheme for childhood cancer. Int J Cancer. 1987;40:620–624.

[3] Steliarova-Foucher E, Stiller C, Lacour B, Kaatsch P. International Classification of Childhood Cancer. Third Edition. © 2005 American Cancer Society. DOI 10.1002/cncr.20910. Published online 14 February 2005 in Wiley InterScience (www.interscience.wiley.com).

[4] Fritz A, Percy C, Jack A, Shanmugaratnam K, Sobin Let, Parkin DM, Whelan S., editors. International Classification of Diseases for Oncology. 3rd ed. Geneva: World Health Organization, 2000.

[5] Vargas L. Cáncer infantil en Chile. 10 años. Programa PINDA. Santiago de Chile: Ministry of Health (CL); 2000

[6] Tsubono Y, Hisamichi S. A Halt to Neuroblastoma Screening in Japan (en inglés). New England Journal of Medicine. 350. 19: 2010-2011 (2004). PMID 15128908

[7] Schilling, Freimut H.; y col. (2002). «Neuroblastoma Screening at One Year of Age» N Engl J Med. Vol. 346. n.° 14. pp. 1047-1053. Consultado el 4 de abril de 2009.

[8] Priscila Torres, MD, Yaima Galán, MPH, Juan Lence, MD, MPH, Mariela García, DDS, MPH, Martha Lezcano, Leticia Fernández, MD, PhD. Childhood Cancer Incidence in Cuba, 2001 to 2003. MEDICC Review, Spring 2010, Vol 12, No 2

[9] Eric Bouffet, David C. Hodgson, and ENG- SIEW KOH. Pediatric Cancers. In UICC. Prognostic Factors in Cancer. Mary K. Gospodarowicz, Brian O'Sullivan, Leslie H. Sobin. 3ed. Chapter 45. pp 317-318. 2006

[10] Lorenzo Alfonso Hernández. Oncología. Preguntas y respuestas. Instituto Nacional de Oncología y Radiobiología. Cuba. Copyright Proas Science, S. A., 2001. Provenza 388, 08025 Barcelona, España. Pp 749-754.

[11] Hiyama E, Yokohama T, Hiyama K, et al.: Multifocal neuroblastoma. Biologic behavior and surgical aspect. Cancer 2000; 88(8):1955-1963.

[12] Shimada H, Umehara S, Monobe Y.International neuroblastoma pathology classification for prognostic evaluation of patients wishes peripheral neuroblastic tumors: a report from the Children s Cancer Group.Cancer 2001; 92:2451'61
[13] Schwab M. Amplified MYCN in human neuroblastoma-paradigm for the translation of molecular genetics to clinical oncology. Ann N Y Acad Sci 2002; 963:63-73.
[14] Neuroblastoma. Medline Plus. Enciclopedia Médica [homepage on the internet]. Maryland: US National Library of Medicine [updated 2008 Oct 6; cited 2009 Jan 29]. Available from:
http://www.nim.nih.gov/medlineplus/spanish/ency/article/001408.htm
[15] Breslow N, McCann B. Statistical estimation of prognosis for children with neuroblastoma. Cancer Res 2003; 31:2092-2103.
[16] Grosfeld J.et al.: Metastasic neuroblastoma: factors influencing survival. J Pediatr Surg 2003; 13:59.
[17] Jerev B, Bretsky SS, Vogel R.Age and prognosis in neuroblastoma.Am J Pediatr Hematolo Oncol 2000; 6:233-138.
[18] Roberts S, Creamer K, Shoupe B, et al: Unique management of stage 4S neuroblastoma complicated by Massive hepatomegaly: case report and review of the literature. J Pediatr Hematol Hero B, Simon T, and Horz S, Berthold F. Metastatic neuroblastoma in infancy: what does the pattern of metastases contribute to prognosis? Med Pediatr Oncol 2000; 35:683-7
[19] Kramer K, Kushner B, et al.: Neuroblastoma metastatic.The Memorial Sloan- Kettering Cancer Center experience and a literature review.Cancer 2001; 91(8):1510-1519.
[20] Nowicki M, Miskowiak B: Prognostic value of stage IV neuroblastoma metastatic immuophenotype in the bone marrow: preliminary report. Journal of Clinical Pathology 2006;59:150-152
[21] Weinstein JL, Katzenstein HM, Cohn SL: Advances in the diagnosis and treatment of neuroblastoma. Oncologist 2003; 8(3): 278-92 Medline
[22] Anne L, Jean M, Olivier H, et al.: High-Dose chemotherapy fallowed by locoregional irradiation improves the outcome of patients with International Neuroblastoma Staging System Stage II and III Neuroblastoma with MYCN Amplification.Cancer 2004;101:1081-9
[23] Castel V, Cañete C, Melero T, et al. Results of the Cooperative Protocol(N-III-95) for metastatic relapses and refractory neuroblastoma. Med Pediatr Oncol. 2000; 35:724-26
[24] Stram DO, Matthay KK, O Leary M: Consolidation chemoradiotherapy and autologous bone marrow transplantation versus continued chemotherapy for metastasic neuroblastoma: a report of two concurrent Children s Cancer Group Studies. J Clin Oncol 2003; 13(8):2417- 2426.
[25] Howman-Giles R, Shaw PJ, Uren RF, Chung DK (2007). «Neuroblastoma and other neuroendocrine tumors» Semin Nucl Med. Vol. 37. n.º 4. pp. 286–302. DOI 10.1053/j.semnuclmed.2007.02.009. PMID 17544628.

13

Fertility and Fecundity After Chemotherapy for Childhood Cancer

C. Berger[1], S. Thouvenin[1], O. Richard[2] and J.L. Stephan[1]
[1]*Pediatric Departments of Hematology and Oncology,*
[2]*Pediatric Departments of Endocrinology,*
CHRU Hôpital Nord, Saint-Etienne Cedex,
France

1. Introduction

In 2011, the regular increase in survival of childhood cancer (overall survival [OS] 72% at 10 years) (Berger 2006) suggests that one of every 850 adults in Europe has had pediatric cancer. As these children become adults, their concerns with possible long-term disease complications and risks associated with therapy received increase. Adverse effects of cancer therapies include disorders of the endocrine system, cardiac and pulmonary dysfunction, renal and hepatic impairment, secondary malignant disease, and psychosocial difficulties. Significant deliberation must also be given to the potential effects of a treatment regimen on the future fertility of pediatric patients with cancer. We review the literature regarding fertility and chemical risk factors for hypofertility in these patients to increase awareness of and avoid long-term clinical consequences of chemical therapies.

2. Gonadic toxicity

Gonadic toxicity results from systemic chemotherapy or irradiation of the spinal axis, pelvis, or entire body.

In boys, toxicity affects the somatic cells, i.e., the Sertoli and Leydig cells and germinal lineage. Sertoli cells assure the support, nutrition, and protection of germ cells, synthetizing numerous proteins, including inhibin and androgen-binding protein (ABP), and Leydig cells secrete testosterone. Chemotherapeutic toxicity primarily involves spermatogenesis, rise in follicle-stimulating hormone (FSH), and decline in inhibin.

Anti-Müllerian hormone (AMH) is the earliest Sertoli cell-specific protein expressed by the male gonad and is secreted by the testes from the eighth week of gestation and at high levels until puberty, when its decreasing production characterizes maturation of the Sertoli cells. The decline in AMH expression during puberty coincides with increased androgen secretion by Leydig cells and is considered a clear marker of the elevated intratesticular androgen concentration that inhibits AMH production by Sertoli cells at this time. The high level of AMH production before puberty allows its measurement to serve as a reliable marker for the presence of testicular tissue in childhood, when testosterone levels are very low.

Chemotherapy alone does not alter Leydig incapacity, as evidenced by a normal secretion of testosterone and declining levels of AMH during puberty. Puberty occurs normally even if involvement of the germinal lineage decreases testicular volume (A La Marca 2010).

Although female reproduction requires a functioning hypothalamic-pituitary-gonadal axis, ovaries, and uterus, reproductive potential in women is mainly limited by available oocytes. The process of oogenesis begins before birth with a peak in oocyte number (6 to 7 million) at 20 weeks' gestation followed by progressive atresia and drop in number of oocytes to one to 2 million at birth and 300,000 at puberty. Oocytes remain arrested as primordial follicles until puberty, a stage postulated to be less sensitive to gonadotoxins. At the initiation of puberty, a monthly cohort of follicles is recruited, one becomes dominant, and the others undergo atresia. Accelerated atresia coincides with a decrease in the quantity and quality of oocytes, raising the risk of infertility, aneuploidy, and spontaneous miscarriage. A rise in serum FSH often indicates accelerated atresia and impending ovarian failure. Before age 40 years, persistent FSH concentrations above 30 IU/L in the setting of amenorrhea, regardless of inciting events, suggest a diagnosis of premature ovarian failure (Rebar 2009).

Levels of anti-Müllerian hormone may represent the ovarian pool and could be a useful marker of ovarian reserve (A La Marca 2010). AMH is produced and secreted into the circulation by the gonads and can be measured in the serum of men and women. Nonsignificant variations in AMH levels have been reported throughout the menstrual cycle. In women, AMH levels seem to be unmodified under conditions in which endogenous gonadotropin release is subtantially diminished, such as during pregnancy, treatment with gonadotropin-releasing hormone (GnRH) agonist, and short-term oral contraceptive administration, indicating that non-cyclic FSH-independent ovarian activity persists even when pituitary FSH secretion is suppressed. However, sometimes damage to the ovarian reserve cannot predict ability to conceive.

Lie Fong and associates compared serum AMH levels in 185 adult female survivors of childhood cancer (excluding brain tumors) and 42 control subjects. Median follow-up was 18.1 years (range, 4.1 to 43.2 years). Median AMH concentrations were not significantly different between the analyzed cohort (1.7 μg/L) and controls (2.1 μg/L). However, in 27% of survivors, AMH levels were lower than the tenth percentile of normal values, and in 43%, they were lower than 1.4 μg/L, a previously established cut-off value for predicting ongoing pregnancy after assisted reproduction. AMH levels did not differ significantly in subgroups classified according to disease but were significantly lower in survivors who underwent 3 or more cycles of chemotherapy containing procarbazine than in controls (median 0.5 μg/L). AMH levels were also significantly lower in survivors who had been treated with abdominal or total body irradiation than in controls (median < 0.1 μg/L). AMH can be used to identify subgroups of survivors of childhood cancer who are at risk for decreased fertility or premature ovarian failure. In these survivors with high risk of hypofertility, the capacity for fertility preservation should be considered prior to starting assisted reproductive treatment because they may have a poor chance of achieving or maintaining pregnancy after treatment (Lie Fong 2009).

3. Which chemotherapies contribute to decline in fertility?

Alkylating agents, including cyclophosphamide, ifosfamide, chlormethine, busulfan, melphalan, procarbazine, and chlorambucil, are the primary chemotherapies that carry a high risk for gonadic dysfunction (Wallace 2005).

Boys frequently experience a passing rise in luteinizing hormone (LH) with azoospermia in the period just after receiving chemotherapy (2 to 8 years). In a series of patients affected by non-Hodgkin lymphomas, Pryzant describes an 83% recovery of spermatogenesis in patients receiving less than 9.5 g/m^2 of cyclophosphamide compared to 43% recovery in those receiving a higher dose (Pryzant 1993). A reduction of cyclophosphamide dose to less than 7.5 g/m^2 is associated with up to 70% conservation of fertility in survivors of Ewing's sarcoma.

A recent study including 6224 survivors aged 15 to 44 years who were not surgically sterile found a decline in fertility in men who had received childhood doses of procarbazine greater than 4.2 g/m^2 or cyclophosphamide greater than 9.3 g/m^2. Those who received cytarabine were more likely to ever sire a pregnancy than those who were not exposed to this agent. There is no clear explanation of this observation. The likelihood of siring a pregnancy was greater for men whose cancer was diagnosed and treated before age 4 years than those diagnosed between 15 and 20 years and did not differ for those diagnosed between 5 to 9 years or 10 to 14 years relative to those 15 to 20 years (Green 2010). Cyclophosphamide administration has been associated with impaired spermatogenesis after treatment of children for nonmalignant and malignant disease. Azoospermia has been reported after cumulative cyclophosphamide doses as low as 6 g/m^2 (Kenney 2001). In survivors of osteosarcoma, there is an implied risk of azoospermia from ifosfamide, with doses between 42 and 60 g/m^2 (Longhi 2003).

Byrne and colleagues evaluated fertility in male long-term survivors of acute lymphoblastic leukemia (ALL) diagnosed during childhood (Byrne 2004). Mean age at diagnosis was 10.9 years, and average age at interview was 22.8 years. Controls were siblings (average age, 24 years). Only 33% of male survivors had married or had a live-in relationship compared to 49% of male controls, and though the age in each group was similar for first fathering a pregnancy, fewer survivors than controls had become fathers. The relative risk (RR) for fertility was 0.80 for survivors aged 18 to 21 years when they first sired a pregnancy compared with sibling controls and 1.02 for survivors older than 21 years at the time they first sired a pregnancy. Men who received cranial radiotherapy (RT) without spinal RT before age 9 were less likely to become fathers than controls; their fertility was only 9% that of controls.

Ovarian function may be impaired after chemotherapy that includes an alkylating agent, such as nitrogen mustard, procarbazine, chlorambucil, or cyclophosphamide. The risk of ovarian failure appears to correlate directly with cumulative dose but inversely with age at exposure (Schilsky 1981, Andrieu 1983). Six cycles of combined nitrogen mustard, vincristine, procarbazine, and prednisone expose a patient to 8.4 g/m^2 of procarbazine and 72 mg/m^2 of nitrogen mustard. Such therapy carries a high risk of premature ovarian failure that may lead to precocious menopause. Green examined the fertility status of 5149 female survivors of childhood cancer aged 15 to 44 years who were not surgically sterile and noted that fertility decreased with increasing doses received of lomustine (CCNU) (from 360 mg/m^2) or cyclophosphamide (from 3.7 g/m^2). A low risk of pregnancy was also associated with increasing doses received of alkylating agents, such as those administered for Ewing's sarcoma (8.4 g/m^2 of cyclophosphamide and 63 g/m^2 of ifosfamide) (Green 2009). Chemotherapies administered before autologous stem cells that include high doses of alkylating agents, such as the busulfan (600 mg/m^2) or melphalan, are a very important cause of premature ovarian failure (Teinturier 1998).

Byrne's group reported a significantly lower unadjusted fertility rate for female survivors of ALL than their siblings but could not demonstrate an effect of treatment with an alkylating agent or spinal irradiation on fertility rates (Byrne 2004).

4. Fecundity of survivors of childhood cancer

Fecundity, the capacity for producing offspring, is affected by various factors, including marital status, emotional disorders, endocrine or neurological disorders, and others.

A recent Italian study analyzes the marital (or living in couples) status of survivors of childhood cancer and compares it to that of the general Piedmontese population. At an average age of 28 years, 75% of survivors are not in couples, but the proportion is reversed after age 40 years, with 75% living in couples. On average, the wedding rate of survivors of childhood cancer is 32% lower than that of the general population for men and 18% lower for women. The discrepancy is very sharply marked for survivors of brain tumors, who are affected by endocrine and neurological complications as well as emotional disorders (Dama 2009).

For the Childhood Cancer Survivor Study, 20,720 patients were eligible for study, 17,561 questionnaires were sent (3159 lost to follow-up), and 3209 patients declined participation. At contact, 12,220 were aged 15 to 44 years (female, 5665; male, 6555). Five hundred and sixteen female survivors were surgically sterile, and 1372 indicated they had been pregnant 5 or more years after the date of their primary cancer diagnosis. Female survivors of the CCSS cohort were less likely than their sibling cohort to become pregnant (relative risk for survivors of ever being pregnant was 0.81 compared with female siblings). Pregnancy was more likely among those who had completed less than a high school education or were African American or married, findings that reflected the general population, or those in the youngest group at diagnosis (Green 2009).

We are conducting a study of fertility and quality of life of women treated in France for childhood cancer (except ALL) between 1948 and 1992 and sent 1261 survivors a self-assessment questionnaire that included an SF36 quality-of-life survey and questions on social outcomes, health, family, and fertility. Of 944 (75%) who answered, 489 had conceived at least one child, 29 adopted, and 94 could not bear a child despite their desire. There was no significant difference in quality of life between women with at least one child and women without children. By itself, the mental score of the SF36 appeared to correlate with growth deficiency, locomotive and psychological late effects, and age at diagnosis but did not correlate with initial tumor, gonadic deficiency, or fertility; the physical score correlated with neither fertility nor gonadic insufficiency. So, the SF36 findings seemed to indicate that the hypofertility experienced by patients treated for childhood cancer did not alter their quality of life. Future study could refine the psychological, social, and professional profile (personal data).

5. Knowledge of fertility?

The varied nature of gonadal insult after chemo- or radiotherapy often makes it difficult to predict whether treatment a patient is about to undergo will impair fertility. However, Wallace has proposed a classification of subfertility risk according to type of malignant disease and associated treatment (Table 1) (Wallace 2005), and protocols for malignant disease are continually evolving to improve survival and reduce late effects, as seen, for example, in the intensification of treatment for ALL but less intensive management of Hodgkin disease over the last 10 years.

Low risk (< 20%)
Acute lymphoblastic leukemia
Wilm's tumor
Soft tissue sarcoma: stage I
Germ-cell tumors (with gonadal preservation and no radiotherapy)
Retinoblastoma
Brain tumor: surgery only, cranial irradiation < 24 Gy

Medium risk
Acute myeloblastic leukemia (difficult to quantify)
Hepatoblastoma
Osteosarcoma
Ewing's sarcoma nonmetastatic
Soft tissue sarcoma: stage II or III
Neuroblastoma
Non-Hodgkin lymphoma
Hodgkin's disease: alternating treatment
Brain tumor: craniospinal radiotherapy, cranial irradiation > 24 Gy

High risk (> 80%)
Whole-body irradiation
Localized radiotherapy: pelvic or testicular
Chemotherapy conditioning for bone marrow transplantation
Hodgkin's disease: treatment with alkylating drugs
Soft tissue sarcoma: stage IV (metastatic)
Ewing's sarcoma: metastatic

Table 1. Best assessment of risk of subfertility after current treatments for common cancers in childhood and adolescence (Wallace 2005)

A study in California (Zebrack 2004) noted that 59% of young adult survivors of childhood cancer from Los Angeles do not know whether they will be fertile. More than half indicate that neither their relatives nor doctors spoke to them of potential consequences of treatments received during the care of their cancer. Others received vague information concerning risks. Such findings suggest that health care providers who come into contact with long-term survivors of childhood cancer need to be prepared to provide them with accurate information about potential reproductive problems and risks for infertility based upon knowledge of their past treatment.

Van den Berg sent short questionnaires to parents of 159 male survivors of childhood cancer diagnosed and treated with chemotherapy in the Emma Children Hospital of Amsterdam (Van den Berg 2008), inquiring about year of birth, age at initial diagnosis, type of malignancy, and whether there was relapse. The remaining questions asked whether information given at initial diagnosis included discussion of possible secondary infertility, if sperm was analyzed after treatment in pubertal boys, and if the parents expected their child to be infertile. Questionnaires were returned by 63%. Of these, 50% of parents recalled statements concerning an effect on fertility, 36% indicated that this had not been the case, and the remainder were unsure. Sperm analysis had been performed after treatment in 4 cases and semen collected prior to start of therapy in 14 cases; in 2 cases, the parent was uncertain in this regard. Nine percent of parents thought their son's infertility was a fact, 31% expected normal fertility, and 60% were uncertain.

Actual infertility influences not only procreation; even the suspicion of its risk profoundly affects body image, dating, and marriage (Schover 1999, Byrne 1989, Thaler-DeMers 2001, Zevon 1990). In long-term survivors of childhood cancer, at least 53% of men and 65% of women worry whether they can have children (Langeveld 2003). Limited knowledge of the effects of their treatment from inadequate processing of information given at diagnosis or failed memory of its content is a major contributing factor to these concerns. Parents are often an important source of information when a child suffers from a malignancy, and as children grow older, parents give them age-specific information. Data in this study indicate that despite the medical teams' certainty that parents were informed, half the parents could not recall receiving information concerning fertility. Care providers and/or parents might also withhold such information. Half the care providers stated that it is inappropriate to provide this information at the time consent is being given for treatment, considering it more important to offer information about fertility when therapy is finished (Goodwin 2007). The literature indicates that at least part of the poor recall of survivors of childhood cancer regarding issues of fertility is that the information was not provided by health care workers. Other contributing factors include the turmoil of unexpected events in the first weeks of illness in a case of childhood malignancy that often overloads parents with information on subjects with which they are unaccustomed and their withholding of information to shield their child from future burden or to avoid the child's reaction. It is highly recommended that medical providers check whether parents have received adequate information on their child's future fertility after they have had time to cope with the problems and emotions at initial diagnosis or relapse.

6. Fertility preservation

6.1 Male patients

Semen cryopreservation is an established and successful technique for men, and though its value has been shown in adolescent patients, it may be difficult to achieve. Treatment of malignant pediatric disease should be started as soon as possible after diagnosis, but teenagers at this early point in the disease process might be too distressed to discuss fertility and subsequently unlikely to produce a semen sample. Discussions should be dealt with sensitively in language understood by the patient. As well, it is important that sperm banking be practiced near pediatric oncology centers.

Boys sufficiently mature might produce semen samples by masturbation, or penile vibratory stimulation or rectal electrostimulation under anaesthetic can be considered if this method is not possible (Schmiegelow 1998). Alternatively, if spermatogenesis is established, sperm can be retrieved after testicular or epididymal aspiration.

Methods of storing sperm have improved significantly, and technological advances in assisted reproductive technology using intracytoplasmic sperm injection (ICSI) increase the likelihood of successful pregnancies using banked sperm.

Prepubertal boys pose additional challenges for fertility preservation because they cannot produce semen for cryopreservation. Germline cells of the prepubertal testes include spermatogonial stem cells, but mature spermatozoa are not yet present. A novel approach to circumvent this problem is cryopreserving the boy's testicular tissue. When he is ready to begin a family years after undergoing cancer treatment, the cryopreserved tissue is thawed and the banked germ cells reimplanted into the patient's testes to enable full maturation and reproductive potential (Brinster 2007). Unfortunately, a typical testicular biopsy contains insufficient numbers of stem cells to restore fertility, and a large supply of stem cells is required to ensure that no remaining cancer cells contaminate the transplanted cell population. Therefore, culturing methods must be developed to remove unwanted cancer cells and increase the number of biopsied stem cells to restore fertility through autotransplantation procedures. A novel approach is to employ a cryopreserved testicular sample to enrich for spermatogonial stem cells that are subsequently matured into viable spermatids *in vitro* through innovative culturing procedures. Use of this strategy could then achieve fertilization by ICSI (Ginsberg 2009).

6.2 Female patients

Oocyte cryopreservation is a feasible method of fertility preservation for young girls. Oocytes are fragile, and ovarian tissue consisting of germ cells can be removed and stored before gonadotoxic treatment. The ovarian cortex is utilized because it is rich in primordial follicles (Poirot 2002-2007). After the patient is cured, this tissue might be either returned to the patient via autotransplantation or matured *in vitro* to produce offspring by *in vitro* fertilization, similar to the technique proposed for male patients at this age. *In vitro* maturation is highly desirable because it obviates the concern of reimplanting cancer cells into the patient. Accordingly, the development of methodologies for obtaining human oocytes from primordial follicles is undergoing intensive laboratory investigation (Smitz 2010). However, ovarian transplantation may not be indicated in female patients with blood-borne malignancy because cancer cells circulating within the blood could remain in cryopreserved ovarian tissues (Dolmans 2010). Because ovarian biopsy is invasive and experimental, this option should only be considered for female patients at high risk of infertility. The most appropriate pediatric female candidates are patients undergoing stem cell transplantation, in whom there is a high likelihood of acute ovarian failure. In contrast, pediatric patients with cancer exposed to high doses of alkylating agents as part of their chemotherapy regimen, who often have a window of fertility following treatment and are more prone to premature ovarian failure, may have the opportunity as adults to undergo successful fertility preservation interventions.

Thus , ovarian cryopreservation, including transplantation, is now a clinical option available for children. Transplanted frozen/thawed tissue may be highly effective in restoring ovarian function and maintain function for prolonged periods of time. The many follicles present in children's ovaries could be used to induce puberty and possibly provide fertility later on. Although tissue can be transplanted to restore fertility, this method's efficacy is limited and requires refinement. Results are encouraging for continued research efforts and may have far reaching possibilities that we must begin to address. Current research focuses on the possibility of hormonal protection of the gonad, long-term storage of testicular or ovarian material, and xenotransplantation into a host species. Transplanted material may subsequently be reintroduced into the patient, or gametes may be extracted for assisted reproductive techniques, such as *in vitro* fertilization.

7. Offspring among survivors of childhood cancer

7.1 Low birth weight in offspring after pelvic irradiation

One CCSS study included 1915 females who reported 4029 pregnancies (63% live births, 1% still4births, 15% miscarriages, 17% abortions, 4% unknown or in gestation). Pregnancy outcome did not differ significantly by treatment. There was a higher, but not statistically significant, risk of miscarriage among women whose ovaries were in the field of radiation therapy (RR = 1.86, P = 0.14), near the field (RR = 1.64, P = 0.06), or shielded (RR = 0.90, P = 0.88). The rate of live birth was not lower for patients treated with any particular chemotherapeutic agent. The offspring of patients who received pelvic irradiation were more likely to weigh less than 2500 g at birth (RR = 1.84, P = 0.03). This large study did not identify adverse pregnancy outcomes for female survivors treated with most chemotherapeutic agents but did indicate that the offspring of women who received pelvic irradiation are at risk for low birth weight (Green 2002).

7.2 No genetic anomalies among offspring

Drugs used to treat cancer are designed to interfere with DNA, cell division, and cellular metabolism, processes essential to embryogenesis and fetogenesis. A cohort study described by Byrne and associates (Byrne 1998) found genetic anomalies in 3.2% of 2198 offspring of survivors of childhood cancer compared to 3.1% in controls (4544 newborns). Similar results are reported in a Danish cohort (Winther 2004). Thus, there appear to be no genetic anomalies in offspring of survivors who underwent chemotherapy for childhood cancer.

7.3 Congenital anomalies among offspring

The large series described by Byrne (Byrne 1998) found congenital anomalies in 3.4% of 2198 offspring of childhood survivors compared to 3.1% in controls. Similarly, an international study (United States and Denmark) described by Boice and associates found no significant difference in relative risk of congenital anomalies among offspring of 25,000 survivors of childhood cancer who either fathered or gave birth to around 6000 children compared with their sibling controls (Boice 2003). Hawkins also reported only 46 congenital anomalies in 1033 (4.4%) newborns of cancer survivors, which is similar with the general population (Hawkins 1988).

However, an increased risk of congenital anomalies has been reported in the offspring of female survivors of cancer previously diagnosed with Wilms' tumor and treated with flank radiation. The mechanism underlying this risk has not been identified but may involve radiation damage to the female gamete (Green 2002 *JCO*)

7.4 No excess risk of cancer among offspring

In the Nordic cohort, including 14,652 survivors of cancer in childhood or adolescence diagnosed since the 1940s and 1950s, only 22 sporadic cancers, excluding retinoblastoma (17 cases) and other hereditary cancers, were observed among 5847 offspring. The standardized incidence ratio is 1.3 (95% confidence interval [CI], 0.8 to 2.0). No neoplasms were observed among the children of survivors of leukemia, neuroblastoma, or hepatic tumors. The overall standardized ratio for nonretinoblastoma neoplasms was 3.9 (95% CI, 2.1 to 6.7) for offspring whose parents were younger than 10 years at diagnosis and 1.1 (95% CI, 0.6 to 1.8) for those with parents diagnosed at age 10 or older. All but one offspring with cancer were born at least 8 years after cancer was diagnosed in their mother (Sankila 1998).

There seems to be no increase in childhood malignancies in offspring of survivors, with the exception of cancers arising as a result of inherited syndromes, including familial adenomatous polyposis, hereditary nonpolyposis colon cancer, retinoblastoma, Li-Fraumeni syndrome, and others.

7.5 No modification of sex ratio

Some researchers have assessed the sex ratio of fetuses born to cancer survivors after treatment compared with the general population and noted no difference, ensuring that cancer treatment does not increase incidence of X-linked mutations (Winther 2003)

8. Conclusion

Infertility is an important issue arising as a late effect of childhood cancer treatment and should be discussed at initial cancer diagnosis if therapy may carry some risk. Although the topic may be difficult for parents, it is necessary to consider some method of protecting fertility at an early stage, even in young children. Although it is very difficult to predict fertility after treatment, there is much interest in potential markers of gonadal damage that can be used in adolescents and young adults.

Beyond the possible precautionary measures in assessing issues surrounding fertility in survivors of childhood cancer, it is necessary to review the history of the patient's disease and treatment regimen, clarifying chemotherapies, surgeries, and irradiation, and biologic markers may also be measured (FSH, testosterone, estradiol, AMH). Knowledge of these data will elucidate how to care better for the patient, and if there is a risk to fertility, a couple can be referred for consultation with a health center for assisted reproduction.

9. Acknowledgement

We would like to thank Rosalyn Uhrig, M.A. for her editorial assistance in the preparation of this manuscript.

10. References

Andrieu JM, Ochoa-Molina ME. Menstrual cycle, pregnancies and offspring before and after MOPP therapy for Hodgkin disease. Cancer 1983, 52, 435-438.

Aubier F, Flamant F, Brauner R, Caillaud JM, Chaussain JM, Lemerle J. Male gonadal function after chemotherapy for solid tumors in childhood. J Clin Oncol 1989, 7, 304-309.

Berger C, Trombert-Paviot B, Mitton N, et al. [Childhood cancer incidence and survival rates in the Rhône-Alpes regional paediatric registry 1987-1999]. Arch Pediatr 2006, 13, 121–129. [Article in French]

Boice JD Jr, Tawn EJ, Winther JF, et al. Genetic effects of radiotherapy for childhood cancer. Health Phys 2003, 85, 65-80.

Brinster RL. Male germline stem cells: from mice to men. Science 2007, 316, 404-405.

Byrne J, Fears TR, Mills JL, et al. Fertility of long-term male survivors of acute lymphoblastic leukemia diagnosed during childhood. Pediatr Blood Cancer 2004, 42, 364-372.

Byrne J, Fears TR, Steinhorn SC, et al. Marriage and divorce after childhood and adolescent cancer. JAMA 1989, 262, 2693-2699.

Byrne J, Rasmussen SA, Steinhorn SC, et al. Genetic disease in offspring of long-term survivors of childhood and adolescent cancer. Am J Hum Genet 1998, 62, 45-52.

Dama E, Maule MM, Mosso ML, et al. Life after childhood cancer: marriage and offspring in adult long-term survivors - a population-based study in the Piedmont region, Italy. Eur J Cancer Prev 2009, 18, 425-430.

Dolmans MM, Marinescu C, Saussoy P, Langendonckt A, Amorim C, Donnez J. Reimplantation of cryopreserved ovarian tissue from patients with acute lymphoblastic leukemia is potentially unsafe. Blood 2010, 116, 2908-2914.

Ginsberg JP, Carlson CA, Lin K, et al. An experimental protocol for fertility preservation in prepubertal boys recently diagnosed with cancer: a report of acceptability and safety. Hum Reprod 2010, 25, 37-41.

Goodwin T, Elizabeth Oosterhuis B, Kiernan M, Hudson MM, Dahl GV. Attitudes and practices of pediatric oncology providers regarding fertility issues. Pediatr Blood Cancer 2007, 48, 80-85.

Green DM, Kawashima T, Stovall M, et al. Fertility of female survivors of childhood cancer: a report from the Childhood Cancer Survivor Study. J Clin Oncol 2009, 27, 2677-2685.

Green DM, Kawashima T, Stovall M, et al. Fertility of male survivors of childhood cancer: a report from the Childhood Cancer Survivor Study. J Clin Oncol 2010, 28, 332-339.

Green DM, Peabody EM, Nan B, Peterson S, Kalapurakal JA, Breslow NE. Pregnancy outcome after treatment for Wilms tumor: a report from the National Wilms Tumor Study Group. J Clin Oncol 2002, 20, 2506-2513.

Green DM, Whitton JA, Stovall M, et al. Pregnancy outcome of female survivors of childhood cancer: a report from the Childhood Cancer Survivor Study. Am J Obstet Gynecol 2002, 187, 1070-1080.

Hawkins MM, Smith RA, Curtice LJ. Childhood cancer survivors and their offspring studied through a postal survey of general practitioners: preliminary results. J R Coll Gen Pract 1998, 38, 102-105.

Kenney LB, Laufer MR, Grand FD, Grier H, Diller L. High risk of infertility and long term gonadal damage in males treated with high dose cyclophosphamide for sarcoma during childhood. Cancer 2001, 91, 613-621.

Langeveld NE, Ubbink MC, Last BF, Grootenhuis MA, Voûte PA, De Haan RJ. Educational achievement, employment and living situation in long-term young adult survivors of childhood cancer in the Netherlands. Psychooncology 2003, 12, 213-225.

Lie Fong S, Laven JS, Hakvoort-Cammel FG, et al. Assessment of ovarian reserve in adult childhood cancer survivors using anti-Müllerian hormone. Hum Reprod 2009, 24, 982-990.

Longhi A, Macchiagodena M, Vitali G, Bacci G. Fertility in male patients treated with neoadjuvant chemotherapy for osteosarcoma. J Pediatr Hematol Oncol 2003, 25, 292-296.

Poirot C, Vacher-Lavenu MC, Helardot P, Guibert J, Brugières L, Jouannet P. Human ovarian tissue cryopreservation: indications and feasibility. Hum Reprod 2002, 17, 1447-1452.

Poirot CJ, Martelli H, Genestie C, et al. Feasibility of ovarian tissue cryopreservation for prepubertal females with cancer. Pediatr Blood Cancer 2007, 49, 74-78.

Pryzant RM, Meistrich ML, Wilson G, Brown B, McLaughlin P. Long-term reduction in sperm count after chemotherapy with and without radiation therapy for non-Hodgkin's lymphomas. J Clin Oncol 1993, 11, 239-247.

Rebar RW. Premature ovarian failure. Obstet Gynecol 2009, 113, 1355-1363.

Sankila R, Olsen JH, Anderson H, et al. Risk of cancer among offspring of childhood-cancer survivors. Association of the Nordic Cancer Registries and the Nordic Society of Paediatric Haematology and Oncology. N Engl J Med 1998, 338, 1339-1344.

Schilsly RL, Sherins RJ, Hubbard SM, Wesley MN, Young RC, DeVita VT. Long term follow up of ovarian function in women treated with MOPP chemotherapy for Hodgkin's disease. Am J Med 1981, 71, 552-556.

Schmiegelow ML, Sommer P, Carlsen E, Sønksen JO, Schmiegelow K, Müller JR. Penile vibratory stimulation and electroejaculation before anticancer therapy in two pubertal boys. J Pediatr Hematol Oncol 1998, 20, 429-430.

Schover LR. Psychosocial aspects of infertility and decisions about reproduction in young cancer survivors: a review. Med Pediatr Oncol 1999, 33, 53-59.

Smitz J, Dolmans MM, Donnez J, et al. Current achievements and future research directions in ovarian tissue culture, in vitro follicle development and transplantation: implications for fertility preservation. Hum Reprod Update 2010, 16, 395-414.

Teinturier C, Hartmann O, Valteau-Couanet D, Benhamou E, Bougneres PF. Ovarian function after autologous bone marrow transplantation in childhood: high-dose busulfan is a major cause of ovarian failure. Bone Marrow Transplant, 1998, 22, 989-994.

Thaler-DeMers D. Intimacy issues: sexuality, fertility, and relationships. Semin Oncol Nurs 2001, 17, 255-262.

Wallace WH, Anderson RA, Irvine DS. Fertility preservation for young patients with cancer: who is at risk and what can be offered? Lancet Oncol 2005, 6, 209-218. Review. Erratum in: Lancet Oncol 2005, 6, 922.

Winther JF, Boice JD Jr, Mulvihill JJ, et al. Chromosomal abnormalities among offspring of childhood-cancer survivors in Denmark: a population-based study. Am J Hum Genet 2004, 74, 1282-1285.

Winther JF, Boice JD Jr, Thomsen BL, Schull WJ, Stovall M, Olsen JH. Sex ratio among offspring of childhood cancer survivors treated with radiotherapy. Br J Cancer 2003, 88, 382-387.

Zebrack BJ, Casillas J, Nohr L, Adams H, Zeltzer LK. Fertility issues for young adult survivors of childhood cancer. Psychooncology 2004, 13, 689-699.

Zevon MA, Neubauer NA, Green DM. Adjustment and vocational satisfaction of patients treated during childhood or adolescence for acute lymphoblastic leukemia. Am J Pediatr Hematol Oncol 1990, 12, 454-461.

14

Fatigue in Pediatric Oncology Patients

Hatice Bal Yılmaz
Ege University, Nursing Faculty,
Turkey

1. Introduction

Cancer-related fatigue in children is defined as a deliberate sense of being weak or having difficulty in moving extremities or even opening eyes. Fatigue may be resulted from environmental, individual/social or treatment-related factors and cause further problems such as playing with other children, lack of concentration or developing negative feelings (anger or sadness) (Hockenberry-Eaton&Hinds, 2000).

National Comprehensive Cancer Network also defines cancer-related fatigue as "a constant and subjective symptom of cancer treatment that affects general functions, perception of physical energy, mental state and psychosocial conditions, and cancer-related weariness" (Mock et al. 2000).

North American Nursing Diagnosis Association (NANDA), on the other hand, classifies fatigue as a self-reported diagnosis in an individual unrelieved by rest which manifests itself with a chronic and tiring exhaustion and a reduced physical and mental performance. In order to prevent adverse effects of fatigue, an effective management is attainable with a careful evaluation and designing individual-specific activities (Erdemir, 2005).

While cancer is now agreed to be a curable disease, especially with the rapid developments in medicine and technology, the prevalence and types of treatment-related side effects have been shown to correspondingly increase (Bal Yılmaz et al. 2010).

A literature analysis on the symptoms in children with cancer illustrated that early studies on pediatric cancer symptoms could be summoned in three main themes, which are treatment related pain; treatment related nausea-vomit and psychosocial symptoms associated with adaptation to being diagnosed with cancer (Allen et al. 1997; Bashore, 2004; Eiser et al. 1997). Enskar et al. (1997) added fatigue and feeling of sickness to these symptoms. Enskar et al. (1997) interviewed adolescents diagnosed with cancer and reported that they felt constantly weary and exhausted and they had occasional complaints of vomit, which eventually caused a feeling of sickness.

Fatigue is a universal symptom reported in cytotoxic chemotherapy, radiation therapy, and bone marrow transplant and with biological response modifiers. Despite being a common symptom among cancer patients, it has gradually increased to almost acute levels with the use of multidimensional treatment applications (Anderson et al. 2003; Mock et al. 2000). It has also been maintained that fatigue, unless supervised, adversely influences daily life activities and quality of life (Taş&Bal Yılmaz, 2008). Fatigue seemingly lies at the core of the current debates since it proves to be a subjective condition with individually differing degrees of duration and characteristics (Yurtsever, 2000).

On account of its subjective nature and multifarious causes, defining and evaluating fatigue remain to be a challenge and it has been formulated within a wide array of medical disciplines. Physiologists understand fatigue as "reduced physical performance" while pathologists define it as "a physical and mental incapacity stemmed from neuromuscular and metabolic disorders".

Nursing researchers commonly conceive fatigue as "a subjective symptom with overall effects ranging from slight exhaustion to unbearable weariness which impedes a person from accomplishing regular daily tasks and functions. Four different aspects of fatigue have been consistently focused on in medical and nursing literature and accordingly fatigue has been defined as:

- An experience affecting all bodily functions induced by emotional, cognitive and physical factors
- An unpleasant perception caused by distress
- A chronic and implacable phenomenon
- A subjective experience based on self-perception (Yurtsever 2000)

Considering that fatigue is primarily perceived by the patient, it is best defined with self-report besides physical examination, laboratory findings, reports from family members and health care professionals (HCPs) on patient's condition and behaviors as additional sources of information (De Nijs et al. 2008).

Fatigue can be observed in a variety of ways. Some of the determinant characteristics of fatigue are:

Major characteristics

- Constant verbal expression of the loss of energy
- Incapacity in sustaining routine activities

Minor characteristics

- A need for extra energy for fulfilling routine daily tasks
- Increase in physical complaints
- Being emotionally unsteady or sensitive
- Loss of concentration skills
- Reduced performance
- Lethargy or indisposition
- Indifference to environment
- Incapacity to fulfill social activities
- Inability to muster up enough energy despite having proper sleep (Yurtsever 2000).

2. Causes of fatigue

Potential causes of fatigue are enlisted as follows:

2.1 Pathophysiological factors

- Infections:
- Acute infections; hepatitis
- Chronic infections; endocarditis
- Secondary to the situations below, associated with reduced tissue oxygenation; congestive heart failure, chronic obstructive pulmonary disease, anemia, peripheral vascular disease
- Secondary to the situations below, associated with biochemical alterations;
- Endocrine disorders; diabetes mellitus, Addison's disease, hypothyroidism, chronic diseases; kidney failure, cirrhosis
- Secondary to the situations below, associated with muscle weakness;
- Neuromuscular diseases; Parkinson, multiple sclerosis
- Secondary to the situations below, associated with the changes in food metabolism or nutritional deficiency; nausea, vomit, diarrhea, side effects of medicines…
- Obesity
- Electrolyte imbalance
- Eating disorders; Fe, B12 vitamin deficiency
- AIDS

2.2 Treatment related factors

- Associated with chemotherapy
- Associated with radiotherapy and immunotherapy
- Associated with side effects of certain medicines (long term use of corticosteroids, beta blockers…)
- Associated with surgical tissue damage and anesthesia

2.3 Situational factors

- Secondary to the situations below, associated with reduced activity and prolonged loss of condition
- Depression, anxiety, fever, diarrhea, pain, social isolation, nausea/vomit
- Associated with the intensity of role systems
- Associated with intense-excessive distress
- Associated with sleeping disorders (Yurtsever, 2000).

3. Factors that may increase or decrease the intensity of fatigue

Identifying fatigue in children also permitted children and parents to identify the factors that may increase or decrease the intensity of fatigue

3.1 Factors that may increase the intensity of fatigue

- Environmental factors; noise, hospitalization, hospital procedures, waiting at the hospital lounge, interpersonal relations, interrupted daily tasks

- Personal/behavioral factors; dynamism, sadness, changes in sleep patterns, waking up at night, having a bad sleep, changes in resting patterns
- Family and social factors, realizing family's anxiety
- Treatment/treatment related factors; onset of treatment, pain, lowering blood test results, stop eating, interventions, infection therapy

3.2 Factors that may decrease the intensity of fatigue

- Personal/behavioral factors; naps/lethargy, providing a comfortable sleep
- Personal/behavioral factors; encouraging participation in activities, supporting pastime activities, interacting with children
- Family and social factors; having visitors, participation in entertainment/pastime activities, ensuring comfort, changes in family life
- Treatment/treatment related factors; nutrition (Hinds et al. 1999A).

4. Cancer-related fatigue in children

Although adult oncology literature provides substantial data on fatigue and chronic fatigue, certain data still remain inadequate for the influences of cancer and cancer treatment on children (Langeveld et al. 2003). Studies on fatigue are narrow in scope in pediatric oncology literature which implies that health care researchers seemingly have underestimated cancer-related fatigue in children when compared to the studies of adult oncology. Cancer and chemotherapy related fatigue definitely possess different characteristics in children. The cancer treatment for children follows an intensive program in the first place in which the prime target is to ensure a high-dose therapy as much as possible. Curative approaches towards pediatric cancers achieved 70% rate of recovery in late 1990's. In contrast to adult treatment programs, fatigue hasn't been considered as a side effect in limiting dosages in pediatric programs because, first of all, fatigue is usually disregarded as a symptom that can possibly lead to dosage changes due to its diagnosis based on self-report. Secondly, unlike adults, children often fail to express their experiences with side effects of the treatment and they may be incapable of noticing the changes in their physical power and daily routines. Adolescents, on the other hand, may assume the loss of energy and fatigue as a natural consequence of having cancer. Thirdly, parents may not be well informed about fatigue as a side effect of the treatment and thus they may be unaware of the urgency for intervention. Most parents are inclined to oversee their children's changing patterns of activity so as not to discuss the matter with health care experts (Hockenberry-Eaton&Hinds, 2000).

Below is the report of a child experiencing fatigue:

Johny T. is a ten years old child with cell lymphoma taking chemotherapy. He remembers his agility before diagnosis. He frequently complains about weakness and fatigue and often wishes to lie down. As he can hardly run, he can't play baseball any more. He misses the school every so often because he needs help a lot and fatigue prevents him from concentrating on the lessons. Johny feels that resting all day may sometimes soothe the intense fatigue. Furthermore, he repeatedly experiences anger and sadness for being so tired as not to be able to play with his friends (Hockenberry-Eaton&Hinds, 2000).

Researches on the significance of fatigue in pediatric population have become prominent within the last 10 years. These studies mainly suggest that;

- Adolescents and children with cancer experience fatigue
- Developing a better insight into the function of fatigue in pediatric population ascertains a more accurate and thorough evaluation of the symptom
- Developmental levels of the children undertaking the treatment should be taken into consideration for an understanding of the symptom in pediatric population
- Understanding fatigue in pediatric population will certainly ensure a holistic approach by eliciting patients' and parents' perspective (Hockenberry et al. 1998; Hockenberry-Eaton&Hinds, 2000).

The analysis of fatigue primarily commenced with the definition of the symptom and its fundamental characteristics, which eventually facilitated establishing a model for understanding fatigue in children. Children with cancer suffer from symptoms of the illness as well as the side effects of chemotherapy. Moreover, they withstand physiological and psychological developmental changes characteristic of their age. They may be adversely affected by physiological and psychological side effects of chemotherapy during their daily routines and activities. These effects may further include nausea and vomit, loss or gain of weight, electrolyte imbalance, weakness and lethargy. These symptoms can be assessed in pediatric patients in a different manner with comparison to adult oncology patients. As a result, it is of utmost importance that fatigue be evaluated in children with cancer as a symptom in consideration of characterizing its outset, prevalence, severity and natural history (Hockenberry et al. 1998; Hockenberry-Eaton&Hinds, 2000).

Fatigue is a subjective experience and children and adults may differ in expressing a subjective experience. Accordingly, data gathered from adults and pediatric patients should be evaluated interdependently. Hinds and Hockenberry (2001) defined the characteristics of fatigue and factors that may increase or decrease the intensity of the symptom. They additionally reported that patients and parents tend to have different personal approaches and proposed that fatigue assessment should be conducted simultaneously for the multidimensional nature of the evaluation process and interventions (Hinds& Hockenberry-Eaton, 2001).

Mock (2000) stated that fatigue is widely regarded as a subjective experience in a majority of studies and that establishing a database for fatigue requires serious efforts to measure subjective experiences in an objective manner, which is to measure physical and cognitive variables. He also explained that a comprehensive definition of fatigue necessitates handling both subjective and objective indicators.

Children, parents or HCPs may have different ideas about the causes of the symptom, which urges an overall evaluation on the interventions to reduce fatigue. A number of scales have been developed to evaluate fatigue so far and some examples are Visual Analogue Scale Fatigue (VAS-F), Symptom Distress Scale, Yoshitake's Fatigue Scale, Rhoten Fatigue Scale and Pearson and Byar's Fatigue Scale (Hart, 1990). However, none of these scales have been peculiarly designed for children and adolescents, which surely hinder a proper evaluation. Linder (2005) reviewed the literature evaluating the measurements of physical symptoms and noted that fatigue was measured in only five different studies (Linder, 2005).

Hockenbery et al. (2003) developed the only scale particularly designed for measuring fatigue in children with cancer Fatigue was commonly considered as an element of the quality of life. The first scales that measured cancer related fatigue in children were developed by Hockenberry et al. (2003). Theoretical guidelines of these scales were basically the results of their studies particularly focusing on cancer related fatigue in children and adolescents (Hinds et al. 1999B; Hockenberry et al. 1998). These studies defined fatigue as a subjective symptom referring to physical, emotional and mental perceptions and resulted in developing different scales for measuring cancer related fatigue in children, which are Children's Fatigue Scale, Childhood Cancer Fatigue Scale for Mothers and Fatigue Scale for 7-12 years old Pediatric Oncology Patients: Health Care Provider's Form. These scales were developed to determine the intensity, prevalence and causes of cancer related fatigue in children within the last week (Hockenberry et al. 2003). Evidently enough, the assessment of fatigue has been carried out by not only children themselves but also care provider family members and nurses in pediatric oncology literature (Bal Yılmaz et al. 2009; Bal Yılmaz et al. 2010; Baraud et al. 2003; Genç&Conk, 2008; Gibson et al. 2005; Gibson et al. 2006; Hindset al. 1999A; Hinds et al. 1999B; Hinds&Hockenberry-Eaton, 2001; Hinds et al. 2007A; Hinds et al. 2007B; Hinds et al. 2007C; Hinds et al. 2010; Hockenberry et al. 2003; Perdikaris et al. 2008; Perdikaris et al. 2009;Yeh et al. 2008).

Fatigue is a perceptive symptom and requires a multidimensional approach. Therefore, researchers are suggested to use other forms in combination while developing the scale and enable parents and HCPs to assess the symptom in addition to patient children (Hinds et al. 2007). It is considered to be imperative that perceptive symptoms should be evaluated by more than one single observer as in the design of the quality of life scales (Taş & Bal Yılmaz, 2008). Each individual may attribute different meanings to wellness in respect to physical, psychological, social and personal traits and consequently experiences the process of illness in a different way, which underscores the significance of an evaluation for both objective and subjective symptoms. Evaluation for objective symptoms entails the capabilities of children and adolescents, life conditions, functionality of environment and school and social relations while evaluation for subjective symptoms essentially comprises physical, emotional and social functionality of children and adolescents (Memik et al. 2007).

5. Management of fatigue

National Comprehensive Cancer Network maintained that fatigue should be rapidly defined, evaluated, controlled and treated with a multidisciplinary approach in each stage of the illness both during and after the treatment.

5.1 Care standards in fatigue management

- Fatigue is a subjective experience identified with self-reports of the patient and other sources of information
- Fatigue is an observable, diagnosable and curable symptom in line with the practice guidelines of clinics
- Fatigue can be characterized on first day of hospitalization and with regular visits later on

- Fatigue should be predominantly characterized, evaluated and reported during and after the treatment
- HCPs should request a timely consultation in evaluating and managing fatigue .
- Institution-specific standards should be developed by multidisciplinary committees for fatigue management
- HCPs should organize education programs to enhance professional knowledge and skills in defining and managing fatigue
- Families and patients should regard fatigue management as a part of holistic health care
- Health care outcomes should include data on cancer related fatigue
- A qualified fatigue care also reflects the institutional effort to enhance the quality of health care

Fatigue care must be contained in medical care expenses (Mock et al. 2000).

5.2 Role of nurses in fatigue management

Pediatric care services have deliberately reiterated the significance of supporting children's emotional and developmental needs for the last 30 years. In pediatric oncology, nurses undertake substantial responsibilities in assisting children and parents to adjust to the illness and the treatment procedures. Nurses can avert acute or delayed effects of the treatment and decrease the intensity of the symptoms by accomplishing considerable tasks such as monitoring, providing care, educating, consulting, conducting researches and pursuing patient's advocacy.

5.3 Nursing Interventions for fatigue

- Ensuring plenty of liquid intake
- Controlling the pain (medicines, relaxing, hot/cold application)
- Treating anemia (with the help of medical team)
- Controlling nausea and vomit (with medicine and relaxation)
- Controlling constipation (with medicines, diet and activities)
- Infection Control
  - *Regular bath*
  - *Regular mouth care*
  - *Washing hands before and after using toilet*
  - *Refraining from any contact with the crowds and people with contagious disease*
  - *Following asepsis-antisepsis principles in invasive interventions*
  - *Limiting visitors for neutropenic children*
- Planning Regular Diet
  - *Sharing the mealtimes with friends and family*
  - *Having nutritious snacks during the day.*
  - *Keeping food variety*
  - *Ensuring protein intake everyday*
  - *Resting before meals*
  - *Cooperating with the dietician*
- Ensuring Enough Sleep and Rest
  - *Planning activities and resting periods on a rotation basis*

- *Limiting naps with 20-30 minutes*
- *Avoiding activities or stimulants before sleep*
- *Maintaining regular sleep*
- *Doing relaxation exercises before sleep*
- *Assuring a quality night sleep*
- Exercise
  - *Wearing comfortable clothes and shoes*
  - *Jogging and exercises starting in a slow tempo and increasing gradually*
  - *Starting with 5-10 minute exercises and extending the sets 1-2 minutes every week.*
  - *Accentuating the significance of stopping exercises before getting exhausted*
- Conservation of Energy
  - *Designing activity programs as "work out-rest, work out-rest" sets*
  - *Ensuring having rest before getting exhausted*
  - *Avoiding hastiness as much as possible*
  - *Replacing hard exercises with soft exercises*
  - *Focusing on favorite exercises*
  - *Avoiding lifting heavy weights*
  - *Arranging play times with friends*
- Maintaining interaction with family and friends
  - *Informing patients and families about asking for help from family members, friends and HCPs* (De Nijs et al. 2008).

6. Conclusion

It was demonstrated that cancer-related fatigue in pediatric patients was perceived to be a significant problem by both parents and HCPs (Gibson et al., 2005; Bal Yılmaz et al. 2009; Bal Yılmaz et al. 2010). The studies mentioned above indicate that fatigue is an important clinical problem that is experienced by children undergoing cancer treatments. By better understanding the factors that cause fatigue, HCPs may be able to perform interventions that either reduce fatigue or make it easier for children with cancer to accept it (Magnusson et al., 1997). The effective diagnosis and treatment of fatigue not only enhances patients' quality of life, but it also improves the quality of care that HCPs are able to provide (Tiesinga et al. 2000). It is thought that to prevent fatigue from having a negative impact on children, all the factors contributing to their fatigue should be identified, then the signs of fatigue should be recognized, and finally, effective interventions should be planned to relieve their symptoms of fatigue (Knowles et al. 2000).

7. References

[1] Allen, R., Newman, S.P., Souhami, R. L., (1997). Anxiety and Depression in Adolescent Cancer: Findings in Patients and Parents at the Time of Diagnosis. *Europan Joumal of Cancer*, 33(8): 1250-1255.

[2] Anderson, K.O., Getto, C.J., Mendoza, T.R., Palmer, S.N., Wang, X.S., Reyes-Gibby, C.C., Cleeland, C.S. (2003). Fatigue and sleep disturbance in patients with cancer, patients with clinical depression, and community-dwelling adults, *J Pain Symptom Manag*ement, 25(4): 307-18.

[3] Bal Yılmaz, H., Muslu, G.K., Taş, F., Başbakkal, Z., Kantar, M. (2009). Parental views regarding symptoms in children with cancer and recognition of cancer-related fatigue. Türk Onkoloji Dergisi, 24(3):122-127.

[4] Bal Yılmaz, H., Taş, F., Muslu, G.K., Başbakkal, Z., Kantar, M. (2010). Health Professionals' Estimation of Cancer-Related Fatigue in Children. Journal of Pediatric Oncology Nursing, 27(6):330–337.

[5] Bashore, L. (2004). Childhood and Adolescent Cancer Survivors' Knowledge of Their Disease and Effects of Treatment, *Journal of Pediatric Oncology Nursing*, 21(2): 98-102.

[6] Braud A.C., Genre D., Leto C., Nemer V., Cailhol J.F., Macquart-Moulin G., Maraninchi D., Viens P. (2003). Nurses' repeat measurement of chemotherapy symptoms: feasibility, resulting information, patient satisfaction. Cancer Nurs, 26(6):468-75.

[7] De Nijs E.J., Ros W., Grijpdonck M.H. (2008). Nursing intervention for fatigue during the treatment for cancer. Cancer Nurs, May-Jun; 31(3):191-206.

[8] Eiser, C., Havermans, T., Craft, A., et al. (1997). Validity of the Rotterdam Symptom Checlist in Paediatric Oncology, *Medical and Pediatric Oncology*, 28: 451-454.

[9] Enskär, H., Carlsson, M., Golsäter, M., et. al. (1997). Symptom Distress and Life Situation in Adolescents with Cancer, *Cancer Nursing*, 20(1): 23-33.

[10] Erdemir, F. (2005). Hemşirelik Tanıları El Kitabı. Nobel tıp kitapevi, "Carpenito-Moyet. Handbook of Nursing Diagnosis".

[11] Genç, R.E., Conk, Z. (2008). Impact of Effective Nursing Interventions to the Fatigue Syndrome in Children Who Receive Chemotherapy, *Cancer Nursing*, 31(4): 312-317.

[12] Gibson, F., Edwards, J., Sepion, B., Richardson, A. (2006). Cancer-related fatigue in children and young people: Survey of healthcare professionals' knowledge and attitudes, European *Journal of Oncology Nursing*, 10:311-316.

[13] Gibson, F., Garnett, M., Richardson, A., Edwards, J., Sepion, B. (2005). Heavy to carry: A survey of parents' and healthcare professionals' perceptions of cancer-related fatigue in children and young people, *Cancer Nursing*, 28(1): 27-35.

[14] Hart, L.K. (1990) Fatigue, *Nursing Clinics of North America*, 25(4):967-977.

[15] Hinds, P.S., Hockenberry, M, Rai, S.N., Zhang, L., Razzouk, B.I., Cremer, L., McCarthy, K., Carlos Rodriguez-Galindo, K. (2007A). Clinical Field Testing of an Enhanced-Activity Intervention in Hospitalized Children with Cancer, *Journal of Pain and Symptom Management*, 33(6): 686-697.

[16] Hinds, P.S., Hockenberry, M., Gattuso, J.S., Srivastava, D.K., Tong, X., Jones, H., West, N., McCarthy, K.S., Sadeh, A., Ash, M., Fernandez, C., Pui, C. (2007B). Dexamethasone Alters Sleep and Fatigue in Pediatric Patients with Acute Lymphoblastic Leukemia, *Cancer*; 110:2321–30.

[17] Hinds, P.S., Hockenberry, M., Quargnenti, A., Burleson, C., Gilger, E., Randall, E., O'Neill, J.B. (1999B). Fatigue in 7 to 12 Year Old Patients with Cancer from Staff Perspective: An Exploratory Study, Onf, 26(1): 37-44.

[18] Hinds, P.S., Hockenberry-Eaton, M. (2001). Developing a research program on fatigue in children and adolescents diagnosed with cancer, *Journal of Pediatric Oncology Nursing*, 18(2): 3-12.

[19] Hinds, P.S., Hockenbery, M., Gilger, E., Kine, N., et al. (1999A). Comparing Patient, Parent and Staff Descriptions of Fatigue in Pediatric Oncology Patients, *Cancer Nursing*, 22: 277-289.

[20] Hinds, P.S., Yang, J., Gattuso, J.S., Hockenberry, M., Jones, H., Zupanec, S., Li, C., Crabtree, V.M., Mandrell, B.N., Schoumacher, R.A., Vallance, K., Sanford, S., Srivastava, D.K. (2010). Psychometric and clinical assessment of the 10-item reduced version of the Fatigue Scale-Child instrument, *J Pain Symptom Management*. 39(3):572-8.

[21] Hinds,P.S., Hockenberry, M. Rai, S.N., Zhang, L., Razzouk, B.I., McCarthy, K. Cremer, L., Rodriguez-Galindo, C. (2007C). Nocturnal Awakenings, Sleep Environment Interruptions, and Fatigue in Hospitalized Children with Cancer, *Oncology Nursing Forum*, 34(2): 393-402.

[22] Hockenberry, M., Hinds, P.S., Alcoser, P., O'Neill, J.B., Euell, K., Howard, V., Gattusu, J.S., Taylor, J. (1998). Fatigue in Children and Adolescent with Cancer, *Journal of Pediatric Oncology Nursing*, 15(3): 172-182.

[23] Hockenberry, M.J., Hinds, P.S., Barrera, P., Bryant, R., Adams-McNeill, J., Hooke, C., Rasco-Baggott, C., Patterson-Kelly, K., Gattuso, J.S., Manteuffel, B. (2003). Three instruments to assess fatigue in children with cancer: the child, parent and staff perspectives, *Journal of Pain and Symptom Management*, 25(4): 319-28.

[24] Hockenberry-Eaton, M., Hinds, P.S. (2000). Fatigue in children and adolescents with cancer: evolution of a program of study, *Seminars in Oncology Nursing*, 16(4): 261-278.

[25] Knowles, G., Borthwick, D., McNamara, S., Miller, M., & Leggot, L. (2000). Survey of nurses' assessment of cancer related fatigue. European Journal of Cancer Care, 9:105-113.

[26] Langeveld, N.E., Grootenhuis, M.A., Voûte, P.A., de Haan, R.J., Van den Bos, C. (2003). No excess fatigue in young adult survivors of childhood cancer. Eur J Cancer, 39(2):204-14.

[27] Linder, A.L. (2005). Measuring Physical Symptoms in Children and Adolescents with Cancer, *Cancer Nursing*, 28(1): 16-26.

[28] Magnusson, K., Karlsson, E., Palmblad, C., Leitner, C., & Paulson, A. (1997). Swedish nurses' estimation of fatigue as a symptom in cancer patients report on a questionnaire.European Journal of Cancer Care, 6:186-191.

[29] Memik, N.Ç., Ağaoğlu, B., Çoşkun, A., Üneri, Ö.Ş., Karakaya, I. (2007). Çocuklar İçin Yaşam Kalitesi Ölçeğinin 13-18 Yaş Ergen Formunun Geçerlik ve Güvenilirliği, *Türk Psikiyatri Dergisi*, 18(4): 353-363.

[30] Mock, V., Atkinson, A., Barsevick, A., Cella, D., Cimprich, B., Cleeland, C., Donnelly, J., Eisenberger, M.A., Escalante, C., Hinds, P., Jacobsen, P.B., Kaldor, P., Knight, S.J., Peterman, A., Piper, B.F., Rugo, H., Sabbatini, P., Stahl, C. ; National Comprehensive Cancer Network. (2000). NCCN Practice Guidelines for Cancer-Related Fatigue, *Oncology*, 14(11A):151-61.

[31] Perdikaris, P., Merkouris, A., Patiraki, E., Papadatou, D., Vasilatou-Kosmidis, H., Matziou, V. (2008). Changes in children's fatigue during the course of treatment for paediatric cancer, *International Nursing Review*, 55: 412-419.

[32] Perdikaris, P., Merkouris, A., Patiraki, E., Papadatou, D., Vasilatou-Kosmidis, H., Matziou, V. (2009). Evaluating cancer related fatigue during treatment according to children's, adolescents' and parents' perspectives in a sample of Greek young patients.Europan Journal of Oncology Nursing. 13(5):399-408.

[33] Taş, F., Bal Yılmaz, H. (2008). Quality of life concept in pediatric oncology patients. Türk Onkoloji Dergisi, 23(2):104-107.

[34] Tiesinga, L.J., Dijkstra, A., Dassen, T.W.N., Halfens, R.J.G., & Van Den Heuvel, W.J.A. (2000). Are nurses able to assess fatigue, exertion fatigue and types of fatigue in residential home patients? Scandinavian Journal of Caring Sciences, 16:129-136.

[35] Yeh C.H., Chiang, Y.C., Lin, L., Yang, C.P., Chien C.L., Weaver, M.A., Chuang, H.L. (2008). Clinical factors associated with fatigue over time in paediatric oncology patients receiving chemotherapy, *British Journal of Cancer*, 99: 23-29.

[36] Yurtsever, S. (2000). Kronik Hastalıklarda Yorgunluk ve Hemşirelik Bakımı, *CÜHYO Dergisi*, 4(1).

15

Cancer Illness in Children and the Socioeconomic Resources of Parents

Astri Syse
Cancer Registry of Norway,Oslo, Norway

1. Introduction

Cancer during childhood may have severe consequences for the children affected (1-5). It may, however, also influence entire families adversely: In order to care for a child with cancer, roles might be altered and family functioning may need to change for shorter or longer periods of time. Parents' work situations and/or relationships may thus be affected by increased psychological stress short- and long-term (6-8), but also by an increased parental care burden associated with chronic illness in children in general (9). As a consequence, the household's income may be reduced (10;11), and this may affect the family's welfare negatively. In addition, these factors alone or in combination may create strain on the family as a system. In line with this, a meta-analysis on the influence of pediatric cancer on parent and family functioning demonstrated that these mothers report a relatively small but significant increased level of family conflicts compared to healthy controls (12). This may negatively affect children's and parents' adjustment and thus affect various aspects of family life. This chapter will summarize existing research on how cancer illness in a child may impact on parental employment and earnings, and thus affect the economic situation of households affected by cancer. It will also present findings on how cancer in a child may affect parents' relationships and divorce rates. Empirical results from Norway on these matters will thereafter be presented (11;13). Knowledge of common outcomes may help families plan their lives, and serve as an important basis for societal attempts to assist.

There is also little knowledge about the impact of parental socioeconomic resources on childhood cancer survival in developed countries (14-19). As diagnostic procedures and treatment protocols for these diseases are largely standardized and centralized (20), childhood cancer survival is often assumed to be fairly equal across different social groups. For children with cancer and their families, it is important to ensure that treatment outcomes are maximized. If there are survival differences across social groups, clinical interventions ought to be targeted to ensure optimal care for all. The chapter will therefore also summarize and discuss research on the influence of parental resources or socioeconomic status more generally on mortality after childhood cancer in a society with presumably equal access to high quality cancer care. Empirical findings from a recent Norwegian study will then follow (21). Lastly, a summary of the current status of knowledge in this field is provided, and areas where further research is warranted are highlighted.

2. Childhood cancer and family effects

Survival rates have improved substantially over the last decades for most childhood cancers (3). These cancers represent, however, diverse diseases treated differently and with dissimilar risks for poor outcomes such as death or long-term adverse effects (3;22-24). Also the burden associated with modern pediatric oncological treatment varies considerably, as certain cancers are treated by one modality for a short period of time while others involve active treatment for years in terms of multi-modal treatments often associated with potential life-threatening complications. The latter treatments also require prolonged and more frequent hospitalizations in which one of the parents generally accompanies the child. Treatment will therefore in varying degrees affect the family, and specifically the parents who will need to care for their child, care for other children, as well as maintain their jobs and personal relationship. Complicated childhood cancers (central nervous system (CNS) tumors, acute myeloid leukemia (AML) and bone tumors) have for instance a significantly more negative effect upon various aspects of parents' mental health than the less complicated acute lymphoblastic leukemia (ALL) (25). Psychologically, perceived uncertainties regarding outcomes have been demonstrated to be particularly stressful (8;25;26). More specific effects of cancer in a child on employment and earnings as well as possible effects on parents' relationship are presented below.

2.1 Existing research on economic consequences of having a child with cancer

Cancer in a child may adversely affect parents' work opportunities due to enlarged care burdens and/or altered priorities: In order to care for a child with cancer, parental roles might be altered and family functioning may need to change for shorter or longer periods of time (6;27;28). Parents' work opportunities may thus be affected by increased psychological stress short- and long-term (6-8), but also by an increased parental care burden associated with chronic illness in children in general (9). In addition, parents' work priorities may change (26). As a consequence, households' incomes may be reduced. Few studies on parents' work force participation exist, however. No reviews on parental employment and/or earnings after cancer or other chronic illness in children could be identified. Published studies are relatively small and may reflect policies and labor markets in particular geographic areas (10;28-35), and only a few utilizes a comparison group (29-31). Existing studies suggest that parental employment and/or earnings are affected by a child's cancer, and that the households' reported incomes may be reduced, at least short-term (10;28;31;33;35). Mothers' employment and earnings appear particularly affected (33;34). The studies indicate that there may be country-specific or regional differences with regard to work opportunities and also that the various features of children's cancer may influence family employment and earnings. Population-based, longitudinal studies from different settings are needed on this topic.

2.2 Existing research on cancer in a child and parents' relationships and the risk of divorce

It is likely a strong normative pressure not to leave a family in times of serious illness in a child, even in today's individualistic society. A low divorce rate could thus perhaps be expected shortly after diagnosis and during critical periods in which the child is hospitalized and/or very ill or there is great uncertainty about survival. Along the same lines, elevated divorce rates could be expected as the child either has recovered fully or died. Also the age of the child at diagnosis could be hypothesized to influence parents' relationships to varying degrees, as parents of younger children may be hypothesized to experience the greatest care burdens (36). Few parental risk factors are known that are strongly associated with the development of cancer in a child (37). Over time, however, certain behaviors and environmental exposures that may be important for the incidence of various childhood cancers have changed, and there have also been socioeconomic and ideational changes with implications for marital stability. Calendar period might thus also influence divorce rates. Spouses' age affect their divorce rates, reflecting in part the link between current age, age at marriage, and duration of marriage, all of which are strong determinants of divorce (38). Educational attainment is an important factor with regards to divorce risk in general. The educational gradient in divorce rates has been found to be strong and negative in many countries, but there is variation in the effect of wives' education on divorce rates, depending on the welfare system and gender relations in countries (39-41). Further, cancer in a child may reduce incomes by interfering with work capabilities and opportunities (10). Lower incomes, especially among men, are likely to increase the chance of divorce (42). For women, it will depend on whether the relationship is tuned towards specialization or pooling of resources (43;44). When higher incomes are taken into account, one would expect that highly educated persons experience would lower divorce rates due to non-economic effects of education (40;41). The presence of siblings could be hypothesized to necessitate a division of parental care between sick and healthy child(ren), thus increasing parental strain and stress (45).

Most of the published studies on divorce are small and from the 1970s (46-48). Only one utilized a comparison group (46). Studies of couples with *disabled* children show, however, increased divorce rates (49;50). Reviews on parental stress and marital adjustment after cancer or other chronic illness in children conclude that population-based, longitudinal studies are needed (6;8;12;26;36;51), as existing myths about cancer in children resulting in increased divorce rates may add to the burden already experienced by couples with a (chronically) sick child (36).

3. Empirical findings on parents' income and divorce rates after cancer in children in Norway

The findings presented here are described in more detail in two articles published in 2010 (11;13).

Detailed registry and census data on the entire Norwegian population with children was used in all analyses. The *Norwegian Population Register* provided information on date of birth, death or migration, dates of changes in marital status from 1974 onwards, and dates of birth of all children. Unique family numbers enabled us to link information on children and spouses. Educational levels were extracted from the *population censuses* of 1970, 1980, 1990, and 2001, and from the *Registry of Education*. The *Norwegian Directorate of Taxes* provided information on yearly gross labor earnings. The *Cause-of-Death Registry* provided information on cause of death for the children who died. Information on cancer in children was drawn from the *Cancer Registry of Norway*, which has registered all cancer diagnoses nationwide since 1953. Mandatory reporting from clinicians, pathologists, and death certificates ensures quality and completeness (52).

It was hypothesized that employment and earnings would be adversely affected by cancer, and that the most pronounced effects would be observed for cancers characterized by intense treatment over long time-periods and/or cancers that result in chronic health problems that persist after treatment is terminated. Similarly, it was hypothesized that the divorce rate would be elevated compared to that of the general population, and that the highest rates would be observed for the parents of children most adversely affected.

3.1 Parental employment and earnings after cancer in a child

3.1.1 Material and methods

Data on the entire Norwegian population of working age (27-66 years old) with children under the age of 20 in 1990-2002 (N=1.2 million) was retrieved from national registries. *The Norwegian Directorate of Taxes* provided information on employment status (yes/no) and yearly gross labor earnings for all citizens, hereafter referred to as earnings. Public benefits (i.e. nursing and care allowances) due to chronic illness in children are limited to US $45 000/year until 18 years of age and were not included in the earnings variable prior to 2002. Parents' first year sick leaves are similarly limited, but these benefits are included in the earnings variable. Employment rates for parents of 3263 children with cancer were compared to those of parents with children without cancer by means of logistic regression models. Log-linear regression models were used to explore childhood cancer's effect on annual parental earnings for the large majority who remained employed.

Employment probabilities in 2002 were assessed by means of logistic regression models. Altogether, 1644 mothers and 1619 fathers had children with cancer between 1991 and 2001. Around 92 % of the fathers and 87 % of the mothers were employed at the end of follow-up in 2002. How cancer in a child the preceding years affected their earnings was assessed by means of log-linear regression models. Overall effects and effects of different common childhood cancer forms, child death, the age of the child at diagnosis, and time elapsed from diagnosis were explored.

Parental age, the number of children, educational level, and prior employment status or earnings were included as covariates in all models. Additional models including interaction terms explored potential modifying effects of the covariates, with a particular focus on educational level, marital status, and presence of siblings. Only mothers' educational level and fathers' marital status appeared to have a modifying effect, and models stratified on these two variables were thus set up.

3.1.2 Results

Cancer in a child was in general *not* associated with a reduced risk of employment, although some exceptions exist among both mothers and fathers. For employed mothers, CNS cancers, germinal cell cancers, and unspecified leukemia were associated with significant reductions in earnings (10%, 21%, and 60%, respectively). Reductions were particularly pronounced for mothers with a young and alive child, and became more pronounced with time elapsed from diagnosis. Fathers' earnings were not affected significantly, and are thus not shown.

3.1.2.1 Overall effects and effects of specific cancer forms on employment

Descriptive characteristics of the population are shown in Tables 1 and 2. The overall adjusted odds ratio (OR) for being employed in 2002 was higher for both mothers and fathers of children with cancer compared to those of the control group, but not statistically significant.

	Mothers			Fathers		
	N	OR[a]	95 % CI[b]	N	OR	95 % CI
Cancer status						
Child without cancer	621439	1.00	(ref)	606469	1.00	(ref)
Child with cancer	1644	1.15	0.96-1.37	1619	1.12	0.90-1.39
Parent's age[c]						
< 35 years	203692	1.19	1.16-1.21	133919	2.76	2.65-2.89
35-39 years	146102	1.00	(ref)	129381	1.00	(ref)
40-44 years	133280	1.06	1.03-1.09	132581	0.71	0.69-0.74
45-49 years	93233	1.04	1.01-1.07	113744	0.55	0.53-0.57
50-54 years	36911	0.82	0.79-0.85	64253	0.41	0.39-0.42
55-59 years	9162	0.58	0.55-0.61	25346	0.27	0.26-0.29
>= 60 years	703	0.43	0.36-0.53	8864	0.10	0.09-0.11
Parent's education[d]						
Elementary school	193894	1.00	(ref)	163175	1.00	(ref)
High school	192797	5.12	5.01-5.22	169307	6.28	6.11-6.46
College education	225835	9.07	8.88-9.26	242818	14.97	14.55-15.41
Master degree	10557	13.67	12.75-14.67	32788	25.95	24.10-27.94
Prior work status[e]						
Employed	455337	1.00	(ref)	523546	1.00	(ref)
Not employed	167746	0.25	0.24-0.25	84542	0.17	0.17-0.17
# of children						
1 child	138201	0.86	0.84-0.88	129347	0.65	0.63-0.67
2 children	273062	1.00	(ref)	269180	1.00	(ref)
>= 3 children	211820	0.83	0.82-0.85	209561	1.08	1.05-1.11

[a]Odds Ratio. [b]Confidence interval. [c]Age ar the end of follow-up. [d]Educational status 1990. [e]Work status 1990.

Table 1. Fully asjusted model of the effect of a child's cancer illnes on parent's employment probability

None of the common childhood cancer forms were associated with significantly reduced employment probabilities parents. The point estimates of employment varied somewhat across cancer sites, and tendencies of both increased and reduced probabilities were observed. No cancer form increased the employment probability among fathers.

3.1.2.2 Overall effects and effects of specific cancer forms on earnings

Median earnings for employed parents are shown in Figure 1. A child's cancer did not impact on fathers' earnings overall, nor for any of the common cancer forms. It resulted in a non-significant 4 % reduction in mothers' earnings. The percentage change in earnings varied somewhat across cancer sites, and tendencies towards both increased and reduced earnings were observed. CNS tumors, germinal cell cancers, and unspecified leukemia were associated with significant reductions in mothers' earnings of 10%, 21% and 60%, respectively.

	Mothers' employment			Mothers' earnings		Fathers' employment		
	N[b]	OR[c]	95 % CI[d]	% change[e]	95 % CI	N	OR	95 % CI
No cancer	621439	1.00	(ref)	(ref)	(ref)	606469	1.00	(ref)
Cancer form								
CNS cancer	459	1.07	0.77-1.49	-9.7	-18.2,-1.8	455	1.04	0.70-1.56
Leukemias (ALL, AML and nos[f])	454	1.17	0.83-1.65	-3.2	-11.6,4.5	448	1.13	0.72-1.76
Lymphomas	173	1.45	0.82-2.56	0	-13.3,11.9	170	1.95	0.91-4.19
Germinal cell cancer	100	0.85	0.45-1.62	-20.8	-44.4,-1.8	98	0.90	0.41-1.97
Neuroblastoma	94	0.62	0.33-1.17	5.6	-12.6,21.1	93	1.19	0.40-3.51
Bone cancer	77	9.20	2.13-39.80	6.7	-12.1,22.4	76	1.27	0.51-3.15
Renal cancer[g]	67	1.21	0.49-2.99	1.6	-20.9,19.9	67	3.08	0.40-23.49
Soft tissue cancer	60	1.02	0.44-2.34	4.7	-18.5,23.6	59	0.87	0.33-2.35
Malignant melanoma	28	1.45	0.38-5.50	-34.7	-95.0,0.03	25	2.81	0.31-25.02
Endocrine cancer[h]	21	0.62	0.19-2.04	7.3	-38.1,38.4	20	0.99	0.27-3.64
Eye cancer[i]	12	1.62	0.20-13.25	-8.9	-55.8,38.8	12	>999.99	NA
Vital status								
Child with cancer, alive	1315	1.04	0.86-1.27	-5.7	-10.7,-0.9	1296	1.15	0.89-1.47
Child with cancer, dead	329	1.70	1.10-2.62	2.5	-6.8,10.9	323	1.01	0.63-1.62
Time since diagnosis								
Cancer 0-4 yrs prior	554	1.01	0.76-1.35	-0.3	-7.8,6.7	542	0.94	0.65-1.35
Cancer >=5 yrs prior	1090	0.80	0.64-1.00	-5.8	-11.2,-0.6	1077	0.87	0.66-1.15
Age at diagnosis								
Child 0-4 yrs	708	1.02	0.78-1.34	-4.7	-11.5,1.6	699	1.33	0.88-2.00
Child 5-9 yrs	352	1.14	0.77-1.69	-12.6	-23.2,-3.0	349	0.83	0.54-1.29
Child 10-14 yrs	307	1.24	0.84-1.83	0.5	-9.5,9.7	300	1.05	0.67-1.63
Child >= 15 yrs	277	1.38	0.90-2.12	3.1	-7.0,12.4	271	1.29	0.80-2.07

[a]Only the effect of the disease variable are shown, but all covariates from table1 were included. In the analysis of earnings, work status 1990 was substituted by earnings in 1990. [b]Number of cancer cases in the respective categories. [c]Odds Ratio. [d]Confidence interval. [e]Change in percent. [f] Not otherwise specified. For these cancers, a statistically significant 59.8% reduction in eamings was observed. [g] Primarily Wilm's tumor. [h]Primarily thyroid cancer. [i]Primarily retinoblastoma.

Table 2. Parents' employment probability and earnings by the child's cancer type, vital status, time from diagnosis and age at diagnosis.

3.1.2.3 The importance of cancer severity and prognosis

Length and severity of treatment regimens may influence parents' care burden and thus their ability to work regular hours. Analyses based on standardized treatment protocols for common childhood cancers did not, however, reveal significant differences. There were also no differences in employment and/or earnings for the different cancer stages at diagnosis.

A significantly elevated employment probability was seen for mothers who lost a child to cancer (OR 1.70). Child death was not associated with inclines or declines in earnings, but a 10% reduction in earnings was observed for those with living children, and the reductions became more pronounced with the time elapsed from diagnosis. Fathers' employment and earnings were not statistically significantly affected by their child's status.

3.1.2.4 Children's age at diagnosis

Children's age at diagnosis may be hypothesized to influence parents' work ability. Among mothers, children's age at diagnosis was not significantly associated with the probability of being employed. A young age at diagnosis (<10 years old) did, however, adversely affect mothers' earnings by around 9%. The effect was most pronounced for those with children 5-9 years old. Children's age did not affect fathers' overall employment or earnings.

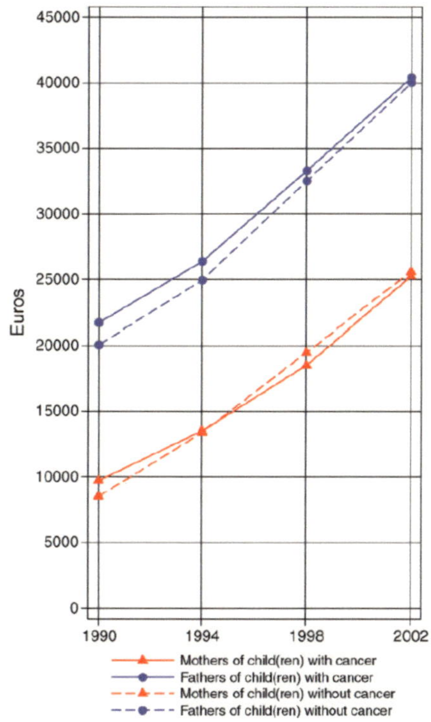

Fig. 1. Median gross labor earnings

3.1.2.5 Impact of siblings, marital status, and household level effects

The presence of healthy siblings was hypothesized to further increase parental strain and stress, imposing a division of parental care between the sick child and its healthy siblings, perhaps impacting negatively on parents' work ability. No difference was, however, observed in employment or earnings for persons with and without also healthy children ($p_{interaction}$ 0.12 for mothers and 0.11 for fathers). There was also no difference in cancer's effect on employment or earnings in married versus unmarried persons overall ($p_{interaction}$ 0.87 for mothers and 0.89 for fathers). Subanalyses did, however, reveal that the married fathers were more likely to remain employed and to maintain their earnings compared to the not married fathers. The effect was particularly pronounced for fathers with children 10 years and older at time of diagnosis and for fathers who lost a child to cancer ($p_{interaction}$ 0.001 and 0.01).

Among married couples with a child with cancer there was an increased probability of either spouse working, as the OR for household employment was 2.30 (95% confidence interval (CI) 1.32-4.00). It was particularly pronounced the first five years after diagnosis (OR 4.91, CI 1.44-16.72) and after child death (OR 3.40, CI 1.00-12.38). There was no significant difference in the employment probabilities for the different cancer forms. Household earnings were not reduced overall among the married couples after child cancer, but the household earnings were reduced around 7% for those with children age 5-9 (p 0.05).

3.1.2.6 Effects of parents' education

Educational level did not affect fathers' employment or earnings differently ($p_{interaction}$ 0.81). As shown in Table 3, however, mothers with a lower education were less likely to stop working when experiencing cancer in their child (OR 1.31), and the probability of employment was further increased five years after diagnosis (OR 1.47). Employment was most likely after leukemia (OR 1.54) and after child death (OR 1.94). The earnings of mothers with a lower education were not affected more adversely than the earnings of mothers with a higher education. Mothers with a higher education did not experience any significant changes in their employment, but their earnings were reduced 6% overall provided their child did not die. A highly significant 26% reduction was observed after germinal cell cancer.

	Low education[b]				High education[c]			
	Employment		Earnings		Employment		Earnings	
Cancer status	**OR[d]**	**95 % CI[e]**	**% change[f]**	**95 % CI**	**OR**	**95 % CI**	**% change**	**95 % CI**
No cancer	1.00	(ref)	NA	(ref)	1.00	(ref)	NA	(ref)
Any cancer, any time	1.31	1.07-1.60	-2.9	-10.0,3.8	1.00	0.73-1.37	-4.5	-10.1,0.9
Cancer form								
Any leukemia	1.54	1.02-2.34	1.2	-12.8,13.5	0.73	0.44-1.23	-4.8	-15.4,4.8
Acute lymphoblastic leukemia	*1.34*	*0.85-2.11*	*4.9*	*-10.8,18.6*	*0.68*	*0.39-1.17*	*-7.0*	*-19.1,3.8*
Acute myelogenous leukemia	*3.71*	*0.86-16.10*	*5.8*	*-28.6,31.3*	*1.03*	*0.24-4.33*	*7.7*	*-17.5,27.8*
CNS tumor	1.08	0.75-1.57	-9.6	-24.9,3.8	1.62	0.80-3.31	-8.7	-19.9,1.5
Lymphomas	1.51	0.82-2.76	6.2	-14.4,23.2	1.35	0.42-4.29	-7.0	-26.4,9.3
Germinal cell cancer	0.80	0.39-1.63	-10.0	-50.0,18.5	3.14	0.43-22.98	-26.2	-57.3,-3.6
Neuroblastoma	0.84	0.40-1.78	16.4	-11.3,38.1	0.49	0.19-1.26	-2.0	-28.3,18.7
Bone cancer	13.32	1.79-98.94	9.6	-18.2,31.4	1.60	0.22-11.80	-3.0	-33.9,20.1
Renal cancer[g]	0.93	0.31-2.79	-12.2	-60.0,20.0	1.12	0.26-4.78	10.4	-16.0,31.4
Child status								
Child with cancer, alive	1.18	0.94-1.48	-4.5	-12.9,3.2	0.93	0.67-1.30	-6.4	-12.8,-0.4
Child with cancer, dead	1.94	1.20-3.14	2.4	-12.2,15.2	1.44	0.63-3.28	3.6	-8.9,14.7
Time since diagnosis								
Cancer 0-4 yrs prior	1.05	0.76-1.46	2.1	-10.6,13.4	0.99	0.59-1.68	-2.3	-11.9,6.4
Cancer >= 5 yrs prior	1.47	1.14-1.90	-5.1	-14.0,3.0	1.01	0.69-1.48	-5.6	-12.7,1.0
Age at diagnosis								
Child 0-4 yrs	1.31	0.94-1.84	-6.1	-18.5,5.1	0.85	0.57-1.29	-2.0	-10.0,5.5
Child 5-9 yrs	1.40	0.88-2.23	-15.4	-34.1,0.4	0.81	0.44-1.50	-10.4	-23.7,1.4
Child 10-14 yrs	1.14	0.76-1.70	7.3	-7.5,20.1	1.64	0.60-4.47	-9.4	-24.7,3.9
Child >= 15 yrs	1.42	0.90-2.22	3.5	-11.6,16.6	2.13	0.67-6.76	1.4	-13.8,14.5

[a]Only the effect of the disease variable are shown, but all covariates from table 2 exept mother's education were included. Prior work status was included in analyses of employment whereas prior earnings was included in analyses of earnings. [b]Unknown/low, elementary or high school education, accounting for 279192 (45%) of the cohort, of which 791 encountered child cancer. [c]College education or above, accounting for 343891 persons in total, of which 853 encountered child cancer. The percentage employed in the respective groups were 78% and 95%, respectivly. [d]Odds Ratio. [e]Confidence interval. [f]Change in perecent. [g]Primarily Wilm's tumor.

Table 3. Mother's employment probability and changes in earnings by cancer in a child and educational level[a]

3.1.3 Summary of main findings

Parents' employment is not adversely affected by a child's cancer in Norway. Earnings are reduced in certain instances, but the overall effects are minor. In line with traditional caregiving responsibilities, reductions in earnings were most pronounced for mothers.

3.2 Parents' risk of divorce after cancer in a child

3.2.1 Material and methods

Data on the entire Norwegian married population aged 17-69 with children under the age of 20 in 1974-2001 (N=1.04 million couples) was retrieved from national registers. The divorce rates for 4590 couples with a child (age <20 years) with cancer were compared to the divorce rate of otherwise similar couples not affected by childhood cancer by means of discrete-time hazard regression models. Couples were followed for an average of 12 years, and the total number of divorces was 168 110. Of these, 535 divorces occurred among couples with a child with cancer. Expected outcomes and the length and severity of treatments may influence parents' relationships, and effects of time elapsed, common childhood cancer types, spread, and death were thus explored. The child's age at diagnosis, the number of siblings, parents' age, earnings and educational level, the duration of marriage, and calendar period, were all included as covariates (Table 4). Additional stratified models and models including interaction terms were also set up to explore potential modifying effects of covariates.

3.2.2 Results

Cancer in a child was not associated with an increased risk of parental divorce rate overall, or for any of the more common cancer forms among children. A tendency towards an increased divorce risk (OR 1.34, CI 1.00-1.81) was observed for parents' of children with renal cancers (primarily Wilms tumor). Neither age, time from diagnosis, nor prognosis influenced the estimates adversely. The death of a child with cancer did not influence the divorce rates significantly in either direction. The couples in which the mothers' education was above high school level did, however, display significantly increased divorce rates (OR 1.19, CI 1.05-1.36). The risk was particularly high shortly after diagnosis. Other risk factors for these couples were CNS cancers, age 5-9 years, and death of the child.

3.2.2.1 Overall effects and site-specific effects

Parents of a child with a cancer of any form, diagnosed at any time, had a divorce rate similar to that of parents of children without cancer (OR 1.04, CI 0.95-1.13). As is shown in Table 5, only renal cancer was statistically significantly associated with an increased risk of parental divorce. The point estimates varied somewhat across cancer sites, and tendencies of both increased and reduced rates were observed. CNS, renal, and endocrine cancer yielded OR estimates above 1.00, whereas malignant melanomas, bone, and hepatic cancers resulted in OR estimates below 1.00. Lymphoma, leukemia, retinoblastoma, soft-tissue, and germinal cell cancer yielded OR estimates close to 1.00. No significant difference in the effect of AML and ALL was observed.

3.2.2.2 The importance of prognosis and cancer stage

No significant differences were observed between cancers with and without spread at time of diagnosis. The point estimate was highest for metastatic cancer (1.16), but statistical significance was not achieved. Likewise, almost identical estimates were obtained for parents with a child who died and for parents with children who remained alive.

	Divorces/pyrs[a]	OR[b]	95 % CI[c]
No cancer	192722/17.94 mill	1.00	(ref)
Child with cancer (any time)	*624/64829*	*1.05*	*0.97-1.14*
Time from diagnosis			
Cancer 0-5 yrs prior	248/17542	1.11	0.98-1.26
Cancer > 5 yrs prior	376/47287	1.01	0.91-1.12
Age group			
17-19 years	328/10918	1.42	1.27-1.59
20-24 years	10653/393128	1.00	(ref)
25-29 years	29994/1.50 mill	0.61	0.60-0.62
30-34 years	39896/2.35 mill	0.46	0.45-0.47
35-39 years	38921/2.52 mill	0.39	0.38-0.40
40-44 years	31700/2.43 mill	0.32	0.31-0.33
45-49 years	21471/2.31 mill	0.22	0.21-0.23
50-54 years	11752/2.23 mill	0.13	0.12-0.13
55-59 years	5499/1.86 mill	0.07	0.06-0.07
60-64 years	2214/1.39 mill	0.03	0.03-0.04
65-69 years	918/987625	0.02	0.02-0.02
Educational level			
Low or unknown	1510/74657	1.51	1-43-1.59
Elementary school	43068/5.45 mill	1.00	(ref)
High school	104984/9.03 mill	0.92	0.90-0.93
College education	39207/3.13 mill	0.86	0.85-0.87
Master degree	4577/325929	0.92	0.89-0.95
Duration of marriage			
0-2 years	10090/1.04 mill	0.64	0.62-0.65
3-4 years	14183/1.00 mill	1.00	(ref)
5-6 years	29179/1.91 mill	1.25	1.22-1.27
7-8 years	25075/1.78 mill	1.36	1.34-1.39
9 years or more	114819/12.27 mill	1.39	1.36-1.42
Calendar period			
1974-1980	30802/3.74 mill	0.96	0.94-0.97
1981-1985	33233/3.28 mill	1.00	(ref)
1986-1990	36707/3.42 mill	1.25	1.23-1.27
1991-1995	39861/3.28 mill	1.57	1.54-1.59
1996-2001	52743/4.28 mill	1.75	1.72-1.78
Number of children			
One child only	43248/3.23 mill	1.30	1.28-1.31
Two children	91496/7.76 mill	1.00	(ref)
Three or more children	58602/7.01 mill	0.90	0.89-0.91
Married in 1974	58602		
Yes	102058/5.35 mill	1.00	0.99-1.02
No	91288/12.65 mill	1.00	(ref)
Remarried			
Yes	7275/248514	3.10	3.02-3.18
No	186071/17.75 mill	1.00	(ref)

[a]Number of divorces per person-year. [b]Odds Ratio. [c]Confidence interval.

Table 4. Fully adjusted model of the effect of a child's cancer illnes on a parents' devorce probability

Cancer type	Divorces/pyrs[b]	OR[c]	95 % CI[d]
No cancer	192722/19.94 mill	1.00	(ref)
Any leukemia	181/17239	1.02	0.88-1.18
Leukemia, nos[e]	14/1273	1.26	0.74-2.13
Acute lymphoblastic leukemia	139/12983	0.99	0.84-1.17
Acute myelogenous leukemia	28/2983	1.07	0.74-1.56
CNS tumor	162/15523	1.11	0.95-1.29
Lymphomas	57/6460	1.12	0.86-1.45
Germinal cell cancer	38/4303	1.24	0.90-1.70
Bone cancer	23/3733	0.78	0.52-1.18
Renal cancer[f]	44/3297	1.34	1.00-1.81
Eye cancer[g]	24/2599	0.91	0.61-1.37
Soft tissue cancer	23/2548	1.01	0.67-1.52
Malignant melanoma	15/2536	0.82	0.49-1.36
Endocrine cancer[h]	8/1004	1.20	0.60-2.41
Hepatic cancer	7/920	0.75	0.36-1.59
Other or unknown	42/4667	0.97	0.71-1.31
Local cancer[i]	520/53748	1.04	0.97-1.15
Regional cancer	82/9798	1.03	0.83-1.28
Metastatic cancer	22/1283	1.14	0.75-1.74
Stage unknown	62/7448	1.01	0.78-1.29
Child with cancer, alive	365/34688	1.05	0.95-1.17
Child with cancer, dead	259/30141	1.04	0.92-1.18
Child 0-4 yrs at diagnosis	300/25315	1.04	0.92-1.16
Child 5-9 yrs at diagnosis	133/12595	1.08	0.91-1.28
Child 10-14 yrs at diagnosis	86/10734	1.03	0.83-1.28
Child >= 15 yrs at diagnosis	105/16185	1.07	0.88-1.30

[a]Only the effect of the disease variable are shown, but all covariates from table 4 were included in the model. [b]Number of divorcing per person-year. [c]Odds Ratio. [d]Confidence interval. [e]Not otherwise specified. [f]Primarily Wilm's tumor. [g]Primarily retinoblastoma. [h]Primarily thyroid cancer. [i]Including blood, lymph, and brain tumors for which no stage is recorded.

Table 5. Devorce probability by children's type, stage, vital status and age[a]

3.2.2.3 Effects of time from diagnosis

Duration of disease did not influence parental divorce risk significantly. Parents of children with a relatively recent cancer diagnosis (0-5 years earlier) had a slightly higher divorce rates than those with children with a cancer diagnosed further back in time (>5 years), but the estimates were not significantly different from those of parents with children without cancer, or from each other (OR 1.10, CI 0.97-1.25 v OR 0.98, CI 0.88-1.10).

3.2.2.4 Effects of age at diagnosis

Cancer in a child 0-9 years old yielded an OR of 1.05 (CI 0.95-1.15), whereas the corresponding estimate for an older child was 1.00 (CI 0.84-1.19). A further subdivision of this age span did not reveal significant differences between parents of younger versus older children.

3.2.2.5 Presence of sibling

No difference was observed between divorce rates for couples with and without also healthy children (OR 1.04, CI 0.96-1.13 v 0.90, 0.63-1.26).

3.2.2.6 Effects of parents' education

The inclusion of an interaction term between cancer and mothers' educational level in the original model suggested a differential effect of cancer depending on the mother's educational level ($p_{interaction}$ <0.01). Stratified analyses confirmed that couples in which the mothers had an education beyond high school displayed a 16% higher divorce rate overall compared to couples with mothers with a lower education, as is shown in Table 6. The risk was particularly high the first five years after diagnosis (OR 1.23, CI 1.02-1.50), due to a 35% increase in the divorce rate the first few years after diagnosis. A significantly elevated rate was also observed for young children (OR 1.20, CI 1.03-1.41), and for CNS cancer (32%), Wilms tumor (64%), and child death (31%). A similar inclusion of an interaction term between cancer and father's educational level did not suggest a differential effect of cancer ($p_{interaction}$ 0.25), and further stratified analyses were thus not undertaken.

	High education[b]		Low education[c]	
Cancer status	OR[d]	95 % CI[e]	OR	95 % CI
No cancer	1.00	(ref)	1.00	(ref)
Any cancer, any time	1.19	1.05-1.36	0.97	0.87-1.07
Cancer 0-2 yrs prior	1.32	1.01-1.76	0.91	0.70-1.19
Cancer 3-5 yrs prior	1.21	0.93-1.57	1.08	0.87-1.33
Cancer 6-7 yrs prior	1.10	0.81-1.50	0.81	0.62-1.05
Cancer 8-10 yrs prior	1.23	0.81-1.86	1.11	0.83-1.50
Cancer > 10 yrs prior	1.14	0.90-1.45	0.96	0.82-1.14
Child 0-4 yrs at diagnosis	1.17	0.98-1.40	0.93	0.80-1.08
Child 5-9 yrs at diagnosis	1.32	1.01-1.74	0.95	0.76-1.19
Child 10-14 yrs at diagnosis	1.04	0.72-1.73	1.02	0.78-1.32
Child >= 15 yrs at diagnosis	1.22	0.86-1.73	1.05	0.83-1.32
Child with cancer, alive	1.11	0.94-1.31	1.01	0.88-1.15
Child with cancer, dead	1.35	1.10-1.65	0.92	0.79-1.07
Acute lymphoblastic leukemia	1.18	0.91-1.53	0.88	0.71-1.10
Acute myelogenous leukemia	1.03	0.54-2.00	1.09	0.69-1.72
CNS tumor	1.35	1.04-1.73	0.99	0.81-1.20
Lymphomas	1.15	0.75-1.75	1.09	0.78-1.52
Germinal cell cancer	1.45	0.87-2.41	1.09	0.72-1.65
Renal cancer[f]	1.52	0.95-2.42	1.21	0.82-1.79
Eye cancer[g]	0.93	0.48-1.80	0.85	0.51-1.41
Local cancer	1.16	0.99-1.35	0.99	0.88-1.11
Regional cancer	1.19	0.82-1.73	0.97	0.74-1.26
Metastatic cancer	1.19	0.61-2.29	1.04	0.60-1.80

[a]Only the effects of the disease variable are shown, but all covariates from table 6 were included in the model. [b]High school education or above. [c]Elementary education only. [d]Odds Ratio. [e]Confidence interval. [f]Primarily Wilm's tumor. [g]Primarily retinoblastoma.

Table 6. Divorce probability by cancer in children and mother's educational level[a]

3.2.3 Summary of main findings

Parents' divorce rates are not generally adversely affected by a child's cancer in Norway. Possible negative long term effects on the parents may be balanced by strengthened parental bonds. An exception exists for couples with a child with highly educated mothers, and further studies are warranted to understand the background for this increase in divorce risk.

4. Discussion of findings from empirical studies on economic consequences and divorce in families after cancer in a child

This large registry-based study has shown that contrary to existing myths, cancer in a child is not associated with substantive reductions in parental employment or earnings, nor in an increase in parental divorce rates.

4.1 Expected outcomes and extent of treatments provided

It was perhaps surprising that employment rates were increased for mothers who lost their child, as other studies have shown that bereavement may interfere with parents' work ability (53;54). Caregiving tasks associated with cancer illness in children eventually subside in cases of child death, and bereavement as an exposure may thus not be a relevant proxy for the cancer form, stage, or treatment endured. Cancer death in children has been shown to be unrelated to parents' social class (15;17), and mothers who experience child death are likely to have endured pronounced, long-term care burdens in the past (12;26), which in turn may have impacted negatively on their working abilities. As the mothers' care burdens are eliminated, they may find opportunities to rejoin the work force. Similarly, mothers' earnings were negatively affected by cancer in their child only when the child remained alive, and their earnings actually appeared to increase beyond that of the comparison group after child death. As the data recordings for employment and earnings come in yearly intervals, it is primarily longer-term effects that are assessed here. Short-term consequences may be different and highly relevant for families in different settings. It was also surprising that divorce was no more or less likely for parents who lost their child (53).

In general, no cancer form reduced the overall employment probability for either parent, and neither overall nor specific childhood cancer forms impacted on fathers' earnings overall.

CNS cancer during childhood may be quite debilitating and alter physical, psychological, and social functioning dramatically (55;56). This could be predicted to increase the care load for parents and have lifelong consequences for the family, including reductions in parental employment and earnings as well as elevated divorce rates. In line with this, a modest but statistically significant reduction in mothers' earnings was observed. Similarly, higher divorce rates were expected after CNS cancer, but this was not observed. Along the same lines, AML was expected to affect employment, earnings and divorce rates more strongly than ALL due to differences in treatment intensities and expected outcomes. This was not observed, but unspecified leukemia was associated with a significant reduction in mothers' earnings.

In line with what has been reported previously, couples with a child with cancer have similar divorce rates as couples with children without cancer (36) An increased risk of divorce was observed only after renal cancer. This may be a chance finding due to the large number of tests performed, and further explorations with a clearly stated a priori hypothesis are needed. Parental divorce risk thus appears unrelated to cancer form, stage, and prognosis in Norway.

4.2 Family orientation, obligations and gender

Encountering and 'conquering' cancer illness in a child has been suggested to increase parents' family orientation (6;26). This may affect work force participation, as parents (and mothers in particular) may choose to work less. In addition, parents' abilities to undertake their usual chores and obligations in family and working life may also be affected, temporarily or permanently. In practical terms, one person may need to stay for prolonged periods in hospitals with the sick child, and either spouse may thus experience a 'role overload' (12), which could affect employment or earnings adversely. In addition, the quality of the marital interactions may be enhanced. A child's illness is often considered by the couple as a common experience, and may thus result in a strengthening of existing bonds between them, perhaps especially if the relationship was good at the outset (8;57) Also their values may change in such a way that divorce becomes less likely: Persons encountering a serious disease in a family member may become more conscious about whatever quality there is in the relationship (58;59), and later marital conflicts may tend to be seen as small compared to what have been endured previously (36). It is also possible that cancer may affect the quality of the relationship adversely. Poor health in a child may lead to parental behavioral and mood changes, and thus yield smaller emotional rewards from the relationship.(36) Spouses' abilities to undertake their usual chores and obligations in marital relationships may be affected (12;41;60). This could pertain in particular to highly educated mothers. Studies have shown that mothers in general take on the greatest parental care burden in case of illness in a child (26), and that fathers thus may be less involved. Remaining engaged in working life and/or upholding a social life may thus be more difficult for mothers than fathers. The relevance of these mechanisms may depend on the age of the child at diagnosis, time elapsed since diagnosis, cancer site and stage, and the type and extent of necessary treatment. Many treatment regiments have become less aggressive over the last few decades, both as a result of technological innovations and an increased awareness and recognition of childhood cancer survivors' overall functioning, possibly accounting for the effects of the earlier time periods.

A meta-analysis on the influence of pediatric cancer on parent and family functioning demonstrated that mothers in particular report a significant increased level of family strain and stress compared to healthy controls (12), whereas other studies show that this is most markedly seen among families who were vulnerable at the outset (8). Reductions in work hours may be a way to decrease stress, and this could be what is picked up here in terms of tendencies towards reduced incomes for mothers in particular. Studies have shown that mothers in general take on the greatest parental care burden in case of illness in a child (26), and remaining engaged in working life may thus be more difficult for mothers than fathers. The gender difference observed corresponds well with the general perceptions of gendered parental caregiving roles and parental care for sick children to a larger extend being undertaken by women, and are in line with what has been observed previously (33;34). To compensate for declines in mothers' work hours, fathers may need or choose to work more to uphold the household's overall income.

Marital status per se did not modify the overall effect of a child's cancer on employment or earnings. Fathers with children with cancer were, however, particularly likely to remain employed after child death and when they were parenting older children. This may reflect compensations at a household level to maintain previous income levels. The likelihood of either spouse experiencing unemployment was, however, greatly reduced among married couples, and these couples may be in a better situation than for instance single parents in case of cancer illness in a child.

4.3 The importance of education

Analyses stratified on parents' educational level showed that mothers with a low education remained employed and/or increased their employment relative to other mothers. This was contrary to what was expected, as occupations only requiring a low education in general are believed to be less flexible. On the other hand, these mothers may "need" to work for economic reasons, and they may thus not have the choice to dedicate themselves to caregiving. At a national level, single Norwegian mothers hold on average a lower education than married and/or cohabitant mothers, and this issue thus needs further exploration. No modifying effect was seen for the fathers' educational level. Cancer may also affect employment and earnings differently across different baseline educational levels and incomes, but the cancer estimates remained nearly identical with and without the inclusion of these factors.

Independent of education, neither husbands nor wives' earnings did influence divorce rates in this study. Elevated divorce rates were, however, observed for couples in which the wives had an above average educational level. No modifying effect was seen for the husband's education. In case of parental divorce, shared parental responsibility is more common among Norwegian couples in which the mother has a high education, but whether this can account for the elevated divorce rate among these couples has not been established.

4.4 Generalisability and implications of results

Cancer incidence in children is very hard to predict, and few well known risk factors have been established (26). Cancer in children thus affects persons randomly across social strata (15), and a cancer diagnosis in a child is therefore not associated with the same stigma as illnesses more obviously resulting from families' life-styles or lack of socioeconomic resources. Possible observed effects are thus likely consequences of cancer.

Norway is a welfare state with public health care available to all citizens, free of charge. The direct parental costs associated with cancer in children, i.e. diagnostic work-up and treatment, are thus minimal, in contrast to what is observed in other countries (33;35). In addition, leaves-of-absence and various economic welfare benefits are commonly yielded parents with chronically ill children. As previously stated, some of the compensatory measures cannot be assessed as they are included in the earnings variable. The existing welfare system, compensating for losses in ordinary labor market incomes and providing health services free of charge, may result in families' financial situations being only modestly affected in Norway compared to countries with less extensive welfare systems. I therefore consider it likely that the observed findings apply to countries with similar health and welfare options, employment rates, and earnings, as for instance Canada and the other Nordic and Western European countries. The relevance of these findings for other populations remains largely unexplored.

4.5 Summary of discussion

This large, methodologically rigorous registry-based study has shown that cancer in children is not associated with reductions in parents' employment probabilities, and that cancer in children is associated with only minor reductions in parents' earnings overall. The latter finding may be due to the extensive welfare options in the Nordic countries in case of illness in children. Contrary to what has been reported previously, parents' employment is not found to be generally adversely affected by cancer in children in this study. Earnings of certain subgroups of parents are, on the other hand, negatively affected, and this is in line with what has been reported previously (10;28;31;33;35). The magnitude overall is, however, minor. Reductions in earnings are mainly seen for mothers who have a high(er) education level, for mothers with living children, and for mothers with children diagnosed at young ages.

Exceptions exist for employed mothers with children with CNS cancers, germinal cell cancers, and unspecified leukemia, for whom significant reductions in earnings were observed. Reductions were particularly pronounced for mothers with young and living children, and became more pronounced with time elapsed from diagnosis. Additional studies are warranted to understand the background for these observed findings, as well as to identify possible interventions to reduce the adverse financial impact on these households. In line with traditional caregiving responsibilities, the adverse effects observed on earnings were most pronounced for mothers. Single mothers' earnings may be particularly affected, and research targeting this specific subgroup is necessary.

Contrary to existing myths, cancer in a child is not associated with an increase in parental divorce rates. Possible negative long term effects on the parents are perhaps balanced by strengthened parental bonds. Couples with highly educated mothers are exempted, and further studies are warranted to understand the background for their increased divorce risk.

A child's cancer illness was expected to increase divorce rates through an increased parental care burden and an increase in the psychological stress experienced by parents. However, except for couples with highly educated mothers, it seems that the divorce-reducing effects dominate or at least balance the opposite contributions, or that both types of effects are weak. Increased parental stress has, however, been documented in other studies, particularly for families who were vulnerable at the outset (8;57), and more research on the relationship between parental stress and divorce is needed.

5. The impact of family resources on childhood cancer

The general inverse association between childhood mortality and socioeconomic status is well established (61). As previously mentioned, the Norwegian public health care system offers all residents free cancer diagnosis and treatment. Private health services that exist typically handle less critical conditions and provide neither primary nor follow-up treatment for cancer. Further, because of highly standardized procedures conducted within centralized designated pediatric hospital departments (62), children supposedly receive the same initial and subsequent treatment regardless of where in the country they live and independent of their parents' resources and personal initiatives vis a vis health personnel. Thus, if there were no other determinants of the survival from these cancers, one would expect to see small differentials in survival by, for example, parents' education or other socio-demographic characteristics.

However, reality may be more complex. Treatments may perhaps be less standardized than widely assumed, and there may be socio-demographic variations in families' abilities to comply with the recommendations for follow-up assessments and treatment, in developed countries as well as in poorer settings (18;63). This might be of particular relevance in out-patient hospital settings or community-based primary care settings, where patients in general have to take on more responsibility to achieve appropriate care. Cancer may also be diagnosed earlier in some social groups than others, which may be important for survival. In addition, some children may have poorer health than others at time of diagnosis, with consequences for survival prospects, or they may develop diseases after diagnosis that are unrelated to the malignancy but increase the chance of dying from it. These so-called 'host factors' are probably influenced by, for example, families' socio-economic resources, as is all-cause mortality in this age group (61).

There is also limited knowledge about the importance of parents' socioeconomic resources from other countries, where effects also may be expected to be dissimilar because of inherent differences in the health care and welfare systems. One study from New Zealand showed that cancer survival was significantly reduced if a parent did not have a registered occupation or if a parent was unemployed, and an adverse effect of low education was also weakly indicated, while single parenthood had no impact (14). Similarly, ethnicity did not play a role (16). A relatively small, older study from the Netherlands concluded that parents' educational level only had a minor impact on childhood leukemia survival in the period 1973-79 (17). A Korean study from 2009 found that parental resources played a minor role (15), whereas a more recent study by the same authors found a clear inverse relationship between childhood cancer mortality and parental socioeconomic position (19). In developing countries, parental resources have been documented to have a significant beneficial effect (18;64).

Survival rates have improved substantially over the last decades for most childhood cancers (3). Childhood cancers represent, however, diverse diseases treated differently and with dissimilar risks for poor outcomes (3;22-24). The burden associated with modern pediatric oncology treatment thus varies considerably, as certain cancers are treated by one modality for a short period of time while others involve active multi-modal treatments for many years often associated with potential life-threatening complications (65). The latter treatments also require prolonged and more frequent hospitalizations in which one of the parents generally accompanies the child, and socio-demographic variation in survival might be expected to be more pronounced.

6. Findings from an empirical study on the impact of family resources on childhood cancer

Diagnostic and treatment protocols for childhood cancer are generally standardized, and survival ought therefore be fairly equal across social strata in societies with free public health care readily available. This study explores whether there nevertheless are disparities in mortality after childhood cancer in Norway depending on parents' socioeconomic status. As shown above, limited knowledge on mortality differentials exist from earlier analyses. Effects of the mother's age, education, and marital status, the mother's and father's combined annual labor earnings, and whether they have additional children, were therefore assessed.

6.1 Material and methods

Data on all Norwegian children diagnosed with cancer at age 0-19 from 1974 through 2007 (N=6280) and their parents were extracted from national registers. Cancer data at time of diagnosis was obtained from the Cancer Registry of Norway, but information on initial and subsequent courses of treatment was not available (52).

Discrete-time hazard regression models for all-cause mortality the first ten years following diagnosis were estimated. For each child, a series of one-month observations were created, starting at time of diagnosis and ending at time of death or emigration, when a second cancer was diagnosed, after ten years had passed since diagnosis, or on December 31st 2007. Each observation included various characteristics of the child, its disease, and its parents. The outcome variable was whether the child died within the month or not. Almost all deaths (i.e. >95%) were registered as due to cancer. In total, there were 1619 deaths within 500 837 person-months of observation. On average, each child contributed 6.7 observation years.

All models included time from diagnosis, child's age at diagnosis, calendar year, whether the parents were married to each other at time of diagnosis, number of siblings, mother's age when the child was born, her education at time of diagnosis, and average combined earnings of mothers and fathers during the last three years prior to diagnosis. Father's educational level could not be included in addition to that of the mother, because of a high degree of educational homogamy in Norway (66). Substituting mothers' education with those of fathers yielded fairly similar estimates. For the same reason, only mothers' age was included.

Some cancer types are more aggressive than others. In case these also occur more frequently in some groups than others, cancer type was controlled for in all models. It turned out, however, that this adjustment was unnecessary, i.e. the distribution of the cancer cases is fairly random. Stage at diagnosis was included in one model to assess its importance as a causally intermediate factor. Lastly, models were estimated separately for mothers with a high versus a low education, for children with and without siblings at diagnosis, for cancer forms anticipated to create long-lasting care burdens versus the remaining, and for an early (<1990) versus later (≥1990) diagnostic period. The cancer forms anticipated to involve long-term care burdens were CNS tumors, leukemias (AML excluded), neuroblastomas, and bone cancers (65).

6.2 Results

6.2.1 Descriptive statistics

Tables 7 show descriptive characteristics of children with cancer and their families. The most common cancer forms among children were CNS tumors, leukemias, lymphomas, germ cell cancers and neuroblastomas. Around 45% of the cancers were diagnosed at a localized stage, and only 6% had metastases at time of diagnosis. Cancer was most common among children older than 15 (36%) and younger than 5 (29%). The annual number of childhood cancer cases has been quite stable (67).

6.2.2 Mortality differentials after childhood cancer

Mortality increases from the first to the second half year after diagnosis (from OR 1.24 CI 1.04-1.49 to OR 1.42 CI 1.18-1.70) and then declines gradually to 0.13 (CI 0.10-0.16). As expected, the estimates also showed that there has been a substantial improvement in survival over time (OR 2.55 CI 2.03-3.19 in 1974-79 and OR 0.60 CI 0.50-0.74 in 2000-07). The lowest mortality was seen for children diagnosed before age 15 (a 22% advantage compared to the oldest children), those with no siblings (a 20% advantage), and those having mothers with a tertiary education (a 17% advantage). Parents' marital status did not affect survival, and neither did mother's age nor the parents' earnings. Mortality was highest for leukemia, bone cancer, hepatic cancer, soft-tissue cancer, neuroblastoma and CNS tumors. As expected, the outcome after localized cancer was clearly superior to that of more advanced cancer (OR 3.59 CI 2.88-4.49 and 6.59 CI 5.09-8.53 for regional and metastatic cancers, respectively). When stage was included in the model, the effects of number of siblings and mother's education remained virtually unchanged (OR 0.80 v 0.82 and 0.83 v 0.86, respectively).

Children				Parents			
Child categories	**N[b]**	**%[c]**	**Deaths/pmo[d]**	**Parental categories**	**N**	**%**	**Deaths/pmo**
Cancer form				**Mothers' age at birth[i]**			
CNS tumor	1524	24.3 %	434/115541	< 20 years old[j]	830	13.2 %	226/69280
Any leukemia	1520	24.2 %	474/115675	20-24 years old	2757	43.9 %	775/221698
Acute lymphoblastic leukemia (ALL)	*940*	*15.0 %*	*281/85342*	25-29 years old	1965	31.3 %	467/157315
Acute myelogenous leukemia (AML)	*210*	*3.3 %*	*124/12118*	30-34 years old	579	9.2 %	118/44792
Leukemias, nos[e]	*370*	*5.9 %*	*69/18215*	> 34 years old	149	2.4 %	33/11198
Lymphomas	742	11.8 %	130/62166				
Germinal cell cancer	509	8.1 %	61/47449	**Mothers' education**			
Neuroblastoma	360	5.7 %	104/27822	High school or below[j]	4614	73.5 %	1317/376515
Bone cancer	352	5.6 %	151/23928	College education or above	1666	26.5 %	302/127768
Soft tissue cancer	256	4.1 %	74/20094				
Malignant melanoma	246	3.9 %	28/25232	**Parents' marital status**			
Renal cancer[f]	219	3.5 %	28/20616	Married	4296	68.4 %	1120/352229
Endocrine cancer[g]	118	1.9 %	2/12198	Not married[j]	1984	31.6 %	499/152054
Hepatic cancer	86	1.4 %	33/5544				
Other or unknown	348	5.5 %	100/28018	**Number of siblings**			
				0[j]	991	15.8 %	222/81367
Cancer stage at diagnosis				1	2514	40.0 %	647/203095
Local cancer	2822	44.9 %	630/243078	>=2	2775	44.2 %	750/219821
Regional cancer	670	10.7 %	202/48911				
Metastatic cancer	350	5.6 %	124/22827	**Parents' earnings[k]**			
Unknown[h]	2438	38.8 %	663/189467	< $10 000[f]	992	15.8 %	381/75510
				$10 000-$19 999	837	13.3 %	304/69029
Age at diagnosis				$20 000-$39 999	1415	22.5 %	380/127093
Child 0-4 yrs	1791	28.5 %	448/145376	$40 000-$59 999	1054	16.8 %	236/93447
Child 5-9 yrs	1165	18.6 %	321/92103	$60 000-$79 999	821	13.1 %	151/67797
Child 10-14 yrs	1088	17.3 %	307/85511	$80 000-$99 999	520	8.3 %	79/35778
Child >= 15 yrs	2236	35.6 %	543/181293	>= $100 000	641	10.2 %	88/35629

[a]Only the time invariant characteristics are shown here. [b]Number of children or parents in the respective categories. [c]Percentage of children or parents in the respective categories. [d]Number of child deaths per person-month. [e]Not otherwise specified. [f]Primarily Wilm's tumor. [g]Primarily thyroid cancer. [h]Including CNS tumors and around 60% of the lymphomas for which no stage is recorded. [i]Age at birth of child later diagnosed with cancer. [j]Including also those with massing values. [k]Three-year avarage of parents' combined gross annual labor earning priot to diagnosis. Excluding parents with missing earnings gave a median combined earningsat diagnosis of $47 000.

Table 7. Characteristics of children with cancer and their families at time of diagnosis is and deaths per person - month[a]

Results from stratified analyses are portrayed in Table 8. Stratifying the children by their mothers' educational level (high, i.e. above high school level, versus low, i.e. high school level or below) resulted in a statistically significant advantage of 22% of being an only child for children with mothers with a low educational level. This was, however, not observed for children with mothers with a high education. A non-significant protective effect was also suggested for children with married mothers with a high education.

When stratifying the children by having sibling(s) versus being an only child, similar results were obtained. The mother's educational level was unimportant for children with cancer without siblings. Children with cancer with sibling(s) at time of diagnosis had, however, a 21% lower death probability if their mothers had a high education.

For children with cancers that require long-term treatments, having no siblings or better-educated mothers was associated with a statistically significant mortality advantage of around 18-19%. This relationship was present but not significant for those with other cancers. A mortality disadvantage of 42% was observed for the oldest children with chronic cancers, whereas an advantage was seen for other cancers in this age group.

	Mothers' educational level				Only child or siblings at diagnosis				Chronic or resolving disease			
	Low education[b]		High education[c]		No siblings[d]		Siblings[e]		Chronic[f]		Resolving[g]	
	OR[h]	95 % CI[i]	OR	95 % CI	OR	95 % CI	OR	95 % CI	OR[d]	95 % CI	OR	95 % CI
Current calendar period												
1974-1979	**2.26**	1.78-2.88	**2.34**	1.21-4.50	1.69	0.90-3.19	**2.42**	1.90-3.08	**2.02**	1.53-2.66	**3.26**	2.22-4.77
1980-1984	**1.56**	1.25-1.94	**2.22**	1.31-3.75	1.37	0.78-2.41	**1.70**	1.36-2.11	**1.47**	1.14-1.89	**2.29**	1.63-3.22
1985-1989	**1.24**	1.01-1.52	1.44	0.88-2.37	1.26	0.75-2.13	**1.27**	1.04-1.56	1.19	0.95-1.51	**1.51**	1.09-2.08
1990-1994	1.00	ref	1.00	ref	1.00	ref	1.00	ref	1.00	ref	1.00	ref
1995-1999	0.83	0.66-1.03	1.21	0.76-1.91	1.02	0.60-1.70	0.87	0.70-1.07	0.92	0.72-1.16	0.84	0.60-1.19
2000-2007	**0.61**	0.49-0.77	0.95	0.60-1.52	0.61	0.36-1.03	**0.69**	0.56-0.86	**0.62**	0.48-0.79	0.84	0.60-1.17
Age at diagnosis												
Child 0-4 yrs	1.00	ref	1.00	ref	1.00	ref	1.00	ref	1.00	ref	1.00	ref
Child 5-9 yrs	1.11	0.94-1.31	0.97	0.68-1.38	0.91	0.60-1.38	1.10	0.93-1.30	1.12	0.95-1.33	0.82	0.61-1.11
Child 10-14 yrs	1.09	0.91-1.31	1.21	0.84-1.74	1.11	0.66-1.87	1.11	0.94-1.32	1.13	0.94-1.37	0.98	0.74-1.28
Child >= 15 yrs	**1.19**	1.01-1.41	1.42	0.98-2.04	1.47	0.91-2.37	**1.22**	1.04-1.44	**1.42**	1.19-1.69	**0.68**	0.54-0.86
Parents' marital status[j]												
Married	1.04	0.91-1.19	0.86	0.65-1.14	1.16	0.85-1.59	0.99	0.87-1.13	0.96	0.83-1.11	1.03	0.84-1.26
Not married[k]	1.00	ref	1.00	ref	1.00	ref	1.00	ref	1.00	ref	1.00	ref
Number of siblings[j]												
0 siblings	**0.78**	0.64-0.94	0.93	0.65-1.33	N/A	N/A	N/A	N/A	**0.81**	0.66-0.99	0.83	0.61-1.13
1 sibling	1.00	ref	1.00	ref	N/A	N/A	N/A	N/A	1.00	ref	1.00	ref
2 or more siblings	0.98	0.87-1.11	0.86	0.66-1.11	N/A	N/A	N/A	N/A	0.91	0.79-1.05	1.11	0.92-1.33
Mothers' educational level[j]												
High school or less[k]	N/A	N/A	N/A	N/A	1.00	ref	1.00	ref	1.00	ref	1.00	ref
College and above	N/A	N/A	N/A	N/A	1.03	0.71-1.50	**0.79**	0.68-0.93	**0.82**	0.69-0.98	0.81	0.64-1.03

[a]All covariates were included in the respective models, cancer form exempted (chronic/resolving cancers, time since diagnosis, parents' earnings and mother age not shown). [b]Low education at or below high school level and includes missing. [c]High education refers to any education beyond high school level. [d]No siblings at time of diagnosis. [e]One or more siblings at time of diagnosis. [f]Includes CNS tumors, leukemias (AML excluded), neuroblastoma and bone cancers. [g]Includes the remaining cancer forms. [h]Odds Ratio. [i]Confidence interval. [j]Refers to the situation at time of diagnosis. [k]Including those with missing values.

Table 8. A child;s death probability stratified according to mother's educational level, number of siblings, and the expected chronicity of treatment and adverse long-term effects[a]

6.2.3 Summary of main findings

This large registry-based study shows that survival after childhood cancer depends on the family's resources: Mortality was reduced by about 15-20% for children without siblings and children whose mother has tertiary education. Stratified analyses suggest, however, that these effects are restricted to cancers that involve long-term treatment. The parents' earnings seem to have no effect above and beyond education, and there is also no or minor impact of parents' age or marital status.

6.3 Discussion

Survival after childhood cancer in Norway depends on the family's resources. Similar studies, based on smaller data sets for other countries, have not shown such a clear relationship between parental education and survival from childhood cancer (14;17;18;68), but the results are in line with those from a recent, large Korean study (19). No earlier investigation has addressed the possible importance of siblings. The lack of effect of marital status accords well with the literature. Income effects have been reported by some authors (14;15), but comparison to studies from different countries is complicated due to dissimilar health care and welfare systems.

6.3.1 Effects of being an only child at time of diagnosis

Stage at time of diagnosis turned out to be relatively unimportant, and in principle two main channels remain for the various socio-demographic factors to operate through in affecting cancer survival: Treatment (the primary and follow-up treatment that is offered and the family's ability to make good use of it), and 'host factors' (the child's health at the time of diagnosis and later health problems unrelated to the malignancy). The presence of siblings may have the consequence that the parents can devote less time to assisting the sick child, which could have effect through both pathways (69). While it may well be the case that every child in Norway is offered the same cancer treatment, regardless of any personal initiatives from eager parents vis a vis the health personnel, mothers and fathers with additional family obligations might be less likely to comply with the recommended procedures for follow-up and less attentive to any unforeseen problems that they ideally should seek help for. When there are more children, there is also less to spend on each (70), given the family income, but the lack of effect of parents' earnings suggests that such economic factors are generally unimportant. It is also possible that having more siblings that compete for parents' time increases the chance of comorbidities before or after diagnosis, though there is little evidence for such effects in developed countries. The above arguments are particularly relevant for cancers that require long-term treatment and thus develop into rather chronic health conditions. It is thus reasonable that I see the sharpest effects of the number of siblings in these instances.

6.3.2 Effects of parents' education

The better survival among children with a better-educated mother, and thus also usually a better-educated father, may partly be the result of these parents having a higher level of health literacy, i.e. being better able to communicate and interact with health care personnel and navigate the health care system. Further, parents who have high education generally hold more flexible jobs that make it easier to spend time in hospitals with their children. All this may increase the chance of the child receiving adequate follow-up treatment. For similar reasons, children of better-educated parents may also have better health at diagnosis and thus avoid later comorbidities. It thus appears reasonable that the observed effects are sharpest for the cancers that require long-term treatment.

6.3.3 The lack of effect of parents' earnings and marital status

It would not be unreasonable to expect an effect of the parents' income, even within a public health care setting. Couples with higher incomes might, for instance, find it easier to reduce their working hours to provide extra care for their child, with implications for the child's follow-up treatment as well as the chance of avoiding comorbidities. Children from richer families may also have better health at time of diagnosis. However, the lack of effect suggests that these mechanisms on the whole are of little importance in Norway. The effect of parents' marital status, net of the other variables included in the model, might be expected to affect the survival largely through time constraints: To the extent that a child with non-married parents lives with only one parent, there may be less time available to help and care for the child, in particular if the other parent is less involved and/or supportive. This might seem to be an important factor in light of the previously discussed sibling-effect. No effect is, however, observed of parents' marital status, and the reason may be that most of the non-married parents are cohabitants, or that also the non-resident parent contributes in case of a child's cancer illness.

6.3.4 Summary of discussion

This large, registry-based study suggests that parents' time constraints and various non-economic rewards from their education impact on childhood cancer survival. It may be that children with resourceful parents are healthier at the outset and/or more likely to avoid later health problems that are unrelated to the malignancy but that weaken the survival prospects. It may also be that children of well-informed and strongly involved parents actually may be *offered* better initial and/or subsequent treatment, even within a universal health care setting with limited private alternatives and supposedly highly standardized treatment protocols in place (18). Alternatively, such parents may be better able to *make use of* what is offered, for instance by adhering more closely to recommendations for out-patient follow-up care (71). The possibility of such differentials in offered and actual treatment should be addressed in future research.

7. Conclusions from Norway in a comparative perspective

7.1 Employment and earnings

Parents' employment is not adversely affected by a child's cancer in Norway. Earnings are reduced in certain instances, but the overall effects are minor. Generous welfare options and flexible labor markets typical for Nordic welfare states may account for this. In line with traditional caregiving responsibilities, mothers' reductions in earnings were most pronounced.

Few studies from other countries on parents' work force participation exist, and no reviews on parental employment and/or earnings after cancer or other chronic illness in children could be identified. The existing studies are relatively small and are likely to reflect policies and labor markets in particular geographic areas (10;28-35), and only a few utilizes a comparison group (29-31). Overall, the results from Norway are more positive and suggest lesser declines in earnings than what has been reported previously (10;28;31;33;35), perhaps due to Norway's extensive welfare system. The negative impact on mothers' employment and earnings are, however, similar in Norway and other countries (33;34). In conclusion, existing knowledge indicate that there may be country-specific or regional differences with regard to work opportunities and also that the various features of children's cancer may influence family employment and earnings differentially.

7.2 Divorce

Parents' divorce rates are not adversely affected by a child's cancer in general in Norway. Possible negative long term effects on the parents may be balanced by strengthening of parental bonds. An exception exists for couples with highly educated mothers, and further studies are warranted to understand the background for this increase in divorce risk.

The overall finding of no effect of cancer in a child on parents' divorce risk is in line with results from earlier studies (46-48). To my knowledge, earlier studies have not been large enough to account for differential effects of mothers' educational level, and this finding needs to be confirmed in future studies. Regional differences in health and welfare systems may also play a role, and studies from diverse settings are warranted.

7.3 Survival

Mortality was reduced by about 15-20% for children with highly educated mothers and children without siblings. These effects were most pronounced for cancers predicted to encompass intense, long-lasting treatments resulting in chronic health problems. Neither parents' earnings nor their marital status affected children's survival.

There is limited knowledge about the importance of parents' socioeconomic resources from other countries, where effects also may be expected to be dissimilar because of inherent differences in the health care and welfare systems. A study from New Zealand showed that cancer survival was significantly reduced if a parent did not have a registered occupation or if a parent was unemployed, and an adverse effect of low education was also weakly indicated, while single parenthood had no impact (14). A relatively small, older study from the Netherlands concluded that parents' educational level only had a minor impact on childhood leukemia survival (17).Likewise, a Korean study from 2009 also found that parental resources played a minor role (15). The Norwegian findings are, however, in line with a more recent Korean study where a clear inverse relationship between childhood cancer mortality and parental socioeconomic position was seen (19). In developing countries, parental resources have been documented to have a significant beneficial effect (18;64), but more research from developed countries is clearly needed.

8. Current state of the knowledge and future directions

Empirical findings from Norway show that cancer in a child adversely affects women's earnings, but that it does not, in general increase divorce rates. Although research shows that parenting a child diagnosed with cancer is burdensome, it does not appear to impact strongly on parental incomes or divorce rates in welfare states. Findings may be different in countries with less extensive welfare systems, be it health care or compensatory benefits to parents in case of illness of children. More research is thus needed to establish how valid these results are for persons in different cultures and societies, as there is conflicting evidence on how cancer in a child affects family life in the published literature.

Further, childhood cancer mortality in Norway varies with parents' education and family size. Low education, especially among mothers, and a larger family size are both associated with increased mortality. There is much evidence from developing countries on that mortality is dependent upon parental socioeconomic status. I find that this is the case also in modern welfare states, and suggest that the situation will be even worse in less extensive welfare states, like for instance the US. Given the widely accepted idea that the health care system should reach well out to everyone and the suspicion that this perhaps is not quite the case after all, a careful analysis of possible treatment differentials utilizing longitudinal directly measured treatment data should be welcome in future studies. While a key concern would be that everyone is offered the same treatment, attention should also be given to the degree of compliance, as it might be argued that this is not solely an individual responsibility but resides within the domain of public policy. Should no such differences in treatment be revealed in future studies, the observed effects must be due to differences in general health (behavior), which would indicate the need for health policy initiatives of a different type. It is obviously challenging to generalize to other settings, and in particular with respect to the effects of economic resources. They could, presumably, be expected to be even more pronounced in most other countries with less generous health and welfare systems.

To summarize, cross-national research on treatment decisions, health care delivery, and utilization across social groups to further comprehend discrepancies in outcomes for both families and children after childhood cancer appears warranted. Larger samples sizes and more studies utilizing control groups are also clearly needed. Lastly, longitudinal designs to assess family dynamics and consequences in a longer-term perspective would be welcome. The great advances in childhood cancer survival over the last decades are positive, but may also have some negative implications that are beginning to surface and needs to be considered.

9. References

[1] Langeveld NE, Stam H, Grootenhuis MA, Last BF. Quality of life in young adult survivors of childhood cancer. Support Care Cancer 2002 Nov;10(8):579-600.
[2] Tonorezos ES, Oeffinger KC. Survivorship after childhood, adolescent, and young adult cancer. Cancer J 2008 Nov;14(6):388-95.
[3] Nathan PC, Greenberg ML, Ness KK, Hudson MM, Mertens AC, Mahoney MC, et al. Medical care in long-term survivors of childhood cancer: a report from the childhood cancer survivor study. J Clin Oncol 2008 Sep 20;26(27):4401-9.
[4] Langeveld NE, Ubbink MC, Last BF, Grootenhuis MA, Voute PA, de Haan RJ. Educational achievement, employment and living situation in long-term young adult survivors of childhood cancer in the Netherlands. Psychooncology 2003 Apr;12(3):213-25.

[5] Diller L, Chow EJ, Gurney JG, Hudson MM, Kadin-Lottick NS, Kawashima TI, et al. Chronic Disease in the Childhood Cancer Survivor Study Cohort: A Review of Published Findings. J Clin Oncol 2009 Apr 13.
[6] Grootenhuis MA, Last BF. Adjustment and coping by parents of children with cancer: a review of the literature. Support Care Cancer 1997 Nov;5(6):466-84.
[7] Kazak AE, Baxt C. Families of infants and young children with cancer: a post-traumatic stress framework. Pediatr Blood Cancer 2007 Dec;49(7 Suppl):1109-13.
[8] Vrijmoet-Wiersma JCM, van Klink JM, Kolk AM, Koopman HM, Ball LM, Maarten ER. Assessment of parental psychological stress in pediatric cancer: a review. J Pediatr Psychol 2008 Aug;33(7):694-706.
[9] Raina P, O'Donnell M, Schwellnus H, Rosenbaum P, King G, Brehaut J, et al. Caregiving process and caregiver burden: conceptual models to guide research and practice. BMC Pediatr 2004 Jan 14;4:1.
[10] Limburg H, Shaw AK, McBride ML. Impact of childhood cancer on parental employment and sources of income: a Canadian pilot study. Pediatr Blood Cancer 2008 Jul;51(1):93-8.
[11] Syse A, Larsen IK, Tretli S. Does cancer in a child affect parents' employment and earnings? A population-based study. Cancer Epidemiol 2010 Sep 3.
[12] Pai AL, Greenley RN, Lewandowski A, Drotar D, Youngstrom E, Peterson CC. A meta-analytic review of the influence of pediatric cancer on parent and family functioning. J Fam Psychol 2007 Sep;21(3):407-15.
[13] Syse A, Loge JH, Lyngstad TH. Does childhood cancer affect parental divorce rates? A population-based study. J Clin Oncol 2010 Feb 10;28(5):872-7.
[14] Blakely T, Atkinson J, Kiro C, Blaiklock A, D'Souza A. Child mortality, socioeconomic position, and one-parent families: independent associations and variation by age and cause of death. Int J Epidemiol 2003 Jun;32(3):410-8.
[15] Kim J, Son M, Kawachi I, Oh J. The extent and distribution of inequalities in childhood mortality by cause of death according to parental socioeconomic positions: a birth cohort study in South Korea. Soc Sci Med 2009 Oct;69(7):1116-26.
[16] Douglas NM, Dockerty JD. Survival by ethnicity for children diagnosed with cancer in New Zealand during 1990-1993. J Paediatr Child Health 2007 Mar;43(3):173-7.
[17] Coebergh JW, van der Does-van den Berg, Hop WC, van Weerden F, Rammeloo JA, van Steensel HA, et al. Small influence of parental educational level on the survival of children with leukaemia in The Netherlands between 1973 and 1979. Eur J Cancer 1996 Feb;32A(2):286-9.
[18] Mostert S, Sitaresmi MN, Gundy CM, Veerman AJ. Attitude of health-care providers toward childhood leukemia patients with different socio-economic status. Pediatr Blood Cancer 2008 May;50(5):1001-5.
[19] Son M, Kim J, Oh J, Kawachi I. Inequalities in childhood cancer mortality according to parental socioeconomic position: A birth cohort study in South Korea. Soc Sci Med 2011 Jan;72(1):108-15.
[20] Mertens AC. Cause of mortality in 5-year survivors of childhood cancer. Pediatr Blood Cancer 2007 Jun 15;48(7):723-6.
[21] Syse A, Lyngstad TH, Kravdal O. Is mortality after childhood cancer dependent on social or economic resources of parents? A population-based study. Int J Cancer 2011 May 26.

[22] Hudson MM, Mulrooney DA, Bowers DC, Sklar CA, Green DM, Donaldson SS, et al. High-Risk Populations Identified in Childhood Cancer Survival Study Investigations: Implications for Risk-Based Surveillance. J Clin Oncol 2009 Mar 16.
[23] Mody R, Li S, Dover DC, Sallan S, Leisenring W, Oeffinger KC, et al. Twenty-five-year follow-up among survivors of childhood acute lymphoblastic leukemia: a report from the Childhood Cancer Survivor Study. Blood 2008 Jun 15;111(12):5515-23.
[24] Mulrooney DA, Dover DC, Li S, Yasui Y, Ness KK, Mertens AC, et al. Twenty years of follow-up among survivors of childhood and young adult acute myeloid leukemia: a report from the Childhood Cancer Survivor Study. Cancer 2008 May 1;112(9):2071-9.
[25] Hoven E, Anclair M, Samuelsson U, Kogner P, Boman KK. The influence of pediatric cancer diagnosis and illness complication factors on parental distress. J Pediatr Hematol Oncol 2008 Nov;30(11):807-14.
[26] Klassen A, Raina P, Reineking S, Dix D, Pritchard S, O'Donnell M. Developing a literature base to understand the caregiving experience of parents of children with cancer: a systematic review of factors related to parental health and well-being. Supportive Care in Cancer 2007 Jul;15(7):807-18.
[27] Franck LS, Callery P. Re-thinking family-centred care across the continuum of children's healthcare. Child Care Health Dev 2004 May;30(3):265-77.
[28] Dockerty JD, Skegg DC, Williams SM. Economic effects of childhood cancer on families. J Paediatr Child Health 2003 May;39(4):254-8.
[29] Piachaud D, Bradshaw J, Weale J. The income effect of a disabled child. J Epidemiol Community Health 1981 Jun;35(2):123-7.
[30] Baldwin S, Godfrey C, Staden F. Childhood disablement and family incomes. J Epidemiol Community Health 1983 Sep;37(3):187-95.
[31] Heath JA, Lintuuran RM, Rigguto G, Tikotlian N, McCarthy M. Childhood cancer: its impact and financial costs for Australian families. Pediatr Hematol Oncol 2006 Jul;23(5):439-48.
[32] Barr RD, Sala A. Hidden financial costs in the treatment for childhood cancer. J Pediatr Hematol Oncol 2003 Nov;25(11):842-4.
[33] Eiser C, Upton P. Costs of caring for a child with cancer: a questionnaire survey. Child Care Health Dev 2007 Jul;33(4):455-9.
[34] Miedema B, Easley J, Fortin P, Hamilton R, Mathews M. The economic impact on families when a child is diagnosed with cancer. Curr Oncol 2008 Aug;15(4):173-8.
[35] Cohn RJ, Goodenough B, Foreman T, Suneson J. Hidden financial costs in treatment for childhood cancer: an Australian study of lifestyle implications for families absorbing out-of-pocket expenses. J Pediatr Hematol Oncol 2003 Nov;25(11):854-63.
[36] Sabbeth BF, Leventhal JM. Marital adjustment to chronic childhood illness: a critique of the literature. Pediatrics 1984 Jun;73(6):762-8.
[37] Johnson KJ, Carozza SE, Chow EJ, Fox EE, Horel S, McLaughlin CC, et al. Parental Age and Risk of Childhood Cancer: A Pooled Analysis. Epidemiology 2009 Apr 15.
[38] Booth A, Edwards JN. Age at Marriage and Marital Instability. Journal of Marriage and the Family 1985;47(1):67-75.
[39] Jalovaara M. The Joint Effects of Partners Socio-economic Positions on Divorce Risk. Demography 2003;40(1).

[40] Lyngstad TH. The Impact of Parents' and Spouses' Education on Divorce Rates in Norway. Demographic Research 2006 Apr 15;10(5):121-42.
[41] White LK. Determinants of Divorce: A Review of Research in the Eighties. Journal of Marriage and the Family 1990;52(11):904-12.
[42] Becker GS, Landes EM, Michael RT. An Economic Analysis of Marital Instability. Journal of Political Economy 1977;85(6):1141-87.
[43] Oppenheimer VK. Women's Rising Employment and the Future of the Family in Industrial Societies. Population and Development Review 1994;20(2):293-342.
[44] Becker GS. A Treatise on the Family. Cambridge, MA: Harvard University Press; 1991.
[45] Ross-Alaolmolki K, Heinzer MM, Howard R, Marszal S. Impact of childhood cancer on siblings and family: family strategies for primary health care. Holist Nurs Pract 1995 Jul;9(4):66-75.
[46] Lansky SB, Cairns NU, Hassanein R, Wehr J, Lowman JT. Childhood cancer: Parental discord and divorce. Pediatrics 1978 Aug;62(2):184-8.
[47] Kaplan DM, Grobstein R, Smith A. Predicting the impact of severe illness in families. Health Soc Work 1976 Aug;1(3):71-82.
[48] Stehbens JA, Lascari AD. Psychological follow-up of families with childhood leukemia. J Clin Psychol 1974 Jul;30(3):394-7.
[49] Reichman NE, Corman H, Noonan K. Effects of child health on parents' relationship status. Demography 2004;41(3):569-84.
[50] Mauldon J. Children's risks of experiencing divorce and remarriage:do disabled children destabilize marriages? Population Studies 1992;46(2):349-62.
[51] Shudy M, de Almeida ML, Ly S, Landon C, Groft S, Jenkins TL, et al. Impact of pediatric critical illness and injury on families: a systematic literature review. Pediatrics 2006 Dec;118 Suppl 3:S203-S218.
[52] Larsen IK, Smastuen M, Johannesen TB, Langmark F, Parkin DM, Bray F, et al. Data quality at the Cancer Registry of Norway: an overview of comparability, completeness, validity and timeliness. Eur J Cancer 2009 May;45(7):1218-31.
[53] Rogers CH, Floyd FJ, Seltzer MM, Greenberg J, Hong J. Long-term effects of the death of a child on parents' adjustment in midlife. J Fam Psychol 2008 Apr;22(2):203-11.
[54] Kreicbergs U, Valdimarsdottir U, Onelov E, Bjork O, Steineck G, Henter JI. Care-related distress: a nationwide study of parents who lost their child to cancer. J Clin Oncol 2005 Dec 20;23(36):9162-71.
[55] Johannesen TB, Langmark F, Wesenberg F, Lote K. Prevalence of Norwegian patients diagnosed with childhood cancer, their working ability and need of health insurance benefits. Acta Oncol 2007;46(1):60-6.
[56] Aarsen FK, Paquier PF, Reddingius RE, Streng IC, Arts WF, Evera-Preesman M, et al. Functional outcome after low-grade astrocytoma treatment in childhood. Cancer 2006 Jan 15;106(2):396-402.
[57] Sloper P. Predictors of distress in parents of children with cancer: a prospective study. J Pediatr Psychol 2000 Mar;25(2):79-91.
[58] Neff LA, Karney BR. Gender differences in social support: a question of skill or responsiveness? J Pers Soc Psychol 2005 Jan;88(1):79-90.
[59] Thompson L. Conceptualizing gender in marriage: The case of marital care. J Marriage Fam 1993;55(August):557-69.

[60] Booth A, Johnson DR. Declining Health and Marital Quality. Journal of Marriage and the Family 1994;56(2):218-23.
[61] Botting B. Mortaility in childhood. In: Drever F, Whitehead M, editors. Health Inequalities.London: Office for National Statistics; 1997.
[62] Gatta G, Corazziari I, Magnani C, Peris-Bonet R, Roazzi P, Stiller C. Childhood cancer survival in Europe. Ann Oncol 2003;14 Suppl 5:v119-v127.
[63] Mostert S, Sitaresmi MN, Gundy CM, Janes V, Sutaryo, Veerman AJ. Comparing childhood leukaemia treatment before and after the introduction of a parental education programme in Indonesia. Arch Dis Child 2010 Jan;95(1):20-5.
[64] Kiani MF. Differentials in child mortality and health care in Pakistan. Pak Dev Rev 1992;31(4 Pt 2):1051-8.
[65] Pizzo PA, Poplauck DG. Principles and practice of pediatric oncology. 6 ed. Philadelphia: Lippincott Williams & Wilkins; 2010.
[66] Birkelund GE, Heldal J. Who marries whom? Educational homogamy in Norway. Demographic Research 2003 Sep 1;8(1):1-30.
[67] Cancer in Norway 2008. Oslo: Kreftregisteret. www.kreftregisteret.no; 2009.
[68] Shaw C, Blakely T, Atkinson J, Crampton P. Do social and economic reforms change socioeconomic inequalities in child mortality? A case study: New Zealand 1981-1999. J Epidemiol Community Health 2005 Aug;59(8):638-44.
[69] Patterson JM, Holm KE, Gurney JG. The impact of childhood cancer on the family: a qualitative analysis of strains, resources, and coping behaviors. Psychooncology 2004 Jun;13(6):390-407.
[70] Foster EM. How economists think about family resources and child development. Child Dev 2002 Nov;73(6):1904-14.
[71] Miller AR, Condin CJ, McKellin WH, Shaw N, Klassen AF, Sheps S. Continuity of care for children with complex chronic health conditions: parents' perspectives. BMC Health Serv Res 2009;9:242.

Part 5

Pediatric Infectious Diseases

16

Fungal Infections in Patients of Paediatric Age

Giuseppina Caggiano
and Maria Teresa Montagna
*Department of Biomedical Science
and Human Oncology, Hygiene Section,
University of Bari "Aldo Moro", Bari,
Italy*

1. Introduction

In recent decades, fungi have emerged as important causes of human infection, due primarily to the increased numbers of patients subjected to severe immunosuppression, so the demand for information on the pathogenic role of these microorganisms and the diseases they cause is growing.

Despite the development of more active, less toxic antifungal agents and the use of antifungal prophylaxis, the mycoses (especially those invasive) continue to be a serious infective complication in several patients' outcomes, resulting in high mortality rates (Lehrnbecher et al., 2010). Both paediatric and adult patients are exposed to fungal infections, even if important differences of epidemiology, diagnostic approaches and therapeutic management have to be considered. To date, globally, these infections have been well studied in different populations of adult patients while thorough epidemiological analyses in paediatric patients, including immunocompromised subjects, e.g. children with haematological malignancies and preterm neonates, are fairly sparse.

1.1 General characteristics of fungi

Fungi are ubiquitous organisms that live as environment saprophytes or as commensal microorganisms of humans and animals.

They morphologically are distinguished in yeasts (unicellular organisms) and moulds (multicellular organisms). Most fungi are found in morphological organization as yeasts or moulds but some species, known as dimorphic fungi, can be found as yeasts or moulds depending on the temperature and substrate on which they develop. They grow in environment as moulds and in humans as yeasts.

Of the more than 100,000 species of fungi identified to date, only few species can infect man and of them only a few are sufficiently virulent to infect a healthy host.

On the basis of their pathogenic role, fungi can be divided into:

- *primary pathogens* (dimorphic fungi, such as *Histoplasma, Blastomyces, Coccidioides*) which can also infect immune-competent subjects. They are microorganisms endemic to America, Africa and Asia.
- *opportunistic pathogens* (yeasts and moulds, such as *Candida* spp., *Cryptococcus* spp, *Aspergillus* spp, *Zygomycetes* and *Fusarium* spp) which can cause damage to the host if the immune system is compromised.

According to the site of infection and degree of tissue involvement, fungi can cause superficial, cutaneous, subcutaneous and deep mycoses (Kern & Blenvins, 1997).

The superficial mycoses are limited to the stratum corneum and essentially elicit no inflammation response; they are caused specially by fungi dermatophytes that produce keratinase and live on human keratin (skin, hair and nails). The cutaneous infections involve the integument and its appendages. The sub-cutaneous mycoses affect the subcutaneous tissues usually at the point of traumatic inoculation of the etiological agent. The deep infections involve systems and organs stimulating high immune response. The Table 1 shows the classification of most fungal infections.

Pattern of infection	Fungal infection	Etiological agent
Superficial and cutaneous	Pityriasis versicolor	*Malassetia furfur*
	Tinea nigra	*Exophiala werneckii*
	White piedra	*Trichosporon beigelii*
	Black piedra	*Piedraia hortae*
	Dermatophytosis	*Microsporum spp* *Trichophyton spp* *Epydermophyton floccosum*
	Candidiasis of skin, nail, mucosa	*Candida spp*
Sub- cutaneous	Chromoblastomycosis	*Fonsecaea pedrosoi* *Phialophora verrucosa etc.*
	Mycetoma	*Madurella mycetomatis* *Acremonium, Pseudallescheria, Exophiala, Curvularia, Fusarium, Aspergillus, etc.*
	Sporotrichosis	*Sporothrix schenckii*
Deep by dimorphic fungi	Blastomycosis	*Blastomyces dermatitidis*
	Coccidioidomycosis	*Coccidioides immitis*
	Histoplasmosis	*Histoplasma capsulatum*
	Paracoccidioidomycosis	*Paracoccidioides brasiliensis*
Deep by opportunistic pathogen fungi	Aspergillosis	*Aspergillus spp*
	Sistemic Candidiasis	*Candida spp*
	Cryptococcosis	*Cryptococcus neoformans/gattii*
	Zygomycoses	*Rhizopus, Absidia, Mucor etc.*

Table 1. Classification of most fungal infections and their principal etiological agents.

The deep mycoses are those of highest concern for the life-threatening consequences. They can be identified in:

Invasive Mycoses: deep fungal infection with predominant deep tissue invasion in the absence of blood dissemination.

Disseminated Mycoses: deep fungal infection involving multiple organs or systems that do not touch each other and without being transported by blood or lymph.

Systemic Mycoses: deep fungal infection confined to a single organ or system achieved by blood.

Infecting fungi may be either exogenous or endogenous so, according to the route of acquisition, a mycoses may be designated as exogenous or endogenous in origin.

The moulds have their natural habitat in the environment so they always originate exogenous infections caused mainly by the inhalation of air widespread conidia . This kind of infections are often correlated to environmental contamination especially during construction works. Given the ubiquitous nature of fungal spores, in particular of *Aspergillus* spp, in the external environment, numerous sources have been identified also in hospitals: unfiltered air; conditioned air systems with poorly maintenance; persistent construction works. Therefore, the presence of *Aspergillus* spp in the hospital setting is the major extrinsic risk factor for the occurrence of nosocomial invasive aspergillosis mainly among neutropenic patients.

On the contrary, the yeasts can be endogen and exogenous. The endogen yeasts colonize the mucosa and in particular conditions (immunocompromise, mucosite post-chemotherapy) can invade the organism and cause the disease. The exogenous yeasts are commensal of skin, they can invade the organism *via percutaneum*, such as parenteral nutrition or intravascular catheter contamined especially by the hands of health care workers. Many of these invasive mycoses are difficult to diagnose early, yet the patient's outcome depends, other than restoration of host defences, on fast and correct etiological diagnosis and so on early and proper antifungal treatment.

2. Paediatric patients at risk of fungal infection

At the beginning century, fungal infections were quite rare, but in the last years the paediatric and adult populations at risk of mycoses continue to expand so also the spectrum of opportunistic fungal pathogens continue to increase.

Even if both children and adults are exposed to these significant infections, important differences between the two populations are documented as predisposing factors and epidemiology.

The main paediatric patients at risk of invasive fungal infections are pre-term neonates, children with congenital immune deficiencies, with acquired immune deficiencies associated with HIV infection, cancer and patients in treatment with corticosteroids or who have chronic destructive lung diseases.

Generally, functional defects of phagocytes cells predispose to invasive infections by opportunistic fungi (*Candida* spp, *Aspergillus* spp, *Fusarium* spp), while alterations of T lymphocytes function are correlated to muco-cutaneous candidiasis and invasive infection by *Cryptococcus neoformans*. In addition, a large variety of non-immunological factors are recognized as predisposing to fungal infection, such as the presence of intravascular catheter, *Candida* colonization, use of broad-spectrum antibiotics, parenteral nutrition and abdominal surgery (Table 2).

Predisposing conditions, patterns of infection, etiological agents and therapeutic treatment are different among diverse paediatric populations.

RISK FACTORS	
Immunological	Non-immunological
Functional defects of phagocytes cells	Intravascular catheter
Alterations of T lymphocytes function	*Candida* colonization
	Use of broad-spectrum antibiotics
	Parenteral nutrition
	Abdominal surgery

Table 2. Classification of some immunological and non-immunological risk factors for invasive fungal infections.

3. Neonate patients

At birth, neonates can be colonized by *Candida* spp at the level of muco-cutaneous surfaces, so also healthy babies can have fungal oral thrush and diaper rash. The thrush is a typical *Candida* oral infection by the mouths of babies. It is caused generally by *Candida albicans,* and more rarely by *Candida glabrata* or *Candida tropicalis.* The infection can develop suddenly and appears as white plaques on mucosa of oral cave (including palate, tongue). In general, candidal trush does not cause fever and the predisposing factors are antibiotics therapy, corticosteroids (especially if inhaled). This infection can be treated with topical antifungal drugs, such as nystatin, miconazole, Gentian violet or amphotericin B. Gentian violet is a dye with antifungal activity that can be used for breastfeeding thrush, but its use is not recommended in large quantities because it can cause mouth and throat ulcerations in nursing babies.

Yeast diaper rash is a reaction of the skin that can appear around anus, on the thighs, genital creases and the infected area is usually red and elevated. It is estimated that 15-20% of diaper rash are due to yeast and in particular to *C. albicans.*

On the contrary of health babies, in pre-term and in critically ill neonates *Candida* spp is often the cause of life-threatening invasive infections. Generally, the incidence of invasive candidiasis is higher in the paediatric population than adult and with the higher risk in neonates. In critically ill neonates, *Candida* spp is the third most common agent of late-onset infections, with an incidence ranging from 2.6-10% among very low birth weight (1001-1500 g) babies and from 5.5-20% among extremely low birth weight (<1000 g) infants (Benjamin et al., 2006; Chapman et al., 2007; Cotten et al., 2006; Levy et al., 2006). The crude mortality associated with these infections ranges from 15-30% and an attributable mortality of 6-22% despite appropriate therapy (Benjamin et al., 2006; Zautis et al.,2007) but these values can increase to 60% (Castagnola & Buratti, 2009). The high mortality rate can be related to the difficulty in making an early diagnosis. In fact, the reduced sensitivity of diagnostic tests, non-specific clinical signs and inadequate or delayed treatments can condition the outcome of patients (Brecht et al., 2009; Stronati & Decembrino, 2006).

Whereas in paediatric patients the risk factors may differ according to the underlying disease and the consequent specific immunodeficiency, in neonates the primary risk factors are prematurity and colonization. In particular *Candida* colonization, originating from the endogenous flora inhabiting the gastrointestinal tract, is considered a prerequisite for the development of invasive candidiasis. Manzoni et al. (Manzoni, et al., 2006) showed that *Candida* colonization in multiple body sites is an important predictor of progression to invasive mycoses, emphasizing the need of systematic surveillance cultures in the preterm infants. It is important to underline that the preterm infants are commonly infected by *C. albicans* and *C. parapsilosis*, the children aged younger than 1 year are infected most often by *C. parapsilosis*, while in the adolescents the incidence of *C. glabrata* exceeds that of *C. parapsilosis* (Sai et al, 2011). Besides, *C. albicans* and *C. parapsilosis* are by a long time recognized as causative agent of infections related to the intravascular catheters and drains that can be contaminated by the hands of health care workers (Velasco et al. 2011, Weems et al., 1986). The relatedness between the strains isolated from the patients and those isolated from the hands of health care workers, strongly suggests person to person transmission and supports the widely held view that the hands of personnel are the route of transmission of some *Candida* spp, in particular *C. parapsilosis*. Also *Malassetia* spp, a commensal lipophilic yeast that colonizes the human skin can cause systemic infection in premature babies. The transmission of infection is liable to contamination of vascular catheters by the hands of healthcare workers or contamination of intravenous solution (Chang et al., 2006; Oliveri et al., 2011).

Recently Montagna et al. (Montagna et al., 2010) evaluated the epidemiology of invasive fungal infections among infants admitted to Neonatal Intensive Care in southern Italy by the multicenter surveillance "Aurora Project". They observed that overall incidence was 1.3% and crude mortality was 23.8%. Infants weighing 1500 g (4.3%) showed a significantly higher incidence than those 2500 g (0.2%). *C. parapsilosis* (61.9%) was the most frequent isolated species. The outcomes for neonates differ markedly from those in older patients. Even if the mortality is generally lower in neonates, they frequently have serious complications as meningoencephalitis.

The neonatal patients rarely show the infections caused by filamentous fungi, such as *Aspegillus* and *Zygomycetes*, however they can cause skin infection after necrotizing skin lesions and gastrointestinal tract infection after mucositis induced by enterocolitis. The filamentous fungi infections are mainly correlated to contaminated water and ventilation systems (Abdul Salam et al., 2010; Robertson et al., 1997). The neonates admitted to intensive care units may be predisposed to aspergillosis because of their immature phagocytic capacity, the frequent administration of corticosteroids and prolonged hospitalization. In a study carried out by Groll et al. (Groll et al., 1998a) on the cases of aspergillosis documented in babies < 3 months of age, 32% had disseminated aspergillosis, 25% had primary cutaneus aspergillosis and 23% had invasive pulmonary aspergillosis. At least 41% of the patients had received corticosteroid therapy before diagnosis and only one patient had been neutropenic, while the prematurity was the major underlying condition (43%), only 14% had proven chronic granulomatous disease. Among different species of *Aspergillus* responsible for invasive aspergillosis, *A. fumigatus* was the species most frequently recovered in babies, followed by *A. flavus* , *A. terreus* and *A. niger*.

Regarding neonatal zygomycosis, poor data are available. Roileds et al. (Roileds et al., 2009) analyzed the documented cases in literature. The prematurity was a major underlying factor among neonatal cases, the most common manifestations of zygomycosis were gastrointestinal (54%) and cutaneous (36%) and the overall mortality was 64%.

3.1 Children patients

Although healthy children have strong natural immunity against fungal infections, some superficial mycoses such as *Tinea* frequently occur. *Tinea,* caused by dermatophyte fungi such as *Trichophyton, Epydermophyton, Microsporum,* is a skin infection that transmit by direct skin-to-skin contact with an infected person, or by contact with contaminated surface such as floors in shower and locker rooms (Andrews et al., 2008). The infection can involve the body in particular trunk, arms and leg, known as *Tinea corporis*; while *Tinea capitis* is a scalp infection, it is frequent among children of age 3–9 years that live in overcrowded areas; *Tinea pedis* is an infection of foot known as *the athletes' foot,* it is acquired by walking barefoot on contaminated surface (including carpet, floors in shower) (Jain et al., 2010).

In children and adolescents with cancer the most important risk factors for fungal infections are the intravenous catheter, the mucositis induced by chemotherapy, broad spectrum antibiotics, and the therapeutic use of corticosteroids, especially in patients with acute leukaemia. *Candida* spp and *Aspergillus* spp are the most common etiological agents. In the neutropenic children, in particular in children with leukaemia or bone marrow transplantation, the frequency of the invasive candidiasis (candidemia, disseminated candidiasis etc.) is 8-10% with a crude mortality until to 100% in patients with persistent neutropenia or after hematopoietic stem cell transplantation (HSCT) (Castagnola et al. 2008; Finco et al. 2011; Klingspor et al., 1997).

Even if *Candida albicans* is recognized as the most common agent of such infections, other species are progressively increasing, such as *Candida glabrata, Candida parapsilosis, Candida krusei* and *Candida tropicalis*. In many locations in USA, in Asia and Latin America, *C. glabrata,* after *C. albicans,* is the second most frequent species, while in Europe *C. parapsilosis* is the most prevalent. *Candida parapsilosis* is a commensal of human skin and often causes exogenous systemic infection related to i.v. catheter use (Barchiesi et al., 2004; Velasco et al. 2011). *Candida parapsilosis,* as well as *C. albicans,* can form a biofilm on the plastic surface of the catheter so it becomes a continuative source of infection. In this regard the Infectious Diseases Society of America (IDSA) guidelines recommend removing the catheter, if at all possible (Pappas et al., 2009). In general the catheter removal is associated with shorter duration of candidemia and reduced mortality in neonates, adults and neutropenic patients, although the management of intravascular catheters in these subjects with candidemia is more complicated than with others. As it is observed in adult patients, the therapy with corticosteroids is one of the most frequent features that increase the risk of fungal infection in children immunocompromised for solid organ transplantation, engraftment after bone marrow transplantation or for immunological disorders (Fonseca et al., 2006).

Other than *Candida* spp infections, in immunocompromised children *Aspergillus* spp infections are also documented. *Aspergillus* spp can cause invasive, saprophytic or allergic diseases. The saprophytic affliction includes *Aspergillus* spp otomycosis and pulmonary aspergilloma; the allergic conditions include allergic sinusitis and allergic bronchopulmonary aspergillosis (APBA). APBA is a hypersensitivity disease of the lungs associated with inflammatory destruction of airways in response to *Aspergillus* spp. It can increase for clinical stages of asthma managed with corticosteroid for a long time. It can be defined through primary diagnostic criteria (episodic bronchial obstruction, asthma, peripheral eosinophilia, elevated serum IgE concentrations, central bronchiectasis) and secondary diagnostic criteria (repeated detection of *Aspergillus* spp in sputum samples, Arthus reaction -late skin reactivity- to *Aspergillus* antigen) (Walsh et al., 2008). ABPA also affects a significant proportion of cystic fibrosis patients because of prolonged colonization with *Aspergillus* spp, this fact has been associated with accelerated deterioration of lung function.

The invasive aspergillosis (IA) represents an important cause of morbidity and mortality in children with haematological malignancies or those undergoing bone marrow transplantation. In fact its frequency is estimated to be 4.5-10% with crude mortality of 40-94% (Steinback, 2005a). The Antimicrobial Availability Task Force (AATF) of the Infectious Diseases Society of America has identified *Aspergillus* spp among the particularly problematic pathogens for which an early treatment is urgently needed, together with other microorganisms, such as *Acinetobacter baumannii*, ESBL-producing *Enterobacteriaceae*, vancomycin-resistant *Enterococcus faecium* (VRE), *Pseudomonas aeruginosa*, and *methicillin resistant Staphylococcus aureus* (MRSA) (Talbot et al., 2006). IA is typical of neutropenic patients and it is usually absent in children in treatment for solid tumours. The most frequent species are *A. fumigatus*, *A. flavus* and *A. terreus.* The infection occurs by inhalation of conidia, of about 2-5 microns in size, small enough to be inhaled and deposited in the lungs of immunocompromised patients, in particular, of subjects exposed to prolonged and severe neutropenia. To date, it is not yet well defined what is the concentration of conidia that exposes the patient to risk of infection, especially for child patients. The concentration of spores in the air depends on several factors: weather, winds, seasonal factors, type of vegetation. So because of the ubiquitous spread of *Aspergillus* spp, environmental control measures, especially in the presence of construction works, are necessary to prevent infections in hospitals. In this regard, to avoid these fungal infections, some prevention measures are needed, such as:

- high efficiency filters (High-Efficiency Particulate Air: HEPA) (Cornet et al., 1999);
- horizontal laminar flow systems (Laminar Air Flow: LAF) (Barnes & Rogers, 1989), although the protection conferred by the LAF systems is still debated;
- hospital rooms with positive pressure (Humphreys, 2004).

In according to the European Organization for Research and Treatment of Cancer/Mycoses Study Group (EORTC/MSG) (De Paw et al, 2008) the diagnosis of invasive fungal infection can be classified as proven, probable and possible. It is considered *proven* when a histopathological documentation of infection and a positive result of culture of a specimen from a normally sterile site are available. It is defined *probable* when there are existing host factors, clinical manifestations (symptoms, signs and radiological features) and microbiological evidence; it is defined *possible* when there are only existing host factors and clinical manifestations. Early initiation of antifungal therapy in patients with strongly suspected invasive aspergillosis is required while a diagnostic evaluation is conducted (Cornely et al., 2007; Greene et al., 2007). With regard to aspergillosis, in addition to children with haematological malignancy, children with primary immunodeficiency, chronic granulomatous disease and cystic fibrosis, are at high risk of IA (Steinbach, 2005a).

4. Laboratory diagnosis of fungal infection

One of the most difficult challenges of medical mycology is still the early initiation of an effective antifungal therapy to improve the outcome of patients, especially if affected by deep mycoses, but this fact is strongly related to a fast and proper etiological diagnosis.

Despite the scientific progress and newer available diagnostic tools, the fungal infection diagnosis is still complex. Actually, the microscopic and cultural investigations remain the gold standard of mycological diagnosis, even if it is difficult to obtain appropriate specimens, the cultures have long duration and often the results are negative. In fact, in neonates with candidemia, the blood cultures have difficulty in providing positive results because only a small quantity of blood can be taken. Besides, blood cultures result positive for *Candida* spp only in 24-60% of cases and the fungal strains grow slowly (Connell et al., 2007; Montagna et al., 2009), this fact is incompatible with an early diagnosis.

Besides the serological assays results are difficult to interpret because, for example, the circulating antibodies to *Candida* spp may occur in healthy subjects for the colonization of mucosal surfaces and their production in the immunocompromised patients can vary according to immune status (Ellepola & Morrison, 2005).

Although, in neonatal patients the detection of mannan antigen, it is an antigen of membrane of *Candida* spp can show a sensitivity and specificity of 94.4% and 94.2% respectively, repetitive sampling is required because of the transient nature of mannan antigen. Besides, the literature data report a very low sensitivity of the *Candida* antigen test in patients with *C. parapsilosis* infection (Oliveri et al., 2008; Montagna et al., 2011a). In recent years, other important serum markers have been studied, such as the 1→3-β-D-glucan (BDG), so it has been included among the relevant diagnostic criteria by the European Organization for Research and Treatment of Cancer/Mycoses Study Group (EORTC/MSG) (De Pauw et al., 2008). BDG is a component of the cell wall of a wide variety of fungi except for *zigomycetes* and *Cryptococcus* spp (Mancini et al., 2010; Odabasi et al., 2006). This test has been studied in adult patients, while in paediatric population only a few reports in particular describe the clinical relevance of BDG in preterm infants or onco-haematological paediatrics, yet this test seems to be very promising especially for the diagnosis of invasive candidiasis (Mularoni et al., 2010). However, it is important to consider that glucan is ubiquitous in the environment, so some medical sources of BDG can lead to a false positive result in the absence of deep mycoses: dialysis membranes and filters made from cellulose, cotton gauze employed during surgery, specific fractionated blood products, such as serum albumin and immunoglobulins, are reported to contain BDG, as well as exposure to some antitumor polysaccharides and certain parenteral antimicrobials (Chandrasekar, 2010; Marty et al., 2006). Montagna et al. (Montagna et al., 2011a) evaluated the performance of the BDG, individually and in comparison with the *Candida* mannan antigen, in preterm infants and onco-haematological paediatric patients with *Candida* BSI already proven by positive culture. The serum levels of BDG resulted positive on the same day as one positive blood culture in all examined patients, while *Candida* mannan antigen was negative in a child with *C. albicans* BSI and in all patients with *C. parapsilosis* fungemia.

Generally, in adults patients, the diagnosis of invasive pulmonary aspergillosis avails of radiology and galactomannan assay, on the contrary in the paediatric population the subjects with invasive pulmonary aspergillosis do not exhibit a "halo" sign and the galactomannan test specificity and sensitivity are very low. Galactomannan is a polysaccharide found within the cell wall of *Aspergillus* spp. It is released into the extracellular fluids (serum, urine, bronchoalveolar lavage, cerebrospinal fluid and other specimens) during hyphal growth and cell wall turnover. The detection of galactomannan in serum have been approved by the US Food and Drug Administration and have been included in the consensus criteria for diagnosis of invasive fungal infections (De Pauw et al., 2008). In a study, overall positive predictive value of galactomannan was calculated to be 92.1% for adult HSCT recipients and 15.4% for children (Herbrecht et al., 2002). The specificity of this test may be compromised during therapy with some antibiotics, such as piperacillin-tazobactam, amoxicillin or amoxicillin with clavulanic acid, because these drugs contain the galactomannan so lead to false positive results. Besides, often the neonates are colonized in the intestinal tract by *Bifidobacterium bifidum* that may interfere with the galactomannan test and load the false-positive test, as well as the food or water containing galactomannan (Mennink-Kersten et al., 2004).

The table 3 shows the advantage and disadvantage of major diagnostic methods.

METHODS	ADVANTAGES	DISADVANTAGES
Cultural investigations	Golden standard Accurate Specific	Fungi strains grow slowly Needs of invasive techniques to obtain appropriate specimen Results may be falsely negative
Galactomannan test	High specificity Non-invasive	Possible false-positives/ Possible false-negatives
1→3-β-D-glucan test	Non-invasive High negative-predictive value for most fungi	Possible false-positives
Candida mannan antigen	Non-invasive Sensitivity Specificity	Transient nature Very low sensitivity in C. parapsilosis infection Possible false-positives
Polymerase chain reaction	Identification genus / species High specificity	Not standardized Not commercially available

Table 3. Advantages and disadvantages of major diagnostic methods.

Another possible marker of invasive fungal infections is the Procalcitonin (PCT), a 116-amino acid protein synthesized in the C cells of the thyroid gland. It is virtually undetectable in healthy subjects (<0.5 ng/mL), but its concentration may increase up to 1000 ng/mL in patients with systemic bacterial infections or septic shock. Some authors have considered the PCT value as a potential biological marker of fungal sepsis (Christofilopoulou et al., 2002; Charles et al., 2009; Martini et al., 2010), but to date its role in diagnosis of these diseases has not yet been elucidated. In particular, the newborns may exhibit elevated PCT levels because of a physiological increase in the first days of life perhaps caused by birth trauma or host response to the initial establishment of the normal intestinal bacterial flora, but 3–4 days after birth the PCT levels revert to normal (Montagna, et al. 2011b; Turner et al., 2006).

Several molecular methods have also been described for the diagnosis of opportunistic mycoses. However, they have not been standardized and have only been used in experimental cases, in the study of phylogenesis or for epidemiological purposes to investigate an epidemic cluster (Wise et al., 2007). The low application of this method in routine investigations can be explained with the very high sensibility of PCR methods (up to 10 fg of nucleic acid, equivalent to 1-10 cells), so it is difficult to distinguish the fungal colonization or contamination from the real infection.

5. Antifungal therapy

Whilst several antibiotics are available, the number of antifungal drugs is relatively low. The slow progress in discovering new drugs could be elucidated by the fact that fungi are eukaryotic cells like mammalian cells, so the antifungal agents that have as target the biosynthesis of protein, RNA or DNA, result in being toxic for humans, especially at the level of liver and kidney. Nevertheless, over recent decades the number of antifungal agents has increased and new molecules with new mechanisms of action have been discovered, such as Echinocandins that act on the cell wall of the fungi. Although, today we have several therapeutic options, the treatment of deep mycoses in the paediatric population is still limited (Steinbach, 2005b; Zautis, 2010).

To date four major categories of antifungal agents are available in clinical use: Polyenes, Azoles, Fluoro-pyrimidines and Echinocandins. Some of these molecules have existed for a long time; others have been introduced into clinical practice only recently (i.e. caspofungin , posaconazole or voriconazole) (Table 4).

The Polyenes are fungicidal drugs with a broad spectrum of activity against the most common yeasts and moulds, even if *Aspergillus terreus, Aspergillus versicolor, Aspergillus lentulus,* some strains of *Aspergillus flavus, Scedosporium* spp and *C. lusitaniae* result in being resistant. These drugs integrate with ergosterol of membranes and form the channels trans-membrane that, increasing the permeability, cause leakage of cytoplasmic contents and cell death. This class includes Nystatin and Amphotericin B (AmB).

Nystatin is used to treat cutaneous, vaginal, mucosal infections caused by *Candida* spp and it may be given orally as well as applied topically. In the UK its licence for treating neonatal oral thrush is restricted to those over the age of one month.

Amphotericin B is available other than in deoxycholate formulation (D-AmB), in three lipid formulations (LFAmBs) approved for use in humans: AmB lipid complex (ABLC), colloidal dispersion (ABCD), and in liposome (L-AmB). The lipid formulations are licensed for patients with invasive mycoses refractory or intolerant of D-AmB, in fact the infusion related reactions and nephrotoxicity often limit therapy with D-AmB. However, D-AmB at dosage of 1 mg/kg daily is recommended for neonates with disseminated candidiasis. If the urinary tract is not involved, L-AmB can be used at the dosage of 3–5 mg/kg daily. Even if not actually licensed, LFAmBs are frequently used as the first-line therapy for treatment of invasive aspergillosis, invasive candidiasis and zygomicosis (Cornely et al., 2007; Kuse et al., 2007).

CLASS AND COMPOUND	MECHANISM OF ACTION	CLINICAL USE
POLYENES	Integrate with ergosterol of membrane and form the channels trans-membrane causing leakage of cytoplasmic contents and cell death	
Amphotericin B		Invasive aspergillosis, invasive candidiasis and zygomycosis
Nystatin		Nongenital muco-cutaneous candidiasis, oro-pharyngeal candidiasis. In the UK the licence for treating neonatal oral thrush is restricted to those over the age of one month.
AZOLES	Interact with cytochrome P-450, during the biosynthesis of ergosterol at the step of synthesis by lanosterol to ergosterol, causing ergosterol depletion and accumulation of sterols in the membrane	
Econazole		inea, pityriasis versicolor
Ketoconazole		Superficial infections such as athlete's foot, ringworm, candidiasis
Fluconazole		Secondary treatment of invasive candidiasis; prophylaxis in neonates whose birth weight is <1000g.
Itraconazole		Invasive aspergillosis in patients who are refractory to standard therapy and in patients with ABPA
Miconazole		Superficial infections (athlete's foot, ringworm), oral or vaginal thrush, lip disorder angular cheilitis. It is used in treatment of neonatal oral thrush. It is an alternative to nystatin for babies of age under one month.

CLASS AND COMPOUND	MECHANISM OF ACTION	CLINICAL USE
Posaconazole		Recommended for prevention of invasive aspergillosis in neutropenic patients with haematological disease; active also against Zygomycetes
....Voriconazole		Primary treatment of invasive aspergillosis; prevention of invasive aspergillosis in neutropenic patients
FLUORO-PYRIMIDINES	Inhibits the biosynthesis of both RNA and DNA	
5-Flucytosine		Rarely administered as a single drug, usually given in combination with AmB for patients with invasive diseases, such as *Candida* endocarditis or meningitis.
ECHINOCANDINS	Inhibit beta 1, 3 D-glucan, block the formation of cell wall of fungi	
Anidulafungin		In neonatal candidiasis should be used with caution and limited to situations in which resistance or toxicity precludes the use of Fluconazole or AmB
Caspofungin		In neonatal candidiasis should be used with caution and limited to situations in which resistance or toxicity precludes the use of Fluconazole or AmB
Micafungina		Approved as first-line therapy against invasive and oropharyngeal candidiasis in the newborn and older children

Table 4. Mechanisms of action of some antifungal agents and their utility in clinical practice.

The Azoles have fungistatic activity and take effect against major yeasts and filamentous fungi. They inhibit the enzymes necessary to convert lanosterol to ergosterol, causing ergosterol depletion and accumulation of sterols in the membrane. The disruption of the structure and many functions of membrane lead to inhibition of fungal growth.

This class includes a major number of molecules. Some drugs are used for the treatment of superficial and cutaneous infections such as Miconazole that is mainly used externally for the treatment of superficial infections (athlete's foot, ringworm) and for treatment of oral or vaginal thrush, for the lip disorder angular cheilitis. It is used in treatment of neonatal oral thrush and it can be an alternative to nystatin for babies of age under one month.

Econazole is used to treat skin tinea, pityriasis versicolor; ketoconazole is usually prescribed for topical infections such as athlete's foot, ringworm, candidiasis.

The azoles principally used in invasive mycoses are Fluconazole, Itraconazole, Posaconazole and Voriconazole.

Fluconazole is rapidly cleared in children, so the daily dose is doubled from 6 to 12 mg/kg for children of all age and neonates. Fluconazole can be used for Neonatal Candidiasis as an alternative to treatment with AmB, besides prophylaxis with Fluconazole may be considered in neonates whose birth weight is <1000 g (Manzoni et al., 2011).

Itraconazole is used for treatment of invasive aspergillosis in patients who are refractory to standard therapy. In combination with corticosteroids, it is recommended for the treatment of allergic bronchopulmonary aspergillosis while there are few data that examine the use of Itraconazole in the treatment of invasive candidiasis.

Posaconazole is recommended for prevention of invasive aspergillosis in neutropenic patients with haematological disease and is active also against zygomycetes. Posaconazole is not indicated for paediatric age.

Voriconazole is approved by FDA for the primary treatment of invasive aspergillosis, and has also been proven effective against *Fusarium* spp and *Scedosporium apiospermum*, it is the first and only drug ever specifically indicated for their treatment by the FDA. Voriconazole is licensed for children over 2 years old.

The class of Fluoro-pyrimidines only represents the 5-Fluoro cytosine, a molecule that inhibits the biosynthesis of both RNA and DNA. Very low birth weight neonates may accumulate high plasma concentrations because of poor renal function due to immaturity, thus, the use of flucytosine needs careful monitoring of serum drug levels in this group of patients. The role of flucytosine in neonates with *Candida* meningitis is questionable and is not routinely recommended (Benjamin et al., 2006). Besides, rapidly the strains can develop resistance to flucytosine, so it is rarely administered as a single agent, but usually in combination with AmB for patients with invasive diseases.

The Echinocandins are the newer antifungal drugs. 1,3 beta-D-glucan and block the formation of the cell wall of the fungi, but some strains such as *Candida guilliermondii* and *Candida parapsilosis, Zygomycetes, Cryptococcus, Trichosporon, Fusarium* and *Scedosporium* are intrinsically less sensitive or even resistant. This class includes Anidulafungin, Caspofungin and Micafungin, they are available only as parenteral preparations. Echinocandins should be used with caution in treatment of neonatal candidiasis and generally limited to situations in which resistance or toxicity precludes the use of Fluconazole or AmB. Micafungin is the only drug that has been authorized for by the EMA (European Medicines Agency) (Manzoni et al, 2011) and approved as first-line therapy against invasive and oropharyngeal candidiasis in the newborn and older children, it has recently been introduced into clinical onco-haematology Practice (Mikulska & Viscoli, 2011).

To date the resistance to the antifungal agents most commonly used in clinical practice is relatively rare, nevertheless the frequent use of antifungal drugs as prophylactic in long-term treatments or empiric and pre-emptive therapy, might select resistant strains. In general the opportunistic fungi have variable susceptibilities to currently available antifungal drugs. For example *Candida krusei* is intrinsically resistant to Fluconazole, *Candida glabrata* is less susceptible than other *Candida* species, *Candida lusitaniae* and *Aspergillus terreus* are resistant to AmB, thus the need for prompt identification at level of genera and species and *in vitro* susceptibility testing is more and more pressing.

The Clinical and Laboratory Standards Institute (Clinical and Laboratory Standards Institute, 2008a, Clinical and Laboratory Standards Institute, 2008b) has developed a reference microdilution broth method for antifungal susceptibility testing of yeasts and moulds, but it is not easy for routinely use in the clinical laboratory. Alternatively, more simplified and efficient approaches also have been developed such as YeastOne Colorimetric Antifungal plate and E-test. At regarding, it is important to underline that antifungal susceptibility testing have some limitations as an imperfect clinical correlation, so the drug susceptibility *in vitro* does not guarantee clinical success or failure.

In every case, the proper antifungal treatment and the patient's outcome depend on an accurate identification of the aetiological agent at the level of genera and species. In fact, although in recent years some fungal strains have become resistant to common drugs, generally the susceptibility of fungi to the currently available antifungal agents is predictable if the species of the infecting isolate is known (Pappas et al., 2009). However, to know the susceptibility *in vitro* and the local epidemiology of drug resistance can help the clinicians to choose the most appropriate therapy and therefore to guide the management of fungal infection.

6. Conclusion

Despite recent advances in diagnostic field and the current armamentarium of antifungal agents with widespread use of prophylaxis in high-risk groups, the mycoses (especially the deep mycoses) are yet a persistent public health problem of difficult management particularly in pediatric age. In these patients the epidemiology of fungal infections is complex and different in various ages, for example: in the children the risk factors may differ according to the specific pathology of the base and the consequent specific immunodeficiency while in neonates the primary risk factors are prematurity and colonization; some drugs are licensed only for children of age > 2 years etc.

To date these fungal infections have been well studied in different populations of adult patients while a thorough analyses of predisposing factors, diagnostic methods and therapeutic options in pediatric age have not been well described. Infact, several studies have been carried out to know the fungal infections and improve the patients' outcome, but most of them have exclude the pediatirc population. This fact has limited the knowledge of the epidemiology and management of pediatric fungal disease, so we often extrapolate from adult data, information for children and neonates. Therefore, diagnostic tests standardized for adult patients or antifungal therapies licensed for adults are often used improperly in pediatric age .The future hope of medical science is to have new tools to improve the immune system of immunocompromised patients to control the opportunistic infections. Besides, the most difficult challenge of medical mycology is still the early initiation of an effective antifungal therapy to improve the patient's outcome, so it is essential to have a fast and proper aetiological diagnosis. In addition, because studies among the paediatric populations affected by fungal infections are few, it would be important in the future that clinical and laboratory investigations are focused in tandem on fungal infections in pediatric age to have an optimal diagnoses and appropriate antifungal treatment.

7. References

Abdul Salam, Z.H.; Karlin, R.B.; Ling, M.L. et al. (2010) The impact of portable high-efficiency particulate air filters on the incidence of invasive aspergillosis in a large acute tertiary-care hospital. *Am J Infect Control,* 38(4): 1-7

Andrews MD, Burns M. (2008). Common tinea infections in children. Am Fam Physician. 77(10):1415-1420.

Benjamin, D.K. Jr; Stoll, B.J.; Fanaroff, A.A., et al. (2006). Neonatal candidiasis among extremely low birth weight infants: risk factors, mortality rates, and developmental outcomes at 18 to 22 months. *Pediatrics,* 117: 84-92.

Barchiesi, F.; Caggiano, G.; Falconi Di Francesco, L., et al. (2004) Outbreak of fungemia due to Candida parapsilosis in a pediatric oncology unit. *Diagn Microbiol Infect Dis,* 49(4):269-271.

Barnes, R.A.; Rogers, T.R. (1989) Control of an outbreak of nosocomial aspergillosis by laminar air-flow isolation. *J Hosp Infect,* 14: 89-94

Brecht, M.; Clerihew, L.; McGuire, W. (2009). Prevention and treatment of invasive fungal infection in very low birth weight infants. *Arch Dis Child Fetal Neonatal Ed,* 94: 65-69.

Castagnola, E.; Buratti, S. (2009). Clinical aspects of invasive candidiasis in paediatric patients. *Drugs,* 69(1):45-50.

Castagnola, E.; Faraci, M.; Moroni C et al. (2008). Invasive mycoses in children receiving hemopoietic SCT. Bone Marrow Transplant, 41 Suppl 2:107-111.

Castagnola E, Franceschi A, Natalizia AR, et al. (2007). Combined antifungal therapy for persistent central venous catheter-related candidemia in extremely low birth weight neonates. J Chemother 21:234-235.

Chandrasekar, P. (2010). Diagnostic challenges and recent advances in the early management of invasive fungal infection. *Eur. J. Haemat,* 84, 281-290.

Chang, H.J.; Miller, H.L.; Watkins, N.; et al. (1998). An epidemic of Malassezia pachydermatis in an intensive care nursery associated with colonization of health care workers' pet dogs. *N Engl J Med,* 338:706-711

Chapman, R.L. (2007). Prevention and treatment of Candida infections in neonates. *Semin Perinatol,* 31:39-46.

Charles, P.E.; Castro, C.; Ruiz-Santana, S.; et al. (2009). Serum procalcitonin levels in critically ill patients colonized with Candida spp: new clues for the early recognition of invasive candidiasis? Intensive CareMed, 35: 2146-2150.

Chiou, C.C.; Wong, T.T.; Lin, H.H.; et al. (1994). Fungal infection of ventriculoperitoneal shunts in children. *Clin Infect Dis,* 19: 1049-1053

Christofilopoulou, S.; Charvalos, E.; Petrikkos, G. (2002). Could procalcitonin be a predictive biological marker in systemic fungal infections? Study of 14 cases. Eur J Intern Med, 13(8): 493-495.

Clinical and Laboratory Standards Institute. (2008). Reference method for broth dilution antifungal susceptibility testing of yeast. Approved standard M27-A3, 3rd ed. Clinical and Laboratory Standards Institute, Wayne, PA.

Clinical and Laboratory Standard Institute. Reference method for broth dilution antifungal susceptibility testing of filamentous fungi; Approved standard—2nd edn. CLSI Document M38-A2. Wayne, PA. Clinical and Laboratory Standard Institute, 2008

Connell, T.G.; Rele, M.; Cowley, D.; et al. (2007). How reliable is a negative blood culture result? Volume of blood submitted for culture in routine practice in a children's hospital. *Paediatrics*, 119 (5): 891-896.

Cornely, O.A.; Maertens, J.; Bresnik, M.; et al. &; AmBiLoad Trial Study Group. (2007) Liposomal amphotericin B as initial therapy for invasive mold infection: a randomized trial comparing a high-loading dose regimen with standard dosing (AmBiLoad trial). *Clin Infect Dis*, 44: 1289–1297.

Cotton, C.M.; McDonald, S.; Stoll, B.; et al. (2006). National Institute for Child Health and Human Development Neonatal Research Network. The association of third-generation cephalosporin use and invasive candidiasis in extremely low birth-weight infants. *Pediatrics*, 118: 717-722.

Cornet, M.; Levy, V; Fleury, L.; et al. (1999). Efficacy of prevention by high-efficiency particulate air filtration or laminar airflow against Aspergillus airborne contamination during hospital renovation. *Infect Control Hosp Epidemiol*, 20: 508-513

De Pauw, B.; Walsh, T.J.; Donnelly, J.P.; et al. (2008). Revised definitions of invasive fungal disease from the European Organization for Research and Treatment of Cancer/Invasive Fungal Infections Cooperative Group and the National Institute of Allergy and Infectious Diseases Mycoses Study Group (EORTC/MSG) Consensus Group. *Clin. Infect. Dis.*, 46, 1813–1821.

Ellepola, A.N.; Morrison, C.J. (2005). Laboratory diagnosis of invasive candidiasis. *J. Microbiol.*, 43, 65-84.

Finco G, Sanna D, Evangelista M, Mura P, Musu M. (2011) Fungal infections in pediatric intensive care units. J Matern Fetal Neonatal Med. 24 Suppl 2:21-3.

Fonseca-Aten, M.; Michaels, M.G. (2006). Infections in pediatric solid organ transplant recipients. *Semin Pediatr Surg*, 15:153-161

Groll, A. H.; Jaeger, G.; Allendorf, A.; et al. (1998). Invasive Pulmonary Aspergillosis in a Critically Ill Neonate: Case Report and Review of Invasive Aspergillosis During the First 3 Months of Life. *Clin. Infect. Dis.*, 27:437–452

Greene, R.E.; Schlamm, H.T.; Oestmann, J.W. et al. (2007) Imaging findings in acute invasive pulmonary aspergillosis: clinical significance of the halo sign. *Clin Infect Dis*, 44:373–9.

Humphreys, H. (2004). Positive pressure isolation and the prevention of invasive asprgillosis. What is the evidence? *J Hosp Infect*, 56: 93-100

Herbrecht, R.; Letscher-Bru, V.; Oprea, C. et al. (2002). *Aspergillus* galattomannan detection in the diagnosis of invasive aspergillosis in cancer patients. *J Clin Oncol*, 20: 1898-1906

Jain A, Jain S, and Rawat S. (2010) Emerging fungal infections among children: A review on its clinical manifestations, diagnosis, and prevention .J Pharm Bioallied Sci. 2(4): 314–320.

Kaufman, D.; Fairchild, K.D. (2004). Clinical microbiology of bacterial and fungal sepsis in very-low-birth-weight infants. *Clin Microbiol Rev*, 17:638-680.

Kern, M.E.; Blevins K.S. (1997). *Medical Mycology: A self-Instructional Text*. 1th edn. Philadelphia, PA: FA Davis Co;

Klingspor, L.; Stintzing, G.; Tollemar, J. (1997). Deep Candida infection in children with leukemia: clinical presentations, diagnosis and outcome. *Acta Paediatr*, 86:30-36.

Kuse, E.R.; Chetchotisakd, P.; da Cunha, C.A.; et al. & Micafungin Invasive Candidiasis Working Group (2007). *Lancet*, 369(9572):1519-1527.

Lehrnbecher, T.; Frank, C.; Engels, K.; et al. (2010). Trends in the postmortem epidemiology of invasive infections at a university hospital. *J. Infect.*, 61(3), 259-265

Levy, I.; Shalit, I.; Askenazi, S. et al. (2006). Duration and outcome of persistent candidaemia in newborn infants. *Mycoses*, 49:197-201.

Malani, P.N.; Brandley, S.F.; Little, R.S.; et al. (2001).Trends in species causing fungaemia in a tertiary care medical centre over 12 years. *Mycoses*, 44: 446-449

Mancini, N.; Carletti, S.; Ghidoli, N.; et al. (2010). The era of molecular and other non-culture-based methods in diagnosis of sepsis. *Clin. Microbiol. Rev.*, 23: 235-251.

Manzoni, P.; Farina, D.; Leonessa, M., et al. (2006) Risk factors for progression to invasive fungal infection in preterm neonates with fungal colonization. *Pediatrics*; 118: 2359-2364

Manzoni P, Benjamin DK, Hope W, Rizzollo S, Del Sordo P, Stronati M, Jacqz-Aigrain E, Castagnola E, Farina D. (2011). The management of Candida infections in preterm neonates and the role of micafungin. J Matern Fetal Neonatal Med.; 24 Suppl 2:24-27

Marty, F.M.; Lowry, C.M.; Lempitski, S.J.; et al. (2006). Reactivity of (1,3)-beta-d-glucan assay with commonly used intravenous antimicrobials. *Antimicrob. Agents Chemother.*, 50: 3450-3453.

Martini, A.; Gottin, L.; Menestrina N. (2010). Procalcitonin levels in surgical patients at risk of candidemia. *J Infect.*, 60(6): 425-430.

Mennink-Kersten, M.; Klont, R.R.; Warris, A. et al. (2004). *Bifidobacterium lipoteichoic* acid and false ELISA reactivity in *Aspergillus* antigen detection. *Lancet*, 363: 325-327.

Mikulska M, Viscoli C. (2011). Current role of echinocandins in the management of invasive aspergillosis. *Curr Infect Dis Rep*, 13(6):517-527

Montagna, M.T.; Caggiano, G.; Borghi, E.; et al. (2009). The Role of the Laboratory in the Diagnosis of Invasive Candidiasis. *Drugs*, 69 (1): 59-63

Montagna, M.T.; Lovero G.; De Giglio O.; et al. and "Aurora Project Group" (2010). Invasive fungal infections in Neonatal Intensive Care Units of Southern Italy: a multicentre regional active surveillance (AURORA Project). *J Prev Med Hyg.* 51: 125-130

Montagna, M.T.; Coretti, C.; Lovero, G. et al (2011) Diagnostic Performance of 1,3-beta-D-Glucan in Neonatal and Paediatric Patients with Candidemia. *Int. J. Mol. Sci.*, 12 (9): 5871-5878

Montagna, M.T.; Coretti, C.; Caggiano, G. (2011) Procalcitonin: a possible marker of invasive fungal infection in high risk patients? *J Prev Med Hyg.* 52(1): 38-39.

Mularoni, A.; Furfaro, E.; Faraci, M.; et al. (2010). High Levels of beta-D-glucan in immunocompromised children with proven invasive fungal disease. *Clin. Vaccine Immunol.*, 17: 882-883.

Oliveri, S.; Trovato, L.; Betta, P.; et al. (2008). Experience with the Platelia Candida ELISA for the diagnosis of invasive candidosis in neonatal patients. *Clin. Microbiol. Infect*,14: 391-393

Oliveri, S., Trovato, L., Betta, P., et al. (2011). Malassezia furfur fungaemia in a neonatal patient detected by lysis-centrifugation blood culture method: first case reported in Italy. *Mycoses*, 54, 638-640

Odabasi, Z.; Paetznick, V.L.; Rodriguez, J.R.; Chen, E.; et al. (2006). Differences in beta-glucan levels in culture supernatants of a variety of fungi. *Med. Mycol.*, 44, 267-272.

Robertson, A.F.; Joshi, V.V.; Ellison, D. et al. (1997). Zygomycoses in neonates. *Pediatr Infect Dis J.*, 21 16: 812-815

Pappas, P.G.; Kauffman, C.A.; Andes D.; et al. (2009). Clinical Practice Guidelines for the Management of Candidiasis: 2009. Update by the Infectious Diseases Society of America. *Clin Infect Dis,* 48: 503-535

Roilides, E.; Zaoutis, T.E.; Walsh, T.J. (2009). Invasive zygomycosis in neonates and children. *Clin Microbiol Infect.,* 15 (5):50-54.

Sai, S.; Holland, L.M.; McGee, C.F., et al. (2011). Evolution of mating within the *Candida parapsilosis* species group. *Eukaryot Cell.* 10(4):578-587.

Steinbach, W.J. (2005). Pediatric aspergillosis: disease and treatment differences in children. *Pediatr. Infect. Dis. J.,* 24(4), 358-364.

Steinbach, W.J. (2005). Antifungal agents in children. *Pediatr Clin North Am,* 52: 895–915

Stronati, M.; Decembrino, L. (2006). Neonatal invasive candidiasis. *Minerva Pediatr,* 58: 537-549.

Talbot, G.H.; Bradley, J., Edwards, J.E. Jr, et al. (2006). Antimicrobial Availability Task Force of the Infectious Diseases Society of America. Bad bugs need drugs: an update on the development pipeline from the Antimicrobial Availability Task Force of the Infectious Diseases Society of America. *Clin Infect Dis.,* 42(5): 657-668.

Turner, D.; Hammerman, C.; Rudensky, B.; et al. (2006). The role of procalcitonin as a predictor of nosocomial sepsis in preterm infants. *Acta Paediatr.,* 95(12): 1571-1576.

Velasco, E., Portugal, R.D. (2011). Factors prompting early central venous catheter removal from cancer patients with candidaemia. *Scand J Infect Dis.* 43(1): 27-31.

Weems, J.J. Jr; Chamberland, M.E.; Waerd, J.; et al. (1987). *Candida parapsilosis* fungemia associated with parenteral nutrition and contaminated blood pressure transducers. *J Clin Microbiol,* 25: 1029-1032.

Wise, M.G.; Healy, M.; Reece, K.; et al. (2007). Species identification and strain differentiation of clinical Candida isolates using the Diversi Lab system of automated repetitive sequence based PCR. *J Med Microbiol,* 56: 778-787.

Walsh, T.J.; Anaissie, J.E.; Denning, D.W., et al. Guidelines of the Infectious Diseases Society of America . *Clin Infect Dis,* 46, 327-370.

Zaoutis T. Candidemia in children. (2010) *Curr Med Res Opin.* 26(7):1761-8.

Zaoutis, T.E; Walsh, T.J. (2007). Antifungal therapy for neonatal candidiasis. *Curr Opin. Infect. Dis.* 20 (6), 592-597.

17

Infantile Chronic Recurrent Parotitis (ICRP): Analysis of Changes in the Expression of Parotid Salivary Proteins Associated with the Disease

Irene Morales-Bozo, Blanca Urzúa Orellana and Mirtha Landaeta Mendoza
University of Chile, Faculty of Dentistry and San Juan de Dios Hospital, Chile

1. Introduction

Infantile chronic recurrent parotitis (ICRP) affects life quality from early childhood to adolescence.

ICRP is an inflammatory disease usually associated to a non-obstructive sialectasis of parotid glands. It is characterized by recurrent episodes of inflammatory volume increase of one or both glands. Occasionally, the episode is accompanied by fever and with the patient feeling unwell. During alternate interepisode periods of normality, lasting from weeks to months, the glands are clinically asymptomatic (Baurmash, 2004; Chitre & Premchandra, 1997). The first episode occurs at ages between 3-months and 13-years old. More frequently, however, the disease appears between 2 and 6 years-old. The number of recurrences varies from one subject to another but an episode every 3 to 4 months is a representative frequency. The highest occurrence frequency is at the first year of school. Then the frequency decays and follows an unpredictable pattern that varies from patient to patient until adolescence. The episodes are manifested by a varying degree of general ill-feeling with moderate fever. Sometimes, this ill condition may oblige to hospitalize the patient for as long as a week (Landaeta et al., 2003). The episodes of gland swelling are associated with upper respiratory conditions, such as a cold, amigdalitis, pneumonia and bronchitis (Landaeta et al., 2003; Vinagre et al., 2003). The incidence rate by sex appears to be identical. Frequently, ICRP occurs unilaterally and among bilateral patients one of the glands is more affected. The increase in parotid volume is quite painful and marked skin redness occurs in the corresponding area. Salivary flow in the affected gland decreases significantly and the corresponding salivary secretion becomes viscous, whitish and mucopurulent (Baurmash, 2004; Chitre & Premchandra, 1997; Vinagre et al., 2003). The inflammatory increase in gland volume may last for 24-hours, 1-2 weeks or, sometimes, several months. After an apparent regression to normality, the gland becomes quiescent until a new inflammatory episode. After puberty symptoms diminish and may fully disappear spontaneously although sometimes the disease may last until adulthood (Baurmash, 2004; Chitre & Premchandra, 1997; Vinagre et al., 2003; Concheiro et al., 2000).

2. The etiology of ICRP is unknown

Several causing factors have been invoked, namely, congenital duct malformations, genetic factors, allergies, local manifestations of autoimmune diseases, immunodeficiencies, maxillary disfunction due to tooth misalignment, etc. (Baurmash, 2004; Chitre & Premchandra, 1997; Bernkopf et al., 2008). None of these factors has been unequivocally demonstrated as a causing agent and to date the etiopathogenesis of the disease remains an enigma. In attempts to elucidate the origin of this clinical condition, a number of microbiological analyses of parotid secretion have been carried out. By direct analysis of parotid saliva from ICRP patients, parotitis virus and several respiratory virus have been discarded as eventual causing agents (Landaeta et al., 2003). Bacteriological analyses by Concheiro et al. (2000) have shown the presence of a mixed flora of Gram-positive cocci. Giglo et al. (1997) have shown that 80% of patients display *Streptococcus pneumoniae, Haemophilus influenzae, Streptococcus viridans* y/o *Moraxella catarrhalis*. Despite the relevance of these insights into the disease, several characteristics of the disease challenge its infectious origin. Among them we can remark that the glandular process is mainly of inflammatory nature, that the general health condition of the patient is just moderately affected, the unilateralness of the condition among patients carrying the above-mentioned flora and, finally, the occurrence of a number of cases in which cultures for bacterial microorganisms give negative results. In the specialized literature expressions like "At the present there is a tendency to consider a multifactorial origin of the disease" have become quite usual. According to this undemonstrated view, sialectasis would be the ICRP-triggering factor. Thus, due to partial malformations of the duct system, iterated ascending infections would result in symptomatic episodes and reinforced the duct alterations (Baurmash, 2004; Chitre & Premchandra, 1997; Rostion et al., 2004; Nahlieli et al., 2004; Nazar et al., 2001). In our view, much more data are still necessary to put forward a consistent hypothesis on the origin of this disease.

3. Sialography and ultrasonography confirm diagnosis of ICRP and allow assessing the degree of glandular involvement

Diagnosis of ICRP is based on the clinical history and is confirmed by both complementary imaging procedures. Sialography demands the introduction of iodinated contrast media via the Stenon's duct in order to opacify the gland ducts and put in evidence the duct dilatations as a typical radiographic flowering pump appearance (Fig. 1). According to images of glandular filling, sialectasis may be punctate, globular, cavitary, destructive or combinations between them (Chitre & Premchandra, 1997; Ramírez et al., 1996). These images would be a reflection of the inflammatory condition affecting the glandular tissue. Histopathological analysis of glandular tissue dissected from ICRP patients shows lymphocyte infiltration tending to organize lymphoid follicles around dilated interlobular ducts (sialectasia) (Chitre & Premchandra, 1997; Nahlieli et al., 2004; Shimizu et al., 1998). Besides confirming diagnosis, sialography is also useful to assess the progression of the gland condition. Thus, sialographic changes tend to decrease or even disappear when the disease becomes inactive, either at puberty or after a successful medical treatment (Chitre & Premchandra, 1997). Thus, Landaeta et al. (2003) have reported that sialograms show recovery of the secondary and tertiary duct systems in the glands of 15 patients who had been recovered from the clinical condition although other 9 patients displayed persistent altered images even without presenting clinic recurrences. On the other hand, there seems to be a correlation between the type of sialectasis, as shown by sialography, and the degree of glandular involvement. Thus, at the beginning sialectasis would be punctate whereas it would be globular once the gland has reached a more advanced degenerative condition. The other types of sialectasis would be very rare in this pathology (Baurmash, 2004).

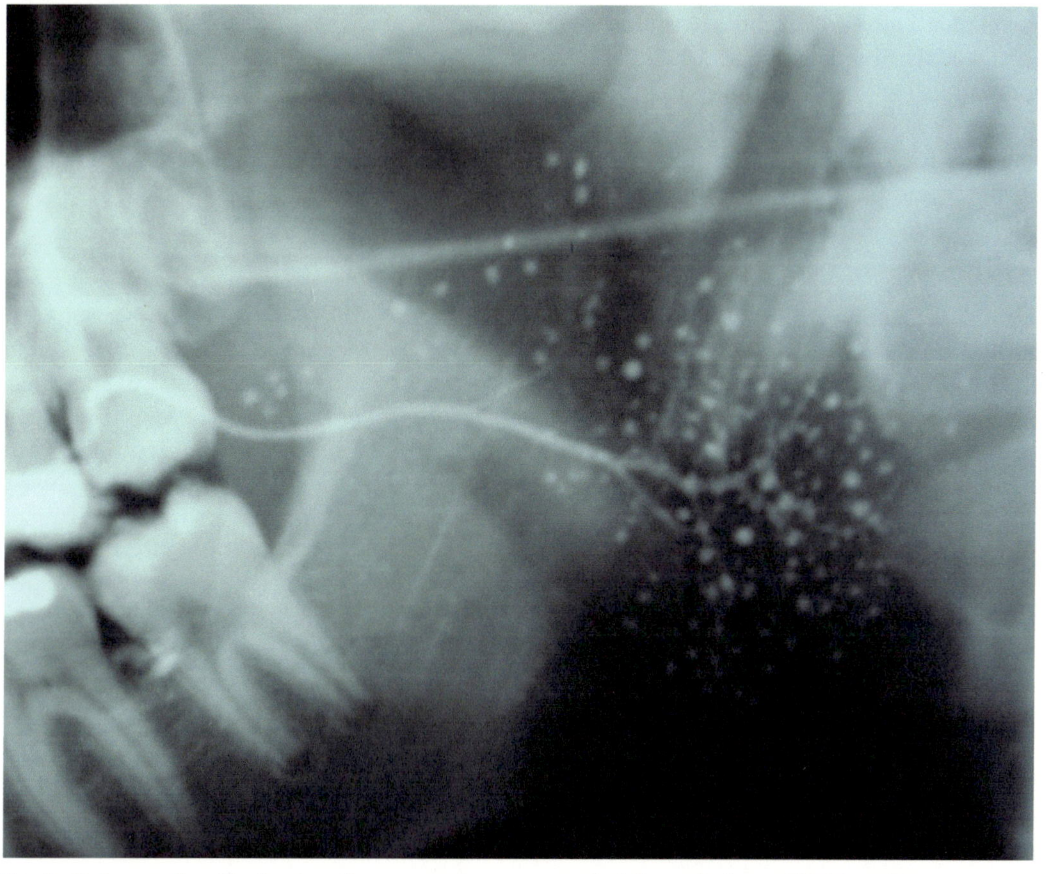

Fig. 1. Sialography displaying the punctate pattern of sialectasis in an ICRP patient.

In a different study on 17 patients a correlation between sialographic findings and duration of the disease has been postulated (Ramírez et al., 1996). After multiple recurrences the gland may experience a permanent destruction. Those altered glands, as evidenced by sialography, and those patients would experience more frequent and more prolonged episodes than patients displaying less accumulated glandular damage (Baurmash, 2004). Surprisingly, altered sialography is usually bilateral although the clinical condition may be unilateral. There is no clear explanation for the fact that only one of the glands undergoes clinical inflammation (Baurmash, 2004; Concheiro et al., 2000; Chitre & Premchandra, 1997;

Nazar et al., 2001). This evidence suggests that a subclinical glandular alteration may occur previous to the clinical condition associated to the increase in gland volume.

In the past few years, the use of ultrasonography as support for ICRP diagnosis has increased. A main advantage of ultrasonography over sialography is its lower invasiveness. Ultrasonographic images of ICRP glands show a diffuse volume increase of the gland, a decreased gland ecogenicity and numerous nodular images on the parenchyma, which may represent sialectasis and lymphocyte infiltrates (Encina et al., 1996; Isaacs et al., 2002; Mandel & Bijoor, 2006; Miziara et al., 2005; Nahlieli et al., 2004; Nazar et al., 2001; Sitheeque et al., 2007; Shacham et al., 2009; Shimizu et al., 1998). Most of the clinical reports indicate a correlation between both imaging studies (Encina et al., 1996; Mandel & Bijoor, 2006; Nazar et al., 2001; Shimizu et al., 1998). However, in some cases sialography has not been compatible with ICRP diagnosis but ultrasonography has shown bilateral glandular involvement (Isaacs et al., 2002). Some authors suggest that ultrasonography would be more sensitive for detecting glandular involvement and therefore advantageous for diagnostic purposes and for monitoring the disease (Shimizu et al., 1998).

4. ICRP treatment is a controversial and confounding issue

Because the etiology of ICRP is unknown and because its clinical manifestations are unpredictable, there is no agreement on the therapeutic management of the disease. As observed in the specialized literature, patients receive car from multiple medical specialists who prescribe different therapies for the same pathological entity. Sometimes, with the aim of increasing the salivary flow, several physical maneuvers are recommended: local heat, gland massages, gum chewing and consumption of acidic sweets (Nahlieli et al., 2004; Nazar et al., 2001). Usually, these maneuvers are recommended for preventing recurrences although gland swelling is abrupt and volume increase occurs within a few hours. In other studies, recurrences are treated with non-steroidal antiinflammatories (Rostion et al., 2004; Nazar et al., 2001), which may be combined with sialogogues, antihistaminics, lisozyme and antibiotics (Concheiro et al., 2000). Based on positive experience with mucolytics in the treatment of a variety of pathologies, such as Sjögren's síndrome and xeroftalmia, at the Surgery Department of the Hospital Roberto del Río the ICRP patients are treated with 4 mg of bromhexina every 8 hours during recurrences (Rostion et al., 2004). By contrast, also based on own experience that following sialography the symptoms of ICRP fully disappear in an important number of patients, and assuming that the contrast medium would have antiseptic activity, at the Child Maxillofacial Unit of the Hospital San Juan de Dios the treatment consists in regular intraglandular washings with an iodinated antiseptic via the excretory duct of the parotid gland (Fig. 2). Such a treatment is repeated until the gland displays a sialographic image that is consistent with normality. In case the patient is ill-feeling the treatment is combined with amoxicillin therapy (Landaeta et al., 2003). In a recent pilot study, the authors treat the jaw malfunctioning due to misocclussion in order to prevent ICRP recurrences. Those authors observed a decrease in the symptoms of 9 out of 13 cases although three of the patients were refractory to the treatment (Bernkopf et al., 2008). Another study recommends treating ICRP patients during the active stage of the condition by an inspection of the Stenon's duct with a sialendoscope and a simultaneous washing of the gland with saline solution under general anesthesia. Once the duct has been washed, the treatment is completed by an intraglandular injection of 100 mg hydrocortisone and intravenous amoxicillyn-clavulanic acid (Issacs, 2002; Shacham et al., 2009). In cases of severe non reversible glandular damage derived from prolonged acute episodes, ligation of the excretory duct of the gland to provoke its atrophy has been recommended (Baurmash, 2004; Nahlieli et al., 2004). As a last resource to deal with severe ICRP conditions, which is recommended when the other treatments have proven unsuccessful, partial or total parotidectomy is performed despite the complexity derived from the facial nerve proximity (Baurmash, 2004; Nahlieli et al., 2004). There are reports in the literature describing bilateral parotidectomy in a 11-year old boy affected by an extreme condition (Moody et al., 2000).

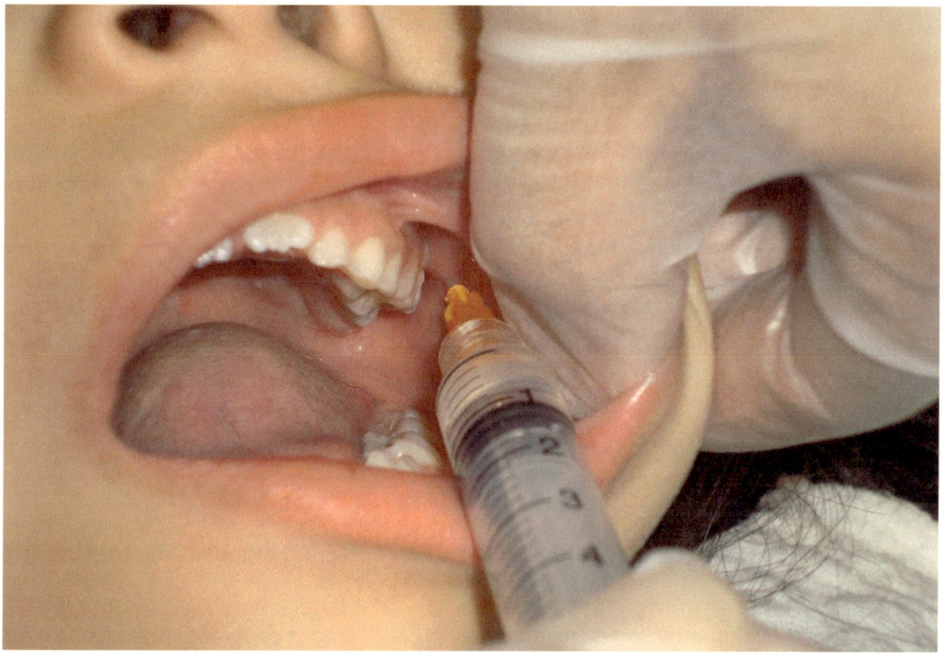

Fig. 2. Intraglandular washing via the excretory duct of the parotid gland in ICRP patient.

Despite the pathological process in ICRP is basically of inflammatory nature, as shown by histopathologicall assessment, most of the reports show that the therapeutical trials include the use of antibiotics. The most frequently used antibacterial drugs are amoxicillin or amoxicillyn combined with clavulanic acid (oral or systemic) or first generation cefalosporines (Baurmash, 2004; Concheiro et al., 2000; Chitre & Premchandra, 1997; Nahlieli et al., 2004; Nazar et al., 2001). Clearly, these therapeutic schemes are oriented to deal with the general ill-condition and so to prevent its worsening. However, it is necessary to bear in mind the risk of microbial resistance derived from the iterative use of drugs to treat a disease whose origin may be other than bacterial. Thus, in some studies topic penicillin or topic chloramphenicol is used for gland lavages during acute episodes. Such a wide spectrum of treatments is a clear reflection of the lack of a minimum consensus on ICRP therapy. Although most of the reports indicate a variable degree of success, none of them claims a full prevention of the recurrences. Furthermore, the general tendency of current therapies seems to be focused on alleviating symptoms, shortening the time of the acute episodes and extending the quiescent periods, preventing a worsening of the general ill-feeling and avoiding as much as possible a damage of the glandular parenchyma due to inflammatory recurrences (Baurmash, 2004; Concheiro et al., 2000; Rostion et al., 2004; Nahlieli et al., 2004; Nazar et al., 2001).

5. Parotid gland as an organ with endocrine functions

Besides its well known role in saliva production and so in the lubrication and protection of the soft tissues that are bathed in it, mounting evidence point to this gland as responsible of some endocrine and metabolic functions. Thus, some studies suggest that this gland plays an active role in nitrite and nitrate metabolism and that its experimental destruction in laboratory animals leads to an unbalance between those molecular species (Xia et al., 2003a). Human parotid saliva presents higher levels of nitrate compared with urine and blood serum. Patients with Sjögren's syndrome (an inflammatory autoimmune exocrinopathy) show a decreased level of nitrate in saliva and a highly increased level of this chemical in urine (Xia et al., 2003b). Experimental bilateral parotidectomy in laboratory animals results in a reduction of dentin apposition in developing molars. Parotin, a protein that has been isolated from porcine parotid glands (Tieche et al., 2005), has been shown to produce hypocalcemia and leucocytosis, to affect bone, cartilage and connective tissue homeostasis and to increase dentinary mineralization (Leonora et al., 2002). Recent evidence suggests that parotin is a proline-rich protein that is biologically active in producing displacement of dentinary fluid (Zhang et al., 2005). In consequence, the effect that the partial or total loss of this organ may have for the human organism, particularly among growing children, is mostly unknown. On that perspective, the control of the accumulative damage of this organ may be more relevant than previously suspected.

6. Contraindication of parotid biopsy among ICRP patients has limited the study of this disease

Parotid biopsy is restricted to some pathologies with a proper cost/benefit ratio. Restriction is explained by the close proximity of facial nerve branches passing through the gland. In this pathology, minor salivary glands remain unaffected. Accordingly, studies involving tissular, cellular or molecular assessments of the parotid gland are extremously rare. Most of the studies on ICRP consist either in clinical assessment, imaging and hematological studies or, alternatively, deal with the outputs of various treatment strategies (Concheiro et al., 2000; Rostion et al., 2004; Miziara et al. 2005; Nahlieli et al., 2004; Nazar et al., 2001; Sitheeque et al., 2007; Shacham et al., 2009). In this context, the analysis of the fluid secreted by the affected parotid gland would constitute a valuable noninvasive tool for the indirect assessment of the physiopathological condition of the gland. Although several studies on ICRP coincide in concluding that parotid saliva is qualitatively altered (Baursham, 2004; Chitre & Premchandra, 1997; Landaeta et al. 2003; Nazar et al., 2001), studies on the chemical properties of this fluid are rare. Sialochemical analysis has been performed in regard to other medical conditions affecting this organ, such as Sjögren's syndrome and therapeutical irradiation of the maxillofacial territory, a condition resulting in chronic inflammation of salivary glands (Asatsuma et al., 2004; Hanemaaijer et al., 1998; Kaufman & Lamster, 2002; Streckfus & Bigler, 2002; Vuotila et al., 2002). Taback in 1978 and Erikson in

1996 reported that parotid saliva from ICRP patients have increased levels of albumin, lactoferrin, kallicrein and IgA, as compared to healthy controls (Ericson & Sjöbäck, 1996; Tabak et al., 1978). On this background, in addition to the observation of a variety of physical changes in saliva from ICRP patients, our research group started in 2005 to analyze chemical properties of parotid saliva from ICRP patients with the aim of identifying molecular alterations, which may be of value in the understanding of the etiology and/or physiopathology of this condition.

7. Occurrence of molecules associated with extracellular matrix turnover in the salivary secretion

Metalloproteinases (MMPs), a family of macromolecules involved in normal and pathological extracellular matrix remodelling, have been observed in saliva of patients with various inflammatory conditions. This observation has contributed to get insights into the pathological process affecting the gland (Asatsuma et al., 2004; Hanemaaijer et al., 1998; Vuotila et al., 2002, Wu et al., 1997). These calcium- and zinc-dependent endopeptidases, whose expression is regulated by growth factors, cytokines, hormones and extracellular matrix components (Sternlicht & Werb, 2001), are initially synthesized as zymogens that are proteolyzed at the extracellular space to become active MMPs (Nagase & Woessner, 1999). Gelatinases MMP-2 and MMP-9 have been involved in a variety of pathological conditions in adults, such as Sjögren's syndrome, Diabetes mellitus and periodontitis (Asatsuma et al., 2004; Collin et al., 2000; Pozo et al., 2005). They have also been observed in inflammatory pathologies of the child, as in chronic suppurative otitis media and in chronic lung diseases (Ekekezie et al., 2004; Jang et al., 2006). Both gelatinases have ben found in a variety of body fluids, namely, caphaloraquid fluid, tracheal secretion, middle ear secretion, gingival fluid, blood plasma and saliva (Ekekezie et al., 2004; Jang et al., 2006; Kettlun et al., 2003; Schulz et al., 2004; Valenzuela, 2000; Wu et al., 1997). Patients subjected to therapeutical irradiation of the maxillofacial territory have active and inactive forms of MMP-2 and MMP-9 in saliva and irradiation would increase the MMP-9 activity (Vuotila et al., 2002). Patients with Sjögren's syndrome have an increased activity of MMP-9 in saliva as well as an altered MMP-9 / TIMP-1 (a tissular inhibidor of MMPs 1) ratio, as compared to healthy control subjects (Asatsuma et al., 2004; Hanemaaijer et al., 1998; Wu et al., 1997). More recent studies in biopsies of minor salivary glands of patients with Sjögren's síndrome have shown alterations in tissular metalloproteinases that coincide with those observed in saliva (Pérez et al., 2005).

The occurrence of these enzymes in saliva has also been tested in relation to pathologies affecting organs and systems other than salivary glands. Levels of MMP-9 and TIMP-1 in saliva of patients with adult periodontitis are higher than in healthy control subjects (Ingman et al., 1996). In a study with patients displaying taste disorders the levels of MMP-9 in saliva were not different compared to the respective controls. However, this study also showed that MMP-9 does occur in saliva of healthy subjects (Watanabe et al., 2005). In a similar observation, Raitio et al. (2005) reported that non-smoker control subjects presented both latent and active forms of MMP-9 whereas the smokers exhibited higher concentrations of latent MMP-9. Concerning systemic conditions, saliva of healthy control subjects has lower levels of the active and latent forms of MMP-2, MMP-9, TIMP-1 and TIMP-2 than saliva of VIH-positive patients (Mellanen et al., 1998). In another study, saliva of control non-pregnant women was found to display lower concentrations of MMP-9 compared to saliva of pregnant women with premature membrane rupture (Miller et al., 2006).

Considering that ICRP is an inflammatory alteration producing damage of the glandular tissue it would be reasonable to suspect that metalloproteases are present in parotid saliva. In a recent study dealing with molecular analysis of parotid saliva from 33 ICRP patients we reported changes in the salivary composition as compared to 33 healthy control subjects. In that study we scored the frequency of subjects having MMP-2 and MMP-9 activities in parotid saliva and found that only two healthy subjects presented these enzymes in saliva whereas 18 and 10 ICRP patients were positive for MMP-9 and MMP-2, respectively (Morales-Bozo et al., 2007). A later study showed a positive association between degree of sialographic damage of single parotid glands and the occurrence of those gelatinases in the corresponding parotid saliva. Zymographic analysis showed that saliva from 32 and 21 parotid glands displaying altered sialographies also exhibited MMP-9 and MMP-2, respectively. When this analysis was performed on glands with no sialographic damage, only 2 of the glands presented MMP-9 and none of them showed MMP-2 (Morales-Bozo et al., 2008). These were the first reports on the occurrence of metalloproteases in saliva of ICRP patients, thus suggesting their involvement in the mechanism of parotid damage.

In a recent study with 32 ICRP patients we assessed the presence of both the active and latent forms of those gelatinases in parotid saliva from ill and unaffected glands of the same patients (Table 1). We found latent MMP-9 in 15 healthy and in 46 affected glands and latent MMP-2 in 9 healthy and in 36 affected glands. We found the active form of MMP-2 only in 2 healthy glands and in 14 ill glands.

	ProMMP-9		*ProMMP-2*		*MMP-2*	
Salivary Gland	-	+	-	+	-	+
Unaffected	1	15	7	9	14	2
ICRP	2	46	12	36	34	14

Table 1. Presence of salivary metalloproteinases MMP-2 and -9 in salivary glands of ICRP patients.

In this study, the affected glands presented higher levels of all the gelatinase forms compared with the healthy glands although differences were not statistically significant. However, in this study we observed a high molecular weight gelatinase (130 kDa) in saliva obtained from 61 parotid glands. Besides, saliva of 15 healthy glands showed 1.75 ± 2.3 ng of this gelatinase per ml of parotid saliva versus 9.6 ± 2.3 ng of the enzyme per ml de saliva obtained from 46 ill glands (p=0.418) (Pinochet, 2008).

Gelatinases interact with a wide variety of molecules to form complexes like MMP-2/TIMP, MMP-2/glycosaminoglicans, MMP-9 dimers, MMP-9/MMP-1, MMP-9/NGAL (Neutrophyl gelatinase-associated lipocalin), MMP-9/Haptoglobuline, MMP-9/ proteoglycans, etc. (51). These complexes may play important roles under physiological and pathological conditions (Malla et al., 2008). The molecular size of the gelatinase complex that we have observed in parotid saliva of ICRP patients suggests that it would correspond to a MMP-9/NGAL complex. The molecular weight of the active form of this complex is 125-130 kDa and is comprised by MMP-9 covalently bonded with NGAL of human neutrophiles (Yan et al., 2001). Through this interaction, MMP-9 becomes protected from degradation, thus breaking the balance between synthesis and degradation (Yan et al., 2001; Devarajan et al., 2007). This complex has been involved in pathogenic mechanisms of a variety of conditions, such as cancer, osteoarthritis, rheumatoid arthritis and renal damage (Devarajan et al., 2007; Gupta et al., 2007; Katano et al., 2009; Zhang et al., 2009). NGAL or lipocalin 2 (25 kDa) is a protein that binds siderophores with a high affinity, thus taking part of the innate immune system against bacterial infections in tissues that are exposed to the external environment (respiratory, gastrointestinal and urinary tracts). Its expression rises up during infection or inflammation (Xu et al., 2009). In submandibular glands of 10 patients having chronic sialadenitis NGAL has been found to be overexpressed in inflammatory infiltrates and in duct cells, as compared to gland tissue from control subjects (Woo et al., 2007). In lip salivary gland of patients with amyloid polyneuropathy, both mRNA NGAL and a 130 kDa form of MMP-9 have been found to be overexpressed compared to lip biopsies from healthy controls (Sousa et al., 2005). To date there are no reports on the presence of either NGAL or complexes between MMP-9 and other molecules in parotid gland or in parotid saliva under normal or pathological conditions.

8. The search for ICRP-associated salivary molecules should be performed in parotid saliva

Excepting the report of Wu et al. (1997), all the studies dealing with the assessment of metalloprotease levels in saliva have been performed in whole saliva. Whole saliva is a complex mix of diverse salivary fluids, plus components of the gingival crevicular fluid, exfoliated cells from the oral mucose, microbial flora and food remnants. In this fluid, the occurrence of MMP-2, MMP-9, TIMP-1 and TIMP-2 has been reported under conditions of gingival normality as well as in periodontal disease (Pozo et al., 2005). Thus, it would be hard to define the origin of those molecules present in whole saliva. In order to elucidate the point, Mäkelä et al. (1994) analyzed parallel samples of parotid saliva, submandibular/sublingual saliva, whole saliva and gingival crevicular fluid, all of them taken from 17 healthy control subjects. Those authors observed that total saliva and the crevicular fluid displayed similar levels of MMP-9 whereas only trace levels of those molecules were observed in glandular salivas. Collin et al. (2000) reported that MMP-9 activity in whole saliva from edentulous subjects, that is, without gingival crevicular fluid, was significantly lower than in whole saliva from dentulous subjects. Both observations suggest that MMP-9 in whole saliva would be provided by the periodontus. Hystolochemical studies on slices of parotid and submandibular glands indicate that MMP-2 and MMP-9 would be mostly located in the duct system and absent from the acinar system (Ogbureke & Fisher, 2004; Nagel et al., 2004; Teymoortash et al., 2004). Similar studies on lip salivary glands have shown the presence of MMP-2 and MMP-9 in duct cells and at the basal region of acinar cells (Pérez et al., 2000, 2005). These observations would suggest that those molecules would not be released from the gland to the oral cavity under normal conditions. On these evidence it becomes necessary that the identification of parotid-produced molecules would require analysis of parotid secretion and that much care should be taken to collect this fluid free of contaminants from other salivary components. To this end, we have designed an *ad hoc* device to collect with high efficiency and comfort very pure parotid saliva (Morales et al., 1998). In addition we have developed an objective method to assess the purity of samples of parotid saliva. Protein fractionation of salivary samples from individual subjects of different ages and genders (N = 190) using unidimensional gel electrophoresis in SDS-polyacrylamide gels has shown that submandibular / sublingual saliva present two polypeptide bands (19 and 18 kDa) that are not present in other types of saliva, excepting whole saliva. Those polypeptide markers should not be present in samples of parotid saliva (Morales et al., 1998; Morales-Bozo et al., 2006).

9. Proteomic analysis of saliva as a tool for investigating ICRP-associated molecules

Parotid saliva comprises a wide variety of protein families whose characterization has been the product of diverse experimental approaches. In the past few years, proteomics of this body fluid has provided a large amount of compositional data in normality (Denny et al., 2008; Hardt et al., 2005; Walz et al., 2006). Changes in the proteome of parotid saliva have also been reported in some pathological conditions. A recent study compares the proteome of parotid saliva of elderly patients displaying root caries with the one of healthy controls (Preza et al., 2009). In 2006, Ryu et al. identified biomarkers in parotid saliva among patients with Sjogren's syndrome. That study comprised 41 patients and 21 control subjects and showed that the proteomic profiles of those patients displayed a marked increase in inflammatory proteins compared with the profiles of control subjects. Particularly, significant increases in β-2 microglobuline, lactoferrin, kappa light chain immunoglobulin, polymeric immunoglobulin receptor, lisozyme C and cystatin C, were observed, in parallel, with a significant decrease in acinar cell proteins, such as amylase, carbonic anhydrase VI and two putative proline-rich proteins (Ryu et al., 2006).

In previous studies from our laboratory we have shown changes in the polypeptide profiles of parotid saliva from ICRP patients as compared to the ones of healthy paired controls. Such alterations were represented by an increase in the frequency of individuals displaying polypeptides of 43, 37, 33, 29, 26, 16 and 10 kDa in parotid saliva produced by clinically affected glands (Morales-Bozo et al., 2007). In a complementary study by protein fingerprinting and MALDI-TOF mass spectrometry of the 26 kDa polypeptide, which is present with no exception in the saliva of all the enrolled ICRP patients, we have found that it corresponds to the C-region of the kappa light chain immunoglobulin, thus suggesting its participation in the pathological process (Werner, 2008). Currently, we are defining bidimensional electrophoretic profiles of parotid saliva from healthy control subjects in order to set a standard profile to contrast the varying profiles of ICRP patients.

10. The problem

There are no studies on the prevalence of ICRP either in Chile or the rest of the world. At the Hospital San Juan de Dios in Santiago, Chile, there are currently around 300 children affected by ICRP and under medical care. Bibliographic references show that this is a world-wide distributed disease. From 1991 to date, the following cases have been reported: **1991**:20 children in Sweden; **1996:** 16 children in Chile and 17 children in Sweden; **1997:** 56 children in

Chile; **1998:** 14 children in Japan; **1999:** 3 children in Germany; **2000:** two children in Germany and 30 children in Spain; **2001:** 16 children in Chile and 12 children in Switzerland; **2002:** one child in Australia; **2003:** 50 children in Chile; **2004:** one child in Israel and 38 children in Chile; **2005:** 26 children in Israel,133 children in Finland, 23 in Austria, 53 in Australia and 5 in Brasil; **2006:** 12 children in Taiwan and one child in USA; **2007:** 26 children in Sri Lanka; **2008:** 10 children in France and 33 children in Chile; recently in **2009:** 13 children in Italy and 76 children in Israel (Bernkopf et al. 2008; Concheiro et al., 2000; Encina et al., 1996; Ericson et al., 1991, Fazekas et al., 2005; 1996; Giglio et al. , 1997; Huisman et al., 2001; Isaacs et al., 2002; Kolho et al., 2005; Leerdam et al., 2005; Mandel & Bijoor, 2006; Menauer et al., 1999; Miziara et al., 2005; Nazar et al., 2001;Nahlieli et al., 2004; Quenin et al., 2008; Rostion et al., 2004; Shacham et al., 2009; Shimizu et al. 1998; Shkalim et al., 2004; Sitheeque et al., 2007; Usmüller, 1999; Vinagre et al., 2003; Wang et al., 2006; Wittekindt et al., 2000).

ICRP is a complex disease given the lack of knowledge about its etiology and pathogenic mechanism and because of the lack of medical treatment leading to a definite cure. On the other hand, systemic effects derived from a prolonged parotid dysfunction, especially among growing infants, are also unknown. On our own experience, most of the patients are initially diagnosed for Viral Parotitis. Once recurrences start to occur, the child patients deambulate through medical and dental care centers until they are derived to reference centers for this disease. Since current medical treatments are only palliative in nature, patients are treated for several years, from preschool age to adolescence or even young adulthood, thus affecting life quality and overusing medical resources. Diagnosis is confirmed by means of sialography, an invasive complementary examination involving the local injection of a contrast medium that may remain in the gland even for years. Possibilities of substituting sialography by ultrasonography are remote due to the lack of equipment and trained professionals in the public health services in Chile.

Although ICRP is not an infectious disease, it uses to be confounded with a bacterial parotitis because salivary secretion becomes thick and whitish and then patients are treated with systemic antibiotics. Thus, despite the diagnosis of ICRP, most of the therapeutical schemes include associated antibiotherapy with a subsequent risk of bacterial resistance (Burmash, 2004; Chitre & Premchandra, 1997; Concheiro et al., 2000; Nahlieli et al., 2004; Nazar et al., 2001). The scarce histological studies on ICRP suggest that it involves an inflammatory condition with lymphocytary infiltration (Ericson, 1995; Ussmüller & Donath, 1999). Because of the high risk of biopsying parotid glands, this maneuver is contraindicated in ICRP. Thus, the compositional analysis of saliva secreted by this gland represents an advantageous noninvasive tool to get insights into the functioning of the affected gland tissue.

Pioneering sialochemical studies indicate that parotid saliva of ICRP patients has higher concentrations of albumin, lactoferrin, kallicrein and IgA, as compared to control subjects (Ericson & Sjöbäck, 1996; Tabak et al., 1978). Lactoferrin, kallicrein and IgA are proteins that are normally present in parotid saliva and play defensive roles. Albumin seems to be passively contributed by blood plasma due to inflammatory processes affecting permeability of the glandular epithelia. Most of these data derive from studies with low numbers of patients (N = 1 and N = 17) whose main aim was to search for specific proteins.

Studies from our laboratory have shown that regardless unilaterality or bilaterality of the clinical condition, saliva of both parotid glands of ICRP patients present a higher concentration of proteins compared to that of control subjects (Morales-Bozo et al., 2007). We have also shown that parotid saliva of ICRP patients display gelatinase activity, which is absent in parotid saliva of healthy control subjects (Morales-Bozo et al. , 2007). MMP-2 and MMP-9 activities show a positive relation with the degree of damage of the parotid gland, as assessed by sialography (Morales-Bozo et al., 2008). Active and latent forms of MMP-9 and latent form of MMP-2 were observed. No relationship was observed between the clinical involvement of the gland and the levels of the active and latent forms of those metalloproteases. However, the clinically affected ICRP glands displayed a much higher concentration of a high molecular weight gelatinase (130 kDa) (Pinochet, 2008). The molecular size of this gelatinase suggests that it would correspond to a MMP-9/lipocalin 2 complex (Gupta et al., 2007; Malla et al., 2008). In other pathologies, a covalent association between both molecular entities results in an unbalance between synthesis and degradation of MMP-9, thus increasing the enzyme activity of the complex (Devarajan et al., 2007; Yan et al., 2001 52,53). Lipocalin 2 is secreted by neutrophiles in tissues that are exposed to the external environment, as it is the case of the oral cavity. This protein of 25 kDa acts by binding and inactivating bacterial siderophores: in the presence of MMP-9 it becomes bonded covalently to the enzyme thus preventing its degradation (Devarajan et al., 2007). These results suggest that polymorphonuclear neutrophiles may be involved in the pathogenesis of this disease.

With the aim of screening for a wide number of salivary proteins from a single subject at once, we have performed unidmensional electrophoresis analysis in parotid saliva from ICRP patients. Our studies have shown marked changes in parotid saliva of these patients compared with the one from control subjects. Analyses of the most frequent changes in definite polypeptides have shown an increase in a group of seven polypeptide bands compared to control electrophoretograms (Morales-Bozo et al., 2007). A 26 kDa band has been identified by protein fingerprinting and Maldi-TOF mass spectrometry as corresponding to the C-region of the human kappa light chain immunoglobulin according to three different databanks (Werner, 2007). To date, there are no reports on bidimensional electrophoresis profiles of parotid saliva either from healthy control children or ICRP patients. Thus, this experimental approach may additionally increase the spectrum of relevant salivary proteins in ICRP.

11. Conclusions

Altogether, the evidence derived from the molecular analysis of parotid saliva of ICRP patients highly suggests that this body fluid may be used advantageously to identify molecules that are related to pathogenesis of the disease, to monitor the ill-condition and to assess the efficacy of the treatment.

12. Acknowledgments

This study was supported in part by University of Chile Grants DI-MULT 05/35-2, FIOUCH 09-2 and VID-Ayuda de viaje 2011.

13. References

Asatsuma, M.; Ito, S.; Watanabe, M.; Takeishi, H.; Nomura, S.; Wada, Y:, Nakano, M.; Gejyo, F. & Igarashi, A. (2004). Increase in the ratio of matrix metalloproteinase-9 to tissue inhibitor of metalloproteinase-1 in saliva from patients with primary Sjogren's syndrome. *Clinica chimica acta; international journal of clinical chemistry,* Vol.345, N°.1-2, (Julio 2004), pp. 99-104. ISSN 0009-8981

Baurmash, HD. (2004). Chronic recurrent parotitis: a closer look at its origin, diagnosis, and management. *Journal of oral and maxillofacial surgery : official journal of the American Association of Oral and Maxillofacial Surgeons,* Vol.62, N°.8, (August 2004), pp. 1010-1018. ISSN 0278-2391

Bernkopf, E., Colleselli, P.; Broia, V. & de Benedictis, FM. (2008). Is recurrent parotitis in childhood still an enigma? A pilot experience. *Acta paediatrica,* Vol.97, N°4, (April 2008), pp.478-482. ISSN 0803-5253

Collin, HL.; Sorsa, T.; Meurman, JH.; Niskanen, L.; Salo, T.; Ronka, H.; Konttinen, YT.; Koivisto. AM. & Uusitupa, M. (2000). Salivary matrix metalloproteinase (MMP-8) levels and gelatinase (MMP-9) activities in patients with type 2 diabetes mellitus. *Journal of periodontal research,* Vol.35, N°.5, (October 2004), pp. 259-265. ISSN 0022-3484

Concheiro, A.; Bellver, E.; Garrido, R. & Garcia, S. (2000). Chronic recurrent parotitis in childhood. *Anales españoles de pediatría,* Vol.53, N°.5, (November 2000), pp. 418-421. ISSN 0302-4342

Chitre, VV. & Premchandra DJ. (1997). Recurrent parotitis. *Archives of disease in childhood,* Vol. 77, N°.4, (October 1997) pp. 359-363. ISSN 0003-9888

Denny, P.; Hagen, FK.; Hardt, M.; Liao, L.; Yan, W.; Arellanno, M.; Bassilian, S.; Bedi, GS.; Boontheung, P.; Cociorva, D.; Delahunty, CM.; Denny, T.; Dunsmore, J.; Faull, KF.; Gilligan, J.; Gonzalez-Begne, M.; Halgand, F.; Hall, SC.; Han, X.; Henson, B.; Hewel, J.; Hu, S.; Jeffrey, S:, Jiang, J.; Loo, JA.; Ogorzalek Loo, RR.; Malamud, D.; Melvin, JE.; Miroshnychenko, O.; Navazesh, M.; Niles, R.; Park, SK.; Prakobphol, A.; Ramachandran, P.; Richert, M.; Robinson, S.; Sondej, M.; Souda, P.; Sullivan, MA:, Takashima. J.; Than, S.; Wang et al., J.; Whitelegge, JP.; Witkowska, HE.; Wolinsky, L.; Xie, Y.; Xu et al., T.; Yu, W.; Ytterberg, J.; Wong, DT.; Yates, JR 3rd. & Fisher, SJ. (2008). The proteomes of human parotid and submandibular/sublingual gland salivas collected as the ductal secretions. *Journal of proteome research,* Vol.7, N°.5, (May 2008), pp. 1994-2006. ISSN 1535-3893

Devarajan, P. (2007) Neutrophil gelatinase-associated lipocalin: new paths for an old shuttle. *Cancer therapy,* Vol.5, N°.B, pp. 463-470. ISSN 1543-9143

Ekekezie, II.; Thibeault, DW.; Simon, SD.; Norberg, M.; Merrill, JD.; Ballard, RA.; Ballard, PL. & Truog, WE. (2004). Low levels of tissue inhibitors of metalloproteinases with a high matrix metalloproteinase-9/tissue inhibitor of metalloproteinase-1 ratio are present in tracheal aspirate fluids of infants who develop chronic lung disease. *Pediatrics,* Vol.113, N°.6, (June 2004), pp. 1709-1714. ISSN 0031-4005

Encina, S.; Ernst, P.; Villanueva, J. & Pizarro, E. (1996). Ultrasonography: a complement to sialography in recurrent chronic childhood parotitis. *Revue de stomatologie et de chirurgie maxillo-faciale,* Vol.97, N°.5, (October 1996) pp. 258-263. ISSN 0035-1768

Ericson, S.; Zetterlund, B. & Ohman, J. (1991). Recurrent parotitis and sialectasis in childhood. Clinical, radiologic, immunologic, bacteriologic, and histologic study. *The Annals of otology, rhinology, and laryngology*, Vol.100, N°.7, (July 1991), pp. 527-535. ISSN 0003-4894

Ericson, S. & Sjoback, I. (1996). Salivary factors in children with recurrent parotitis. Part 2: Protein, albumin, amylase, IgA, lactoferrin lysozyme and kallikrein concentrations. *Swedish dental journal*, Vol.20, N°.5, (1996), pp. 199-207. ISSN 0347-9994

Fazekas, T.; Wiesbauer, P.; Schroth, B.; Potschger. U.; Gadner, H. & Heitger, A. (2005). Selective IgA deficiency in children with recurrent parotitis of childhood. *The Pediatric infectious disease journal*, Vol.24, N°.5, (May 2005), pp. 461-462. ISSN 0891-3668

Giglio, MS.; Landaeta et al., M. & Pinto, ME. (1997). Microbiology of recurrent parotitis. *The Pediatric infectious disease journal,* Vol.16, N°.4, (April 1997), pp. 386-390. ISSN 0891-3668

Gupta, K.; Shukla, M., Cowland, JB., Malemud, CJ. & Haqqi, TM. (2007). Neutrophil gelatinase-associated lipocalin is expressed in osteoarthritis and forms a complex with matrix metalloproteinase 9. *Arthritis and rheumatism*, Vol.56, N°.10, (October 2007), pp. 3326-3335. ISSN 0004-3591

Hanemaaijer, R.; Visser, H.; Konttinen, YT.; Koolwijk, P. & Verheijen, JH. (1998). A novel and simple immunocapture assay for determination of gelatinase-B (MMP-9) activities in biological fluids: saliva from patients with Sjogren's syndrome contain increased latent and active gelatinase-B levels. *Matrix biology : journal of the International Society for Matrix Biology*, Vol.17, N°.8-9, (December 1998), pp. 657-665. ISSN 0945-053X

Hardt, M.; Thomas, LR.; Dixon, SE.; Newport, G.; Agabian, N.; Prakobphol, A.; Hall, SC.; Witkowska, HE. & Fisher, SJ. (2005). Toward defining the human parotid gland salivary proteome and peptidome: identification and characterization using 2D SDS-PAGE, ultrafiltration, HPLC, and mass spectrometry. *Biochemistry*, Vol.44, N°.8, (March 2005), pp. 2885-2899. ISSN 0006-2960

Huisman, TA.; Holzmann, D. & Nadal, D. (2001). MRI of chronic recurrent parotitis in childhood. *Journal of computer assisted tomography*, Vol.25, N°.2, (March 2001), pp. 269-273. ISSN 0363-8715

Ingman, T.; Tervahartiala, T.; Ding, Y.; Tschesche, H.; Haerian, A.; Kinane, DF.; Konttinen, YT. & Sorsa, T. (1996). Matrix metalloproteinases and their inhibitors in gingival crevicular fluid and saliva of periodontitis patients. *Journal of clinical periodontology*, Vol.23, N°.12, (December 1996), pp. 1127-1132. ISSN 0303-6979

Isaacs, D. (2002). Recurrent parotitis. *Journal of paediatrics and child health*, Vol.38, N°.1, (February 2002), pp. 92-94. ISSN 1034-4810

Jang, CH.; Shin, SH.; Cho, HH.; Moon, SJ. & Cho, YB. (2006). Expression of matrix metalloproteinase-9 and -2 in pediatric chronic otitis media with effusion. *International journal of pediatric otorhinolaryngology*, Vol.70, N°.7, (July 2006), pp. 1155-1158. ISSN 0165-5876

Katano, M.; Okamoto, K.; Arito, M.; Kawakami, Y.; Kurokawa, MS.; Suematsu, N.; Shimada, S.; Nakamura, H.; Xiang, Y.; Masuko, K.; Nishioka, K.; Yudoh, K. & Kato, T. (2009).

Implication of GM-CSF induced neutrophil gelatinase-associated lipocalin in pathogenesis of rheumatoid arthritis revealed by proteome analysis. *Arthritis research & therapy*, Vol.11, N°.1, (January 2009), pp. R3. ISSN 1478-6354

Kaufman, E. & Lamster, IB. (2002). The diagnostic applications of saliva--a review. *Critical reviews in oral biology and medicine : an official publication of the American Association of Oral Biologists*, Vol.13, N°.2, (February 2002), pp. 197-212. ISSN 1045-4411

Kettlun, AM.; Cartier, L.; Garcia, L.; Collados, L.; Vasquez, F.; Ramírez, E. & Valenzuela, MA. (2003). TIMPs and MMPs expression in CSF from patients with TSP/HAM. *Life sciences*, Vol.72, N°.25 (May 2003), pp. 2863-2876. ISSN 0024-3205

Kolho, KL.; Saarinen, R.; Paju, A.; Stenman, J.; Stenman, UH. & Pitkaranta, A. (2005) New insights into juvenile parotitis. *Acta paediatrica*, Vol.94, N°.11; (November 2005), pp. 1566-1570. ISSN 1651-2227

Landaeta, M.; Giglio, MS.; Ulloa, MT.; Martínez, MJ. & Pinto, ME. (2003). Clinical, microbiological aetiology and therapeutic aspects in infantil chronic recurrent parotitis (PCRI). *Revista Chilena de Pediatría*, Vol.74, N°.3, (March 2003), pp. 269-276. ISSN 0370-4106

Leerdam, CM.; Martin, HC. & Isaacs, D. (2005). Recurrent parotitis of childhood. *Journal of paediatrics and child health*, Vol.41, N°.12, (December 2005), pp. 631-634. ISSN 1034-4810

Leonora, J.; Tjaderhane, L. & Tieche et al., JM. (2002). Parotid gland function and dentin apposition in rat molars. *Journal of dental research*, Vol.81, N°.4, (April 2002) pp. 259-264. ISSN 0022-0345

Malla, N.; Sjøli, S.; Winberg, JO.; Hadler-Olsen, E. & Uhlin-Hansen, L. (2008). Biological and pathobiological functions of gelatinase dimers and complexes. *Connective tissue research*, Vol.49, N°.3, (March 2008) pp. 180-184. ISSN 0300-8207

Mandel, L. & Bijoor R. (2006). Imaging (computed tomography, magnetic resonance imaging, ultrasound, sialography) in a case of recurrent parotitis in children. *Journal of oral and maxillofacial surgery : official journal of the American Association of Oral and Maxillofacial Surgeons*, Vol.64, N°.6 (June 2006), pp. 984-988. ISSN 0278-2391

Mäkelä, M.; Salo, T.; Uitto, VJ. & Larjava, H. (1994). Matrix metalloproteinases (MMP-2 and MMP-9) of the oral cavity: cellular origin and relationship to periodontal status. Journal of dental research.Vol.73, N°.8, (August 1994), pp. 1397-1406. ISSN 0022-0345

Mellanen, L.; Salo, T.; Ingman, T.; Konttinen, YT.; La hdevirta, J. & Sorsa, T. (1998). 72-kDa and 92-kDa gelatinases in saliva of patients with human immunodeficiency virus infection. *Acta odontologica Scandinavica*, Vol.56, N°.3, (June 1998), pp. 135-142. ISSN 0001-6357

Menauer, F.; Jäger, L., Leunig, A. & Grevers, G. (1999). Role of diagnostic imaging in chronic recurrent parotitis in childhood. *Laryngo- rhino- otologie*, Vol.78, N°.9, (September 1999), pp. 497-499. ISSN 0935-8943

Miller, CS.; King, CP.; Langub, MC.; Kryscio, RJ. & Thomas. MV. (2006) Salivary biomarkers of existing periodontal disease: a cross-sectional study. *The Journal of the American Dental Association*, Vol.137, N°3; (March 2006), pp. 322-329. ISSN 0002-8177

Miziara, ID. & Campelo, VE. (2005) Infantile recurrent parotitis: follow up study of five cases and literature. *Brazilian journal of otorhinolaryngology*, Vol.71, N°.5 (September 2005), pp. 570-575. ISSN 1808-8694

Moody, AB.; Avery, CM.; Walsh, S.; Sneddon, K. & Langdon, JD. (2000). Surgical management of chronic parotid disease. *The British journal of oral & maxillofacial surgery*, Vol.38, N°.6, (December 2000), pp. 620-622. ISSN 0266-4356

Morales, I.; Domínguez, P. & López R.O. (1998). Dispositivos para colección de saliva de las glándulas salivales mayores. Resultados en sujetos normales. *Revista Médica de Chile*, Vol.126, N° 5, (May 1998), pp. 538-547. ISSN 0034-9887

Morales-Bozo, I.; Urzúa-Orellana, B.; Domínguez P.; Aguilera S. & López-Solís R. Patterns and variability in electrophoretic polypeptide profiles of human saliva in a healthy population. *Journal of physiology and biochemistry*, Vol.62, N°.3, (September 2006), pp. 179-188. ISSN 1138-7548

Morales-Bozo, I.; Urzúa-Orellana, B.; Landaeta, M.; Montalbán, R.; Torres, J., Pinochet, A., Valverde, G. & Muñoz-Martínez, A. (2007). Molecular alterations of parotid saliva in infantile chronic recurrent parotitis. *Pediatric research*, Vol.61, N°.2, (February 2007), pp. 203-208. ISSN 0031-3998

Morales-Bozo, I.; Landaeta, M., Urzúa-Orellana, B. & Retamales P. (2008). Association between the occurrence of matrix metalloproteinases 2 and 9 in parotid saliva with the degree of parotid gland damage in juvenile recurrent parotitis. *Oral surgery, oral medicine, oral pathology, oral radiology, and endodontics*, Vol.106, N°.3, (September 2008), pp. 377-383. ISSN 1079-2104

Nagase, H. & Woessner, JF. (1999). Matrix metalloproteinases. *The Journal of biological chemistry*, Vol.274, N°.31, (May 1999), pp. 21491-21494. ISSN 0021-9258

Nagel, H.; Laskawi, R.; Wahlers, A. & Hemmerlein, B. (2004). Expression of matrix metalloproteinases MMP-2, MMP-9 and their tissue inhibitors TIMP-1, -2, and -3 in benign and malignant tumours of the salivary gland. *Histopathology*, Vol.44, N°.3, (March 2004) pp. 222-231. ISSN 0309-0167

Nahlieli, O.; Shacham, R.; Shlesinger, M. & Eliav, E. (2004). Juvenile recurrent parotitis: a new method of diagnosis and treatment. *Pediatrics*, Vol.114, N°.1, (July 2004), pp. 9-12. ISSN 0031-4005

Nazar, G. ; Iñiguez, F. & Der M, C. Parotiditis aguda recurrente en el niño. *Revista Chilena de Pediatría*, Vol.72, N°.5, (Septiembre 2001), pp. 437-442. ISSN 0370-4106

Ogbureke, KU. & Fisher, LW. (2004). Expression of SIBLINGs and their partner MMPs in salivary glands. *Journal of dental research*, Vol.83, N°.9, (September 2004), pp. 664-670. ISSN 0022-0345

Pérez, P.; Goicovich, E.; Alliende, C.; Aguilera, S.; Leyton, C.; Molina, C., Pinto, R.; Romo, R.; Martinez, B. & Gonzalez, MJ. (2000). Differential expression of matrix metalloproteinases in labial salivary glands of patients with primary Sjogren's syndrome. *Arthritis and rheumatism*, Vol.43, N°.12, (December 2000), pp. 2807-2817. ISSN 0004-3591

Pérez, P.; Kwon, YJ.; Alliende, C.; Leyton, L.; Aguilera, S.; Molina, C.; Labra, C.; Julio, M.; Leyton, C. & Gonzalez, MJ. (2005). Increased acinar damage of salivary glands of patients with Sjogren's syndrome is paralleled by simultaneous imbalance of matrix metalloproteinase 3/tissue inhibitor of metalloproteinases 1 and matrix metalloproteinase 9/tissue inhibitor of metalloproteinases 1 ratios. *Arthritis and rheumatism*, Vol.52, N°.9, (September 2005), pp. 2751-2760. ISSN 0004-3591

Pinochet, A. (2008). Determinación de la frecuencia y actividad enzimática de las formas activas y latentes de las metaloproteinasas 2 y 9 en la saliva parotídea de pacientes afectados por Parotiditis Crónica Recurrente Infantil. Tesis para optar al Título de Cirujano Dentista, Facultad de Odontología, Universidad de Chile.

Pozo, P.; Valenzuela, MA.; Melej, C.; Zaldivar, M.; Puente, J.; Martinez, B. & Gamonal, J. (2005). Longitudinal analysis of metalloproteinases, tissue inhibitors of metalloproteinases and clinical parameters in gingival crevicular fluid from periodontitis-affected patients. *Journal of periodontal research*, Vol.40, N°.3, (June 2005), pp. 199-207. ISSN 0022-3484

Preza, D.; Thiede, B.; Olsen, I. & Grinde, B. (2009). The proteome of the human parotid gland secretion in elderly with and without root caries. *Acta odontologica Scandinavica*, Vol.67, N°.3, (March 2009), pp. 161-169. ISSN 0001-6357

Quenin, S.; Plouin-Gaudon, I.; Marchal, F.; Froehlich, P.; Disant, F. & Faure, F. (2008). Juvenile recurrent parotitis: sialendoscopic approach. *Archives of otolaryngology--head & neck surgery*, Vol.134, N°.1, (July 2008), pp. 715-719. ISSN 0886-4470

Raitio, A.; Tuomas, H.; Kokkonen, N.; Salo, T.; Sorsa, T.; Hanemaaijer, R. & Oikarinen, A. (2005). Levels of matrix metalloproteinase-2, -9 and -8 in the skin, serum and saliva of smokers and non-smokers. *Archives of dermatological research*, Vol.297, N°.6, (December 2005), pp. 242-248. ISSN 0340-3696

Ramírez, J.; Urrutia, H. & Aravena, A. (1996). Correlación entre la duración de la enfermedad y las imágenes sialográficas en casos con parotiditis recurrente unilateral. *Archivos de odonto estomatología*, Vol.12, N°.9, (Septiembre 1996) pp. 517-521. ISSN 0213-4144

Rostion, CG.; Giuliano, C. & Acosta, S. (2004). Parotiditis crónica recurrente en el niño. *Revista Chilena de Pediatría*, Vol.75, N°.1 (Enero 2004), pp. 43-47. ISSN 0370-4106

Ryu, OH.; Atkinson, JC.; Hoehn, GT.; Illei, GG. & Hart, TC. (2006). Identification of parotid salivary biomarkers in Sjogren's syndrome by surface-enhanced laser desorption/ionization time-of-flight mass spectrometry and two-dimensional difference gel electrophoresis. *Rheumatology*, Vol.45, N°.9, (September 2006), pp. 1077-1086. ISSN1462-0324

Shacham, R.; Droma, EB.; London, D.; Bar, T. & Nahlieli, O. (2009). Long-term experience with endoscopic diagnosis and treatment of juvenile recurrent parotitis. *Journal of oral and maxillofacial surgery : official journal of the American Association of Oral and Maxillofacial Surgeons*, Vol.67, N°.1, (January 2009), pp. 162-167. ISSN 0278-2391

Schulz, CG.; Sawicki, G.; Lemke, RP.; Roeten BM.; Schulz, R. & Cheung, PY. (2004). MMP-2 and MMP-9 and their tissue inhibitors in the plasma of preterm and term neonates. *Pediatric research*, Vol.55, N°.5, (May 2004), pp. 794-801. ISSN 0031-3998

Shkalim, V.; Monselise, Y.; Mosseri, R.; Finkelstein, Y. & Garty, BZ. (2004). Recurrent parotitis in selective IgA deficiency. *Pediatric allergy and immunology : official publication of the European Society of Pediatric Allergy and Immunology*, Vol.15, N°.3, (June 2004), pp 281-283. ISSN 0905-6157

Shimizu, M.; Ussmuller, J.; Donath, K.; Yoshiura, K.; Ban, S.; Kanda, S.; Ozeki, S. & Shinohara, M. (1998). Sonographic analysis of recurrent parotitis in children: a comparative study with sialographic findings. Oral surgery, oral medicine, oral pathology, oral radiology, and endodontics, Vol.86, N°.5, (November 1998), pp. 606-615. ISSN 1079-2104

Sitheeque, M.; Sivachandran, Y.; Varathan, V.; Ariyawardana, A. & Ranasinghe, A. (2007). Juvenile recurrent parotitis: clinical, sialographic and ultrasonographic features. *International journal of paediatric dentistry / the British Paedodontic Society [and] the International Association of Dentistry for Children*, Vol.17, N°.2, (March 2007), pp. 98-104. ISSN 0960-7439

Sousa, MM., do Amaral, JB.; Guimarães, A. & Saraiva, MJ. (2005). Up-regulation of the extracellular matrix remodeling genes, biglycan, neutrophil gelatinase-associated lipocalin, and matrix metalloproteinase-9 in familial amyloid polyneuropathy. *The FASEB journal : official publication of the Federation of American Societies for Experimental Biology*, Vol.19, N°.1, (January 2005), pp.124-126. ISSN 0892-6638

Sternlicht, MD & Werb, Z. (2001). How matrix metalloproteinases regulate cell behavior. *Annual review of cell and developmental biology*, Vol.17, (2001), pp. 463-516. ISSN 1081-0706

Streckfus, CF. & Bigler, LR. Saliva as a diagnostic fluid. *Oral diseases*, Vol.8, N°.2, (March 2002), pp. 69-76. ISSN 1354-523X

Tabak, L.; Mandel, ID.; Herrera, M. & Baurmash, H. (1978). Changes in lactoferrin and other proteins in a case of chronic recurrent parotitis. *Journal of oral pathology*, Vol.7, N°.2, (April 1978), pp. 91-99. ISSN 0300-9777

Tieche, JM.; Leonora, J. & Steinman, RR. (1980). Isolation and partial characterization of a porcine parotid hormone that stimulates dentinal fluid transport. *Endocrinology*, Vol.106, N°.6, (June 1980), pp. 1994-2005. ISSN 0013-7227

Teymoortash, A.; Mandic, R.; Schrader, C. & Werner, JA. (2004). Extracellular matrix molecules in chronic obstructive sialadenitis: an immunocytochemical and Western blot investigation. *Journal of oral science*, Vol.46, N°.4, (December 2004), pp. 227-233. ISSN 1343-4934

Ussmüller, J. & Donath, K. (1999). Clinical, histopathologic and immunohistochemical studies of chronic sialectatic parotitis in childhood and adolescence. *Klinische Pädiatrie*, Vol.211, N°.3, (May-Jun 1999), pp.165-171. ISSN 0300-8630

Valenzuela, MA.; Collados, L.; Kettlun, AM.; Gonzalez, F. & Cartier, L. (2000). Increased activity of metalloproteinases and their inhibitors in cerebrospinal fluid of patients with tropical spastic paraparesis. *Revista médica de Chile*, Vol.128, N°.6, (June 2000), pp. 585-592. ISSN 0034-9887

Vinagre, C.; Martínez, MJ.; Avendaño, LF.; Landaeta M. & Pinto, ME. (2003). Virology of infantile chronic recurrent parotitis in Santiago de Chile. *Journal of medical virology*, Vol.70, N°.3, (July 2003), pp. 459-462. ISSN 0146-6615

Vuotila, T.; Ylikontiola, L.; Sorsa, T.; Luoto, H.; Hanemaaijer, R.; Salo, T. & Tjaderhane, L. (2002). The relationship between MMPs and pH in whole saliva of radiated head and neck cancer patients. *Journal of oral pathology & medicine : official publication of the*

International Association of Oral Pathologists and the American Academy of Oral Pathology, Vol.31, N°.6, (July 2002), pp. 329-338. ISSN 0904-2512

Walz, A.; Stühler, K.; Wattenberg, A.; Hawranke, E.; Meyer, HE.; Schmalz, G. Blüggel, M. & Ruhl, S. (2006). Proteome analysis of glandular parotid and submandibular-sublingual saliva in comparison to whole human saliva by two-dimensional gel electrophoresis. *Proteomics*, Vol.6, N°.5, (March 2006), pp. 1631-1639. ISSN 1615-9853

Wang, TC.; Shyur, SD.; Kao, YH. & Huang, LH. (2006). Juvenile recurrent parotitis. *Acta paediatrica Taiwanica*, Vol.47, N°.6, (Nov-Dec 2006), pp. 297-302. ISSN 1608-8115

Watanabe, M.; Asatsuma, M.; Ikui, A.; Ikeda, M.; Yamada, Y.; Nomura, S. & Igarashi, A. (2005). Measurements of several metallic elements and matrix metalloproteinases (MMPs) in saliva from patients with taste disorder. *Chemical senses*, Vol.30, N°.2, (February 2005), pp. 121-125. ISSN 0379-864X

Werner, A. (2008). Identificación de péptidos salivales parotideos asociados a la condición de Parotiditis Crónica Recurrente Infantil. Tesis para optar al Título de Cirujano Dentista, Facultad de Odontología, Universidad de Chile. 2008.

Wittekindt, C.; Jungehülsing, M.; Fischbach. R. & Landwehr, P. (2000). Chronic recurrent parotitis in childhood in monozygotic twins. Magnetic resonance sialography *HNO*, Vol.48, N°.3, (March 2000), pp. 221-225. ISSN 0017-6192

Woo, JS.; Kim, KM.; Kang, JS.; Zodpe, P.; Chae, SW.; Hwang, SJ. & Lee, HM. (2007). Expression of neutrophil gelatinase-associated lipocalin in human salivary glands. *The Annals of otology, rhinology, and laryngology*, Vol.116, N°.8, (August 2007), pp. 599-603. ISSN 0003-4894

Wu, AJ.; Lafrenie, RM.; Park, C.; Apinhasmit, W.; Chen, ZJ.; Birkedal-Hansen, H.; Yamada KM.; Stetler-Stevenson, WG, & Baum, BJ. (1997). Modulation of MMP-2 (gelatinase A) and MMP-9 (gelatinase B) by interferon-gamma in a human salivary gland cell line. *Journal of cellular physiology*, Vol.171, N°.2, (May 1997), pp. 117-124. ISSN 0021-9541

Xia, DS.; Deng, DJ. & Wang, SL. (2003a). Destruction of parotid glands affects nitrate and nitrite metabolism. *Journal of dental research*, Vol.82, N°.2, (February 2003), pp. 101-105. ISSN 0022-0345

Xia, DS.; Deng, DJ. & Wang, SL. (2003b). Alterations of nitrate and nitrite content in saliva, serum, and urine in patients with salivary dysfunction. *Journal of oral pathology & medicine : official publication of the International Association of Oral Pathologists and the American Academy of Oral Pathology*, Vol.32, N°.2, (February 2003), pp. 95-99. ISSN 0904-2512

Xu, S. & Venge, P. (2000). Lipocalins as biochemical markers of disease. *Biochimica et biophysica acta*, Vol.1482, N°1-2, (Oct 2000), pp. 298-307. ISSN 0006-3002

Yan, L.; Borregaard, N.; Kjeldsen, L. & Moses, MA. (2001). The high molecular weight urinary matrix metalloproteinase (MMP) activity is a complex of gelatinase B/MMP-9 and neutrophil gelatinase-associated lipocalin (NGAL). Modulation of MMP-9 activity by NGAL. *The Journal of biological chemistry*, Vol.276, N°.40, (October 2001), pp. 37258-37265. ISSN 0021-9258

Zhang, Q.; Szalay, AA.; Tieche, JM.; Kyeyune-Nyombi, E., Sands, JF.; Oberg, KC. & Leonora, J. (2005). Cloning and Functional Study of Porcine Parotid Hormone, a Novel Proline-rich Protein. *The Journal of biological chemistry*, Vol.280, Nº.23, (June 2005), pp. 22233-22244. ISSN 0021-9258

Zhang, XF.; Zhang, Y.; Zhang, XH.; Zhou, SM.; Yang, GG.; Wang, OC.; Guo, GL.; Yang, GY. & Hu, XQ. (2009). Clinical significance of NGAL mRNA expression in human rectal cancer. *BMC câncer*, Vol.9, Nº1, (May 2009), pp. 134. ISSN 1471-2407